Ophthalmic Drug Delivery Systems

DRUGS AND THE PHARMACEUTICAL SCIENCES

Executive Editor

James Swarbrick

PharmaceuTech, Inc.
Pinehurst, North Carolina

Advisory Board

Larry L. Augsburger
University of Maryland
Baltimore, Maryland

David E. Nichols
Purdue University
West Lafayette, Indiana

Douwe D. Breimer
Gorlaeus Laboratories
Leiden, The Netherlands

Stephen G. Schulman
University of Florida
Gainesville, Florida

Trevor M. Jones
The Association of the
British Pharmaceutical Industry
London, United Kingdom

Jerome P. Skelly
Alexandria, Virginia

Hans E. Junginger
Leiden/Amsterdam Center
for Drug Research
Leiden, The Netherlands

Felix Theeuwes
Alza Corporation
Palo Alto, California

Vincent H. L. Lee
University of Southern California
Los Angeles, California

Geoffrey T. Tucker
University of Sheffield
Royal Hallamshire Hospital
Sheffield, United Kingdom

Peter G. Welling
Institut de Recherche Jouveinal
Fresnes, France

DRUGS AND THE PHARMACEUTICAL SCIENCES

A Series of Textbooks and Monographs

Ophthalmic Drug Delivery Systems

Second Edition, Revised and Expanded

edited by

Ashim K. Mitra

University of Missouri–Kansas City
Kansas City, Missouri, U.S.A.

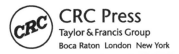

CRC Press
Taylor & Francis Group
Boca Raton   London   New York

CRC Press is an imprint of the
Taylor & Francis Group, an **informa** business

First published 2003 by Marcel Dekker, Inc.
This edition published in 2011 by Informa Healthcare

Published 2019 by CRC Press
Taylor & Francis Group
6000 Broken Sound Parkway NW, Suite 300
Boca Raton, FL 33487-2742

© 2011 by Taylor & Francis Group, LLC (except as otherwise indicated)
CRC Press is an imprint of Taylor & Francis Group, an Informa business

First issued in paperback 2019

No claim to original U.S. Government works

ISBN 13: 978-0-367-44676-5 (pbk)
ISBN 13: 978-0-8247-4124-2 (hbk)

**Visit the Taylor & Francis Web site at
http://www.taylorandfrancis.com**

**and the CRC Press Web site at
http://www.crcpress.com**

A CIP record for this book is available from the British Library.

Library of Congress Cataloging-in-Publication Data available on application

Foreword

For new medications to be used effectively, and for those now available to provide maximal benefit, improvements in ocular drug delivery are essential. Drug delivery is no less vital than drug discovery.

Although many drugs can be safely delivered by eye drops, effective treatment depends on patient compliance. Non-compliance is a major problem, especially in poorly educated patients and patients who are required to apply drops frequently. Lack of compliance frequently results in suboptimal therapeutics, which may lead to blindness. People with chronic conditions or debilitating disease find complicated eye drop regimens to be a serious handicap.

Even when drugs can be delivered through the cornea and conjunctiva, concentrations may be suboptimal and the therapeutic effect minimal. In the past, a variety of approaches to topical drug delivery have been tested, including gelatin wafers or soft contact lenses soaked in drugs and placed on the cornea or in the cul-de-sac, corneal collagen shields, and iontophoresis. The diversity of these approaches is an indication of the need for a superior method of topical drug delivery and a testament to the fact that no uniformly acceptable method has been developed to date. Currently, vehicles and carriers such as liposomes and substances that gel, as well as nanoparticles, are being evaluated. Also, prodrugs, such as medicines that hydrolyze within the eye, are being developed to achieve higher concentrations, prolonged activity, and reduced toxicity of topically applied medications. These important techniques and others are considered in this book.

Perhaps even more important than surface delivery is the need to apply medications to the posterior segment of the eye. Treatment of blinding posterior segment diseases, including uveitis, proliferative retinopathy, and macular degeneration, requires drug delivery to the retina, the choroid, or the ciliary body in a safe and convenient way. Systemic delivery that can localize to the retina may be possible. Improving scleral permeability may be important for periocular delivery, and devices inserted into the vitreous have certainly been valuable. Both nonbiodegradable controlled-release devices and biodegradable implants inserted into both aqueous and vitreous show great promise.

Posterior segment drug delivery is also becoming important for gene therapy. The need to deliver polypeptide medications and DNA inhibitors has become clear. The challenge of understanding the pharmacokinetics of the drug is matched by the challenge of providing a delivery system that can provide optimal duration of drug delivery in therapeutically sufficient concentrations and still be safe and convenient for the patient.

Our approaches to these goals are imperfect at present, but this critically important book describes in vital detail and with great clarity the progress that has been made so far and the course that needs to be pursued in the future. In my pharmacological memory, it does not seem so long ago that we had no treatment for viral diseases, pilocarpine was the only treatment for glaucoma, and antibiotics were crude and relatively ineffective. Similarly, our present achievements in the field of ocular drug delivery may seem equally primitive as we follow the paths to future progress detailed in this book.

Herbert E. Kaufman, M.D.
Boyd Professor of Ophthalmology, Pharmacology, and Microbiology
Louisiana State University Health Sciences Center
New Orleans, Louisiana, U.S.A.

Preface

A major goal of pharmacotherapeutics is the attainment of an effective drug concentration at the intended site of action for a desired length of time. Efficient delivery of a drug while minimizing its systemic and/or local side effects is the key to the treatment of ocular diseases. The unique anatomy and physiology of the eye offer many challenges to developing effective ophthalmic drug delivery systems, but the knowledge in this field is rapidly expanding. Systems range from simple solutions to novel delivery systems such as biodegradable polymeric systems, corneal collagen shields, iontophoresis, and viral and nonviral gene delivery systems, to name a few. An increase in our understanding of ocular drug absorption and disposition mechanisms has led to the development of many of these new systems.

The first edition of this book laid the foundation necessary for understanding barriers to ophthalmic drug delivery and to review the conventional systems available and/or in various stages of research and development. Since then, significant advances have been made in understanding the molecular mechanisms involved in ocular drug transport. The book begins with a brief discussion on the anatomy and physiology of the eye relevant to ocular drug delivery. The latest techniques, such as microdialysis, and models developed to study ocular drug disposition are discussed. A review of both the conventional and novel delivery systems follows. The book stresses the fact that simple instillation of drug solution in the cul-de-sac is not always acceptable and emphasizes the need for the development of newer and more efficient systems. The book concludes with

v

the basic information required for pharmaceutical scientists to protect their inventions.

Part I investigates the fundamental considerations in ocular drug delivery. The three chapters in this part review the relevant ocular anatomy and physiology, the constraints imposed by the eye upon successful delivery, and the associated ion and solute transport processes in the eye. They provide information on the various transport processes as well as recently identified drug efflux pumps, which regulate the transport of endogenous and exogenous substances.

Part II opens with a discussion of pharmacokinetics relevant to ocular drug delivery. The next chapter discusses the pharmacokinetic processes guiding the ocular disposition and expands on the pharmacokinetic/pharmacodynamic modeling processes to determine the appropriate dosage regimen. This chapter is followed by a detailed discussion of the various mathematical models developed to describe the distribution and elimination of drugs from the vitreous. This part also includes chapters dealing with the application of microdialysis technique to study ocular drug delivery and disposition, and the applicability of the microdialysis sampling approach for the examination of ocular pharmacokinetics and dynamics of ophthalmics.

Part III is divided into conventional and advanced drug delivery systems. The first section deals with such conventional systems as collagen shields, iontophoresis, microparticulates, and dendrimers. These chapters have been updated to include advances in ocular drug delivery achieved in the past decade. The second section examines the delivery of macromolecules to treat various ocular pathologies. The reader will find more information on the recent developments in animal models of retino-choroidal diseases. The viral and nonviral gene delivery systems introduced in this section are still in their infancy but have the potential to provide enormous therapeutic benefits. This section also focuses on the advances in treating retinal degenerative diseases. The last chapter in this section discusses the principles and delivery aspects of gene, oligonucleotide, and ribozyme therapy.

Part IV provides information on regulatory and patent considerations. Pharmaceutical scientists will gain knowledge of the regulations governing animal and human testing and ultimately the release of the product commercially for public use. The final chapter conveys the legal issues involved in protecting inventions and the basic legal requirements for obtaining patents.

Ashim K. Mitra

Contents

Contributors

Imran Ahmed, Ph.D. Pfizer Global R&D—Groton Laboratories, Groton, Connecticut, U.S.A.

Hemant Alur, Ph.D. Murty Pharmaceuticals, Inc., Lexington, Kentucky, U.S.A.

James E. Chastain, Ph.D. Alcon Research, Ltd., Forth Worth, Texas, U.S.A.

Yu-Ling Cheng, Ph.D. Department of Chemical Engineering and Applied Chemistry, University of Toronto, Toronto, Canada

Nandita G. Das Department of Pharmaceutical Sciences, Idaho State University, Pocatello, Idaho, U.S.A.

Sudip K. Das, Ph.D. Department of Pharmaceutical Sciences, Idaho State University, Pocatello, Idaho, U.S.A

Surajit Dey Department of Pharmaceutical Sciences, University of Missouri–Kansas City, Kansas City, Missouri, U.S.A

Clapton S. Dias Department of Pharmaceutical Sciences, University of Missouri–Kansas City, Kansas City, Missouri, U.S.A

Stuart Friedrich, Ph.D. Department of Chemical Engineering and Applied Chemistry, University of Toronto, Toronto, Canada

Shiro Higaki, M.D. Department of Ophthalmology, LSU Eye and Vision Center of Excellence, Louisiana State University Health Science Center, New Orleans, Louisiana, U.S.A.

James M. Hill, Ph.D. Department of Ophthalmology, LSU Eye and Vision Center of Excellence, Louisiana State University Health Science Center, New Orleans, Louisiana, U.S.A.

Patrick M. Hughes, Ph.D. Allergan Pharmaceuticals, Irvine, California, U.S.A.

Thomas P. Johnston, Ph.D. Department of Pharmaceutical Sciences, University of Missouri–Kansas City, Kansas City, Missouri, U.S.A

Nelson L. Jumbe Albany Medical College, Albany, New York, and Amgen Inc., Thousands Oaks, California, U.S.A.

Uday B. Kompella, Ph.D. Department of Pharmaceutical Sciences and Ophthalmology, University of Nebraska Medical Center, Omaha, Nebraska, U.S.A

Murali K. Kothuri Department of Pharmaceutical Sciences, Idaho State University, Pocatello, Idaho, U.S.A.

Ramesh Krishnamoorthy, Ph.D. Formulation Development, Inspire Pharmaceuticals, Durham, North Carolina, U.S.A.

D. Scott Krueger, Ph.D. Regulatory Affairs, Alcon Research, Ltd., Fort Worth, Texas, U.S.A.

Thomas Wai-Yip Lee, B. Pharm. School of Pharmacy, University of Wisconsin–Madison, Madison, Wisconsin, U.S.A.

Jeannette M. Loutsch, Ph.D. Department of Ophthalmology, LSU Eye and Vision Center of Excellence, Louisiana State University Health Science Center, New Orleans, Louisiana, U.S.A.

Sreeraj Macha, Ph.D.[*] Department of Pharmaceutical Sciences, University of Missouri–Kansas City, Kansas City, Missouri, U.S.A.

Michael H. Miller Albany Medical College, Albany, New York, U.S.A.

Keith J. Miller Bristol–Myers Squibb Company, Pennington, New Jersey, U.S.A.

Ashim K. Mitra, Ph.D. Department of Pharmaceutical Sciences, University of Missouri–Kansas City, Kansas City, Missouri, U.S.A.

Marvin E. Myles, Ph.D. Department of Ophthalmology, LSU Eye and Vision Center of Excellence, Louisiana State University Health Science Center, New Orleans, Louisiana, U.S.A.

Desiree Ong Department of Ophthalmology, LSU Eye and Vision Center of Excellence, Louisiana State University Health Science Center, New Orleans, Louisiana, U.S.A.

Swathi Pinnamaneni[†] Department of Pharmaceutical Sciences, Idaho State University, Pocatello, Idaho, U.S.A.

Leena Pitkänen, Lic. Med. Department of Pharmaceutics, University of Kuopio, and Department of Ophthalmology, Kuopio University Hospital, Kuopio, Finland

Kay D. Rittenhouse, Ph.D. Nonclinical Drug Safety, Global Research and Development, La Jolla Laboratories, Pfizer Inc., San Diego, California, U.S.A.

Joseph R. Robinson, Ph.D. School of Pharmacy, University of Wisconsin–Madison, Madison, Wisconsin, U.S.A.

Robert E. Roehrs, Ph.D.[‡] Alcon Research, Ltd., Fort Worth, Texas, U.S.A.

---

[*] *Current affiliation*: Boehringer Ingelheim Inc., Ridgefield, Connecticut, U.S.A.
[†] *Current affiliation*: Exploratory Biopharmaceutics and Stability, Bristol-Myers Squibb Company, New Brunswick, New Jersey, U.S.A.
[‡] Retired.

Lotta Salminen, M.D. Department of Ophthalmology, University of Tampere, and Department of Ophthalmology, Tampere University Hospital, Tampere, Finland

Bradley Saville, Ph.D. Department of Chemical Engineering and Applied Chemistry, University of Toronto, Toronto, Canada

Ronald D. Schoenwald, Ph.D. College of Pharmacy, The University of Iowa, Iowa City, Iowa, U.S.A.

Gangadhar Sunkara, Ph.D* Department of Pharmaceutical Sciences, University of Nebraska Medical Center, Omaha, Nebraska, U.S.A.

Joyce Tombran-Tink, Ph.D. Department of Pharmaceutical Sciences, University of Missouri–Kansas City, Kansas City, Missouri, U.S.A.

Arto Urtti, Ph.D. Department of Pharmaceutics, University of Kuopio, Kuopio, Finland

---

* *Current affiliation*: Clinical Pharmacology Division, Novartis Pharmaceuticals, East Hanover, New Jersey, U.S.A.

Ophthalmic Drug Delivery Systems

1

Overview of Ocular Drug Delivery

Sreeraj Macha* and Ashim K. Mitra
University of Missouri–Kansas City, Kansas City, Missouri, U.S.A.

Patrick M. Hughes
Allergan Pharmaceuticals, Irvine, California, U.S.A.

I. INTRODUCTION

Opthalmic drug delivery is one of the most interesting and challenging endeavors facing the pharmaceutical scientist. The anatomy, physiology, and biochemistry of the eye render this organ highly impervious to foreign substances. A significant challenge to the formulator is to circumvent the protective barriers of the eye without causing permanent tissue damage. Development of newer, more sensitive diagnostic techniques and novel therapeutic agents continue to provide ocular delivery systems with high therapeutic efficacy. Potent immunosuppressant therapy in transplant patients and the developing epidemic of acquired immunodeficiency syndrome have generated an entirely new population of patients suffering virulent uveitis and retinopathies. Conventional ophthalmic solution, suspension, and ointment dosage forms no longer constitute optimal therapy for these indications. Research and development efforts to design better therapeutic systems particularly targeted to posterior segment are the primary focus of this text.

The goal of pharmacotherapeutics is to treat a disease in a consistent and predictable fashion. An assumption is made that a correlation exists between the concentration of a drug at its intended site of action and the resulting pharmacological effect. The specific aim of designing a therapeutic system is to achieve an optimal concentration of a drug at the active site for

---

**Current affiliation*: Boehringer Ingelheim Inc., Ridgefield, Connecticut, U.S.A.

the appropriate duration. Ocular disposition and elimination of a therapeutic agent is dependent upon its physicochemical properties as well as the relevant ocular anatomy and physiology (1). A successful design of a drug delivery system, therefore, requires an integrated knowledge of the drug molecule and the constraints offered by the ocular route of administration.

The active sites for the antibiotics, antivirals, and steroids are the infected or inflamed areas within the anterior as well as the posterior segments of the eye. Receptors for the mydriatics and miotics are in the iris ciliary body. A host of different tissues are involved, each of which may pose its own challenge to the formulator of ophthalmic delivery systems. Hence, the drug entities need to be targeted to many sites within the globe.

Historically, the bulk of the research has been aimed at delivery to the anterior segment tissues. Only recently has research been directed at delivery to the tissues of the posterior globe (the uveal tract, vitreous, choroid, and retina).

The aim of this chapter is merely to present the challenges of designing successful ophthalmic delivery systems by way of introduction. The reader is referred to specific chapters within this book for a thorough discussion of the topic introduced in this section.

II. MECHANISMS OF OCULAR DRUG ABSORPTION

Topical delivery into the cul-de-sac is, by far, the most common route of ocular drug delivery. Adsorption from this site may be corneal or noncorneal. A schematic diagram of the human eye is depicted in Figure 1. The so-called noncorneal route of absorption involves penetration across the sclera and conjunctiva into the intraocular tissues. This mechanism of absorption is usually nonproductive, as drug penetrating the surface of the eye beyond the corneal-scleral limbus is taken up by the local capillary beds and removed to the general circulation (2). This noncorneal absorption in general precludes entry into the aqueous humor.

Recent studies, however, suggest that noncorneal route of absorption may be significant for drug molecules with poor corneal permeability. Studies with inulin (3), timolol maleate (3), gentamicin (4), and prostaglandin $PGF_{2\alpha}$ (5) suggest that these drugs gain intraocular access by diffusion across the conjunctiva and sclera. Ahmed and Patton (3) studied the noncorneal absorption of inulin and timolol maleate. Penetration of these agents into the intraocular tissues appears to occur via diffusion across the conjunctiva and sclera and not through reentry from the systemic circulation or via absorption into the local vasculature. Both compounds gained access to the iris–ciliary body without entry into the anterior cham-

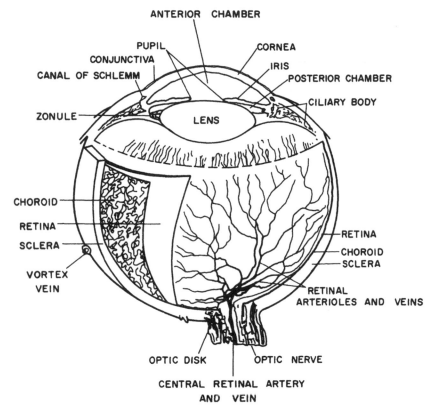

Figure 1   Anatomical structure of the human eye. (From Ref. 12.)

ber. As much as 40% of inulin absorbed into the eye was determined to be the result of noncorneal absorption.

The noncorneal route of absorption may be significant for poorly cornea-permeable drugs; however, corneal absorption represents the major mechanism of absorption for most therapeutic entities. Topical absorption of these agents, then, is considered to be rate limited by the cornea. The anatomical structures of the cornea exert unique differential solubility requirements for drug candidates. Figure 2 illustrates a cross-sectional view of the cornea. In terms of transcorneal flux of drugs, the cornea can be viewed as a trilaminate structure consisting of three major diffusional barriers: epithelium, stroma, and endothelium. The epithelium and endothelium contain on the order of 100-fold the amount of lipid material per unit mass of the stroma (6). Depending on the physiochemical properties of the drug entity, the diffusional resistance offered by these tissues varies greatly (7,8).

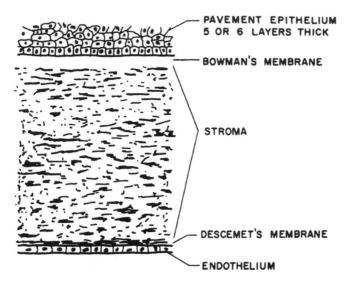

PAVEMENT EPITHELIUM
5 OR 6 LAYERS THICK

BOWMAN'S MEMBRANE

STROMA

DESCEMET'S MEMBRANE

ENDOTHELIUM

Figure 2 Cross-sectional view of the corneal membrane depicting various barriers to drug absorption. (From Ref. 12.)

The outermost layer, the epithelium, represents the rate-limiting barrier for transcorneal diffusion of most hydrophilic drugs. The epithelium is composed of five to seven cell layers. The basement cells are columnar in nature, allowing for minimal paracellular transport. The epithelial cells, however, narrow distal to Bowman's membrane, forming flattened epithelial cells with zonulae occludentes interjunctional complexes. This cellular arrangement precludes paracellular transport of most ophthalmic drugs and limits lateral movement within the anterior epithelium (9). Corneal surface epithelial intracellular pore size has been estimated to be about 60 Å (10). Small ionic and hydrophilic molecules appear to gain access to the anterior chamber through these pores (11); however, for most drugs, paracellular transport is precluded by the interjectional complexes. In a recent review, Lee (10) discusses an attempt to transiently alter the epithelial integrity at these junctional complexes to improve ocular bioavailability. This approach has, however, only met with moderate success and has the potential to severely compromise the corneal integrity.

Sandwiched between the corneal epithelium and endothelium is the stroma (substantia propia). The stroma constitutes 85–90% of the total corneal mass and is composed of mainly of hydrated collagen (12). The stroma exerts a diffusional barrier to highly lipophilic drugs owing to its hydrophilic nature. There are no tight junction complexes in the stroma, and paracellular transport through this tissue is possible.

The innermost layer of the cornea, separated from the stroma by Descermet's membrane, is the endothelium. The endothelium is lipoidal in nature; however, it does not offer a significant barrier to the transcorneal diffusion of most drugs. Endothelial permeability depends solely on molecular weight and not on the charge of hydrophilic nature of the compound (13,14).

Transcellular transport across the corneal epithelium and stroma is the major mechanism of ocular absorption of topically applied ophthalmic pharmaceuticals. This type of Fickian diffusion is dependent upon many factors, i.e., surface area, diffusivity, the concentration gradient established, and the period over which concentration gradient can be maintained. A parabolic relationship between octanol/water partition coefficient and corneal permeability has been described for many drugs (15–19). The optimal log partition coefficient appears to be in the range of 1–3. The permeability coefficients of 11 steroids were determined by Schoenwald and Ward (15). The permeability versus log partition coefficient fit the typical parabolic relationship, with the optimum log partition coefficient being 2.9. Narurkar and Mitra studied a homologous series of 5' aliphatic esters of 5-iodo-2'-deoxyuridine (IDU) (16,17). In vitro corneal permeabilities were optimized at a log partition coefficient of 0.88, as can be seen graphically in Figure 3 and in Table 1, where CMP represents the corneal permeability values as measured by in vitro perfusion experiments on rabbit corneas (I = IDU, II = IDU-propionate, III = IDU-butyrate, IV = IDU-isobutyrate,

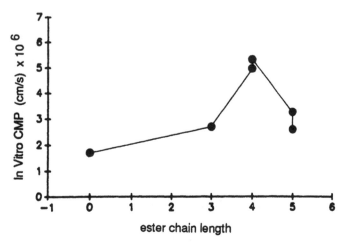

Figure 3 A plot depicting the parabolic relationship between in vitro CMP and ester chain length. (From Ref. 16.)

Table 1 Physicochemical Properties of IDU and Its 5'-Ester Prodrugs

Compound[b]	m.p. (°C)	Solubility[a] in pH 7.4 phosphate buffer, 25°C (M/L ± SD [×10³])	$K^a \pm SD$ (octanol/water)
I	168–171 (dec)	5.65 (0.5)	0.11 (0.02)
II	167–168	3.48 (0.3)	4.77 (0.1)
III	145–146	1.45 (0.1)	7.50 (0.3)
IV	144–145	1.75 (0.3)	6.92 (0.8)
V	142–143	0.40 (0.2)	27.54 (2.0)
VI	106–107	0.44 (0.1)	22.10 (1.5)

[a]N = 3.
[b]See text for compound identification.

V = IDU-valerate, VI = IDU-pivalate). A homologous series of *n*-alkyl-*p*-aminobenzoate esters in a study of Mosher and Mikkelson fit the parabolic relationship displaying optimal permeability at a log partition coefficient of 2.5 (18). Maximizing bioavailability of ophthalmic mediations, then, requires that the active compound be neither extremely hydrophilic nor lipophilic. To this end, the pH of the postinstillation precorneal fluid becomes an important factor. The postinstillation pH time course will be dictated by the buffer concentration of the formulation. Most ophthalmic formulations are formulated in the pH range of 5–6; hence, depending on the pK_a of the drug to be administered, the postinstillation buffering capacity of the formulation may greatly affect the drug's bioavailability. Mitra and Mikkelson studied the effect of varying the concentration of citrate buffer in a pH 4.5 formulation on the miosis versus time profile of a 1% pilocarpine solution (20). The area under the miosis-time profile, maximum pupillary response, and duration of mitotic activity were all decreased with increasing buffer concentrations. Figure 4 displays the effect of increasing buffer concentration on the mitosis-time profiles for different total molar citrate values (0.0, 0.055, 0.075, 0.110). The ratio of pilocarpinium ion to pilocarpine increases with the postinstillation buffering capacity, thus reducing the net transcorneal flux of pilocarpine.

III. CONSTRAINTS TO OCULAR DRUG DELIVERY

Ocular tissues are protected from exogenous toxic substances in the environment or bloodstream by a variety of mechanisms, notably, tear secretion continuously flushing its surface, an impermeable surface epithelium, and a

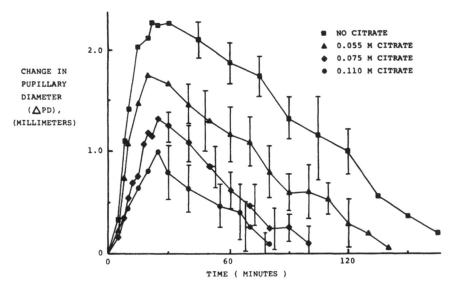

Figure 4 Miosis-time profiles: Plots of the average observed changes in pupillary diameter (ΔPD) as a function of time following the instillation of 25.0 μL of the isotonic 1% pilocarpine nitrate solutions, which contained the different concentrations of citrate buffer. The vertical lines through the data points are ±SD (data points with standard deviation lines omitted is for clarity of the figure). (From Ref. 20.)

transport system actively clearing the retina of agents potentially able to disturb the visual process. However, the same protective mechanisms may cause subtherapeutic drug levels at the intended site. The difficulties can be compounded by the structure of the globe itself, where many of its internal structures are isolated from the blood and the outside surface of the eye. A major goal in ocular therapeutics is to circumvent these structural obstacles and protective mechanisms to elicit desired pharmacological response.

Physiological barriers to the diffusion and productive absorption of topically applied ophthalmic drugs exist in the precorneal and corneal spaces. Anterior chamber factor also greatly influence the disposition of topically applied drugs. Precorneal constraints include solution drainage, lacrimation and tear dilution, tear turnover, and conjunctival absorption. For acceptable bioavailability, a proper duration of contact with the cornea must be maintained. Instilled solution drainage away from the precorneal area has been shown to be the most significant factor reducing this contact time and ocular bioavailability of topical solution dosage forms (21,22). Instilled dose leaves the precorneal area within 5 minutes of instillation in humans (21,23). The natural tendency of the cul-de-sac is to reduce its fluid volume to 7–10 µL (24–26). A typical ophthalmic dropper delivers 30 µL, most of which is rapidly lost through nasolacrimal drainage immediately following dosage. This drainage mechanism may then cause the drug to be systemically absorbed across the nasal mucosa or the gastrointestinal tract (27). Systemic loss from topically applied drugs also occurs from conjunctival absorption into the local circulation. The conjunctiva possesses a relatively large surface area, making this loss significant.

Simple dilution of instilled drug solution in the tears acts to reduce the transcorneal flux of drug remaining in the cul-de-sac. Lacrimation can be induced by many factors, including the drug entity, the pH, and the tonicity of the dosage from (28–30). Formulation adjuvants can also stimulate tear production (20).

Tear turnover acts to remove drug solution from the conjunctival cul-de-sac. Normal human tear turnover is approximately 16% per minute, which can also be stimulated by various factors, as described elsewhere (21,25). These factors render topical application of ophthalmic solutions to the cul-de-sac extremely inefficient. Typically, less than 1% of the instilled dose reaches the aqueous humor (27,31). The low fraction of applied dose (1%) of drug solution reaching the anterior chamber further undergoes rapid elimination from the intraocular tissues and fluids. Absorbed drug may exit the eye through the canal of Schlemm or via absorption through the ciliary body of suprachoroid into the episcleral space (27). Enzymatic metabolism may account for further loss, which can occur in the precorneal space and/or in the cornea (32,33). Age and genetics have been determined to be two important factors in ocular metabolism (34,35).

Clearly, the physiological barriers to topical corneal absorption are formidable. The result is that the clinician is forced to recommend frequent high doses of drugs to achieve therapeutic effect. This pulsatile dosing not only results in extreme fluctuations in ocular drug concentrations but may cause many local and/or systemic side effects. Approaches taken to circumvent this pulsatile dosing and their ramifications on ocular therapies are the subject matter of this text.

For the effective treatment of diseases involving the retina, drugs must cross the blood-ocular barrier in significant amounts to demonstrate therapeutic effect. The blood-ocular barrier is a combination of microscopic structures within the eye, which physiologically separate it from the rest of the body. It is comprised of two systems: (a) blood-aqueous barrier, which regulates solute exchange between blood and the intraocular fluid, and (b) blood-retinal barrier, which separates the blood from the neural retina. Both barriers contain epithelial and endothelial components whose tight junctions limit transport.

A transient increase in the blood-retinal barrier permeability can be achieved by modification of the barrier properties. For instance, opening of the blood-retinal barrier can be achieved by intracarotid infusion of a hyperosmotic solution, such as mannitol or arabinose. Perfusion with such a solution for about 30 seconds is shown to open the blood-retinal barrier reversibly. Osmotically induced shrinkage of the retinal and brain capillary endothelial cells causes opening of the tight junctions. Other methods include perfusion with oleic acid or protamine. These methods, however, produce a nonspecific opening of the blood-retinal barrier, possibly with associated retinal and central nervous system toxicity.

Chemical modification is more commonly employed to enhance drug transport across biological barriers. Lipophilic analogs of the parent drug increase lipid solubility and thereby their blood-retinal barrier permeability. Another approach to enhance transport across the blood-retinal barrier could involve utilizing specific carrier systems on the epithelial membrane. Drugs may be modified in such a way that their structures resemble endogenous ligands for a specific carrier system on the blood-retinal barrier.

Drug delivery through nutrient transport systems has been reported previously with intestinal absorption (36–38). β-Lactam antibiotics and other compounds that share the structural features of the endogenous peptides are recognized by the peptide transporters. Recently valacyclovir (valyl ester of acyclovir) (39,40) and valganciclovir (valyl ester of ganciclovir) (41) were shown to be the substrates for peptide transporters. These prodrugs increased the oral bioavailability of acylclovir and ganciclovir significantly (42,43), thus reducing the daily oral dose requirement.

Various transporters/receptors are reported to be present on the retina and/or the blood-ocular barriers. The reader is referred to specific chapters in this volume for detailed description. However, very few studies have been carried out to explore the transporters present on the retina or the blood-ocular barrier. The transporters/receptors present on the retina or the blood-ocular barrier may be exploited to increase ocular bioavailability of drugs with poor intrinsic permeability.

ACKNOWLEDGMENTS

Supported by NIH grants R01 EY09171 and R01 EY10659.

REFERENCES

1. M. Gibaldi and D. Perrier. Pharmacokinetics. New York: Marcel Dekker, 1982.
2. D. M. Maurice. The eye. In: H. Davsoned, ed. Vegetative Physiology and Biochemistry. New York: Academic Press, 1969.
3. I. Ahmed and T. F. Patton. Importance of the noncorneal adsorption route in topical ophthalmic drug delivery. Invest. Ophthalmol. Vis. Sci. 26:584–587, 1985.
4. S. E. Bloomfield, T. Miyata, M. W. Dunn, N. Bueser, K. H. Stenzel, and A. L. Rubin. Soluble gentamicin ophthalmic inserts as a drug delivery system. Arch. Ophthalmol. 96:885–887, 1978.
5. L. Z. Bito and R. A. Baroody. The penetration of exogenous prostaglandin and arachidonic acid into, and their distribution within, the mammalian eye. Curr. Eye Res. 1:659–669, 1981.
6. D. G. Cogan and E. D. Hirch. Cornea: Permeability to weak electrolytes. Arch. Ophthalmol. 32:276, 1944.
7. V. E. Kinsey. Physiology of the eye. In; F. Adler, H., eds. St. Louis: Mosby, 1965.
8. H. S. Huang, R. D. Schoenwald, and J. L. Lach. Corneal penetration behavior of beta-blocking agents II: Assessment of barrier contributions. J. Pharm. Sci. 72:1272–1279, 1983.
9. G. M. Grass and J. R. Robinson. Mechanisms of corneal drug penetration. II: Ultrastructural analysis of potential pathways for drug movement. J. Pharm. Sci. 77:15–23, 1988.
10. V. H. L. Lee. Mechanisms and facilitation of corneal drug penetration, J Controlled Rel, 11:79 (1990).
11. S. D. Klyce and C. E. Crosson. Transport processes across the rabbit corneal epithelium: a review. Curr. Eye Res. 4:323–331, 1985.
12. A. K. Mitra. Ophthalmic drug delivery. In: P. Tyle, ed. Drug Delivery Devices. New York: Marcel Dekker, 1988.
13. A. M. Tonjum. Permeability of rabbit corneal epithelium to horseradish peroxidase after the influence of benzalkonium chloride. Acta Ophthalmol. (Copenh.) 53:335–473, 1975.
14. S. Mishima. Clinical pharmacokinetics of the eye. Proctor lecture. Invest. Ophthalmol. Vis. Sci. 21:504–541, 1981.
15. R. D. Schoenwald and R. L. Ward. Relationship between steroid permeability across excised rabbit cornea and octanol-water partition coefficients. J. Pharm. Sci. 67:786–788, 1978.
16. M. M. Narurkar and A. K. Mitra. Prodrugs of 5-iodo-2'-deoxyuridine for enhanced ocular transport. Pharm. Res. 6:887–891, 1989.
17. M. M. Narurkar and A. K. Mitra. Synthesis, physicochemical properties, and cytotoxicity of a series of 5'-ester prodrugs of 5-iodo-2'-deoxyuridine. Pharm. Res. 5:734–737, 1988.

18. G. L. Mosher and T. J. Mikkelson. Permeability of the n-alkyl-p-aminobenzo-ate esters across the isolated corneal membrane of the rabbit. Int. J. Pharm 2:239, 1979.

19. R. D. Schoenwald and H. S. Huang. Corneal penetration behavior of beta-blocking agents I: Physiochemical factors. J. Pharm. Sci. 72:1266–72, 1983.

20. A. K. Mitra and T. J. Mikkelson. Ophthalmic solution buffer systems I. The effect of buffer concentration on the ocular absorption of pilocarpine. Int. J. Pharm. 10:219, 1982.

21. S. S. Chrai, T. F. Patton, A. Mehta, and J. R. Robinson. Lacrimal and instilled fluid dynamics in rabbit eyes. J. Pharm. Sci. 62:1112–1121, 1973.

22. S. S. Chrai, M. C. Makoid, S. P. Eriksen, and J. R. Robinson. Drop size and initial dosing frequency problems of topically applied ophthalmic drugs. J. Pharm. Sci. 63:333–338, 1974.

23. J. W. Sieg and J. R. Robinson. Mechanistic studies on transcorneal permeation of pilocarpine. J. Pharm. Sci. 65:1816–1822, 1976.

24. D. M. Maurice. The dynamics and drainage of tears. Int. Ophthalmol. Clin. 13:103–116, 1973.

25. S Mishima, A. Gasset, S. D. Klyce, Jr., and J. L. Baum. Determination of tear volume and tear flow. Invest. Ophthalmol. 5:264–276, 1966.

26. N. Ehlers. The precorneal film, biomicroscopical, histological, and chemical investigations. Acta Ophthalmol. 81(Suppl.):1, 1965.

27. V. H. Lee and J. R. Robinson. Topical ocular drug delivery: Recent developments and future challenges. J. Ocul. Pharmacol. 2:67–108, 1986.

28. A. Kupferman, M. V. Pratt, K. Suckewer, and H. M. Leibowitz. Topically applied steroids in corneal disease. 3. The role of drug derivative in stromal absorption of dexamethasone. Arch. Ophthalmol. 91:373–376, 1974.

29. J. W. Sieg and J. R. Robinson. Vehicle effects on ocular drug bioavailability II: Evaluation of pilocarpine. J. Pharm. Sci. 66:1222–12228, 1977.

30. J. M. Conrad, W. A. Reay, R. E. Polcyn, and J. R. Robinson. Influence of tonicity and pH on lacrimation and ocular drug bioavailability. J. Parenter. Drug Assoc. 32:149–161, 1978.

31. T. J. Mikkelson, S. S. Chrai, and J. R. Robinson. Competitive inhibition of drug-protein interaction in eye fluids and tissues. J. Pharm. Sci. 62:1942–1945, 1973.

32. V. H. Lee, K. W. Morimoto, and R. E. Stratford, Jr. Esterase distribution in the rabbit cornea and its implications in ocular drug bioavailability. Biopharm. Drug dispos. 3:291–300, 1982.

33. V. H. Lee, H. W. Hui, and J. R. Robinson. Corneal metabolism of pilocarpine in pigmented rabbits. Invest. Ophthalmol. Vis. Sci. 19:210–213, 1980.

34. V. H. L. Lee, J. Stratford, and K. W. Morimoto. Age related changes in esterase activity in rabbit eyes. Int. J. Pharm. 13:183, 1983.

35. H. Shichi and D. W. Nebert. Genetic differences in drug metabolism associated with ocular toxicity. Environ. Health Perspect. 44:107–117, 1982.

36. J. P. Bai, M. Hu, P. Subramanian, H. I. M osberg, and G. L. Amidon. Utilization of peptide carrier system to improve intestinal absorption: target-

ing prolidase as a prodrug-converting enzyme. J. Pharm. Sci. 81:113–116, 1992.

37. M. Hu, P. Subramanian, H. I. Mosberg, and G. L. Amidon. Use of the peptide carrier system to improve the intestinal absorption of L-alpha-methyldopa: carrier kinetics, intestinal permeabilities, and in vitro hydrolysis of dipeptidyl derivatives of L-alpha-methyldopa. Pharm. Res. 6:66–70, 1989.

38. I. Tamai, T. Nakanishi, H. Nakahara, et al. Improvement of L-dopa absorption by dipeptidyl derivation, utilizing peptide transporter PepT1. J. Pharm. Sci. 87:1542–1546, 1998.

39. R. L. de Vrueh, P. L. Smith, and C. P. Lee. Transport of L-valine-acyclovir via the oligopeptide transporter in the human intestinal cell line, Caco-2. J. Pharmacol. Exp. Ther. 286:1166–1170, 1998.

40. M. E. Ganapathy, W. Huang, H. Wang, V. Ganapathy, and F. H. Leibach. Valacyclovir: a substrate for the intestinal and renal peptide transporters PEPTT1 and PEPT2. Biochem. Biphys. Res. Commun. 246:470–5, 475, 1998.

41. M. Sugawara, W. Huang, Y. J. Fei, F. H. Leibach, V. Ganapathy, and M. E. Ganapathy. Transport of valganciclovir, a ganciclovir prodrug, via peptide transporters PEPT1 and PEPT2. J. Pharm. Sci. 89:781–789, 2000.

42. M. D. Pescovitz,J. Rabkin, R. M. Merion, et al. Valganciclovir results in improved oral absorption of ganciclovir in liver transplant recipients. Antimicrob. Agents Chemother. 44:2811–2815, 2000.

43. P. Reusser. Oral valganciclovir: A new option for treatment of cytomegalovirus infection and disease in immunocompromised hosts. Expert. Opin. Invest. Drugs 10:1745–1753, 2001.

2

Membrane Transport Processes in the Eye

Gangadhar Sunkara* and Uday B. Kompella
University of Nebraska Medical Center, Omaha, Nebraska, U.S.A.

I. INTRODUCTION

Epithelial and/or endothelial cells sealed by tight junctions serve as the major membrane barriers for the transport of nutrients, ions, and drugs into intraocular tissues. The principal membrane barriers of the eye are located in the cornea, conjunctiva, iris-ciliary body, lens epithelium, and retina (Fig. 1). Various specialized transport processes in these barriers control the movement of solutes into and out of intraocular chambers. These processes maintain the visual function, control intraocular pressure, provide nutrients to avascular cornea and lens, and protect ocular tissues from xenobiotics. An alteration in the function of these transporters is often the underlying cause of various ocular diseases. In addition, these transport processes can play a role in drug transport.

Drug therapy is useful in the treatment of corneal epitheliopathy, keratitis, conjunctivitis, extracellular infections, glaucoma, iritis, and cataract—diseases that afflict the anterior segment of the eye—and vitreoproliferative disorders, endophthalmitis of bacterial and fungal origins, uveitis, viral retinitis, diabetic retinopathy, and macular degeneration—diseases that afflict the posterior segment of the eye. Ocular drug therapy often involves topical or systemic administration of drugs. Therefore, for effective delivery to intraocular tissues, drugs must penetrate across cornea, conjunctiva, and/ or sclera following topical administration or across endothelial barriers

---

Current affiliation: Novartis Pharmaceuticals, East Hanover, New Jersey, U.S.A.

13

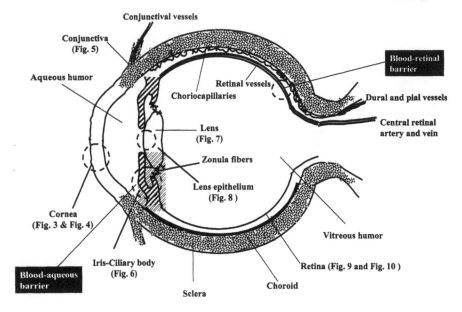

Figure 1   Various epithelial and endothelial barriers of the eye.

along with the epithelial barriers of the iris-ciliary body or retina following systemic administration. However, as these barriers restrict the transport of therapeutic agents, the ocular bioavailability of drugs following topical or systemic administration is low. These barriers also play a role in the drug clearance following periocular or intraocular administration.

This chapter describes the various ocular epithelial and endothelial barriers and the associated ion and solute transport processes in the eye. The discussion includes ocular drug transport processes as well as recently identified drug efflux pumps.

II. GENERAL MECHANISMS AND ROUTES OF TRANSPORT

A. Mechanisms of Transport

The membrane, whether it is plasma membrane or a membrane encompassing cellular organelles, imposes a barrier to the free movement of molecules. Simple diffusion, facilitated diffusion, primary active transport, secondary active transport, transcytosis, and group translocation are six primary mechanisms of solute transport across a membrane (Saier, 2000a). Simple or passive diffusion is a process that does not require cellular energy, but requires a chemical gradient for the solute to be transported. Facilitated diffusion is similar to simple diffusion in not requiring energy and following chemical gradient, but it requires a membrane transporter or carrier to facilitate the transport. Two primary modes of facilitated transport have been recognized in the biological systems: channel type and carrier type. In channel-type facilitated diffusion, the solute passes in a diffusion-limiting process from one side of the membrane to the other via a channel or pore that is lined by appropriately hydrophilic, hydrophobic, or amphipathic amino acyl residues of the constituent proteins. In carrier-type facilitated diffusion, some part of the transporter is classically presumed to pass through the membrane together with the substrate. Carriers usually exhibit rates of transport, stereospecificity, and saturation kinetics in higher magnitude compared to channels. Solute transport processes where energy is required to transport the solutes against a concentration gradient are referred to as active transport processes. In primary active transport, energy is directly expended by the transporter in the form of ATP hydrolysis or electron flow. In secondary active transport, the transporter does not directly expend cellular energy but relies on a primary active transport process for its driving force. Some macromolecules cross the cell bafflers through endocytosis (receptor-mediated, adsorptive, or fluid-phase) followed by exocytosis, a process known as transcytosis. Finally, with group translocation, the transported substance is chemically modified by the membrane transporter during the transport event, which may require energy either directly or indirectly.

B. Routes of Transport

Across any continuous epithelium, a solute can be transported either through the cells or between the cells. The cellular pathway is known as the transcellular route, and the intercellular pathway is known as the paracellular route (Fig. 2). The transport of most of the solutes is contributed by both pathways. Lipophilic molecules and molecules with specialized transport processes prefer the transcellular route, whereas hydrophilic molecules lacking membrane transport processes prefer the paracellular route. However, dissecting the fraction contributed by each pathway is difficult (Ho et al., 1999). One measure of the overall barrier permeability is its electrical resistance, a measure of the resistance of the tissue to ion transport. The electrical resistance of various ocular barriers is summarized in Table 1.

The mechanisms of transcellular transport include simple diffusion, facilitated diffusion, active transport, and endocytosis. The plasma membrane of a cell consists of a lipid bilayer with an array of peripherally and integrally associated proteins, some of which serve as specific transporters or

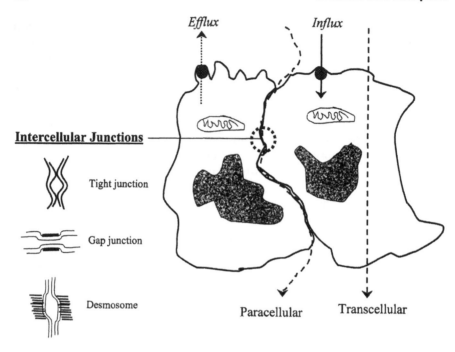

Figure 2   Transcellular and paracellular pathways for drug transport across epithelial and endothelial barriers.

receptors, which allow solute uptake into the cell via active transport, facilitated   diffusion, or receptor-mediated endocytosis. However, for a majority of the currently available drug molecules, no such transporters or receptors exist, and these drugs are transported by passive diffusion through the apical membrane, through the cell proper, and across the basolateral membrane to move across the cell. During transcellular movement, the solute must interact with some components of the cell membrane. The interaction of the solute with the cell is influenced by both the structural characteristics of the solute and the cell itself.

Transport along the paracellular route is passive and is only limited by the size and charge of the intercellular spaces. The paracellular pathway is an aqueous route involving diffusion of the solute between adjacent epithelial cells/endothelial cells restricted by the presence of a series of junctional strands known as tight junctions or *zonula occludens* (ZO), which are joined at the apical pole (Madara and Trier, 1982; Yu, 2000). Freeze-fracture electron microscopy studies demonstrated that ZO forms fusion sites that appear as a complex network of protein strands that seal the intercellular

Table 1 Transmembrane Electrical Resistances of Various Ocular Barriers

Tissue	Rt (ohm-cm^2)	Ref.
Cornea		
Intact rabbit cornea	7500	Marshall and Klyce, 1983
Primary rabbit corneal epithelial cultures (air interface)	5000	Chang et al., 2000
Ciliary body		
Intact rabbit ciliary body	77	Noske et al., 1994
Rabbit nonpigmented epithelial cell cultures	20–30	Cilluffo et al., 1993
Human nonpigmented epithelial cell culture	20	Noske et al., 1995
Conjunctiva		
Excised rabbit conjunctiva	1400	Kompella et al., 1993
Primary rabbit conjunctival cultures (liquid interface)	1900	Saha et al., 1996
Primary rabbit conjunectival cultures (air interface)	1100	Yang et al., 2000
Retina		
RPE-Choroid		
Adult human	79	Quinn and Miller, 1991
Fetal human	206	Quinn and Miller, 1991
Bovine	138	Steinberg et al., 1978
Rabbit	350	Quinn and Miller, 1992
Cat	133–259	Joseph and Miller, 1991
Cultured RPE		
Fetal human	70	Hernandez et al., 1995
Fetal bovine	329	Hernandez et al., 1995
Adult human	225	Hu et al., 1994

space all around the cell perimeter (Lapierre, 2000). The tightness of the barrier increases with an increase in the number of junctional strands. In general, the tight junctions are essentially impermeable to molecules with radii greater than 15 Å. Various proteins that form the tight junctional complex include ZO-l, ZO-2, cingulin. and occludin (Lapierre, 2000). In addition to tight junctions, intercellular spaces possess intermediate junctions or *zonula adherens,* desmosomes, and gap junctions. *Zonula adherens* and desmosomes are sites of firm adhesion between cells that ensure mechanical stability. Gap junctions are responsible for electrical and metabolic coupling between cells (Simon and Goodenough, 1998).

C. Transporters

Transport systems serve the cell by allowing the cellular entry and exit of essential ions and nutrients, and by expelling the toxic metabolites out of the cell. All transmembrane transport processes are mediated by integral membrane proteins, sometimes functioning in conjunction with extracytoplasmic receptors or receptor domains and/or cytoplasmic energy coupling and regulatory proteins or protein domains. These integral membrane proteins and any associated protein or protein domains are referred to as a transport process, transport system, transporter, porter, permease system, or permease (Saier, 2000a). Many transporters are localized in a polarized manner in an epithelium or endothelium to perform vectorial transport of solutes. All transporters are proteins with specific conformations, which makes them unique in their function. Broadly, various types of transporters on the cell membrane can be classified as channels, pumps, uniporters, symporters or cotransporters, and exchangers or antiporters (Table 2) (Saier, 2000a). Some transport proteins having multiple substrate domains are structured so that these domains are arranged in the plane of the membrane in a circle, thereby forming a barrel to transport small solutes such as H^+, Na^+, and K^+ into and out of the cell. When ions or solutes pass through such a transporter by passive diffusion, the transporter is called a channel. Alternatively, the transporter protein may directly utilize energy, usually derived from ATP,

Table 2 Commonly Used Symbols for Various Transporters

Transporter	Symbol	Example
Channel		Na^+, K^+, and Cl^- channels
Cotransporter (symporter)		Na^+-glucose and Na^+-amino acid transporters
Exchanger (antiporter)		Na^+/H^+ and Cl^-/HCO_3^- exchangers
Uniporter		Glucose transporter (GLUT)
Pump		Na^+/K^+-ATPase P-glycoprotein/MRP

to actively drive solutes from one side of the plasma membrane to the other, in which case it is called as a pump. A uniporter transports one solute at a time. A symporter transports the solute and one or more cotransported solutes at the same time in the same direction. An antiporter transports the solute in (or out) and another solute in the opposite direction. Transporter proteins may exist in different isoforms with the same function but with variable affinities, uptake kinetics, and tissue expression profiles. For example, facilitated glucose transport is mediated by a family of glucose transporter (GLUT) proteins, seven isoforms of which are known to date (Thorens, 1996). GLUT1, GLUT2, GLUT3, and GLUT4 are involved in cellular glucose uptake; GLUT1, GLUT3, and GLUT4 are high-affinity glucose transporters, and GLUT2 has a significantly lower affinity. GLUT5 is a high-affinity fructose transporter with poor glucose transport capacity. GLUT7 is closely related to GLUT2, but it is retained in the endoplasmic reticulum and not transported to the plasma membrane. The role of GLUT6 is still unknown. Similarly, various families of transmembrane transporters exist in the mammalian plasma membranes for amino acids and their derivatives (Palacin et al., 1998; Saier, 2000b). Transfer of amino acids across the hydrophobic domain of the plasma membrane is mediated by proteins that recognize, bind, and transport these amino acids, which exhibit broad substrate specificity and stereospecificity. There are three best-known amino acid transport systems present in the plasma membrane of mammalian cells based on the type of amino acid the protein moves and the thermodynamic properties of the transport: (a) zwitterionic amino acid systems (A, ASC, N, BETA, GLY, IMINO, PHE, B^0, L), (b) cationic amino acid systems ($B^{0,+}$, b^+, y^+, y^+L, $b^{0,+}$), and (c) anionic amino acid systems (X^-_{AG}, X^-_C). A detailed description of these transporters is provided elsewhere (Palacin et al., 1998).

III. TRANSPORT BARRIERS IN THE EYE

A. Cornea

While primarily being a refractive element of the eye, the cornea acts as a mechanical and chemical barrier to intraocular tissues. The mammalian cornea, with relatively few exceptions, consists of five to six distinct layers, with a total thickness of 300–500 μm (Pepose and Ubels, 1992). These layers include (Fig. 3): corneal epithelium, underlying basement membrane, acellular Bowman's layer, corneal stroma, Descemet's membrane, and corneal endothelium. Bowman's layer is absent in the cornea of rabbit, a routinely used animal model in eye research (Fig. 3).

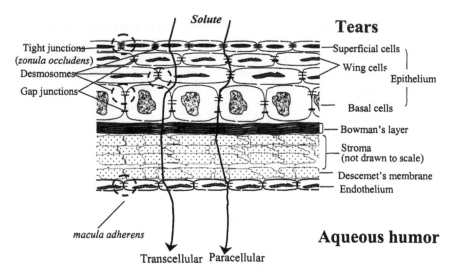

Figure 3 The cornea. Cellular organization of various transport limiting layers.

1. Corneal Epithelium

The corneal epithelium plays critical roles in the maintenance of a barrier against tearborne agents and in maintaining a balanced stromal hydration. The corneal epithelium, with a total thickness of 35–50 µm, is made of five cell layers constituted by superficial, wing, and basal cells and is maintained by several cell-cell and cell-substrate interactions (Pepose and Ubels, 1992). The superficial cells are joined by numerous desmosomes, and the barrier function of these cells is due to the presence of tight junctional complexes that are exclusive to superficial cells in the epithelium. Wing cells are attached to superficial cells and to one another by desmosomes. Large gap junctions are also present between the wing cells, allowing a high degree of intercellular communication in this layer. The basal cells also have desmosomes and gap junctions that are fewer in number. Corneal epithelium overlies on an array of collagen fibrils and glycosaminoglycans (GAGs) known as acellular Bowman's membrane followed by stroma, a hydrated (75–78% water) matrix of collagen fibrils and GAGs, which constitutes 90% of the corneal thickness. This arrangement is followed by Descemet's membrane and corneal endothelium. Descemet's membrane forms the basement membrane for the corneal endothelium (Fig. 3).

The corneal epithelium is considered a "tight" epithelium due to its high shunt resistance, which is in the range of 12–16 kohm-cm^2 (Marshall and Klyce, 1983). The tightness of the corneal epithelium is due to the existence of *zonulae occludens* or tight junctions between the superficial cells. These intercellular junctions maintain the asymmetrical distribution of several receptors for endogenous molecules such as hormones or growth factors and transporters such as Na$^+$/K$^+$-ATPase, Cl$^-$ channel, and Na$^+$– amino acid cotransporter in order to maintain the vectorial transport (Klyce and Crosson, 1985).

The resistance to transport across the cornea is the sum of the resistances to transport across each of the individual corneal layers, i.e., R$_{cornea}$ = R$_{epithelium}$ + R$_{stroma}$ + R$_{endothelium}$. Although the corneal epithelium represents less than 10% of the entire corneal thickness, it contributes 99% of the resistance to solute diffusion across cornea. Of this, the superficial epithelial cells contribute as much as 60%. The stroma and endothelium contribute 3% to the total corneal electrical resistance. The transepithelial or transmembrane resistance of various corneal preparations is summarized in Table 1.

2. Corneal Endothelium

Corneal endothelium is a monolayer of polygonal cells, most of which are hexagonal in shape with about 20 μm diameter and 4–6 μm thickness. These cells play a key role in maintaining corneal transparency through their transport, synthetic, and secretory functions. Contrary to the corneal epithelial cells, *macular occludens,* not entirely occlusive junctions, rather than *zonula occludens* exist between the endothelial cells (McLaughlin et al., 1985). This results in a "leaky" barrier between aqueous humor and stroma. The endothelium has a passive permeability that allows the passage of large molecules up to 70 kDa in size (Pepose and Ubels, 1992). Although the endothelium is leaky, it is the site of the major active ion and fluid transport mechanisms that maintain constant corneal thickness. Gap junctions present on the lateral membranes of the endothelial cells contribute to intercellular communication.

3. Ion and Organic Solute Transport

Corneal surface and stromal hydration is maintained by the movement of Na$^+$, K$^+$, and Cl$^-$ across the apical and basolateral membranes of the epithelium and the corneal endothelium (Fig. 4). The active transport of these ions is responsible for the tear-side negative potential difference of the corneal epithelial cells. The ouabain-sensitive Na$^+$/K$^+$-ATPase on the basolateral side of the epithelium actively transports Na$^+$ out of the cells

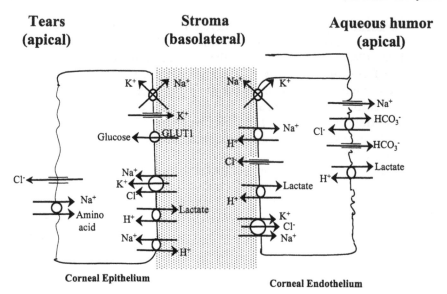

Figure 4 Putative ion and solute transport processes in the mammalian corneal epithelium and endothelium.

in exchange for K^+ (Green, 1970). Cl^- entry across the basolateral membrane of the epithelium is mediated by a loop diuretic–sensitive $Na^+/K^+/Cl^-$ cotransporter (Klyce, 1972; Marshall and Klyce, 1983). This Cl^- entry occurs against an electrochemical potential and is ouabain sensitive, suggesting that Cl^- entry is coupled to the Na^+/K^+-ATPase activity. The $Na^+/K^+/Cl^-$ cotransporter elevates the intracellular Cl^- concentration to three to four times greater than that expected from simple equilibrium, enabling the passive transport of Cl^- through Cl^- channels located on the apical side. K^+ has low paracellular permeability, and it enters the cells through Na^+/K^+-ATPase (Marshall and Klyce, 1983) and exits through K^+ channels located on the basolateral side.

     In endothelial cells, the Na^+/K^+-ATPase is located on the basolateral side (Whikehart and Soppet, 1981; Whikehart et al., 1987). Inhibition of this pump with ouabain stops sodium transport, causes corneal swelling, and eliminates the transendothelial potential difference. Stromal Cl^- concentration is in part determined by Cl^- entry through a Cl^-/HCO_3^- exchanger located on the apical membrane of the endothelial cells and exit through Cl^- channel on the basolateral membrane of the endothelium (Bonanno et al., 1998). Also, $Na^+/K^+/Cl^-$ cotransporter present on the lateral membrane of the corneal endothelium contributes to the transendothelial Cl^- flux (Jelamskii et al., 2000).

In corneal epithelial and endothelial cells, Na^+/H^+ exchanger, Na^+-HCO_3^- symport, and Cl^-/HCO_3^- exchanger are involved in the regulation of intracellular pH (Jentsch et al., 1985; Bonanno et al., 1999). Na^+/H^+ exchanger is present in the basolateral membranes of both epithelial and endothelial cells. Na^+/HCO_3^- transporter is predominantly localized on the basolateral side of the corneal endothelium and is weakly expressed in the corneal epithelium (Sun et al., 2000).

H^+-lactate cotransport is present on the baslolateral side of the rabbit corneal epithelium (Bonanno, 1990) and on both sides of the rabbit corneal endothelium (Giasson and Bonanno, 1994). In addition, the corneal endothelium has a Na^+-lactate cotransport process on the basolateral side (Giasson and Bonanno, 1994). These transport processes efficiently remove lactate from the highly glycolytic cornea, thereby preventing lactate-mediated corneal swelling.

The corneal epithelium is relatively impermeable to water-soluble compounds such as amino acids derived from tears (Thoft and Friend, 1972). The limbal blood supplies less than 20% of the corneal nutrients, with the aqueous humor being the primary source of amino acids (Thoft and Friend, 1972). Indeed, corneal endothelium, the principal barrier between the aqueous humor and the corneal epithelium, transports amino acids from the aqueous humor to the extracellular fluid of the stroma against a concentration gradient in the rabbit cornea (Riley, 1977). Consistent with this, the steady-state concentrations of most free amino acids in the stroma of the rabbit cornea are higher than those in the aqueous humor (Thoft and Friend, 1972; Riley et al., 1973; Riley and Yates, 1977). Similarly, the high glucose requirements of the corneal epithelium are met in part by the facilitated glucose transporter, GLUT 1, present on the basolateral side of the epithelium (Takahashi et al., 1996).

B. Conjunctiva

The conjunctiva is a thin, transparent mucous membrane lining the inside of the eyelids and is continuous with cornea. In rabbits, the conjunctiva occupies 9 times larger surface area, and in humans, it occupies 17 times larger surface area than the cornea (Watsky et al., 1988). The conjunctiva can be divided into three layers: (a) an outer epithelium, a permeability barrier, (b) substantia propria, containing nerves, lymphatics, and blood vessels, and (c) submucosa, which provides a loose attachment to the underlying sclera. The conjunctiva differs from cornea in its rich vasculature, the presence of many goblet cells, and its ability to transdifferentiate.

1. Conjunctival Epithelium

The conjunctival epithelium is similar to the cornea with respect to the organization of epithelial cells—it contains superficial, wing, and basal cells, the three principal corneal epithelial cell types. The epithelium is two to three cell layers thick, nonkeratinized, stratified and sqamous at the eyelids, and columnar towards the cornea. The tight junctions in the apical pole of the conjunctival epithelium render it a relatively impermeable barrier. The epithelial cells of the conjunctiva are attached to one another by means of desmosomes and to the basal lamina through hemidesmosomes.

2. Ion and Organic Solute Transport

The conjunctiva is a tight epithelium with an electrical resistance of 1.4 kohm-cm^2 (Kompella et al., 1993) (Fig. 5). The potential difference of the conjunctiva is lumen-negative like the cornea, suggesting a net secretion of anions and/or a net absorption of cations.

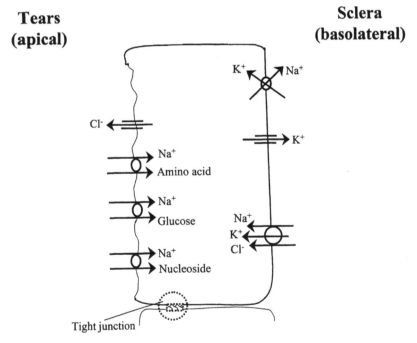

Figure 5 Putative ion and solute transport processes in the mammalian conjunctival epithelium.

The conjunctiva actively secretes Cl^- (Kompella et al., 1993), and about 80% of the conjunctival active ion transport is accounted for by Cl^- secretion through apically localized channels. Cl^- enters the basolateral side via $Na^+/K^+/Cl^-$ cotransport energized by the basolateral Na^+/K^+-ATPase. Conjunctiva secretes fluid secondary to active Cl^- secretion (Shiue et al., 2000). Active Na^+ absorption can counter this fluid secretion. Net fluid secretion rate across the conjunctiva is altered by pharmacological agents known to affect active Cl^- secretion or Na^+ absorption (Shiue et al., 2000).

Evidence exists for the presence of ion-dependent solute transport processes such as Na^+-glucose, Na^+-amino acid, and Na^+-nucleoside transporters in the conjunctival epithelium (Kompella et al., 1995; Hosoya et al., 1996; Hosoya et al., 1998b). After bathing conjunctiva in a glucose-free glutathione bicarbonate Ringer (GBR) solution, mucosal addition of D-glucose elevated short-circuit current (Isc) by a maximum of 20% in a dose-dependent manner. Phlorizin, a specific inhibitor of Na^+-glucose cotransporter, reduced the Isc in a dose-dependent manner, suggesting the possible apical localization of Na^+-glucose cotransporter in the pigmented rabbit conjunctiva (Hosoya et al., 1996). Similarly, mucosal addition of glycine, L-arginine, D-arginine, and L-glutamic acid have increased Isc in the presence but not in the absence of sodium in the medium, suggesting the possible existence of Na^+-amino acid cotransporters on the apical side of the conjunctiva (Kompella et al., 1995). Furthermore, $B^{0,+}$, a sodium-dependent transporter of neutral (L-Glu) and basic amino acids (L-Arg, L-Lys, and N^G-nitro-L-arginine) is present in the conjunctiva (Hosoya et al., 1998a).

Uridine, a nucleoside, is transported preferentially from the mucosal to serosal direction in a temperature- and phlorizin-sensitive manner across the conjunctiva (Hosoya et al., 1998b). At constant Na^+ concentration (141 mM) on mucosal side, uridine increased Isc in a dose-dependent fashion. At constant uridine concentration (10 μM), increasing Na^+ concentration increased Isc with a Hill coefficient of 1.1, suggesting that there is a 1:1 coupling in the transport of Na^+ and uridine. Na^+-dependent uridine transport was inhibited by 10 μM adenosine, guanosine, and inosine, but not by thymidine, suggesting that the transport process may be mainly selective for purine nucleosides.

C. Iris-Ciliary Body

The iris, ciliary body, and choroid comprise the vascular uveal coat of the eye. The anterior iris is immersed in the aqueous humor, which enters the iris stroma through openings or crypts along its anterior surface. The iris receives its blood supply from the major arterial circle, which lies in the stroma of the ciliary body near the iris root. The ciliary body can be divided into the following regions: nonpigmented ciliary epithelium, pigmented ciliary epithelium, stroma, and ciliary muscle. The main arterial blood supply to the ciliary body is through the long posterior and the anterior ciliary arteries. These capillaries are fenestrated (Cunha-Vaz, 1979) and leaky (Stewart and Tuor, 1994).

The ciliary body secretes aqueous humor into the posterior chamber, from where it flows through the pupil into the anterior chamber and leaves the eye in a bulk flow through trabecular and uveo-scleral routes at the angle of the anterior chamber. The aqueous humor is a transparent, aqueous solution, and its composition is different from that of plasma in its low concentration of plasma proteins and 20 to 60-fold higher concentration of ascorbic acid (Caprioli, 1992). The aqueous humor production and the intraocular pressure are maintained by membrane transport processes. For instance, the aqueous humor production can be controlled by agents that directly or indirectly alter the release of Cl^- through basolateral channels of nonpigmented ciliary epithelium, which is the rate-limiting step in the aqueous humor secretion in the eye (Bowler et al., 1996).

1. Blood-Aqueous Barrier

The blood-aqueous barrier restricts the penetration of solutes such as acriflavine (MW 540) into the posterior chamber as well as the anterior chamber (Rodriguez-Peralta, 1975). With the blood-aqueous barrier, inward movement of solutes from the blood to the eye is more restrictive compared to the outward movement. The blood-aqueous barrier is principally constituted by two discrete layers of cells: the endothelium of the iris and ciliary blood vessels and the nonpigmented ciliary epithelium. To pass from the blood vessels of iris into the posterior chamber, a substance has to cross the iris vessels, the stroma, a layer of iris muscle, and the iris epithelium. Transport from the stroma into the anterior chamber is easier because the cellular layer on the anterior surface of the iris is incomplete. In the anterior chamber angle, there is continuous drainage of aqueous humor, which limits the movement of solutes from the anterior chamber to posterior chamber. To pass from the blood vessels of the ciliary body into the posterior chamber, a solute has to cross the ciliary microvessels, the loose connective tissue of the stroma, and the two-layered ciliary epithelium. The capillaries of the iris have a relatively thick wall layered by the continuous-type endothelial cells that are attached to each other by tight junctional complexes (Raviola, 1977; Freddo and Raviola, 1982). The number of strands in the *zonulae occludens* of these cells in the monkey varies from one to eight. As in the blood-brain barrier (BBB), GLUT-1 and P-glycoprotein are present in iris and ciliary vessel endothelial cells, while endothelial antigen PAL-E (Pathologische Anatomie Leiden-Endothelium) and the transferrin receptor are absent (Schlingemann et al., 1998). This suggests a phenotypic similarity of iris and ciliary vessels with brain microvessels. The iris vessels restrict the transport of circulating horseradish peroxidase (HRP) and fluorescein due to the presence of tight junctions between the endothelial cells. In this regard, the vessels of the iris, retina, and brain share a common behavior (Hank et al., 1990; Holash and Stewart, 1993; Stewart and Tuor, 1994). However, ciliary vessels are permeable to circulating HRP, and it is speculated that it reaches ciliary muscle by diffusion from the permeable vessels of the ciliary processes.

The ciliary body epithelium is made of an outer pigmented epithelium (PE) and an inner nonpigmented epithelium (NPE) juxtaposed at their apical surfaces (Fig. 6). The tight junctions between NPE cells impose a diffusion barrier between blood and aqueous humor (Schlingemann et al., 1998). Intravenously injected HRP passes through the fenestrated ciliary endothelial cells and reaches the intercellular spaces around PE cells and those between PE and NPE cells. However, the tight junctions at the apico-lateral

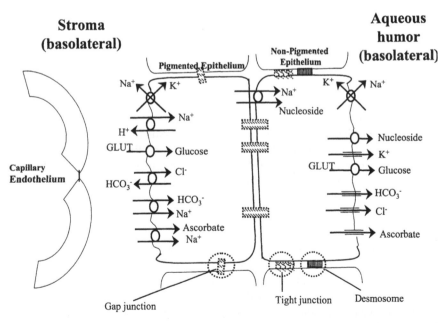

Figure 6 Putative ion and solute transport processes in the mammalian pigmented and nonpigmented epithelial cells of the ciliary body.

fusion points of the NPE cells block further movement of HRP into the posterior chamber (Schlingemann et al., 1998). Gap junctions are ubiquitous in the ciliary body epithelium, connecting PE-to-PE, NPE-to-NPF, and PE-to-NPE cells (Freddo, 1987) (Fig. 6). The gap junctions between PE and NPE cells are permeable to molecules at least as large as 900–1000 daltons (Spray and Bennett, 1985).

In general, the breakdown of the blood-aqueous barrier takes place when the mammalian eye is subjected to painful or irritant stimuli in response to mechanical trauma or by carotid infusion of hyperosmotic agents, leading to the leakage of plasma proteins into the aqueous humor (Butler et al., 1988). This breakdown may be due to shrinkage of the pigmented epithelial cells, degeneration of the junctional complexes, and separation of the two epithelial cell layers. In addition, stimulation of ocular motor nerve, local administration of prostaglandin (PGE 1), and systemic injection of α-MSH causes dilatation of iris and ciliary capillaries and relaxation of afferent vessels, leading to the disruption of the blood-aqueous barrier.

4.   Ion and Organic Solute Transport

Aqueous humor formation was once considered a simple process of diffusion or ultrafiltration of fluid from the plasma across the ciliary epithelia. It is now well established that active transport of certain solutes by the ciliary epithelia is the most important process in the formation of aqueous humor (Caprioli, 1992). Na^+/K^+-ATPase (Usukura et al., 1988; Okami et al., 1989; Martin-Vasallo et at., 1989), H^+/K^+-ATPase (Fain et al, 1988) and active ascorbate transport system (Socci and Delamere, 1988) are present in the ciliary epithelia. Immunoblot analysis revealed the presence of Na^+/K^+-ATPase mainly on the basolateral surfaces of PE and NPE cells, with the labeling density being twofold higher in PE cells relative to NPE cells (Okami et al., 1989). H^+/K^--ATPase is present extensively on the apical membrane of both PE and NPE cells (Fain et al., 1988). In addition, the basolateral membrane of pigmented layer contains the entry step for $Cl^-/Na^+/K^+$ cotransporter, a Cl^-/HCO_3-exchanger, a Na^+/HCO_3^- cotransporter, a Na^+/H^+ exchanger, and a $Na^+/$ascorbate cotransporter (Zadunaisky, 1992). These systems produce low levels of sodium in the two cells, a high level of potassium, and a high ascorbic content and control the intracellular pH. The basolateral membrane of the nonpigmented epithelium contains the channels for the exit of chloride, sodium, bicarbonate, and ascorbate into the posterior chamber and induce the movement of water for the formation of the aqueous humor (Zadunaisky, 1992).

In spite of the tight barrier properties of ciliary epithelium, the concentration of glucose in aqueous humor is kept at a level similar to that in plasma. This is facilitated by GLUT1, a glucose transporter localized in the ciliary epithelial cells (Hank et al., 1990; Takata et al., 1997). The rate of glucose transport into posterior chamber is very high. GLUT 1 at the basal infoldings of NPE cells, which face the posterior chamber, may play a role in the exit of glucose from the NPE cells to the aqueous humor (Fig. 6). Immunocytochemical studies indicated a two fold higher expression of GLUT1 in basal plasma membrane of PE cells compared to NPE cells. From blood, glucose crosses fenestrated ciliary endothelial cells and then enters PE cells by GLUT1 located in the basal infoldings of their plasma membrane. From PE, glucose enters NPE cells by passing through the gap junctions that connect PE and NPE cells. Finally, glucose leaves the NPE cells via GLUT1 at the infolded basal plasma membrane and enters the aqueous humor.

The concentration of most amino acids is higher in the aqueous than in the plasma, possibly due to active transport of amino acids across the ciliary epithelium in several mammalian species (Zlokovic et al., 1992, 1994). In sheep, concentrations of aspartic acid and glutamic acid in the aqueous were 9–13 times higher compared to plasma, and cystine and lysine levels were approximately 1.7 times those in the plasma. For other amino acids, such as alanine, arginine, glycine, isoleucine, leucine, methionine, phenylalanine, serine, threonine, tyrosine, and valine, the aqueous/plasma ratio was greater than 2. A descriptive statistical study of the covariation of the concentration of amino acids and related compounds in human aqueous suggested the existence of six transport systems in the ciliary epithelia: three for neutral amino acids and one each for basic amino acids, acidic amino acids, and urea (Ehlers et at., 1978; Zlokovic et at., 1992). The protein concentration in the aqueous humor is always less than 1% of its plasma concentration, and it consists primarily of lower molecular weight proteins such as albumin and β-globulin. Heavy molecular proteins such as β-lipoproteins and heavy immunoglobulins are present only in trace quantities in the aqueous humor. Diffusion of protein from the stroma of the ciliary body through the iris stroma and into the aqueous humor has been proposed to account for the major fraction of protein in the rabbit aqueous humor (Freddo et al., 1990).

Ciliary epithelium expresses transporters to allow the transmembrane flux of organic acids such as prostaglandins and eicosanoids (Bito, 1986). Organic acids such as iodopyracet are actively removed from the eye when introduced into the vitreous body. The ciliary epithelium contains at least two systems for the transport of organic acids, the liver-like or L-system, and the classical hippurate or H-system. These systems limit the accumulation of eicosanoids in the eye, which are produced in greater amounts under pathological conditions (Bito and Wallenstein, 1977). The concentrative accumulation of prostaglandins by the isolated anterior uvea is energy and sodium dependent (Dibenedetto and Bito, 1980). Prostacycline, 6-keto-PGF1α, and the classical E and F prostaglandins appear to be substrates for the same transport process. Tissues surrounding the anterior chamber and those covering the surface of the eye, such as the cornea, conjunctiva, sclera, and the anterior surface of the iris, do not appear to possess transporters for prostaglandins (Bito, 1986).

In bovine pigment ciliary epithelial cells, Na$^+$-dependent [^{14}C] ascorbic acid accumulation was seen to proceed against a 40-fold intracellular gradient (Helbig et at., 1989). This uptake was inhibited by phloretin, ouabain, amphotcriein, and D-isoascorbate, but not by glucose. The Na$^+$ dependence of the uptake indicated that two or more Na$^+$ ions translocate with each molecule of ascorbate, resulting in an electrogenic transport. In general transport terms, ocular ascorbic acid fits a type of "pump-leak" model: the pump consists of ascorbic acid transport into aqueous humor; the leak is combined loss of ascorbic acid by fluid drainage through the canal of Schlemm and chemical loss through oxidation. The ascorbic acid uptake in excised iris-ciliary body is saturable and can be inhibited by D-isoascorbate, ouabain, and metabolic inhibitors including dinitrophenol, iodoacetate, and cyanide. The iris-ciliary body resembles retina, ileum, and kidney in having an active transport process for ascorbic acid (Socci and Delamere, 1988). Unlike the uptake process, the efflux of [^{14}C]ascorbic acid was not inhibited by ouabain or other above-mentioned metabolic inhibitors (Chu and Candia, 1988).

Endogenous nucleosides enter nonpigmented epithelial cells through a sodium-nucleoside cotransporter localized on the apical side of the nonpigmented layer of the ciliary body facing the pigmented epithelium and exit into the aqueous humor across the basolateral membrane via an equilibrative transport system (Redzic et at., 1998). Knowledge of the transport of nucleosides through the blood-aqueous barrier is now made more important with the increasing use of nucleoside analogs in the treatment of acquired immunodeficiency malignancies and syndrome (AIDS). As synthetic nucleosides are now known to be transported from blood into the aqueous humor (Redzic et at., 1995), such molecules may compete for the carrier systems used by endogenous nueleosides.

D. Lens

The lens is a transparent tissue, with 65% of its weight consisting of water and the remainder principally of proteins. Anteriorly, the lens is in contact with the pupillary portion of the iris, and posteriorly it fits into a hollow depression of the anterior vitreous surface (Paterson and Delamere, 1992). The major components of the lens are capsule, epithelium, and lens fiber cells (Fig. 7). The lens capsule is acellular, transparent, elastic, and acts as an unusually thick basement membrane that encloses the epithelium and lens fiber cells. It is mainly composed of type IV collagen together with 10% glycosaminoglycans (GAGs). The inner portion of the anterior capsule is in immediate contact with lens epithelium, while the posterior capsule is in contact with the most superficial lens fiber cells. A single layer of epithelial cells forms a cap on the inner anterior surface of the lens, and hundreds of thousands of differentiated fiber cells form its bulk. Lens cortex or periphery is composed of fiber cells that are formed from the differentiation of epithelial cells in the equatorial zone. Young and superficial fiber cells contain cytoplasmic inclusions similar to those of epithelial cells. Since the lens does not shed any of its cellular components from embryonic development onward, the older cells of the lens will be displaced towards the center or nucleus of the lens. Most of the cells in the lens nucleus lack nuclei and particulate cytoplasmic contents. Membrane transport proteins in the lens

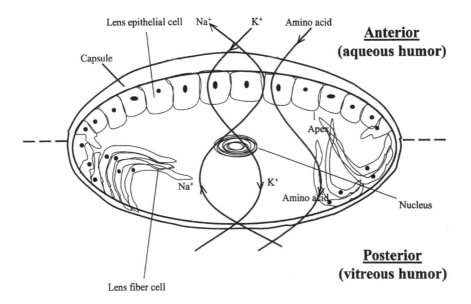

Figure 7 The lens. Representation of pump-leak system and cellular barriers in the movement of ions and nutrients. The fiber cells are distributed through out the lens body.

play an important role in cell volume regulation, nutrient supply, and lens transparency (Goodenough, 1992, Rae, 1994). All cells of the lens are interconnected by gap junctions that form low-resistance pathways between the cytoplasm of adjacent cells.

1. Lens Epithelium

The lens epithelium lies beneath the anterior and equatorial regions of lens capsule, but not under the posterior region of the capsule. The apices of the epithelial cells face the interior of the lens, and their bases face the lens capsule. There are several junctional relationships between the cells of the lens epithelium. The lateral and apical aspects of the plasma membranes have desomosomes for cell adhesion. *Zonula occludens* is also present between epithelial cells in both frog and human lens, and these junctions could restrict the movement of high molecular weight solutes (Lo and Harding, 1986). There is a small number of gap junctions between the lens epithelial cells and the underlying lens fibers, which allow cell-to-cell communication (Brown et al., 1990). The cells of the lens epithelium are anatomically and physiologically polarized, thereby bringing net transport of many essential nutrients. While the lens epithelial cells are selectively permeable to K^+, lens fiber cells have a low and nonselective overall conductance (Robinson and Patterson, 1982).

2. Ion and Organic Solute Transport

In the mammalian lens, the concentration of ions inside the cells plays a major role in the development of cataract. Ions such as Ca^{2+} have been shown to form aggregates with lens α-crystallins, thereby causing opacity (Benedek, 1971; Benedek et al., 1999). Low intracellular calcium is maintained by Na^+/Ca^{2+} exchanger and Ca^{2+}-ATPase (Hightower et al, 1980). Evidence exists for the presence of Na^+/Ca^{2+} exchanger in the apical membrane of lens epithelial cells (Ye and Zadunaisky, 1992a,b). In rabbit, bovine, dog, and rat lenses, while the lack of sodium did not affect the efflux of Ca^{2+} from the cells, inhibitors of Ca^{2+}-ATPase, lanthanum and propranolol inhibited Ca^{2+} efflux (Hightower et al, 1980). ATPase is present in both the lens epithelium and cortex but absent in the nucleus, with the expression being the highest in the epithelium (Ye and Zadunaisky, 1992b) (Fig. 8). Na^+/H^+ exchanger regulates intracellular pH in the lens epithelial cells as well as the lens fiber cells (Wolosin et al., 1988).

Because of lens avascularity, there is a need for the continuous supply of nutrients such as glucose, amino acids, and ascorbic acid for metabolic and synthetic reactions. Lens derives most of its nutrients from aqueous humor. Entry of solutes into the lens occurs by both saturable and nonsa-

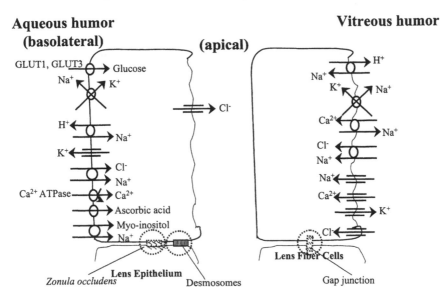

Figure 8 Putative ion and solute transport processes in the mammalian lens epithelial and fiber cells.

turable paths (Merrimann-Smith et al., 1999). While water, chloride, urea, and glycerol are likely to traverse the plasma membrane of the lens epithelial cells by simple diffusion, amino acids are transported actively. The uptake of D-glucose and nonmetabolizable 3-O-methyl-D-glucose into the rat lens was saturable and the capacity of the system for D-glucose was similar at both anterior and posterior surfaces. Transport studies with a variety of sugars indicated that a C-1 conformation and the presence of H or OH on carbon number 1 are critical to transport. Furthermore, the GLUT family of proteins, GLUT 1 and GLUT3, is predominantly responsible for the uptake of glucose in the anterior epithelium (Kern and Ho, 1973; Merrimann-Smith et al., 1999). These transporters are abundant in the lens nucleus and present in the cortex to a lower extent in both human and rat eyes.

Lens contains a higher concentration of amino acids compared to the surrounding aqueous and vitreous humors. In vitro lens uptake studies with labeled amino acids indicated saturation kinetics, energy and temperature dependency, consistent with their active transport (Zlokovic et al., 1992). Furthermore, separate systems exist for the transport of neutral, basic, and acidic amino acids in the lens. Lens expresses A-, L-, Gly-, β-, and Ly^+-systems (Kern et al., 1977). The ASC system, selective for three- or four-carbon neutral amino acids, is present in the lens epithelial cell, and it is the preferred pathway at physiological levels of L-alanine, L-serine, and L-cystein (Kern et al., 1977). The lens behaves like a "pump-leak system" in which the substances actively transported by the epithelium are concentrated in the lens and then diffuse toward the posterior pole and eventually leave the lens across the posterior capsule.

The rate of differentiation of lens epithelial cells into fiber cells is dependent on the synthesis of phosphoinositides from myoinositol (Zelenka and Vu, 1984). Since myoinositol synthesis in the lens is negligible, membrane transport is the major source of cellular myoinositol. The lens allows both sodium-dependent active transport and passive diffusional transport of myo-inositol (Diecke et al., 1995).

The oxidative balance in the lens is maintained by ascorbic acid, whose primary source is aqueous humor (Kern and Zolot, 1987). The active uptake of ascorbic acid by lens epithelium is 20 times greater than L-glucose. Within 7 minutes following systemic administration, [^{14}C]ascorbic acid is concentrated more in the lens epithelium than the aqueous humor.

Nucleotides enter the lens via Na$^+$-dependent transport processes, with the uptake being comparable at the two surfaces of the lens, similar to sugars (Redzic et al., 1998). Saturable uptake was observed for purines such as guanosine, inosine, and adenosine, but not for pyrimidines and adenine.

E. Blood-Retinal Barrier

Fully developed retina is organized into the following layers (Fig. 9): retinal pigment epithelium (RPE), photoreceptor layer, outer limiting membrane, outer nuclear layer, outer plexiform layer, inner nuclear layer, inner plexiform layer, ganglion cell layer, nerve fiber layer, and inner limiting membrane (Wu, 1995). Large retinal vessels are present in the optic nerve fiber layer, and retinal capillaries are present between the inner nuclear layer and the outer plexiform layer. The outer and inner limiting membranes of the retina are quite permeable. The outer limiting membrane has traditionally been described as a layer of *zonulae adherens* that connect Müller cells to photoreceptors, and it is permeable to macromolecules. The inner limiting membrane is a continuous glycoprotein coating identical to the basal lamina of epithelia or endothelia. The inner limiting membrane contains the cell bodies of most neurons and forms a basement membrane for the Müller and glial cells and separates the base of the Müller cells from the vitreous body. The intercellular clefts between the Müller cell processes that abut the inner limiting membrane are open and lack specialized intercellular junctions. Freeze-fracture studies confirmed the absence of *zonulae occludens* between the basal feet of the Müller cells in both humans and monkey. The perme-

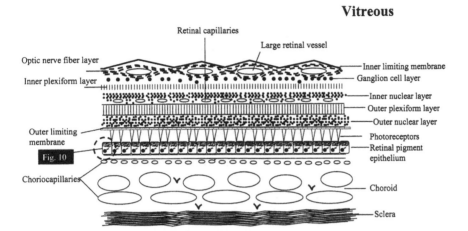

Figure 9 Cellular organization of the retina.

ability properties of inner limiting membrane are likely similar to the basal laminae, which retain particulate matter but allow the transport of molecules up to the size of ferritin (400 kDa) (Wu, 1995). Among all the retinal layers, the principal barrier to solute transport is the blood-retinal barrier (BRB), which includes retinal pigment epithelium and retinal vessels.

The BRB is located at two levels: the outer BRB, consisting of the retinal pigment epithelium (RPE), and the inner BRB, consisting of the endothelial membranes of the blood vessels of the retina. BRB plays a critical role in the homeostatis of the neural retina by limiting the entry of xenobiotics into the extravascular spaces of the retina and by preventing the loss of essential solutes. Blood-retinal barrier breakdown, a key factor underlying pathological conditions such as diabetic retinopathy, is a leading cause of vision loss. In neovascular disorders such as proliferative diabetic retinopathy or age-related choroidal neovascularization, elevation of angiogenic factors such as vascular endothelial growth factor ($VEGF_{165}$) and transforming growth factor ($TGF-\beta$), can disrupt the blood-retinal barrier (Behzadian et al., 2001). Quantification of the degree of damage to blood-retinal barrier can be performed by locating [125]I- and [135]I-albumin tracers (Miyamoto et al., 1999) or Evans blue in the retinal tissue and/or vitreous following their systemic injection (Xu et al., 2001).

1. Retinal Pigment Epithelium

RPE is a monolayer of hexagonal cells separating the outer surface of the neural retina from the choriocapillaries. Many of these cells are multinucleated, and the nuclei are located in the basal portion of the cell. RPE plays a central role in regulating the microenvironment surrounding the photoreceptors in the distal retina, where the phototransduction takes place. The outer segments of rods and cones are closely associated with the RPE via villous and pesudopodial attachments. The RPE phagocytoses distal potions of rod and cone outer segments.

Following intravitreal injection, horseradish peroxidase crosses the inner limiting membrane, ganglion cell layer, inner plexiform layer (synaptic layer), inner nuclear membrane, outer limiting membrane, and the layer of the photoreceptors but blocked by the tight junctions of the retinal pigment epithelial cells (Tornquist et al., 1990). Thus, the retinal pigment epithelium is a principal barrier to solute transport. Macromolecules such as horseradish peroxidase that escape from the permeable vessels of the choriocapillaries, cross Bruch's membrane and penetrate the intercellular clefts of the retinal pigment epithelium. Further progression into the retina is blocked by the junctional complexes of the RPE (Tornquist et al., 1990). In a number of vertebrate species, these junctional complexes consist of *zonula occludens, zonula adherens*, and gap junctions, and their surface specializations are different from those observed in other epithelia (Hudspeth and Yee, 1973). The gap junctions lie apically (vitread), the *zonula adherens* lie basally (sclerad), and the *zonula occludens* overlap the other two junctions. With the presence of tight junctions, RPE forms a polarized monolayer of cells with morphologically and functionally distinct apical and basolateral membranes. The apical membrane of RPE faces the photoreceptor outer segment across the subretinal space, and the basolateral membrane is juxtaposed to the choriocapillaries across Bruch's membrane. Various transporter proteins are distributed in a polarized manner in RPE (Rodriguez-Boulan and Nelson, 1989; Mays et al., 1994).

RPE is extremely restrictive for paracellular transport of solutes due to the presence of tight junctions. However, it is capable of a variety of specialized transport processes (Betz and Goldstein, 1980). To understand the barrier properties of RPE, experimental models such as isolated RPE-choroid preparations (Crosson and Pautler, 1982; Tsuboi and Pederson, 1988; Joseph and Miller, 1991; Quinn and Miller, 1992; la Cour et al., 1994), neural retina-RPE-choroid preparations (Shirao and Steinberg, 1987), and confluent monolayers of cultured RPE (Defoe et al., 1994; Hernandez et al., 1995; Gallemore et al., 1995) can be used. The electrical resistance of various RPE and choroid preparations is summarized in Table 1. The electrical resistance of RPE preparations ranges from 70 to 350 ohm-cm^2 in various species and preparations. The low in vitro resistance of these preparations does not appear to be representative of the formidable in vivo blood-retinal barrier.

2. Retinal Vessels

The studies led by Cunha-Vaz et al. (1979) proposed that the endothelial cells along with their junctional complexes are the main sites of the blood-retinal barrier for substances like thorium dioxide, trypan blue, and fluorescein. Many investigations demonstrated the barrier properties of the retinal endothelium (Tomquist et al., 1990; Xu et al., 2001). Following intravenous injection of thorium dioxide or horseradish peroxidase, tight junctions blocked tracer progression along the clefts between the endothelial cells of the retinal capillaries. Also, the tracer transport into the endothelial cytoplasm was negligible. Compared to several other blood vessels in the body, the retinal vessels have more extensive *zonula occludens*, which render them impermeable to both horseradish peroxidase (MW 40 kDa; hydrodynamic radius ~5 nm) and microperoxidase (MW 1.9 kDa; hydrodynamic radius ~2 nm) (Smith and Rudt, 1975). These junctional complexes restrict solute movement in either direction, as indicated by the inability of vitreal horseradish peroxidase in reaching the lumen of retinal vessels (Peyman and Bok, 1972). These junctions may restrict small solutes differently because fluorescein does not cross the blood-retinal barrier when injected intraperitoneally into rabbits (Cunha-Vaz and Maurice, 1967), but it is easily absorbed by the retinal vessels following vitreal administration, suggesting that the retinal vessels and the pigment epithelium are capable of removing organic anions from the vitreous. Poor permeability into the vitreous was seen for solutes such as urea, sodium, potassium, chloride, phosphate, inulin, sucrose, antibiotics, and proteins such as albumin, myoglobin, and horseradish peroxidase following intravenous injection (Tornquist et al., 1990). Higher quantities were observed in the anterior vitreous following entry from the posterior chamber or ciliary circulation, suggesting that blood-aqueous barrier is more leaky compared to BRB. The BRB permeability of fluorescein with a molecular radius of 5.5 Å was estimated to be about 0.14×10^{-5} cm/s, which is similar to fluorescein permeability across the blood-brain barrier, suggesting that BRB and BBB are functionally similar (Vinores, 1995). The passive transport of solutes across the BRB is 50 times lower than in most other vessels of the body and 10 times lower than in the iris vessels (Tornquist et al., 1990). Lipophilic substances such as rhodamine penetrate freely across the BRB into the vitreous after systemic administration, with the blood-to-vitreous ratio being 1 (Maurice and Mishima, 1984). Indeed, with increasing drug partition coefficients, the vitreal concentrations as well as the rate of vitreal penetration of different antibiotics increased (Bleeker et al. 1968; Lesar and Fiscella, 1985). The low permeability surface area products (PS) for sucrose (0.44×10^{-5} mL/g/s) and mannitol (1.25×10^{-5} mL/g/s) across BRB are similar to that of BBB (Lightman et al., 1987).

3.   Ion and Organic Solute Transport

There is substantial evidence for the vectorial transport of solutes across the BRB. Various solute transport processes present in RPE are shown in Figure 10. Unlike other epithelial tissues and similar to the choroid plexus, RPE expresses Na^+/K^+-ATPase primarily in the apical membrane (Quinn and Miller, 1992). RPE cells secrete Na^+ actively. Indeed, the active ^{22}Na secretion was inhibited by apical ouabain (Miller and Edelman, 1990). RPE cells of human as well as rat origins express tetrodotoxin-sensitive Na^+ channels (Wen et al., 1994; Botchkin and Matthews, 1994). Besides Na^+ secretion, Cl^- absorption is the principal contributor to the active ion transport across the RPE. Cl^- absorption is primarily determined by furosemide- and bumetanide-sensitive $Na^+/K^+/Cl^-$ cotransporter, which allows apical Cl^- entry (La Cour, 1992). Ca^{2+}- cAMP-activated Cl^- channels are present on the basolateral side to allow Cl^- exit (Ueda and Steinberg, 1994; Strauss et al., 1996). Also, patch-clamp studies on single cells demonstrated a swelling-activated Cl^- channel in RPE. Bovine and human RPE express CFTR, a cAMP-regulated Cl^- channel (Miller et al., 1992). Na^+/Ca^{2+} exchanger is also present in the apical membrane of bovine and dogfish RPE cells (Fijisawa et al., 1993).

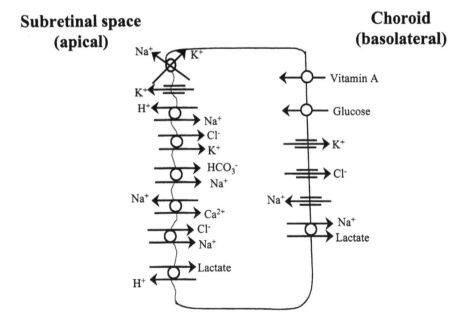

Figure 10   Putative ion and solute transport processes in the mammalian retinal pigmented epithelium.

RPE has a reverse polarization of Na^+/K^+-ATPase, because this pump is localized on the apical membrane as opposed to the basolateral membrane. To determine whether such reverse polarization is also the case with protein trafficking and sorting in RPE cells, Bok et al. (1992) determined the budding of viruses whose progeny bud from specific membrane domains in epithelial cells as directed by the sorting of their envelope glycoprotein. Upon infection of human and bovine RPE with these envoloped viruses, cultured human and bovine RPE exhibited the same pattern of viral budding as has been observed in other polarized epithelia, with the influenza hemagglutinin sorted to the apical membrane and the vesicular stomatitis glycoprotein sorted to the basolateral membrane.

In addition to the above-mentioned ionic transport processes, there are specific transporters that regulate the transport of nutrients and metabolites such as glucose, amino acids, nucleosides, folic acid, lactic acid, ascorbic acid, and retinoids in the retina. A facilitated glucose transporter, GLUT1, a 50 kDa protein, is expressed in various cells, including retinal pigmented epithelial cells, choroidal cells, retinal Müller cells, and the outer segments of the photoreceptor cells in the adult eye. Immunofluorescence and immunogold studies revealed that GLUT1 is present on both apical and basolateral sites of RPE cells (Mantych et al., 1993). Immunoreactivity for GLUT3, a 50–55 kDa protein, was observed in the adult inner synaptic layer of the retina (Mantych et al., 1993).

In the blood-retinal barrier of rats, carrier systems exist for the transport of neutral and basic amino acids (Tornquist and Alm, 1986; Tornquist et al., 1990). Also, taurine and myo- inositol enter RPE cells via carrier-mediated transport mechanisms (Miyamoto et al., 1991). A purine nucleoside transporter is present in RPE cells and retinal neurons, indicated by an increase in the accumulation of [^{3}H]phenylisopropyl adenosine and [^{3}H]adenosine in the presence of nitrobenzylthioinosine, an inhibitor of purine nucleoside transporter (Blazynski, 1991). The localization of these transporters is still not clear. The apical reduced-folate transporter (RFT- 1) and the basolateral folate receptor alpha (FRα) mediate vectorial transfer of reduced folate from choroidal blood to the neural retina in mouse and human RPE cells (Chancy et al., 2000).

To regulate lactate levels in the neural retina, RPE transports lactate between two tissue compartments, the interphotoreceptor matrix and the choriocapillaries. In isolated bovine RPE, Na^+-lactate cotransporter located on the basolateral side moves lactate out of cells and the apically localized H^+-lactate cotransporter moves lactate into the cells (Kenyon et al., 1994). The transport of lactate and other monocarboxylates in mammalian cells is mediated by a family of monocarboxylate transporters (MCTs), a group of highly homologous proteins that reside in the plasma membrane of almost all cells and mediate the 1:1 electroneutral transport of a proton and a lactate ion. MCT3 has been identified in RPE cells with basolateral distribution (Yoon et al., 1997). Unlike GLUT1, MCT1 is highly expressed in the apical processes of RPE and absent on the basal membrane of pigment epithelium (Philip et al., 1998; Gerhart et al., 1999; Bergersen et al., 1999). MCT1 is also associated with Müller cell microvilli, the plasma membranes of the rod inner segments, and all retinal layers between the inner and external limiting membranes. MCT1 functions to transport lactate between the retina and the blood at the level of retinal endothelium as well as the pigment epithelium. MCT2, on the other hand, is abundantly expressed on the inner (basal) plasma membrane of Müller cells and glial cells surrounding retinal microvessels. MCT4 is weekly expressed in RPE cells (Philip et al., 1998).

In primary or subcultured bovine and cat retinal pigment epithelium, ascorbate transport was observed to be coupled to the movement of sodium down its electrochemical gradient (Khatami et al., 1986). In cultured bovine capillary pericytes, ascorbate was transported via facilitated diffusion (Khatami, 1987). The uptake was specific for ascorbate, and this process was not sensitive to metabolic inhibition, the presence of ouabain, or the removal of Na^+ from the bathing medium, consistent with ascorbate entry into the cells by facilitated diffusion.

RPE cells are critical in the maintenance of the visual or retinoid cycle, which involves the back-and-forth movement of vitamin A (retinol) and some of its derivatives (retinoids) between the rods and cones (photoreceptors) and the RPE (Bok et al., 1984). Binding of retinol to retinol-binding proteins such as cellular retinol-binding protein and an interphotoreceptor retinoid-binding protein increases its solubility and delivers it to the RPE by a receptor-mediated process. The presence of cellular retinol binding protein and an interphotoreceptor retinoid-binding protein was shown in human, monkey, bovine, rat, and mouse retinas (Bunt-Milam and Saari, 1983; Bok et al., 1984). Cellular retinol-binding protein is predominantly localized in the space that surrounds the photoreceptor outer segments and the apical surface of RPE cells. It is also present in Müller glial cells. Interphotoreceptor retinoid-binding protein is localized in the space bordered by three cell types—RPE, photoreceptor, and Müller—which is consistent with its proposed role in the transport of retinoids among cells.

IV. DRUG EFFLUX PUMP

Drug efflux pumps belong to a large family of ATP binding cassette (ABC) transporter proteins. These pumps bind their substrate and export it through the membrane using energy derived from ATP hydrolysis. The original concept of multidrug resistance was introduced in 1970s to designate cells resistant to one drug, which develop cross-resistance to unrelated drugs that bear no resemblance in structure or cellular target (Biedler and Riehm, 1970). Multidrug resistance was first associated with the presence of one or more drug efflux transporters such as P-glycoprotein (P-gp) and multidrug resistance–associated protein (MRP) in tumor cells. Current evidence suggests that these transporters are present in the normal tissues, and, therefore, they may play a role in the drug disposition (Lum and Gosland, 1995). In this section, the expression of P-gp and MRP in various ocular epithelia is summarized.

A. P-Glycoprotein

P-gp, a 170 kDa membrane glycoprotein, is expressed in tumor cells as well as various normal tissues associated with the eye, small intestine, liver, kidney, lung, and the blood-brain barrier (Thiebaut et al., 1989). In the eye, P-gp is expressed in retinal capillary endothelial cells, iris, and ciliary muscle cells (Holash and Stewart, 1993), and retinal pigmented (Schlingemann et al., 1998), ciliary nonpigmented (Wu et al., 1996), corneal (Kawazu et al., 1999), and conjunctival epithelial (Saha et al., 1998) cells. P-gp exports a variety of structurally and pharmacologically unrelated hydrophobic compounds such as vinblastine, vincristine, cyclosporin (CsA), glucocorticoids, and lipophilic peptides such as *N*-acetyl-leucyl-leucyl-norleucinal (Sharma et al., 1991; Hunter et al., 1991, Tsuji et al., 1992).

Rhodamine-123 (Rho-123), a flourescent P-gp substrate, is often used to examine the function of P-gp in vitro and in vivo. Kajikawa et al. (1999) determined the contribution of P-gp to rabbit blood-aqueous barrier by analyzing the distribution of Rho-123 in aqueous humor after intravenous injection in the presence or absence of topically administered P-gp inhibitors. Following topical quinidine (12.5 mM eye drops, five applications at 5-minute intervals) and cyclosporin A (12.5 mM eye drops, five applications at 5-minute intervals) treatments, the aqueous humor distribution of intravenously injected Rho-123 was increased 11.2- and 11.3-fold, respectively, compared to controls. This suggests that P-gp is functionally active in the blood-aqueous barrier. Functional studies with other P-gp substrates, such as cyclosporin A, verapamil, and dexamethasone, were also investigated to determine the presence of P-gp activity in the conjunctival epithelium (Saha et al., 1998). The basolateral-apical apparent permeability coefficients of cyclosporin A, verapmil, and dexamethasone were 9.3, 3.4, and 1.6 times that of apical-basolateral permeability coefficients, respectively. Cyclosporin A efflux was reduced by 50–70% in the presence of verapamil and anti-Pgp antibody (4E3 mAb), consistent with P-gp activity in the conjunctival epithelium.

B. Multidrug Resistance–Associated Protein

MRP belongs to a group of mammalian ABC transporters that can be clearly differentiated from others such as P-gp or cystic fibrosis transmembrane regulator (CFTR). The most important difference in MRP and P-gp is that MRP is an organic anion transporter with high activity towards compounds conjugated to glutathione (GSH), glucuronide, or sulfate (Muller et al., 1994; Jedlitschky et al., 1994). Currently, MRP is known to exist in seven isoforms, including MRP1, MRP2, MRP3, MRP4, MRP5, MRP6, and MRP7 (Cole et al., 1992; Flens et al., 1996; Kool et al., 1997, 1999a,b). In polarized epithelial cells, MRP1, MRP3, and MRP5 are usually present on the basolateral side, whereas MRP2 is present on the apical surface.

The expression of MRP 1 has been demonstrated in the human retinal pigment epithelial cell line (ARPE- 19) and in the primary cultures of human retinal pigment epithelium (HRPE) using Western blot analysis and RT-PCR studies (Aukunuru and Kompella, 1999a; Aukunuru et al., 2001). Accumulation of fluorescein, an MRP substrate, was increased in both ARPE-19 and HRPE cells in the presence of MRP inhibitors, including probenecid, verapamil, and indomethacin. Similar observations were made in ARPE-19 cells with benzoylaminophenylsulfonylglycine (BAPSG), an anionic aldose reductase inhibitor intended for diabetic complications (Fig. 11). Thus, MRP inhibition may enhance the drug uptake into RPE cells. MRP1 is present in rabbit conjunctival epithelial cells as indicated by a ~190 kDa protein corresponding to MRP1 in Western blots (Yang and Lee, 2000). The apical to basolateral transport of leukotriene (LTC4), an MRP substrate, was abolished by basolateral probenecid, suggesting that MRP is likely localized on the basolateral side.

V. DRUG TRANSPORT ACROSS OCULAR BARRIERS

The general goal of ophthalmic drug delivery is to maximize drug levels in the target eye tissues while minimizing the levels in the remainder of the body. Ocular delivery can be achieved by topical administration, systemic administration, periocular injections, and intraocular injections. Topical administration of drugs results in higher drug concentrations in the extraocular barriers (conjunctiva, cornea), followed by the anterior chamber and its structures (aqueous humor, lens), with minimal drug entering the poster-

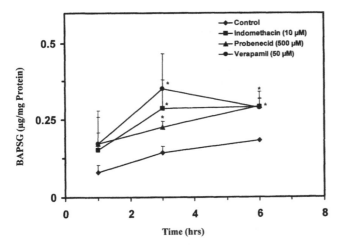

Figure 11 Influence of MRP inhibitors on N-4(benzoylamino)phenylsulfonyl glycine (BAPSG) uptake in ARPE-19 cells ($*P < 0.05$). (From Aukunuru et al., 2001.)

ior ocular structures including vitreous, retina, and choroid. Following systemic administration, the concentration of drug obtained within the eye depends on the blood concentration-time profile of the free drug and the rate of drug clearance from the eye compartments. The blood-ocular barriers, which include the iris blood vessel endothelium, ciliary body epithelium, retinal blood vessel endothelium, and retinal-pigmented epithelium, influence the overall amount of drug entering the anterior and posterior compartments of the eye from blood. As the blood-retinal barrier presents a greater hindrance to drug penetration than does the blood-aqueous barrier, the aqueous humor concentrations are typically higher than vitreous humor concentrations following systemic administration of drugs (Lesar and Fiscella, 1985). Periocular injections such as subconjunctival injections and intravitreal injections place drug more proximal to the target tissues, thereby overcoming some of the ocular barriers. In this section, physiochemical factors that affect the transport across blood-ocular barriers and case reports of drug transport are presented.

Ocular tissue permeability following topical administration can be influenced by the physicochemical properties of the drug. Molecular size restricts paracellular transport in cornea, conjunctiva, and sclera. The paracellular and aqueous penetration routes in cornea, conjunctiva, and sclera were characterized in rabbits using a mixture of polyethyleneglycols (PEGs) with mean molecular weights of 200, 400, 600, and 1000, which display some basic features of peptides and oligonucleotides (hydrophilicity, hydrogen-bonding capacity, and size) (Hamalainen et al., 1997). The conjunctival and scleral tissues were more permeable to PEGs than the cornea. The conjunctival permeability was less influenced by molecular size compared to that of cornea, which is expected because the conjunctiva has 2 times larger pores and 16 times higher pore density than the cornea. The total paracellular space in the conjunctiva was estimated to be 230 times greater than that in the cornea. Conjunctiva is commensurately permeable to hydrophilic molecules up to ~40 kDa. Prausnitiz and Noonan (1998) summarized the corneal, conjunctival, and scleral penetration of various drugs as a function of lipophilicity, molecular size, molecular radius, partition coefficient, and distribution coefficient. They observed an increase in corneal as well as corneal endothelial permeability with an increase in the drug distribution coefficient. Cornea as well as corneal endothelium exhibited molecular size-dependent drug permeability. Conjunctiva did not show clear dependence on distribution coefficient, but it did show a possible dependence on molecular size. Scleral transport was not dependent on either molecular radius or distribution coefficient.

Size is one determinant that influences the transport of molecules across blood-ocular barriers (Bellhorn, 1981). In a systematic study, the permeability of the ocular blood vessels and neuroepithelial layers in neonatal and adult cats was assessed using FITC-dextrans of various sizes. The iris and ciliary vessels were permeable to molecules with effective diffusion radius as large as 85 Å. The choriocapillaries were permeable to molecules with an effective diffusion radius of 32–58 Å. Iris vessels in humans, monkey, rabbit, and rat were not permeable to free and protein–bound sodium fluorescein, whereas marked permeability was observed in cats (Sherman et al, 1978).

Conjunctiva expresses organic cation transport processes (Ueda et al., 2000). The permeability of guanidine and tetramethylammonium in the mucosal-to-serosal direction was temperature and concentration dependent, and it was much greater than that in the serosal-to-mucosal direction. Guanidine transport was also inhibited by dipivefrine (72%), brimonidine (70%), and carbachol (78%). Also, acidification of mucosal fluid, apical exposure of a K^+ ionophore, as well as high K^+ levels reduced the transport of guanidine. However, it was not affected by the serosal presence of 0.5 mM ouabain. These observations suggest that transport of certain amine-type ophthalmic drugs may be driven by an inside-negative apical membrane potential difference.

Propranolol transport was assessed in conjunctival epithelial cells in the presence and absence of P-gp–competing substrates and anti-P-gp monoclonal antibody or a metabolic inhibitor, 2,4-DNP (Yang et al., 2000). Propranolol was transported preferentially in the basolateral-to-apical direction. When exposed apically, inhibitors of P-gp, cyclosporin A, progesterone, rhodamine 123, verapamil, and 2,4-DNP increased propranolol accumulation by 43–66%. These results suggest that P-gp is likely localized on the apical plasma membrane to restrict the conjunctival absorption of some lipophilic drugs.

Cornea, conjunctiva, RPE, and iris pigment epithelial cells exhibit particulate uptake processes (Mayerson and Hall, 1986; Zimmer et al., 1991; Rezai et al., 1997). Zimmer et al. (1991) determined the uptake of 120 nm particles in excised rabbit cornea and conjunctiva. Following 30 minutes of incubation of rhodamine 6G nanoparticle suspension, particle uptake was observed in both tissues. No particles were observed in intercellular junctions probably because the openings for the intercellular space are too small for the 120 nm particles. Also, penetration of fluorescein was not seen in these cells or across the whole cornea when fluorescein solution instead of particles were used, suggesting the superiority of nanoparticles as a drug delivery system. Penetration through whole corneal tissue did not occur either. RPE cells possess nonspecific phagocytic activity and are capable of binding and ingesting latex particles (Mayerson and Hall, 1986; Aukunuru and Kompella, 1999b, 2002). Also, rod outer segments enter RPE via phagocytosis, which involves recognition, attachment, internalization, and degradation of the rod outer segments. With respect to particle uptake, iris pigment epithelial cells are functionally similar to RPE cells (Rezai et al., 1997).

Another important factor that may limit the ocular concentrations of some classes of drugs is the presence of an active transport system that removes drugs from ocular compartments and drains into blood. Barza et al. (1982) determined the kinetics of intravitreally injected carbenicillin, an organic anion antimicrobial, in rabbits following concomitant intraperitoneal administration of probenecid, an organic anion transport inhibitor. Probenecid increased the vitreous half-life of carbenicillin from 5 to 13 hours. In addition, it increased the drug concentrations in cornea, aqueous, and iris. Similar observations were made in rhesus monkeys, wherein probenecid increased the vitreous half-life of carbenicillin and cefazolin from 10 to 20 hours and 7 to 30 hours, respectively (Barza et al., 1983). These findings suggest that a probenecid-sensitive active transport system present in the retinal pigmented epithelium may actively remove organic acids such as penicillins and cephalosporins. Lipid-soluble compounds are also lost through the retina due to their ability to cross the blood-retinal barrier (Barza et al., 1982, 1983). Confounding ocular inflammation results in elimination of nontransported drugs such as aminoglycosides (Barza et al., 1983). However, the effect of inflammation on the loss of actively transported carbenicillin from the vitreous is less due to a decrease in the function of the active transport systems (Lesar and Fiscalle, 1985).

From the drug delivery point of view, monocarboxylate transport processes such as proton or Na^+-coupled lactate systems in epithelial cells may serve as conduits for anionic drugs such as cromolyn, which is used in the treatment of vernal conjunctivitis and flurbiprofen and dicolfenac, which are used in the treatment of herpes conjunctivitis. Evidence exists for a Na^+-dependent carrier-mediated monocarboxylate transport process on the mucosal side of the conjunctival epithelium (Horibe et al., 1998). This process may be used by ophthalmic nonsteroidal anti-inflammatory drugs (NSAIDs) and fluoroquinolone antibacterial drugs. While NSAIDs and fluoroquinolones reduced L-lactate transport across conjunctiva, cromolyn and prostaglandins (PGE_2 and PGF_2) did not affect L-lactate transport, probably because cromolyn is a dicarboxylic acid and the hydrophobicity of PGE2 and PGF2 may hamper their recognition by the monocarboxylate transporter (Nord et al., 1983).

Besides Na^+-lactate transporter, various ion transport processes discussed in Sec. III are likely to influence drug transport. The various ion transport processes can influence cell surface pH, fluid transport, tight junctional permeability, and vesicular trafficking, thereby altering drug transport (Kompella and Lee, 1999). Active transport of ions such as Na^+, K^+, and Cl^- contributes to net fluid transport across various epithelia. For instance, cornea and conjunctiva secrete Cl^- towards tears. In association with this Cl^- secretion, net fluid secretion occurs towards tears. A change in this fluid secretion is likely to affect the transport of hydrophilic solutes. Exposure of nutrients such as amino acids to the apical side of conjunctiva can induce Na^+ absorption in association with fluid absorption. This fluid absorption in conjunction with possible opening of tight junctions by these amino acids can allow increased absorption of hydrophilic solutes across conjunctiva. Elevation of intracellular Ca^{2+} through various transporters such as Ca^{2+} channels and Na^+/Ca^{2+} exchanger is another likely approach to increase paracellular permeability. Function of Cl^- channels such as CFTR correlate with the extent of endocytosis in various cells. Activation of Cl^- channels with 8Br-cAMP and terbutaline have been shown to increase the transport of horseradish peroxidase (Kompella and Lee, 1999).

pH in the microclimate of the cell surface can be different from that in the surrounding fluid bulk. This is due to unstirred water layers and the presence of several surface transporters such as Na^+/H^+ exchanger, Na^+/HCO_3^- cotransporter, and Cl^-/HCO_3^- exchangers. Because transcellular diffusion of drugs is dependent on partitioning, which is dependent on pH, the function of these transporters is likely to influence drug transport. Indeed, inhibition of Na^+/H^+ exchanger with hexamethylene amiloride has been shown to elevate drug transport across conjunctiva (Kompella and Lee, 1999).

VI. CONCLUSIONS

The principal membrane barriers located in the cornea, conjunctiva, iris-ciliary body, lens, and retina express highly specialized transport processes that control the movement of endogenous as well as exogenous solutes into and out of intraocular chambers. Ion transport processes such as Na^+/K^+-ATPase, $Na^+/K^+/Cl^-$ and Na^+/Cl^- cotransporter, K^+, Cl^-, and Na^+ channels are primarily responsible for the maintanence of potential differences and fluid transport across various cellular barriers. Ion transport processes such as Na^+/H^+ exchanger, Cl^-/HCO_3^- exchanger, and Na^+-HCO_3^- cotransporter regulate cellular pH. Transporters such as Na^+/Ca^{2+} exchanger and Ca^{2+}-ATPase regulate the cellular levels of Ca^{2+}, a messenger involved in multiple membrane transport events. By regulating fluid transport, cellular pH, and intracellular Ca^{2+}, ion transport processes are likely to influence drug transport.

The various ocular barriers express transport processes for hydrophilic solutes such as organic anions, glucose, amino acids, and nucleosides in one or both sides of the cell. These transporters may play a role in the transport of structurally related drug molecules. In addition, the ocular barriers express efflux pumps such as MRP and P-gp, which can export several structurally diverse anionic drugs and lipophilic drugs, respectively.

ACKNOWLEDGMENTS

We are thankful to Mr. Jithuan V. Aukunuru for his editorial assistance in the preparation of the manuscript.

REFERENCES

Aukunuru, J. V., Sunkara, G., Bandi, N., Thoreson, W. B., and Kompella, U. B. (2001). Expression of multidrug resistance protein (MRP1) in retinal pigment epithelial cells, and its interaction with BAPSG, a novel aldose reductase inhibitor. *Pharm. Res* 18(5):565–572.

Aukunuru, J. V., and Kompella, U.B. (1999a). Functional and biochemical evidence for the expression of multidrug resistance associated protein (MRP) in a human ertinal pigment epithelial cell line. *PharmSci.*, 1(4):2609.

Aukunuru, J. V., and Kompella, U. B. (1999b). Size- and concentration-dependent uptake of microspheres by human retinal pigment epithelial cells. *PharmSci.*, 1(4):3294.

Aukunuru, J.V., and Kompella, U.B. (2002). In vitro delivery of nano- and micro-particles to retinal pigment epithelial cells. Drug Del. Technol., 2:50–57.

Barza, M., Kane, A., and Baum, J. (1982). The effects of infection and probenecid on the transport of carbenicillin from the rabbit vitreous humor. Invest. Ophthalmol. Vis. Sci., 22:720–726.

Barza, M., Kane, A., and Baum, J. (1983). Pharmacokinetics of intravitreal carbenicillin, cefazolin and gentamicin in rhesus monkeys. Invest. Ophthalmol. Vis. Sci., 24:1602–1606.

Behzadian, M. A., Wang, X., Windsor, J., Ghaly, N., and Caldwell, R. B. (2001). TGF-β increases retinal endothelial cell permeability by increasing MMP-9: possible role of glial cells in endothelial barrier function. Invest. Ophthalmol. Vis. Sci., 42(3):853–859.

Bellhorn, R. W. (1981). Permeability of blood-ocular barriers of neonatal and adult cats to fluorescein-labeled dextrans of selected molecular sizes. Invest. Ophthalmol. Vis. Sci., 21(2):282–290.

Benedek, G. B. (1971). Theory of transparency of the eye. Appl. Optics, 10:459–473.

Benedek, G. B., Pande, J., Thurston, G. M., and Clark, J. I. (1999). Theoretical and experimental basis for the inhibition of cataract. Prog. Retin. Eye Res., 18(3):391–402.

Bergersen, L., Johannsson, E., Veruki, M. L., Nagellius, E. A., Halestrap, A., Sejersted, O., M., and Ottersen, O. P. (1999). Cellular and subcellular expression of monocarboxylate transporters in the pigment epithelium and retina of the rat. Neuroscience, 90(1):319–331.

Betz, A. L., and Goldstein, G. W. (1980). Transport of hexoses, potassium and neutral amino acids into capillaries isolated from bovine retina. Exp. Eye Res., 30(5):593–605.

Biedler, J. L., and Riehm, H. (1970). Cellular resistance to actinomycin D in Chinese hamster cells in vitro: cross-resistance, radioautographic, and cytogenetic studies. Cancer Res., 30(4):1174–1184.

Bito, L. Z. (1986). Prostaglandins and other eicosanoids: their ocular transport, pharmacokinetics and therapeutic effects. Trans. Ophthalmol. Soc. UK, 105(Pt2):162–170.

Bito, L. Z., and Wallenstein, M. C. (1977). Transport of prostaglandins across the blood-brain and blood-aqueous barriers and the physiological significance of these absorptive processes. Exp. Eye Res., 25(suppl):229–243.

Blazynski, C. (1991). The accumulation of [^{3}H]phenylisopropyl adenosine ([^{3}H]PIA) and [^{3}H]adenosine into rabbit retinal neurons is inhibited by nitrobenzylthioinosine (NBI). Neurosci. Lett., 121(1–2):1–4.

Bleeker, G. M., van Haeringen, N. J., Mass, E. R., and Glasius, E. (1968). Selective properties of the vitreous barrier. Exp. Eye. Res., 7(1):37–46.

Bok, D., Ong, D. E., and Chytil, F. (1984). Immunocytochemical localization of cellular retinol binding protein in the rat retina. Invest. Ophthalmol. Vis. Sci., 25(8):877–883.

Bok, D., O'Day, W., and Rodriguez-Boulan, E. (1992). Polarized budding of vesicular stomatitis and influenza virus from cultured human and bovine retinal pigment epithelium. Exp. Eye Res., 55(6):853–860.

Bonanno, J. A. (1990). Lactate-proton cotransport in rabbit corneal epithelium. *Curr. Eye Res.*, 9(7):707–712.

Bonanno, J. A., Yi, G., Kang, X. J., and Srinivas, S. P. (1998). Reevaluation of Cl^-/HCO_3^- exchange in cultured bovine corneal endothelial cells. *Invest. Ophthalmol. Vis. Sci.*, 39(13):2713–2722.

Bonanno, J. A., Guan, Y., Jelamskii, S., and Kang, X. J. (1999). Apical and basolateral CO_2-HCO_3^- permeability in cultured bovine corneal endothelial cells. *Am. J. Physiol.*, 277(3 pt 1):C545–C553.

Botchkin, L. M., and Matthews, G. (1994). Voltage-dependent sodium channels develop in rat retinal pigment epithelium cells in culture. *Proc. Natl. Acad. Sci. USA*, 91:4564–4568.

Bowler, J. M., Peart, D., Purves, R. D., Carre, D. A., Macknight, A. D. and Civan, M. M. (1996). Electron probe X-ray microanalysis of rabbit ciliary epithelium. *Exp. Eye. Res.*, 62(2):131–139.

Brown, H. G., Pappas, G. D., Ireland, M. E., and Kuszak, J. R. (1990). Ultrastructural, biochemical, and immunologic evidence of receptor-mediated endocytosis in the crystalline lens. *Invest. Ophthalmol. Vis. Sci.*, 31(12):2579–2592.

Bunt-Milam, A. H., and Saari, J. C. (1983). Immunocytochemical localization of two retinoid-binding proteins in vertebrate retina. *J. Cell. Biol.*, 97(3):703–712.

Butler, J. M., Unger, W. G., and Grierson, I. (1988). Recent experimental studies on the blood-aqueous barrier: the anatomical basis of the response to injury, *Eye*, 2:S213–S220.

Caprioli, J. (1992). The ciliary epithelia and aqueous humor. In: Adler's Physiology of the Eye. Hart, W. M., Jr. (Ed.). Mosby-Year Book, Inc., St. Louis, pp. 228–247.

Chancy, C. D., Kekuda, R., Huang, W., Prasad, P. D., Kuhnel, J. M., Sirotnak, F., Roon, P., Ganapathy, V., and Smith, S. B. (2000). Expression and differential polarization of the reduced-folate transporter-1 and the folate receptor α in mammalian retinal pigment epithelium. *J. Biol. Chem.*, 275(27):20676–20684.

Chang, J. E., Basu, S. K., and Lee, V. H. (2000). Air-interface condition promotes the formation of tight corneal epithelial cell layers for drug transport studies. *Pharm. Res.*, 17(6):670–676.

Chu, T. C., and Candia, O. A. (1988). Active transport of ascorbate across the isolated rabbit ciliary epithelium. *Invest. Ophthalmol. Vis. Sci.*, 29(4):594–599.

Cilluffo, M. C., Fain, M. J., and Fain, G. L. (1993). Tissue culture of rabbit ciliary body epithelial cells on permeable support. *Exp. Eye Res.*, 57(5):513–526.

Cole, S. P., Bhardwaj, G., Gerlach, J. H., Mackie, J. E., Grant, C. E., Almquist, K. C., Stewart, A. J., Kurz, E. U., Duncan, A. M., and Deeley, R. G. (1992). Overexpression of a transporter gene in a multidrug-resistant human lung cancer cell line. *Science*, 258(5088);1650–1654.

Crosson, C. E., and Pautler, E. L. (1982). Glucose transport across isolated bovine pigment epithelim. *Exp. Eye Res.*, 35:371–377.

Cunha-Vaz, J. G. (1979). The blood-ocular barriers. *Surv. Ophthalmol.*, 23(5):279–296.

Cunha-Vaz, J. G., and Maurice, D. M. (1967). The active transport of fluorescein by the retinal vessels and the retina. *J. Physiol.*, 191(3):467–486.

Defoe, D. M., Ahmad, A., Chen, W., and Hughes, B. A. (1994). Membrane polarity of the Na^+-K^+ pump in primary cultures of Xenopus retinal pigment epithelium. *Exp. Eye Res.*, 59(5):587–596.

Dibeneditto, F. E., and Bito, L. Z. (1980). The kinetics and energy dependence of prostaglandin transport processes. I. In vitro studies on the rate of PGF2 α accumulation by the rabbit anterior uvea. *Exp. Eye Res.*, 30(2):175–182.

Diecke, F. P., Beyer-Mears, A., and Mistry, K. (1995). Kinetics of myo-inositol transport in rat ocular lens. *J. Cell Physiol.*, 162(2):290–297.

Ehlers, N., Kristensen, K., and Scholnheyder, F. (1978). Amino acid transport in human ciliary epithelium. *Acta Ophthalmol.*, 56(5):777–784.

Fain, G. L., Smolka, A., Cilluffo, M. C., Fain, M. J., Lee, D. A., Brecha, N. C., and Sachs, G. (1988). Monoclonal antibodies to the H^+-K^+ ATPase of gastric mucosa selectivity stain the non-pigmented cells of the rabbit ciliary body epithelium. *Invest. Ophthalmol. Vis. Sci.*, 29(5):785–794.

Fijisawa, K., Ye, J., and Zadunaisky, J. A. (1993). A Na^+/Ca^{2+} exchange mechanism in apical membrane vesicles of the retinal pigment epithelium. *Curr. Eye Res.*, 12(3):261–270.

Flens, M. J., Zaman, G. J., van der Valk, P., Izquierdo, M. A., Schroeijers, A. B., Scheffer, G. L., van der Groep, P., de Haas, M., Meijer, C. J., and Scheper, R. J. (1996). Tissue distribution of the multidrug resistance protein. *Am. J. Pathol.*, 148(4);1237–1247.

Freddo, T. F. (1984). Intercellular junctions of the iris epithelia in *Macaca mullata*. *Invest Ophthalmol. Vis. Sci.*, 25(9):1094–1104.

Freddo, T. F. (1987). Intercellular junctions of the ciliary epithelim in anterior uveitis. *Invest. Ophthalmol. Vis. Sci.*, 28(2):320–329.

Freddo, T. F., and Raviola, G. (1982). Freeze-fracture analysis of the interendothelial junctions in the blood vessels of the iris in *Macaca mullata*. *Invest. Ophthalmol. Vis. Sci.*, 23(2):154–167.

Freddo, T. F., Bartles., S. P., Barsotti, M. F., and Kamm, R. D. (1990). The source of proteins in the aqueous humor of the normal rabbit. *Invest. Ophthalmol. Vis. Sci.*, 31(1):125–137.

Gallemore, R. P., Hu, J., Fambach, D. A., and Bok, D. (1995). Ion transport in cultured fetal human retinal pigment epithelium. *Invest. Ophthalmol. Vis. Sci.*, 36:S316.

Gerhart, D. Z., Leino, R. L., and Drewes, L. R. (1999). Distribution of monocarboxylate transporters MCT1 and MCT2 in rat retina. *Neuroscience*, 92(1):367–375.

Giasson, C., and Bonanno, J. A. (1994). Facilitated transport of lactate by rabbit corneal endothelium. *Exp. Eye Res.*, 59(1):73–81.

Gliula, N. B., Reeves, O. R., and Steinbach, A. (1972). Metabolic coupling, ionic coupling and cell contacts. *Nature*, 235(5336):262–265.

Goodenough, D. A. (1992). The crystalline lens. A system networked by gap junctional intercellular communication. *Semin. Cell. Biol.*, 3(1):49–58.

Green, K. (1970). Stromal cation binding after inhibition of epithelial transport in the cornea. *Am. J. Physiol.*, 218(6):1642—1648.

Hamalainen, K. M., Kananen, K., Auriola, S., Kontturi, K., and Urtti, A. (1997). Characterization of paracellular and aqueous penetration routes in cornea, conjunctiva, and sclera. *Invest. Ophthalmol. Vis. Sci.*, 38(3):627–634.

Harik, S. I., Kalaria, R. N., Whitney, P. M., Andersson, L., Lundahl, P., Ledbetter, S. R., and Perry, G. (1990). Glucose transporters are abundant in cells with "occluding" junctions at the blood-eye barriers. *Proc. Natl. Acad. Sci. USA*, 87(11):4261–4264.

Helbig, H., Korbmacher, C., Wohlfarth, J., Berweck, S., Kuhner, D., and Widerholt, M. (1989). Electrogenic Na^+-ascorbate cotransport in cultured bovine pigmented ciliary epithelial cells. *Am. J. Physiol.*, 256(1 Pt 1):C44–C49.

Hernandez, E., Hu, J., Frambach, D., and Gallemore, R. (1995). Potassium conductances in cultured bovine and human retinal pigment epithelium. *Invest. Ophthalmol. Vis. Sci.*, 36:113–122.

Hightower, K. R., Leverenz, V., and Reddy, V. N. (1980). Calcium transport in the lens. *Invest. Ophthalmol. Vis. Sci.*, 19(9):1059–1066.

Ho, N. F. H., Raub, T. J., Burtoon, P. S., Barsutin, C. L., Adson, A., Audus, K. L., and Borchardt, R. T. (1999). Quantitative approaches to delineate passive transport mechanisms in cell culture monolayers. In: *Transport Processes in Pharmaceutical Systems*. Amidon, G. L., Lee, P. I., and Topp, E. M. (Eds.). Marcel Dekker, Inc., New York, pp. 219–316.

Holash, J. A., and Stewart, P. A. (1993). The relationship of astrocyte-like cells to the vessels that contribute to the blood-ocular barriers. *Brain Res.*, 629(2):218–124.

Horibe, Y., Hosoya, K., Kim, K. J., and Lee, V. H. L. (1998). Carrier mediated transport of monocarboxylate drugs in the pigmented rabbit conunctiva. *Invest. Ophthalmol. Vis. Sci.*, 39(8):1436–1443.

Hosoya, K., Kompella, U. B. Kim, K. J., and Lee, V. H. (1996). Contribution of Na(+)-glucose cotransport to the short-circuit current in the pigmented rabbit conjunctiva. *Curr. Eye Res.*, 15(4):447–451.

Hosoya, K. I., Horibe, Y., Kim, K. J., and Lee, V. H. (1998a). Carrier-mediated transport of NG-nitro-L-arginine, a nitric oxide synthase inhibitor, in the pigmented rabbit conjunctiva. *J. Pharmacol. Exp. Ther.*, 285(1):223–227.

Hosoya, K., Horibe, Y., Kim, K. J., and Lee, V. H. (1998b). Nucleoside transport mechanisms in the pigmented rabbit conjunctiva. *Invest. Ophthalmol. Vis. Sci.*, 39(2);372–377.

Hudspeth, A. J., and Yee, A. G. (1973). The intercellular junctional complexes of retinal pigment epithelia. *Invest. Ophthalmol.*, 12(5):354–365.

Hunter, J., Hirst, B. H., and Simmons, N. L. (1991). Transepithelial vinblastine secretion mediated by P-glycoprotein is inhibited by forskolin derivatives. *Biochem. Biophys. Res. Commun.*, 181(2):671–676.

Jedlitschky, G., Leier, I., Buchholz, U., Center, M., and Keppler, D. (1994). ATP-dependent transport of glutathione S-conjugates by the multidrug resistance-associated protein. *Cancer Res.*, 54(18):4833–4836.

Jelamskii, S., Sun, X. C., Herse, P., and Bonanno, J. A. (2000). Basolateral Na^+-K^+-$2Cl^-$ cotransport in cultured and fresh bovine corneal endothelium. *Invest. Ophthalmol. Vis. Sci.*, 41(2):488–495.

Jentsch, T. J., Keller, S. K., and Wiederholt, M. (1985). Ion transport mechanisms in cultured bovine corneal endothelia cells. *Curr. Eye Res.*, 4(4);361–369.

Joseph, D., and Miller, S. (1991). Apical and basolateral membrane ion transport mechanisms in bovine retinal pigment epithelium. *J. Physiol.*, 435:439–463.

Kajikawa, T., Mishima, H. K., Murakami, T., and Takano, M. (1999). Role of P-glycoprotein in distribution of rhodamine 123 into aqueous humor in rabbits. *Curr. Eye Res.*, 18(3):240–246.

Kawazu, K., Yamada, K., Nakamur, M., and Ota, A. (1999). Characterization of cyclosporin A transport in cultured rabbit corneal epithelial cells: P-glycoprotein transport activity and binding to cyclophilin. *Invest. Ophthalmol. Vis. Sci.*, 40(8):1738–1744.

Kenyon, E., Yu, K., La Cour, M., and Miller, S. S. (1994). Lactate transport mechanisms at apical and basolateral membranes of bovine retinal pigment epithelium. *Am. J. Physiol.*, 267(6Pt1):C1561–1573.

Kern, H. L., and Ho, C. K. (1973). Localization and specificity of the transport system for sugars in the calf lens. *Ex. Eye Res.*, 15(6):751–765.

Kern, H. L., and Zolot, S. L. (1987). Transport of vitamin C in the lens. *Curr. Eye Res.*, 6(7):885–896.

Kern, H. L., Ho, C. K., and Ostrove, S. A. (1977). Comparison of transport at the anterior and posterior surfaces of the calf lens. *Exp. Eye Res.*, 24(6): 559–570.

Khatami, M. (1987). Na^+-linked active transport of ascorbate into cultured bovine retinal pigment epithelial cells: heterologous inhibition by glucose. *Membr. Biochem.*, 7:115–130.

Khatami, M., Stramm, L. E., and Rockey, J. H. (1986). Ascorbate transport in cultured cat retinal pigment epithelial cells. *Exp. Eye Res.*, 43(4):607–615.

Klyce, S. D. (1972). Electrical profiles in the corneal epithelium. *J. Physiol.*, 226(2):407–429.

Klyce, S. D., and Crosson, C. E. (1985). Transport processes across the rabbit corneal epithelium: a review. *Curr. Eye Res.*, 4(4);323–331.

Kompella, U. B., Kim, K. J., and Lee, V. H. L. (1993). Active chloride transport in the pigmented rabbit conjunctiva. *Curr. Eye Res.*, 12:1041–1048.

Kompella, U. B., Kim, K. J., Shiue, M. H., and Lee, V. H. (1995). Possible existence of Na) +)-coupled amino acid transport in the pigmented rabbit conjunctiva. *Life Sci.*, 57(15):1427–1431.

Kompella, U. B., and Lee, V. H. L. (1999). Barriers to drug transport in ocular epithelia, In: *Transport Processes in Pharmaceutical Systems*. Amidon, G. L., Lee, P. I., and Topp, E. M. (Eds.). Marcel Dekker, Inc., New York, pp. 317–375.

Kool, M., de Haas, M., Scheffer, G. L., Scheper, R. J., van Eijk, M. J., Jujin, J. A., Baas, F., and Borst, P. (1997). Analysis of expression of cMOAT (MRP2),

MRP3, MRP4, and MRP5, homologues of the multidrug resistance-associated protein gene (MRP1), in human cancer cell lines. *Cancer Res.*, 57(16):3537–3547.

Kool, M., van der Linden, M., de Haas, M., Scheffer, G. L., de Vree, J. M., Smith, A. J., Jansen, G., Peters, G. J., Ponne, N., Scheper, R. J., Elferink, R. P., Baas, F., and Borst, P. (1999a). MRP3, an organic anion transporter able to transport anti-cancer drugs. *Proc. Natl. Acad. Sci. USA*, 96(12);6914–6919.

Kool, M., van der Linden, M., de Haas, M., Baas, F., and Borst, P. (1999b). Expression of human MRP6, a homologue of the multidrug resistance protein gene MRP1, in tissues and cancer cells. *Cancer Res.*, 59(1):175–182.

la Cour, M. (1992). Cl⁻ transport in frog retinal pigment epithelium. *Exp. Eye Res.*, 54(6):921-931.

la Cour, M., Lin, H., Kenyon, E., and Miller, S. S. (1994). Lactate transport in freshly isolated human fetal retinal pigment and epithelium. *Invest. Ophthalmol. Vis. Sci.*, 35:434–442.

Lapierre, L. A. (2000). The molecular structure of the tight junctions. *Adv. Drug Deliv. Rev.*, 41(3):255–264.

Lesar, S. T., and Fiscella, R. G. (1985). Antimicrobial drug delivery to the eye. *Drug Intel. Clin. Pharm.*, 19:642–653.

Lightman, S., Rechthand, E., Latker, C., Plaestine, A., and Rapoport, S. (1987). Assessment of the permeability of the blood-retinal barrier in hypertensive rats. Hypertension, 10(4):390–395.

Lo, W. K., and Harding, C. V. (1986). Structure and distributionof gap junctions in the lens epithelium and fiber cells. *Cell Tissue Res.*, 244(2):253–263.

Lum, B. L., and Gosland, M. P. (1995). MDR expression in normal tissues. Pharmacologic implications for the clinical use of P-glycoprotein inhibitors. *Hematol. Oncol. Clin. North Am.*, 9(2);319–326.

Madara, J. L., and Trier, J. S. (1982). Structure and permeability of goblet cell tight junctions in rat small intestine. *J. Membr. Biol.*, 66(2):145–147.

Mantych, G. J., Hageman, G. S., and Devaskar, S. U. (1993). Characterization of glucose transporter isoforms in the adult and developing human eye. *Endocrinology*, 133(2):600–607.

Marshall, W. S., and Klyce, S. D. (1983). Cellular and paracellular pathway resistances in the "tight– Cl⁻-secreting epithelium of rabbit cornea. *J. Memb. Biol.*, 73:275–282.

Martin-Vasallo, P., Ghosh, S., and Coca-Prados, M. (1989). Expression of Na⁺/K⁺-ATPase alpha subunit isoforms in the human ciliary body and cultured ciliary epithelial cells. *J. Cell. Physiol.*, 141(2):243–252.

Maurice, D. M., and Mishima, S. (1984). Ocular pharmacokinetics. In: Pharmacology of the Eye, Sears, M. L. (Ed.). Springer-Verlag, New York.

Mayerson, P. L., and Hall, M. O. (1986). Rat retinal pigment epithelial cells show specificity of phagocytosis in vitro. *J. Cell Biol.*, 103:299–308.

Mays, R. W., Beck, K. A., and Nelson, J. W. (1994). Organizaton and function of the cytoskeleton in polarized epithelial cells: a component of the protein sorting machinery. *Curr. Opin. Cell Biol.*, 6:16–24.

McLaughlin, B. J., Caldwell, R. B., Sasaki, Y., and Wood, T. O. (1985). Freeze-fracture quantitative comparison of rabbit corneal epithelial and endothelia membranes. *Curr. Eye Res.*, 4(9):951–961.

Merriman-Smith, R., Donaldson, P., and Kistler, J. (1999). Differential expression of facilitative glucose transporters GLUT1 and GLUT3 in the lens. *Invest. Ophthalmol. Vis. Sci.*, 40(13):3224–3230.

Miller, S., and Edelman, J. (1990). Active ion transport pathways in the bovine retinal pigment epithelium. *J. Physiol.*, 4 24:283–300.

Miller, S. S., Rabin, J., Strong, T., Iannuzzi, M., Adams, A. J., Collins, F., Reenstra, W., and McCray, P., Jr. (1992). Cystic fibrosis (CF) gene product is expressed in retina and retinal pigment epithelium. *Invest. Ophthalmol. Vis. Sci.*, 33:1009 (abstr).

Miyamoto, K., Khosrof, S., Bursell, S. E., et al. (1999). Prevention of leukostatis and vascular leakage in streptozotocin-induced diabetic retinopathy via intercellular adhesion molecule-1 inhibition. *Proc. Natl. Acad. Sci. USA*, 96:10836–10841.

Miyamoto, Y., and Del Monte, M. A. (1994). Na^+-dependent glutamate transporter in human retinal pigment epithelial cells. *Invest. Ophthalmol. Vis. Sci.*, 35:3589–3598.

Miyamoto, Y., Kulanthaivel, P., Leibach, F. H., and Ganapathy, V. (1991). Taurine uptake in apical membrane vesicles from the bovine retinal pigment epithelium. *Invest. Ophthalmol. Vis. Sci.*, 32:2542–2551.

Muller, M., Meijer, C., Zaman, G. J., Borst, P., Scheper, R. J., Mulder, N. H., de Vries, E. G., and Jansen, P. L. (1994). Overexpression of the gene encoding the multidrug resistance-associated protein results in increased ATP-dependent glutathione S-conjugate transport. *Proc. Natl. Acad. Sci. USA*, 91(26):13033–13037.

Nord, E. P., Wright, S. H., Kippen, I., and Wright, E. M. (1983). Specificity of the Na^+-dependent monocarboxylic acid transport pathway in rabbit renal brush border membranes. *J. Membr. Biol.*, 72(3):213–221.

Okami, T., Yamamoto, A., Omori, K., Akayama, M., Uyama, M., and Tashiro, Y. (1989). Quantitative immunocytochemical localization of $Na^+, K^+ = ATPase$ in rat ciliary epithelial cells. *J. Histochem. Cytochem.*, 37:1353–1361.

Palacin, C., Tarrago, C., and Ortiz, J. A. (1998). Molecular biology of mammalian plasma membrane amino acid transporters. *Physiol. Rev.*, 78(4):969–1054.

Paterson, C. A., and Delamere, N. A. (1992). The ciliary epithelia and aqueous humor. In: *Adler's Physiology of the Eye.* Hart, W. M. Jr. (Ed.). Mosby-Year-Book, Inc., St. Louis, pp. 412–441.

Pepose J. S., and Ubels, J. L. (1992). The cornea. In: *Adler's Physiology of the Eye.* Hart, W. M., Jr. (Ed.). Mosby-Year Book, Inc., St. Louis, pp. 29–70.

Peyman, G. A., and Bok, D. (1972). Peroxidase diffusion in the normal and laser-coagulated primate retina. *Invest. Ophthalmol.*, 11(1):35–45.

Philip, N. J., Yoon, H., and Grollman, E. F. (1998). Monocarboxylate transporter MCT1 is located in the apical membrane and MCT3 in the basal membrane of rat RPE. *Am. J. Physiol.*, 274 (6 Pt 2):R1824–R1828.

Prausnitz, M. R., and Noonan, J. S. (1998). Permeability of cornea, sclera, and conjunctiva: A literature analysis for drug delivery to the eye. *J. Pharm. Sci.*, 87(12):1479–1488.

Quinn, R. H., and Miller, S. S. (1992). Ion transport mechanisms in native human retinal pigment epithelium. *Invest. Ophthalmol. Vis. Sci.*, 33:3513–3527.

Rae J. L. (1994). Outwardly rectifying potassium currents in lens epithelial cell membranes. *Curr. Eye Res.*, 13(9):679–686.

Raviola, G. (1977). The structural basis of the blood-ocular barriers. *Exp. Eye Res.*, 25:27–63.

Redzic, Z. B., Markovic, I. D., Jovanovic, S. S., Zlokovic, B. V., and Rakic, L. M. (1995). Penetration of [^{3}H]tiazofurin into guinea pig eye by a saturable mechanism. *Eur. J. Ophthalmol.*, 5(2):131–135.

Redzic, Z. B., Markovic, I. D., Vidovic, V. P., Vranic, V. P., Gasic, J. M., Duricic, B. M., Pokrajac, M., Dordevic, J. B., Segal, M. B., and Rakic, L. M. (1998). Endogenous nucleosides in the guinea-pig eye: analysis of transport and metabolites. *Exp. Eye. Res.*, 66:315–325.

Rezai, K. A., Lappas, A., Farrokh-Siar, L., Kohen, L., Widemann, P., and Heimann, K. (1997). Iris pigment epithelial cells of long evans rats demonstrate phagocytic activity. *Exp. Eye Res.*, 65:23–29.

Riley, M. V. (1977). A study of the transfer of amino acids across the endothelium of the rabbit cornea. *Exp. Eye Res.*, 24(1):35–44.

Riley, M. V., and Yates, E. M. (1977). Glutathione in the epithelium and endothelium of bovine and rabbit cornea. *Exp. Eye Res.*, 25(4):385–389.

Riley, M. V., Campbell, D., and Linz, D. H. (1973). Entry of amino acids into the rabbit cornea. *Exp. Eye Res.*, 15(6):677–681.

Robinson, K. R., and Patterson, j. W. (1982). Localizastion of steady currents in the lens. *Curr. Eye Res.*, 2(12):843–847.

Rodriguez-Boulan, E., and Nelson, W. J. (1989). Morphogenesis of the polarized epithelial cell phenotype. *Science*, 245:718–725.

Rodriguez-Peralta, L. (1975). The blood-aqueous barrier in five species. *Am. J. Ophthalmol.*, 80(4):713–725.

Saha, P., Kim, J., and Lee, V. H. (1996). A primary culture model of rabbit conjunctival epithelial cells exhibiting tight barrier properties. *Curr. Eye Res.*, 15(12):1163–1169.

Saha, P., Yang, J. J., and Lee, V. H. (1998). Existence of a P-glycoprotein drug efflux pump in cultured rabbit conjunctival epithelial cells. *Invest. Ophthalmol. Vis. Sci.*, 39(7):1221–1226.

Saier, M. H. (200a). A functional phylogenetic classification system for transmembrane solute transporters. *Microbiol. Mol. Biol. Rev.*, 64(2):354–411.

Saier, M. H., Jr. (2000b). Families of transmembrane transporters elective for amino acids and their derivatives. *Microbiology*, 146:1775–1795.

Schlingemann, R. O., Hofman, P., Klooster, J., Blaauwgeers, H. G., Van der Gaag, R., and Vrensen, G. F. (1998). Ciliary muscle capillaries have blood-tissue barrier characteristics. *Exp. Eye Res*, 66(6):747–754.

Sharma, R. C., Assaraf, Y. G., and Schimke, R. T. (1991). A phenotype conferring selective resistance to lipophilic antifolates in Chinese hamster ovary cells. *Cancer Res.*, 51(11);2949–2959.

Sherman, S. H., Green, K., and Laties, A. M. (1978). The fate of anterior chamber fluorescein in the monkey eye. 1. The anterior chamber outflow pathways. *Exp. Eye Res.*, 27(2);159–173.

Shirao, Y., and Steinberg, R. (1987). MEchanisms of effects of small hyper-osmotic gradients on the chick RPE. *Invest. Ophthalmol. Vis. Sci.*, 280:2015–2025.

Shiue, M. H., Kulkarni, A. A., Gukasyan, H. J., Swisher, J. B., Kim, K. J., and Lee, V. H. (2000). Pharmacological modulation of fluid secretion in the pigmented rabbit conjunctiva. *Life Sci.*, 66(7):PL105–111.

Simon, A. M., and Goodenough, D. A. (1998). Diverse functions of vertebrate gap junctions. *Trends Cell Biol.*, 8(12);477–483.

Smith, R. S., and Rudt, L. A. (1975). Ocular vascular and epithelial barriers to microperoxidase. *Invest. Ophthalomol.*, 14(7):556–560.

Socci, R. R., and Delamere, N. A. (1988). Characteristics of ascorbate transport in the rabbit iris-ciliary body. *Exp. Eye Res.*, 46(6):853–861.

Spray, D. C., and Bennett, M. V. (1985). Physiology and pharmacology of gap junctions. *Ann. Rev. Physiol.*, 47:281–303.

Stewart, P. A., and Tuor, U. I. (1994). Blood-eye barriers in the rat: correlation of ultrastructure with function. *J. Comp. Neurol.*, 340(4):566–576.

Strauss, O., Widerholt, M., Wienrich, M. (1996). Activation of Cl^- currents in cultured rat retinal pigment epithelial cells by intracellular applications of ionositol-1,4,5,-triphosphate: differences between rats with retinal dystrophy (RCS) and normal rats. *J. Membr. Biol.*, 151:189–200.

Sun, X. C., Bonanno, J. A., Jelamskii, S., and Xie, Q. (2000). Expression and localization of Na^+-HCO_3^- cotransporter in bovine corneal endothelium. *Am. J. Physiol. Cell Physiol.*, 279(5):C1648–C1655.

Takahashi, H., Kaminski, A. E., and Zieske, J. D. (1996). Glucose transporter 1 expression is enhanced during corneal epithelial wound repair. *Exp. Eye Res.*, 63(6):649–659.

Takata, K., Hirano, H., and Kasahara, M. (1997). Transport of glucose across the blood-tissue barriers. *Int. Rev. Cytol.*, 172:1–53.

Theibaut, F., Tsuruo, T., Hamada, H., Gottesman, M. M., Pastan, I., and Willingham, M. C. (1989). Immunohistochemical localization in normal tissues of different epitopes in the multidrug transport protein P170: evidence for localization in brain capillaries and crossreactivity of one antibody with a muscle protein. *J. Histochem. Cytochem.*, 37(2):159–164.

Thoft, R. A., and Friend, J. (1972). Corneal amino acid supply and distribution. *Invest. Ophthalmol. Vis. Sci.*, 11(9);723–727.

Thorens, B. (1996). Glucose transporters in the regulation of intestinal, renal, and liver glucose fluxes. *Am. J. Physiol.*, 270(4 Pt 1): G541–G553.

Tornquist, P., and Alm, A. (1986). Carrier-mediated transport of amino acids through the blood-retinal and the blood-brain barriers. *Grafes. Arc. Clin. Exp. Ophthalmol.*, 224(1):21–25.

Tornquist, P., Alm, A., and Bill, A. (1990). Permeability of ocular vessels and transport across the blood-retinal-barrier. *Eye*, 4 (Pt 2):303–309.

Tsuboi, S., and Pederson, J. E. (1988). Effect of plasma osmolality and intraocular pressure on fluid movement across the blood-retinal barrier. *Invest. Ophthalmol. Vis. Sci.*, 29(11):1747–1749.

Tusji, A., Terasaki, T., Takabatake, Y., Tenda, Y., Tamai, I., Yamashima, T., Moritani, S., Tsuruo, T., and Yamashita, J. (1992). P-glycoprotein as the drug efflux pump in primary cultured bovine brain capillary endothelial cells. *Life Sci.*, 51(18);1427–1437.

Ueda, Y., and Steinberg, R. (1994). Chloride currents in freshly isolated rat retinal pigment epithelial cells. *Exp. Eye Res.*, 58:31–342.

Ueda, H., Horibe, Y., Kim, K. J., and Lee, V. H. (2000). Functional characterization of organic cation drug transport in the pigment rabbit conjunctiva. *Invest. Ophthalmol. Vis. Sci.*, 41(3):870–876.

Usukura, J., Fain, G. L., and Bok, D. (1988). [^{3}H]Ouabain localization of Na$^+$-K$^+$ ATPase in the epithelium of rabbit ciliary body pars plicata. *Invest. Ophthalmol. Vis. Sci.*, 29(4):606–614.

Vinores, S. A. (1995). Assessment of blood-retinal barrier integrity. *Histol. Histopathol.*, 10(1):141–154.

Wang, L., Chen, L., Walker, V., and Jacob, T. J. (1998). Antisense to MDR1 mRNA reduces P-glycoprotein expression, swelling-activated CL$^-$ current and volume regulation in bovine ciliary epithelial cells. *J. Physiol.*, 511(Pt 1):33–44.

Watsky, M. A., Jablonski, M. M., and Edelhauser, H. F. (1988). Comparison of conjunctival and corneal surface areas in rabbit and human. *Curr. Eye Res.*, 7:483–486.

Wen, R., Lui, G. M., and Steinberg, R. H. (1994). Expression of a tetrodoxin-sensitive Na$^+$ current in cultured human retinal pigment epithelial cells. *J. Physiol (Lond).*, 475:187–196.

Whikehart, D. R., and Soppet, D. R. (1981). Activities of transport enzymes located in the plasma membranes of corneal endothelial cells. *Invest. Ophthalmol. Vis. Sci.*, 21(6):819–825.

Whikehart, D. R., Montgomery, B., and Hafer, L. M. (1987). Sodium and potassium saturation kinetics of Na$^+$-K$^+$ ATPase in plasma membranes from corneal endothelium: fresh tissues vs. tissue culture. *Curr. Eye Res.*, 6(5):709–717.

Widerholt, M., Jentsch, T. J., and Keller, S. K. (1985). Electrogenic sodium-bicarbonate symport in cultured corneal endothelial cells. *Pflugers Arch.*, 405(suppl 1):S167–171.

Wolosin, J. M., Alvarez, L. J., and candia, O. A. (1988). Cellular pH and Na$^+$-H$^+$ exchange activity in the lens epithelium of Bufo marinus toad. *Am. J. Physiol.*, 255(5 Pt 1):C595–C602.

Wolosin, J. M., Alvarez, L. J., and Candia, O. A. (1990). HCO$_3^-$ transport in the toad lens epithelium is mediated by an electronegative Na(+)-dependent symport. *Am. J. Physiol.*, 258(5 Pt 1):C855–C861.

Wu, G. (1995). Anatomy and physiology of the retina/ocular embryology. In: *Retina: The fundamentals*. W. B. Saunders Company, Philadelphia.

Wu, J., Zhang, J. J., Koppel, H., and Jacob, T. J. (1996). P-glycoprotein regulates a volume-activated chloride current in bovine non-pigmented ciliary epithelial cells. *J. Physiol.*, 491(Pt 3):743–755.

Xu, Q., Quam, T., and Adamis, A. P. (2001). Sensitive blood-retinal barrier breakdown quantitation using evans blue. *Invest. Ophthalmol. Vis. Sci.*, 42(3):789–794.

Yang, J. J., and Lee, V. H. (2000). Role of multidrug resistance protein (MRP) in drug transport in rabbit conjunctival epithelial cells. *PharmSci.*, 2(4):S3168.

Yang, J. J., Kim, K. J., and Lee, V. H. (2000). Role of P-glycoprotein in restricting propranolol transport in cultured rabbit conjunctival epithelial cell layers. *Pharm. Res.*, 17(5):533–538.

Ye, J. J., and Zadunaisky, J. A. (1992a). Ca^{2+}/Na^{+} exchanger and Na^{+}, K^{+}, $2Cl^{-}$ cotransporter in lens fiber plasma membrane vesicles. *Exp. Eye Res.*, 55(6):797–804.

Ye, J. J., and Zadunaisky, J. A. (1992b). Study of the Ca^{2+}/Na^{+} exchange mechanism in vesicles isolated from apical membranes of lens epithelium of spiny dogfish (*Squalas acanthias*) and bovine eye. *Exp. Eye Res.*, 55(2):243–250.

Yoon, H., Fanelli, A., Grollman, E. F., and Philip, N. J. (1997). Identification of a unique monocarboxylate transporter (MCT3) in retinal pigment epithelium. *Biochem. Biophys. Res. Commun.*, 234(1):90–94.

Yu, A. S. (2000). Paracellular solute transport more than just a leak? *Curr. Opin. Nephrol. Hypertens.*, 9(5):513–515.

Zaunaisky, J. A. (1992). Membrane transport in ocular epithelia. In: *Barriers and Fluids of the Eye and Brain*. Segal, M. B. (Ed.). CRC Press, Inc., Ann Arbor.

Zelenka, P. S., and Vu, N. D. (1984). Correlation between phosphatidylinositol degradation and cell division in embryonic chicken lens epithelia. *Dev. Biol.*, 105(2):325–329.

Zimmer, A., Kreuter, J., and Robinson, J. R. (1991). Studies on the transport pathway of PBCA nanoparticles in ocular tissues. *J. Microencapsulation.* 8(4):497–504.

Zlokovic, B. V., Mackic, J. B., McComb, J. G., Kannan, R., and Weiss, M. H. (1992). An in-situ perfused guinea pig eye model for blood-ocular transport studies: application to amino acids. *Exp. Eye Res.*, 54:471–477.

Zlokovic, B. V., Mackic, J. B., McComb, J. G., Kaplowitz, N., Weiss, M. H.,and Kannan, R. (1994). Blood-to-lens transport of reduced glutathione in an in situ perfused guinea pig eye. *Exp. Eye Res.*, 59:487–496.

3
General Considerations in Ocular Drug Delivery

James E. Chastain
Alcon Research, Ltd., Fort Worth, Texas, U.S.A.

I. INTRODUCTION

The use of pharmacokinetic principles has become widespread in the pharmaceutical industry, primarily because of their utility in relating efficacy and toxicity to drug concentrations in plasma or some other appropriate body compartment. In general, pharmacokinetics is the process of absorption, distribution, and excretion of a drug. Excretion is usually coupled with metabolism, which typically converts drug to a more water-soluble form, more amenable to excretion. Most of the pharmacokinetic literature deals with systemically administered drugs that reach their pharmacological target by way of the blood following oral or parenteral administration.

There are various approaches to studying the pharmacokinetics of a drug. Classical pharmacokinetics empirically derives one or more exponentials to mathematically describe concentration versus time data. Physiological pharmacokinetics associates compartments with specific anatomical tissues or organs and usually includes blood flow and drug clearance in individual organs/tissues as part of the model. Noncompartmental pharmacokinetics, as its name implies, makes no assumptions regarding compartments but usually employs statistical moment theory to derive basic parameters such as volume of distribution and clearance. All of these methods can prove useful in describing a drug's pharmacokinetic behavior, an essential step toward determining an appropriate dosing regimen for a drug relative to its efficacy and toxicity profiles.

Ocular pharmacokinetics includes the features of absorption, distribution, and excretion found with systemic administration but applied to the eye. However, owing to the unique anatomy and physiology of the eye and surrounding tissue, ocular pharmacokinetics is considerably more difficult to describe and predict than its systemic counterpart. The task is further complicated by the various formulations, routes, and dosing regimens typically encountered in ophthalmology.

Pharmacodynamics is the measurement of pharmacological response relative to dose or concentration. The pharmacological response induced by a drug can vary greatly from individual to individual due to differences in factors such as eye pigmentation, the pathological state of the eye, tearing, or blink rate. The application of pharmacological endpoints is particularly useful in the study of drugs in the human eye, where the ability to determine the ocular pharmacokinetics based on ocular tissue concentrations is severely limited.

This chapter discusses the ocular pharmacokinetics associated with topical ocular, intravitreal, periocular, and systemic administration. In addition, the pharmacodynamics related to ophthalmic drugs and the role of ocular drug metabolism are reviewed.

II. OCULAR PHARMACOKINETICS

Application of classical pharmacokinetics to ophthalmic drugs is problematic because of the complexities associated with eye anatomy and physiology. As a result, most of the literature is limited to measuring concentrations in ocular tissues over time following single or multiple administration. This approach, while informative, does not easily yield quantitative predictions for changes in formulation or dosage regimen. Compounding the problem is the fact that most studies have been conducted in rabbit eyes, which differ significantly from human eyes in anatomy and physiology (see Table 1). the most obvious differences are in blink rate and the presence or absence of a nictitating membrane. An overall, detailed discussion of these factors and ocular pharmacokinetics as a whole has been presented elsewhere (1–9).

A. Topical Ocular Administration

1. Absorption

The general process of absorption into the eye from the precorneal area (dose site) following topical ocular administration is quite complex. The

Table 1 Comparison of Anatomical and Physiological Factors in the Rabbit and Human Eye

Factor	Rabbit	Human
Tear volume (μL)	5–10	7–30
Tear turnover rate (μL/min)	0.6–0.8	0.5–2.2
Spontaneous blinking rate	4–5 times/h	6–15 times/min
Nictitating membrane	Present	Absent
Lacrimal punctum/puncta	1	2
pH of lacrimal fluids	7.3–7.7	7.3–7.7
Milliosmolarity of tears	305	305
Corneal thickness (mm)	0.40	0.52
Corneal diameter (mm)	15	12
Corneal surface area (cm^2)	1.5–2.0	1.04
Ratio of conjunctival surface and corneal surface	9	17
Aqueous humor volume (mL)	0.25–0.3	0.1–0.25
Aqueous humor turnover rate (μL/min)	3–4.7	2–3

Source: Adapted from Refs. 8, 9.

classical sequence of events involves drug instillation, dilution in tear fluid, diffusion through mucin layer, corneal penetration (epithelium, stroma, endothelium), and transfer from cornea to aqueous humor. Following absorption, drug distributes to the site of action (e.g., iris-ciliary body). Parallel absorption via the conjunctiva/sclera provides an additional pathway to eye tissues but, for most drugs, is minor compared with corneal absorption. Also, nonproductive, competing, and parallel pathways (e.g., nasolacrimal drainage or systemic absorption via the conjunctiva) work to carry drug away from the eye and limit the time allowed for the absorption process. Moreover, in some species, such as the rabbit, nonproductive absorption into the nictitating membrane can occur. Figure 1 presents a summary of these precorneal events, along with a relatively simplified view of the kinetics in the cornea, aqueous humor, and anterior segment.

a. Corneal Penetration. Drug absorption through the cornea into the eye is dependent to a large degree upon a drug's physicochemical properties, such as octanol-water partition coefficient, molecular weight, solubility, and ionization state. In addition, corneal penetration is layer (corneal epithelium, stroma, and endothelium) selective. Schoenwald and Ward demonstrated a parabolic relationship between log corneal

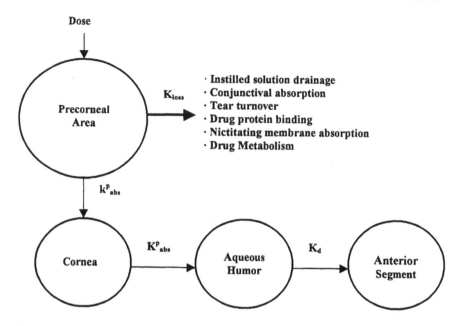

Figure 1 Model showing precorneal and intraocular events following topical ocular administration of a drug. (Adapted from Ref. 2.)

permeability coefficients and log octanol-water coefficients of various steroids (10) (see Fig. 2). The optimum log octanol-water coefficient was 2.9. Schoenwald and Huang showed a correlation between octanol-water partitioning of beta-blocking agents and their corneal permeabilities using excised rabbit corneas (11). Over a fourfold logarithmic range, the best fit was also a parabolic curve. In a refinement of this parabolic relationship, Huang et al. demonstrated in vitro a sigmoidal relationship between permeabiilty coefficient and distribution coefficient (12) (see Fig. 3). In this study, the endothelium offered little resistance and the stroma posed even less. Lipophilic drugs penetrated the cornea more rapidly; however, the hydrophilic stroma was rate limiting for these compounds. Maren et al. studied 11 sulfonamide carbonic anhydrase inhibitors (CAIs) of varied physicochemical characteristics with respect to transcorneal permeability and reduction of intraocular flow (13). In isolated rabbit cornea with a constantly applied drug concentration, the first-order rate constants ranged from $0.1-40 \times 10^{-3}$ h^{-1}, nearly proportional to lipid solubility, with water-insoluble drugs tending to have higher rate constants.

For most drugs, the multicell layered corneal epithelium presents the greatest barrier to penetration, primarily due to its cellular membranes.

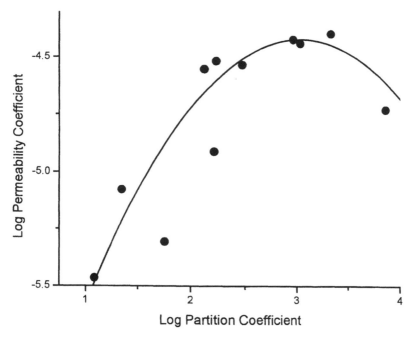

Figure 2 Log-log plot of corneal permeability coefficient (pH 7.65) versus distribution coefficient (pH 7.65). Observed data (●) and predicted curve (—) are presented. (Replotted from Ref. 10.)

Stroma and particularly endothelium offer little resistance, except for highly lipophilic drugs. In fact, these two layers are often lumped together, along with aqueous humor, as a single compartment for purposes of pharmacokinetic modeling. The influence of the epithelium is most clearly demonstrated by studying corneal penetration following removal of the epithelium. Cox et al. showed in rabbits that when the epithelium was intact, no ^{14}C-dexamethasone was detected in cornea or aqueous humor following topical ocular administration (14,15), while detectable levels were observed after removal of the corneal epithelium. Chien et al. studied the relationship between corneal epithelial integrity and prodrug lipophilicity with corneal penetration of a homologous series of timolol prodrugs (16). Deepithelization of the corneal in vitro did not affect corneal permeability of O-acetyl, propionyl, or butryl timolol but reduced penetration of the other prodrugs. In contrast, deepithelization in vivo only reduced timolol aqueous humor concentrations derived from O-propionyl and octanoyl esters. Therefore, factors other than the corneal epithelium may play a role in penetration.

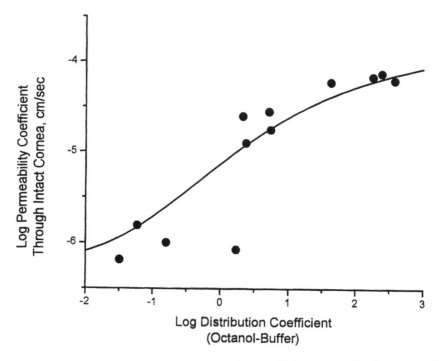

Figure 3 Log-log plot of corneal permeability coefficient versus distribution coefficient (octanol-Sorensen's buffer, pH 7.65). Intact corneal data (●) and computer-generated, model-derived curve (—) are presented. (Replotted from Ref. 12.)

Corneal penetration is also affected by the composition of the drug formulation. Whether a formulation is a solution, suspension, contains a buffer, viscosilating agent, or penetration enhancer, can influence absorption. Burstein and Anderson have reviewed corneal penetration and ocular bioavailability of drugs relative to optimizing formulations for typical ocular use (1). They evaluated the effects of preservatives, vehicles, adjunct agents, and anatomy and developed model systems for selecting the best formulations for preclinical and clinical use. Vehicle pH was one important factor considered. Adjusting the pH so that the drug was mostly in the unionized form greatly enhanced corneal penetration. Furthermore, it was concluded that buffering capacity, which keeps drug mainly in the ionized form, should be minimized to allow for adequate neutralization by tear film.

Other formulation components have been examined for their effect on absorption. Madhu et al. studied the influence of benzalkonium chloride (BAC)/EDTA on ocular bioavailability of ketorolac tromethamine following topical ocular instillation onto normal and deepithelialized rabbit corneas in vitro and in vivo (17). BAC/EDTA caused a statistically significant increase in the ocular bioavailability of ketorolac through deepithelialized cornea but not intact cornea in vitro and in vivo. Jani et al. demonstrated that inclusion of ion exchange resins in an ophthalmic formulation of betaxolol increased the ocular bioavailabilty of betaxolol twofold (18). Hyaluronic acid, which can adhere to the corneal surface, is also capable of prolonging precorneal residence time (19).

b. Noncorneal, Ocular (Productive) Absorption. In addition to the classical corneal pathway, there is a competing and parallel route of absorption via the conjunctiva and sclera, the so-called conjunctival/scleral pathway. For most drugs this is a minor absorption pathway compared to the corneal route, but for a few compounds its contribution is significant. Ahmed and Patton investigated corneal versus noncorneal penetration of topically applied drugs in the eye (20,21). They demonstrated that noncorneal absorption can contribute significantly to intraocular penetration. A "productive" noncorneal route involving penetration through the conjunctiva and underlying sclera was described. Drug can therefore bypass the anterior chamber and distribute directly to the uveal tract and vitreous. This route was shown to be particularly important for drugs with low corneal permeability, such as inulin. In a separate study, Ahmed et al. evaluated in vitro the barrier properties of the conjunctiva, sclera, and cornea (22). Diffusion characteristics of various drugs were studied. Scleral permeability was significantly higher than that in cornea, and permeability coefficients of the β-blockers ranked as follows: propranolol > penbutolol > timolol > nadolol for cornea, and penbutolol > propranolol > timolol > nadolol for the sclera. Resistance was higher in cornea versus conjunctiva for inulin but similar in the case of timolol. Chien et al. studied the ocular penetration pathways of three α_2-adrenergic agents in rabbits both in vitro and in vivo (23). The predominant pathway for absorption was the corneal route, with the exception of *p*-aminoclonidine, the least lipophilic, which utilized the conjunctival/scleral pathway. The results suggest that the pathway of absorption may be influenced in part by lipophilicity and that hydrophilic compounds may prefer the conjunctival/scleral route.

Some investigators have employed a dosing cylinder affixed to the cornea to study corneal and noncorneal absorption. Drug is applied within the cylinder for corneal dosing and outside the cylinder for noncorneal (conjunctival/scleral) dosing. In a study by Schoenwald et al., the conjunctival/scleral pathway yielded higher iris-ciliary body concentrations for all compounds evaluated with the exception of lipophilic rhodamine B (24).

Romanelli et al. demonstrated the absorption of topical ocular bendazac into the retina/choroid via the conjunctival/scleral pathway (25). Absorption by way of this extracorneal route was influenced by physico-chemical features and not by vehicle, while the transcorneal route was affected by vehicle.

   c. Noncorneal, Nonproductive Absorption and Precorneal Drainage. Routes that lead to the removal of drug from the precorneal area and do not result in direct ocular uptake are referred to as nonproductive absorption pathways. These noncorneal pathways, which are in parallel with corneal absorption, include conjunctival uptake and drainage via the nasolacrimal duct. Both lead to systemic absorption by way of conjunctival blood vessels in the former case or via the nasal mucosa and gastrointestinal tract in the latter case. As discussed previously, the conjunctiva can absorb drug and, via the sclera, deliver drug to the eye; however, blood vessels within the conjunctiva can also lead to systemic absorption.

   Nonproductive, noncorneal absorption and drainage loss greatly impact the precorneal residence time and the time for ocular absorption. Drainage, in particular, is very rapid and generally limits ocular contact at the site of absorption to about 3–10 minutes (8). However, the lag time—the time for drug to traverse the cornea and appear in the aqueous humor—is sufficiently long to extend time to maximal concentration in the aqueous to between 20 and 60 minutes for most drugs (8). Due to rapid loss of drug from the precorneal region, less than 10%, and more typically less than 1–2%, of a topical dose is absorbed into the eye. At the same time, systemic absorption can be as high as 100%, indicating that most of the drug dose is unavailable for efficacy. For example, Ling and Combs showed that the ocular bioavailability of topical ocular ketorolac was 4% in anesthetized rabbits, while systemic absorption was complete (26). Ocular tissue levels were about 13-fold higher than those in plasma, and peak concentrations were achieved by 1 hour in both aqueous humor and plasma postdose. Tang-Liu et al. showed that topical ocular levobunolol was rapidly absorbed, with an ocular bioavailability of 2.5% and systemic bioavailability of 46% (27). Patton and Robinson have investigated the contribution of tear turnover, instilled solution drainage, and nonproductive absorption to precorneal loss of drug (28). Instilled solution drainage was shown to be the predominant factor in precorneal loss, while the influence of tear turnover was minor. It was concluded that noncorneal, nonproductive loss was potentially significant due to the large surface area of noncorneal tissue; however, its role was minimal compared to drainage. Ocular (aqueous humor) and systemic bioavailabilities for various drugs are presented in Table 2.

Table 2 Ocular and Systemic Bioavailabilities (Percent of Dose) Following Topical Ocular Administration

Drug	Ocular (%)	Systemic (%)	Test subject	Ref.
Ketorolac	3.7	~ 100	Anes. rabbit	26
Levobunolol	2.5	46	Rabbit	27
Flurbiprofen	7–10	74	Anes. rabbit	46
Imirestat	ND	50–75	Anes. rabbit and dog	120
Propranolol	55, 5.6	ND	Rabbit, dog	51
Pilocarpine nitrate	0.62	ND	Rabbit, duct open	28
	2.12	ND	Rabbit, duct plugged	28
	0.80	ND	Anes. rabbit, duct open	28
	1.87	ND	Anes. rabbit, duct plugged	28
Clonidine	1.6	ND	Rabbit	67
Cortisol	ND	30–35	Rabbit	2
Tetrahydrocannabinol	ND	23	Rabbit	2

ND, Not determined; Anes, anesthetized.

Volume instilled is one factor that can influence drainage and non-corneal absorption. Chrai et al. evaluated the effect of instilled volume on drainage loss using miosis data in albino rabbits (29). A radioisotopic method was used to determine lacrimal volume and tear turnover. Unanesthetized rabbits had lacrimal volume of 7.5 µL, whereas anesthetized rabbits had a slightly larger volume of 12.0 µL. Lacrimal turnover was slower in anesthetized rabbits, in which the rate was negligible. Instilled volume drainage was found to be first order, and drainage was dependent on the volume administered in unanesthetized but not anesthetized rabbits. In a separate study, using ^{99m}Tc (technetium), Chrai et al. demonstrated that drug loss through drainage increased with increasing drop size (30a). Concentration in the precorneal tears was higher, while drainage was increased, following a larger drop volume. An instillation volume of 5–10 µL containing a larger concentration of drug was recommended. For comparison, most commercial ophthalmic droppers deliver 30–70 µL. In addition, it was shown that 5-minute spacing between drops was optimal for minimizing drainage loss. Also, for two drugs given as two separate drops, the second drop will negatively influence the first, arguing for combination therapy. Interestingly, Keister et al. showed that for drugs with high corneal permeability, ocular bioavailability and corneal permeability are relatively unaffected by drug volume (30b). In contrast, for drugs with low corneal permeability, reducing to a small dose volume can increase ocular bioavailability up to fourfold.

It is known that increasing the formulation viscosity has the potential to decrease drainage rate, thereby increasing precorneal residence time and prolonging the time for ocular absorption. Zaki et al. studied the precorneal drainage of radiolabeled polyvinyl alcohol or hydroxymethylcellulose formulations in the rabbit and humans by gamma scintiography (31). Significant retardation of drainage in humans was observed at higher polymer concentrations. Patton and Robinson also used polyvinyl alcohol, along with methylcellulose, to evaluate the relationship between viscosity and contact time or drainage loss (32). The optimum viscosity range was 12–15 centipoise in rabbits; however, the relationship was not direct, presumably due to shear forces acting on the formulation film at the eye surface. Chrai et al. also demonstrated, using methylcellulose vehicle, that increasing viscosity of an ophthalmic solution results in decreased drainage (33). Over the range of 1–15 centipoise, there was a threefold change in drainage rate constant and another threefold change over the range of 15–100 centipoise.

Differences in the anatomical and physiological characteristics of the eye, particularly between species, can also affect drainage and noncorneal absorption. A comparison of attributes between rabbit and human eyes has been presented in Table 1. In vivo evaluations in humans and rabbits by Edelhauser and Maren demonstrated lower permeability of a series of sulfonamide CAIs in humans, possibly due to a greater blinking rate, a twofold greater tear turnover, and a twofold lower corneal-conjunctival area (34). Maurice has shown that corneal penetration is enhanced in the rabbit due to low blink rate (35). This can increase area under the aqueous humor concentration-time curve threefold over that in humans. For many drugs, epithelial permeability is sufficiently high to mitigate effects of blink rate, although blinking may be critical to the proper ocular absorption and distribution of certain other drugs (36).

As one might expect, occlusion of the nasolacrimal duct substantially reduces drainage and prolongs precorneal residence time. As a result, an increase in ocular bioavailability and a decrease in systemic exposure typically occur. Kaila et al. studied the absorption kinetics of timolol following topical ocular administration to healthy volunteer subjects with eyelid closure, nasolacrimal occlusion (NLO), or normal blinking (37). NLO reduced total timolol systemic absorption, although, in some subjects, the initial absorption was enhanced. In another example, Zimmerman et al. showed that there were lower fluorescein anterior chamber levels and a shorter duration of fluorescein in the absence of NLO or eyelid closure (38). Systemic drug absorption in normal subjects was reduced more than 60% with these techniques. Linden and Alm studied the effect of tear drainage on intraocular penetration of topically applied fluorescein in healthy human eyes using fluorophotometry (39). Upper and lower punctal plugs in one eye caused a significant ($p < 0.025$) increase in aqueous humor fluorescein concentrations 1–8 hours postdose of 20 µL of 2% solution of sodium fluorescein in the lower conjunctival sac. Compressing the tear sac and/or closing the eyelids for 1 minute after application had no effect on corneal or aqueous levels of fluorescein. Lee et al. evaluated the effect of NLO on the extent of systemic absorption following topical ocular administration of various adrenergic drugs (40). Table 3 summarizes the results of this study. Hydrophilic atenolol and lipophilic betaxolol, which were not absorbed into the circulation as well as timolol and levobunolol, were not affected in their systemic absorption by 5 minutes of NLO. However, systemic bioavailability decreased 80% by prolonging precorneal retention of the dose to 480 minutes. It was concluded that modest formulation changes will have little effect on systemic absorption for extremely hydrophilic drugs. Drugs similar in lipophilicity to timolol will be well absorbed systemically, while extremely hydrophilic drugs or extremely lipophilic drugs will be absorbed to a lesser extent.

As alluded to earlier in this chapter, the rate and extent of systemic absorption via the conjunctiva relative to corneal absorption is dependent on the physicochemical properties of a drug or its formulation. Ahmed and Patton showed that the conjunctival pathway is particularly important for drugs with low corneal permeability and that noncorneal permeation is limited by nonproductive loss to the systemic circulation (21). Hitoshe et

Table 3 Systemic Bioavailabilities[a] (Percent of Dose) Following Topical Ocular Administration with Various Durations of Nasolacrimal Duct Occlusion

| Drug | Ocular | | |
	0 min	5 min	120 min
Atenolol[b]	41	39	12
Timolol	106	88	36
Levobunolol	82	54	56
Betaxolol	66	56	58

[a] Relative to subcutaneous route.
[b] For atenolol, the duration of occlusion was 480 min.
Source: Ref. 40.

al. demonstrated that drugs and prodrugs could be designed to selectively reduce conjunctival absorption and thus suppress systemic exposure (41). This can be accomplished by taking advantage of the apparently lower lipophilicity of the conjunctiva versus that of the cornea. Ashton et al. studied the influence of pH, tonicity, BAC, and EDTA on conjunctival and cornea penetration of four beta blockers: atenolol, timolol, levobunolol, and betaxolol (42). Isolated pigmented rabbit conjunctiva and cornea were used. The conjunctiva was more permeable than cornea, and formulation changes had greater influence on corneal versus conjunctival penetration. This was particularly true for the hydrophilic compounds; therefore, changes in formulation can effect both ocular and systemic absorption.

d. Absorption Kinetics. As discussed, lag time and drainage severely curtail the absorption process in the eye. These events make it somewhat difficult to estimate absorption kinetics. In particular, an anomaly arises when attempting to derive the absorption rate constant, K_a, in that there is a large discrepancy between the theoretical and actual times during which absorption occurs. For example, phenylephrine has an absorption half-life of 278 hours (43); therefore, the theoretical time to complete absorption would be an enormous 1200 hours (4–5 half-lives). In actuality, the absorption process terminates within 3–10 minutes. Consistent with this, Makoid and Robinson showed that extensive parallel absorption pathways resulted in an apparent K_a one to two orders of magnitude larger than actual for ^{3}H-pilocarpine (44). Aqueous flow accounted for most of the drug elimination. The predominating effects on absorption and elimination, independent of drug structure, suggested that similar pharmacokinetics may be found for a variety of drugs. Table 4 shows absorption half-lives ranging from about 3 hours for pilocarpine to as high as 278 hours for phenylephrine. These values illustrate that corneal absorption is relatively slow and that the theoretically derived times for absorption are substantially longer than the actual 3–10 minutes typically encountered.

Rapid drainage of drug from the precorneal area largely determines the time to peak concentration in the aqueous humor irrespective of a drug's physicochemical properties. As a general rule, virtually all drugs will reach peak concentration in the aqueous humor within 20–60 minutes postinstillation (8). Makoid and Robinson have derived an equation for calculating time to peak (t_p):

$$t_p = \frac{\ln\left(\dfrac{K_{na}}{K_a}\right)}{(K_{na} - K_a)} \tag{1}$$

Table 4 Transcorneal First-Order Absorption Rate Constant (K_a) and Absorption Half-Life ($t_{1/2abs}$) for Corneal Absorption

Drug	$K_a(\text{min}^{-1})$	$t_{1/2abs}(\text{h})$	Ref.
Pilocarpine	4×10^{-3}	2.88	64
6-Hydroxyethoxy-2-benzothiazolesulfonamide	4.2×10^{-3}	5.37	48
Ethoxzolamide	1.5×10^{-3}	7.7	48
Aminozolamide	1.4×10^{-3}	8.25	111
Clonidine	1.4×10^{-3}	8.25	67
2-Benzothiazolesulfonamide	1.3×10^{-3}	8.88	48
Ibuprofen	9.64×10^{-4}	12	121
Ibufenac	6.03×10^{-4}	18.3	121
Phenylephrine	4.15×10^{-5}	278	43

Source: Adapted from Ref. 8.

where K_{na} and K_a are nonabsorptive loss rate constant and the transcorneal absorption rate constant, respectively, and $K_{na} \gg K_a$ (44). Since for most drugs K_{na} is about twofold larger than K_a, this formula is widely applicable. Huang et al. have shown for various β-blockers in rabbits that aqueous humor T_{max} is inversely proportional to corneal permeability coefficient (45), and that C_{max} and area under the concentration-time curve (AUC) for aqueous humor generally correlate with permeability. Table 5 shows

Table 5 Time to Maximal Concentration (T_{max}) in Aqueous Humor Following Topical Ocular Administration

Drug	T_{max} (min)	Ref.
Falintolol	30–60	122
Lincomycin hydrochloride	30–45	123
Bufuralol	10	45
Acebutolol	85	45
Propranolol	30	124
L-662,583[a]	120	125
Timolol	10	126
	25	45
Ketorolac	60	26

[a] 5-(3-Dimethylaminomethyl-4-hydroxy-phenylsulfonyl) thiophene-2-sulfonamide.

times to maximal aqueous humor concentration (T_{max}) for various drugs. T_{max} falls within a range of 10 minutes to 2 hours.

As mentioned, the typical percentage of drug absorbed into the eye following a topical ocular dose is in the range of 1–10%, while systemic bioavailability can be as high as 100% (Table 2). For calculating bioavailability fraction (F), aqueous humor AUC can be determined by intracameral injection (27,46) or topical instillation with plugged drainage ducts (28). In the former case, aqueous humor AUCs, normalized for dose, are compared between topical and intracameral doses to derive F. In the latter case, Patton and Robinson (28) calculated F using the following equation:

$$F = \frac{k_{10} \times V \times AUC}{D} \tag{2}$$

where D is the instilled dose, k_{10} is the loss of drug from the precorneal area, and V is the estimated aqueous humor volume of 0.3 mL.

For some drugs, such as topical anti-infectives, tear bioavailability and not aqueous humor bioavailability is the determining pharmacokinetic factor for efficacy. Unlike aqueous humor, tear film is readily sampled in humans. Depending on the method of collection, analytical sensitivity may be a limiting factor due to small volumes typically collected and the short precorneal residence time typically encountered. Nevertheless, when area under the tear concentration-time curve values are available, bioavailabilities can be calculated and compared between formulations. Tear sampling technique may be an important factor in obtaining this type of data. For example, Ding et al. compared two tear sampling techniques (capillary tubes and Schirmer strips) and one recovery technique (cotton swabs) for suitability for determining precorneal drug levels as a function of time for ophthalmic gels (47). All three methods yielded similar corneal contact times (about 1 hour). Capillary tubes proved effective for tear sampling, while the strip method suffered from gel carry-over. The cotton swab technique was gentle, easy, and nondestructive and yielded recovery of total drug in the cul-de-sac, but failed to provide information for tear film.

2. Ocular Distribution

Compared to absorption and elimination, distribution is generally more difficult to describe kinetically. In the concentration-time curve shown in Figure 4, distribution is associated with the log-linear decline in aqueous humor concentration immediately following peak concentration and before the terminal elimination phase.

  a. Distribution Within the Anterior Segment.   The fundamental parameter to describe distribution is volume of distribution (V_d), which is de-

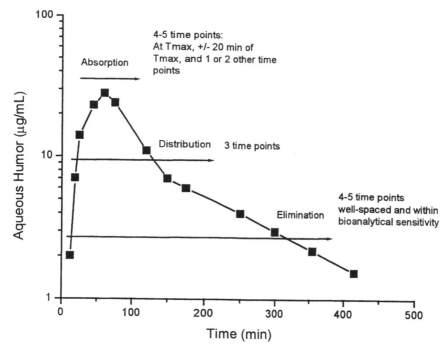

Figure 4 Ideal sampling times for determining the pharmacokinetics of topical ocular drugs. (Adapted from Ref. 8.)

fined as a proportionality constant relating concentration to amount. Volume of distribution at steady-state (V_{ss}) most closely reflects the distribution capacity and, as such, is the most useful measure of V_d. Unlike whole body V_{ss}, determining V_{ss} in the eye is particularly difficult because the amount of drug in the eye at any time is not known following a single topical ocular administration. Two approaches have been developed to overcome this obstacle. The first method uses a well affixed over the cornea of an anesthetized rabbit so that drug solution is in constant contact with the cornea and not the surrounding sclera (48,49). Drug solution remains on the cornea for 90–160 minutes until concentration of drug in the aqueous humor reaches steady state. This so-called topical infusion study, with constant rate input, can yield absorption rate constant, ocular clearance, and V_{ss}.

The second method for determining V_{ss} and distribution involves intracameral injection, which delivers a bolus dose directly into the anterior chamber. Conrad and Robinson used this approach to determined the volume of distribution in albino rabbits (50). Inulin yielded an aqueous humor volume of 287 µL in close agreement with that previously determined by other methods. The apparent volume of distribution of pilocarpine was twofold larger than the assumed apparent volume of 250–300 µL, indicating distribution into surrounding tissues. Rittenhouse et al. examined the ocular uptake and disposition of topical ocular β-adrenergic antagonists in individual dogs and rabbits (51). Radiolabeled (^{3}H) propranolol was administered intracamerally and topically, and microdialysis was performed to monitor concentrations of radioactivity in the anterior chamber. Ocular bioavailability was 5.6% and 55% in anesthetized dog and rabbit, respectively. The value in rabbit was outside the 1–10% range typically observed with topical ocular instillation. The high bioavailability may be related to the use of anesthesia, which can cause a reduction in blinking and precorneal drainage. Table 6 presents ocular V_d values determined using either technique for various drugs.

Reliable estimates of V_{ss} are useful for establishing multiple dose regimens; however, because of the somewhat specialized methods needed to determine V_{ss} in the eye following topical ocular administration, it is not surprising that V_{ss} has been estimated for only a few drugs. An obvious alternative for evaluating distribution is to simply measure directly the concentration of drug in ocular tissues. Researchers have taken this approach

Table 6 Ocular Volumes of Distribution (V_d) for Various Drugs

Drug	V_d (mL)	Method	Ref.
2-Benzothiazolesulfonamide	0.24	SS[a]	48
Ethoxzolamide	0.28	SS	48
6-Hydroxyethoxy-2-benzothiazolesulfonamide	0.33	SS	48
Phenylephrine	0.42	SS	43
Clonidine	0.53	SS	67
Aminozolamide	0.53	SS	111
Pilocarpine	0.58	EXT[b]	50
Flurbiprofen	0.62	EXT	46
Levobunolol	1.65	EXT	27
Dihydrolevobunolol	1.68	EXT	27
Ketorolac tromethamine	1.93	EXT	26

[a] SS = steady-state method. A constant concentration of drug is applied to the cornea of anesthetized rabbit. V_{ss} is calculated from aqueous humor concentration versus time data.
[b] EXT = Extrapolated method. C at t_0 is determined by log-linear extrapolation and divided into the intracameral dose.
Source: Adapted from Ref. 8.

for many years, generating a fairly large database of tissue concentration information. Many of these studies have employed radioactive methods to achieve the detection limits needed to measure the small amounts of drug often encountered with small-sized ocular tissues. Unfortunately, unless amounts are high enough for chromatographic separation or metabolism is known not to occur, the identity of the radioactivity, i.e., parent drug versus metabolite, remains in question. This problem is overcome by the use of highly sensitive and selective bioanalytical methods, such as high-performance liquid chromatography coupled with mass spectrometry (HPLC/MS or HPLC/MS/MS).

Most topical ocular drugs demonstrate a tissue distribution pattern within the eye consistent with corneal penetration, that is, a concentration gradient of cornea > conjunctiva > aqueous humor > iris-ciliary body > lens, vitreous, and/or choroid-retina (8). However, with certain topical ocular drugs, such as clonidine, timolol, dapiprazole, oxymetazoline, and ketorolac tromethamine, iris-ciliary body concentrations are higher than those in aqueous humor (8). A number of explanations have been offered for this phenomenon, but the most plausible appears to involve conjunctival/scleral absorption with direct distribution to the iris-ciliary body. Several studies support this idea as discussed previously in reference to noncorneal, productive absorption (20–25).

Distribution kinetics can be significantly influenced by binding of drug to tissue. In addition, if binding affinity is high, elimination from the tissue will be delayed. A common observation with ophthalmic drugs is binding to pigmented tissues, such as the iris-ciliary body. Binding to melanin is usually evidenced by greater concentrations in pigmented rabbit eyes than nonpigmented, albino eyes. Lindquist has presented a comprehensive review of binding of drugs to melanin (52). Patil and Jacobowitz investigated the accumulation of adrenergic drugs by pigmented and nonpigmented irides (53). At the highest concentration of 10 µM, accumulation of norepinephrine, epinephrine, and phenylephrine by the pigmented iris was twofold higher than that in the nonpigmented iris. Araie et al. demonstrated that β-adrenergic blockers can also bind to melanin-containing tissues and may be slowly eliminated from these tissues (54). Their data suggest that efficacy may be reduced short-term and binding may occur after long-term use in heavily pigmented subjects. Lyons and Krohn demonstrated that pigmented irides and ciliary bodies accumulated two- to threefold more pilocarpine than nonpigmented tissue (55), and Chien et al. showed a pigment binding effect with ^{14}C-brimonidine (56). In a study by Achempoing et al., iris-ciliary body levels of brimonidine peaked at 40 minutes and 1.5 hours and declined with a half-life of 1 hour and 160 hours in albino and pigmented rabbits, respectively (57). These results indicate that elimination from pigmented tissue is prolonged compared to that in nonpigmented tissue. Pigment binding may also reduce efficacy as demonstrated by Nagata et al (58). In vivo, topically applied timolol and pilocarpine lowered intraocular pressure (IOP) in albino but not in pigmented rabbits.

b. Distribution to the Posterior Segment. The aging of the general population, along with the higher incidences of eye diseases, such as age-related macular degeneration or retinal edema, has created a need to deliver drugs to the posterior segment (i.e., retina and choroid). Although treatment of posterior diseases usually involves intraocular or periocular injections, the advantages of topical ocular administration are obvious.

It has generally been observed that drugs applied topically to the eye do not reach therapeutic levels in the posterior segment tissues, except perhaps by way of absorption from the percorneal area into the systemic circulation and redistribution into the retina/choroid (59). However, there are a few studies suggestive of topical ocular drugs reaching the posterior segment by direct distribution. In a study in monkeys, Dahlin et al. estimated the contributions of local ocular versus systemic delivery to posterior-segment concentrations of betaxolol at steady state following multiple topical dosing of Betoptic S (60). Significant levels of betaxolol were found in the retina and optic nerve head. A comparison of dosed versus nondosed eye tissue concentrations revealed that most of the drug in the posterior segment was from local delivery (absorption) with some contribution from the systemic plasma. High concentrations in the iris-ciliary body, choroid, and sclera suggested the presence of a depot, which possibly facilitated transfer to the retina and optic nerve head. In another example, Chien et al. evaluated the ocular distribution of brimonidine in albino and pigmented rabbits following a single topical ocular dose of ^{14}C-labeled drug (56). The results indicated that drug was retained in choroid/retina and optic nerve head. Levels in the nondosed contralateral eyes were much lower than those in the treated eyes for both albino and pigmented rabbits, suggesting that the majority (>99%) of the intraocularly absorbed drug was due to local topical application and not to redistribution from plasma.

The mechanism by which drugs may be locally delivered to the posterior segment from the precorneal area is unknown, but the evidence seems to indicate a noncorneal route, possibly involving conjunctival/scleral absorption followed by distribution to choroid, vitreous, and retina. Romanelli et al. confirmed the existence of a noncorneal alternative route in their investigations of the posterior distribution of drugs (61). Concentrations in retina were lower than those in aqueous for drugs that easily penetrate into the aqueous, while levels in retina were equal or higher for drugs with poor penetration into aqueous. The authors concluded that topically applied drugs reach the retina not by passing through the vitreous or anterior chamber, but possibly by an alternative route of drug penetration into the eye.

3. Elimination

The elimination phase typically appears as the terminal log-linear portion of the concentration versus time plot (see Fig. 4). Elimination rate from the aqueous humor within the anterior chamber is of particular interest. Elimination from the anterior chamber can involve aqueous humor outflow, elimination by distribution into the lens, and/or metabolism.

Elimination rate from the aqueous humor varies little from drug to drug, as shown in Table 7 in terms of half-life. The half-lives fall within a relatively narrow range of about 0.3–6 hours for a wide variety of drugs. Determining the aqueous humor half-life is largely dependent on the sensitivity of the analytical method employed. If the method is insufficiently sensitive, terminal concentrations will be missed and the half-life may be underestimated. On the other hand, if the method reports false concentrations at the low end of analytical sensitivity, the half-life will be overestimated.

Clearance is the most common and useful parameter for expressing elimination and is defined as a proportionality constant relating concentration to rate of drug loss. Ocular clearance (Q_e) can be calculated using any one of the following equations (8):

$$Q_e = K_e \times V_d \tag{3}$$

$$Q_e = \frac{K_0 \times T}{AUC_{inf}} \tag{4}$$

$$Q_e = \frac{D_{ic}}{AUC_{inf}} \tag{5}$$

where K_e is the first-order rate constant for elimination from the aqueous humor, V_d is the apparent ocular volume of distribution, K_0 is the constant rate input into the anterior chamber, T is the duration of constant rate input, D_{ic} is the intracameral dose, and AUC_{inf} is the area under the aqueous humor concentration-time curve extrapolated to infinity. These equations require the accurate determination of K_e and AUC_{inf}. Table 8 shows aqueous humor clearances for a number of drugs.

Table 7 Aqueous Humor Half-Lives[a] of Ophthalmic Drugs Administered to the Rabbit Eye Topically, Subconjunctivally or Intracamerally

Drug	Half-life (h)	Ref.
Dapiprazole	5.8	127
Timolol	4.8	126
Imirestat	4.75	120
6-Mercaptopurine	4.6	85
Ciprofloxacin	3.5	68
Fusidic acid	2.8	128
Suprofen	2.5–2.75	129
Histamine	2.2	130
Cimetidine	2.2	130
Norfloxacin	2.2	131
Ketorolac tromethamine	2.1	26
Benzolamide	2.0	132
I-643,799[b]	1.8	133
Flurbiprofen	1.7	134
Lomefloxacin	1.6	131
Phenylephrine	1.4	43
Timolol	1.2	135
	0.84	45
6-Amino-2-benzothiazolesulfonamide	1.15	111
L-662,583[c]	1.11	125
Acetbutolol	1.1	45
Cefsulodin	1.0	136
5-Fluorouracil	1.0	86
Brimonidine	1.3	57
Dihydrolevobunolol	0.98	27
6-Hydroxyethoxy-2-benzothiazolesulfonamide	0.97	48
6-Acetamido-2-benzothiazolesulfonamide	0.93	111
L-650,719[d]	0.81	133
Trifluoromethazolamide	0.78	132
Tobramycin	0.75	62
Levobunolol	0.67	27
Ethoxzolamide	0.63	48
	0.23	132
Pyrilamine	0.61	130
Methazolamide	0.58	132
Cefotazime	0.57	137
Bufuralol	0.50	45
Clonidine	0.49	67
BCNU[e]	0.38	94
2-Benzothiazolesulfonamide	0.29	48

[a] Half-lives based on terminal phase of log concentration-time curve.
[b] 6-Hydroxybenzothiazide-2-sulfonamide.
[c] 5-(3-Dimethylaminomethyl-4-hydroxy-phenylsulfonyl) thiophene-2-sulfonamide.
[d] 6-Hydroxy-2-benzothiazidesulfonamide.
[e] 1,3-Bis(2-chloroethyl)-1,1-ntirosurea.
Source: Adapted from Ref. 8

Table 8 Ocular Clearances (Q_e) from Aqueous Humor for
Various Drugs

Drug	Q_e (μL/min)	Ref.
Levobunolol	28.7	27
Dihydrolevobunolol	19.7	27
Clonidine	14.9	67
Phenylephrine	14.6	43
Fluriboprofen	14.4	46
Pilocarpine	13.0	138
Ketorolac tromethamine	11.0	26
Ethoxzolamide	9.0	49
6-Hydroxyethoxy-2-benzothiazolesulfonamide	3.0	49
2-Benzothiazolesulfonamide	1.15	49

Source: Adapted from Ref. 8.

4. Ocular Pharmacokinetic Models

Various approaches to modeling pharmacokinetic data from ocular studies
have been developed. These primarily involve (a) classical, empirical compartmental modeling, (b) physiological modeling, and (c) noncompartmental modeling employing statistical moment theory. Critical to pharmacokinetic modeling is an adequate description of the concentration versus
time curve. Unfortunately, the rationale for selecting the number and
timing of sample intervals is not always clear. In many cases, a sampling
scheme may be dictated by bioanalytical sensitivity, practicality, or even
economics. However, Schoenwald (8) has provided general sampling
guidelines that may prove useful in properly designing ocular studies
(Fig. 4).

Not only are an appropriate number of time intervals necessary,
but there should also be a sufficient number of replicates per time
point. Rabbits studies have used as few as 4 and as many as about
20 eyes per time interval, depending on the study objectives. Higher
numbers are preferred for bioequivalence studies. Moreover, because
the animal is typically euthanized for ocular tissue/fluid sampling,
each animal subject (e.g., rabbit or monkey) yields at most two data
points (one/eye) per interval. Mean concentrations, derived from individual animal data, are then used to calculate the pharmacokinetic parameters. A statistical approach to this sparse sampling scheme has been

developed for comparison of area under the concentration-time curves (62,63).

    a. Classical Empirical Pharmacokinetics. Classical modeling uses compartments, representing kinetically homogeneous groups of tissues/organs, linked together by various rate constants. For ocular pharmacokinetics, the simplest model is one employing a single compartment as shown in Figure 5a. However, this model fails to account for precorneal loss. The model in Figure 5b corrects for this but is still very simplified and treats the cornea as a homogeneous tissue, lumping all precorneal

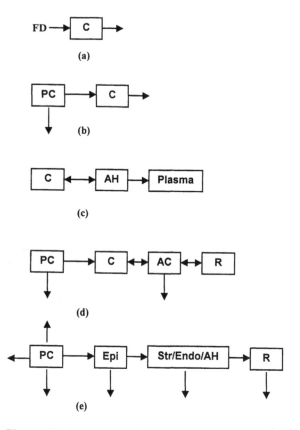

Figure 5 Schematics of various models of topical ocular drug pharmacokinetics FD = Bioavailability times dose; C = cornea; PC = precorneal area; AH = aqueous humor; AC = anterior chamber; R = reservoir; Epi = corneal epithelium; Str = corneal stroma; Endo = corneal endothelium. (Adapted from Refs. 4, 44, 64.)

rate constants together into one. The model in Figure 5c divides the anterior segment of the eye into cornea and aqueous humor, although this still excludes precorneal loss and does not adequately describe disposition beyond entry into the aqueous. Makoid and Robinson proposed a four-compartment caternary model for pilocarpine, as shown in Figure 5d, which combines precorneal loss with differentiation of cornea and anterior chamber (44). However, cornea is still treated as a homogeneous tissue, when the epithelium is known to be the major barrier to ocular uptake. The model in Figure 5e portrays epithelium as one compartment and stroma/endothelium/aqueous humor as a separate lumped compartment and incorporates elimination from each of the compartments (64). An example of one of the more sophisticated models is shown in Figure 6, which includes a conjunctival compartment, along with sclera, intraocular, and systemic circulation compartments, as well as redistribution to the contralateral eye (21).

 b. Physiological Model. Beyond the classical compartmental modeling approach is one that incorporates more realistic physiological components. Physiological pharmacokinetic models are intuitively more predictive by their use of actual anatomical and physiological parameters, such as tissue blood flow and volume (65). Ocular pharmacokinetics appears to be an ideal candidate for physiological modeling, since it is relatively simple to remove the tissue components of the eye for measurement of drug levels. For example, Himmelstein et al. developed

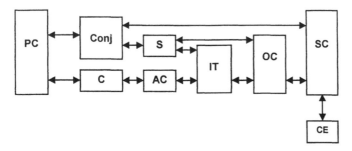

Figure 6 Schematic of an ocular pharmacokinetic model showing precorneal events, absorption into the eye via the cornea or conjunctive/sclera, distribution to the systemic circulation, and redistribution to the contralateral (undosed) eye. PC = Precorneal area; Conj = conjunctiva; C = cornea; S = sclera; AC = anterior chamber; IT = intraocular tissues; OC = ocular circulation; SC = systemic circulation; CE = contralateral eye. (Adapted from Ref. 21.)

a simple physiological pharmacokinetic model, shown in Figure 7, for predicting aqueous humor pilocarpine concentration following topical application to rabbit eyes (66). The model takes into account instilled volume and drug concentration and can predict the effect of precorneal drainage.

Physiological modeling may not be the best approach in all cases. For example, Chiang and Schoenwald determined the concentrations of clonidine in seven different ocular tissues and plasma after a single topical ocular dose of clonidine was administered to rabbits (67). The data were fit to a physiological model and a classical diffusion model with seven ocular tissue compartments and a plasma reservoir. The complex classical model was subdivided into fragmental models. While predicted and observed concentrations profiles closely agreed with the physiological model, the classical model fit the data better than the physiological model.

c. Other Models. A few other modeling approaches have been proposed, including noncompartmental modeling and population pharmacokinetics. Eller et al. applied noncompartmental statistical moment theory to topical infusion data to describe the disposition of various compounds with a range of transcorneal permeabilities within the rabbit eye (48). Morlet et al. used population pharmacokinetics to evaluate pharmacokinetic data in plasma and vitreous of the human eye (68). Gillespie et al. applied principles and methods of linear system analysis to the analysis of ocular pharmacokinetics (69). Using convolution integral mathematics, a

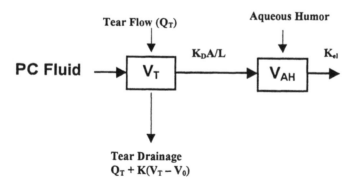

Figure 7 Schematic of a two-compartment model consisting of the precorneal area and the aqueous humor. PC = precorneal; Q_T = normal tear production rate; V_T = total volume in the precorneal area any given time; K = proportionality constant that is a function of instilled drop size; V_0 = normal tear volume; V_{AH} = normal aqueous humor volume A = corneal area; L = corneal thickness; K_{el} = lumped first-order clearance parameter from aqueous humor. (Adapted from Ref. 66.)

mechanistic model of precorneal disposition was used to predict concentration. The authors adequately predicted betaxolol levels resulting from a multiple dose regimen and from single doses of prototype controlled-release ocular inserts. This approach appears to require fewer, less restrictive assumptions than compartmental or physiological model methods.

B. Intravitreal Administration

Intravitreal injection is the most direct approach for delivering drug to the vitreous humor and retina; however, this method of administration has been associated with serious side efects, such as endophthalmitis, cataract, hemorrhage, and retinal detachment (59). In addition, multiple injections are usually required, further increasing the risk. Nevertheless, intravitreal injection continues to be the mode of choice for treatment of acute intraocular therapy.

The kinetic behavior of intravitreally delivered drugs is complicated by the stagnent, nonstirred nature of the normal vitreous. Mechanisms that may influence movement of molecules within the vitreous include diffusion, hydrostatic pressure, osmotic pressure, convective flow, and active transport (70). For small to moderately sized molecules, such as fluorescein or dextran, diffusion is the predominant mechanism of transvitreal movement (4,70). Although low-level convective flow has been observed within the vitreous (71), this flow has only a negligible effect on transvitreal movement in comparison to diffusion. For small to moderately sized molecules, diffusion within the vitreous is generally unimpeded and similar to that observed in water or saline (4,70).

1. Distribution and Elimination

As shown in Figure 8, drug distribution and elimination can occur in two main patterns: diffusion from the lens region toward the retina with elimination via the retina-choroid-sclera or anterior diffusion with elimination via the hyloid membrane and posterior chamber (4). A molecule's path of distribution and elimination in the vitreous largely depends on its physiochemical properties and substrate affinity for active transport mechanisms in the retina. Lipophilic compounds, such as fluorescein (72) or dexamethasone (73), and transported compounds tend to exit mainly via the retina. On the other hand, hydrophilic substances, such as fluorescein glucuronide, and compounds with poor retinal permeability, such as fluorescein dextran, diffuse primarily through the hyloid membrane into the posterior chamber and eventually into the anterior chamber (72). Table 9 shows vitreal half-lives for a variety of drugs and eye conditions. Generally, shorter half-lives are

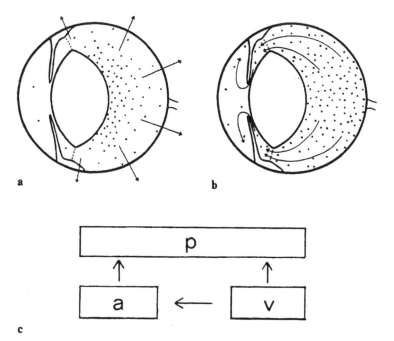

Figure 8 Schematic of exit pathways from the vitreous humor: (a) transretinal, (b) by way of drainage out of the aqueous humor; (c) compartmental model showing kinetic relationships between a, anterior chamber, p, plasma, and v, vitreous. (Reprinted with permission from Maurice, D. M. and Mishima, S. (1984). Ocular pharmacokinetics. In: *Pharmacology of the Eye* (M. L. Sears, ed.). Springer-Verlag, Berlin, p. 73.) (Ref. 4).

associated with elimination through the retina, with its high surface area, while longer half-lives are reflective of elimination through the hyloid membrane and the anterior segment.

Injection volume and position within the vitreous body can also influence the distribution and elimination pattern of a drug. Friedrich et al. demonstrated that these factors had a substantial effect on vitreal distribution and elimination of fluorescein and fluorescein glucuronide (74). Four extreme positions and injection volumes of 15 or 100 μL were considered. The mean concentration of drug remaining in the vitreous 24 hours postdose varied by up to 3.8-fold depending on injection position, and increasing injection volume dampened this effect.

Retinal inflammation (which can cause a breakdown of the blood-retinal barrier) and aphakia are common pathophysiological states that can alter a drug's vitreal kinetics. Friedrich et al. showed that drug diffu-

Table 9 Vitreous Humor Half-Lives of Drugs Administered
Intravitreally

Drug	Species	Half-Life (h)	Ref.
ISIS 2922[a]	Rabbit	62	139
Foscarnet	Rabbit	34	140
Octreotide acetate	Cat	16	141
Vancomycin	Rabbit	12.5–14.5	142
Amphotericin B	Rabbit	6.9–15.1	76
		1.8 days (aphakic)	76
Rifampin	Rabbit (i.v.)	5.59	95
Carbenicillin	Rabbit	5.0	143
	Monkey	10	81
	Monkey	20 (+ probenecid)	81
Gentamicin	Cat	12.6	77
		6.5 (infected)	77
	Monkey	33	81
Dexamethasone	Rabbit	3.0	73
	Rabbit	3.48	144
Ganciclovir[b]	Rabbit	$0.017 \text{ cm}^2\text{hr}^{-1}$	145
	Human	$0.015 \text{ cm}^2\text{hr}^{-1}$	145
Cefazolin	Monkey	7	81
	Monkey	30 (+ probenecid)	81
Ceftizoxime	Rabbit	5.7	78
	Rabbit	9.4 (infected)	78
Ceftriazone	Rabbit	9.1	78
	Rabbit	13.1 (infected)	78
Ceftazidime	Rabbit	20.0	78
	Rabbit	21.5 (infected)	78
Cefepime	Rabbit	14.3	78
	Rabbit	15.1 (infected)	78

[a] Phosphorothioate oligonucleotide.
[b] Half-lives for ganciclovir normalized for volume and retinal surface area.

sivity and retinal permeability are important factors that determine elimination from the vitreous particularly in the case of blood-retinal barrier compromise (75). Furthermore, drug is eliminated faster in aphakic eyes, especially for drugs with low retinal permeability and injected proximal to the lens capsule. Injection close to the primary elimination barrier appears to be a key factor. Wingard et al. showed that intravitreally injected amphotericin B progressively accumulated in the sclera-choroid-retina in control phakic eyes, a phenomenon not observed in aphakic eyes (76). Whole phakic eye half-life was 6.9–15.1 days,while aphakic half-life was only 1.8 days. In the case of infected eyes, Ben-Nun et al. showed, with intravitreal injection of gentamicin, that the elimination rate of drug was greater in infected than normal eyes, presumably due to an alternation in blood-retinal barrier (77). In another evaluation of the vitreal kinetics of ceftizoxime, ceftriazone, ceftazindime, and cefepime in rabbits, $T_{1/2}$ values ranged from 5.7 to 20 hours in rabbits with uninflamed eyes and from 9.4 to 21.5 hours in rabbits with infected eyes (78). The longer $T_{1/2}$ suggested a predominant anterior route of elimination, while the shorter $T_{1/2}$ and low aqueous/vitreous concentration ratios suggested retinal elimination.

As mentioned, some compounds are actively transported out of the vitreous leading to a faster elimination than expected based on physicochemical properties; for example, Mochizuki investigated the transport of indomethacin in the anterior uvea of the albino rabbit in vitro and in vivo (intravitreal injection) (79). An energy-dependent carrier-mediated transport mechanism with low affinity was observed in the anterior uvea of the rabbit that could have accounted for the drug's rapid clearance (30% per hour) from the eye. Yoshida et al. characterized the active transport mechanism of the blood-retina barrier by estimating inward and outward permeability of the blood-retinal barrier in monkey eyes using vitreous fluorophotometry and intravitreally injected fluorescein and fluorescein glucuronide (80). Outward permeability (P_{out}) was 7.7 and 1.7 $\times$ 10^{-4} cm/min, respectively. P_{out}/P_{in} was 160 for fluroescein and 26 for fluorescein glucuronide. Intraperitoneal injection of probenecid caused a significant decrease in P_{out} for fluorescein but had no effect on fluorescein glucuronide P_{out}. The data suggest that fluorescein is actively transported out of the retina. In another example, Barza et al. studied the ocular pharmacokinetics of carbenicillin, cefazolin, and gentamicin following intravitreal administration to rhesus monkeys (81). Vitreal half-lives ranged from 7 to 33 hours. Concomitant intraperitoneal injection of probenecid prolonged the vitreal half-life of the cephalosporins, indicating a secretory mechanism. The results are consistent with the hypothesis that, in primates (as in rabbits), β-lactam antibiotics are eliminated by the retinal route and aminoglycosides by the anterior route.

2. Vitreal Pharmacokinetic Models

Several models have been proposed to describe the kinetics of intravitreally injected drugs. The simplest models assume a well-stirred vitreous body compartment in an effort to reduce the complexity of the mathematics. This may be a closer approximation in studies employing injection volumes of 100 μL or more, where the normally nonstirred vitreous can become agitated; however, injection volumes of greater than 20 μL generally require removal of an equal volume of vitreous to avoid a precipitous rise in intraocular pressure. This act alone may alter the physiology of the vitreous body. More sophisticated modeling takes into account diffusion through the relatively stagnant vitreous humor by employing Fick's law of diffusion. For example, Ohtori and Tojo determined the elimination of dexamethasone sodium *m*-sulfobenzoate (DMSB) following injection in the rabbit vitreous body under in vivo and in vitro conditions (82). The rate of elimination was greater in vivo versus in vitro. A general mathematical model, based on Fick's second law of diffusion, was developed to describe the pharmacokinetics. The model assumed a cylindrical vitreous body with three major elimination pathways: posterior aqueous chamber, retina-choroid-scleral membrane, and lens (see Fig. 9). Concentration in the vitreous decreased rapidly near the posterior aqueous chamber, indicating that the annular gap between the lens and ciliary body

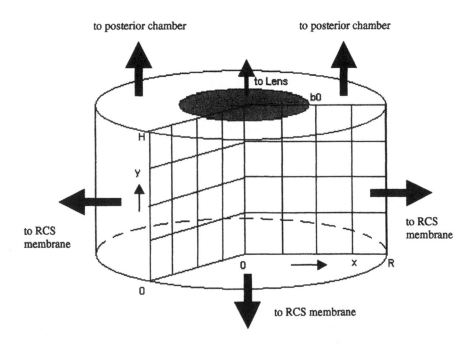

Figure 9 Cylindrical model of the vitreous body of rabbits. The posterior chamber, the retina-choroid-sclera (RCS), and the lens constitute elimination pathways out of the vitreous. (From Ref. 82.)

(posterior chamber) was the major route of elimination. The concentration gradient near the retina was considerable. It was concluded that, because of its large surface area, the retina can be a significant route of elimination. In a seprate study, Tojo and Ohtori used the cylindrical model approach to demonstrate three potential pathways of elimination including the annular gap, the lens, and the retina-choroid-sclera (83). The concentration in the retina was affected by the site of injection or initial distribution profiles, while concentration at the lens was independent of dose site. Drug injected into the anterior segment of the vitreous rapidly exited through the annular gap into the posterior chamber. The authors reasoned that drugs should be injected into the posterior vitreous to prolong therapeutic levels in the retina. Their results also showed that half-life was proportional to molecular weight and elimination into the lens was neglible due to the barrier function of the lens capsule.

Probably the most precise modeling of vitreal pharmacokinetics uses finite element analysis, a method commonly employed in engineering. This approach accounts for the detailed geometry and boundary conditions of the vitreous and precisely predicts the concentration gradients within the vitreous. Friedrich and colleagues adapted finite element modeling to the study of the drug distribution in the stagnent vitreous humor of the rabbit eye after an intravitreal injection of fluorescein and fluorescein-glucuronide (74,75,84). The computer-generated concentration profile in the vitreous humor is shown in Figure 10. Retinal permeability of fluorescein and fluorescein glucuronide were estimated by the model at 1.94×10^{-5} to 3.5×10^{-5} cm/s and from 0 to 7.62×10^{-7} cm/s, respectively. Simulations have also been performed for the human eye (74). In both rabbit and human eyes, the effect of injection position was found to be an important variable, as indicated in Figure 11 (84).

C. Periocular Administration

As previously mentioned in this chapter, while there is some evidence for direct drug delivery via the topical ocular route, drugs usually do not reach therapeutically relevant levels in the posterior segment following topical ocular instillation. If significant concentrations are achieved at the back of the eye, they are usually the result of redistribution from the systemic circulation, not local delivery. Consequently, to treat diseases of the posterior segment, drug must typically be administered intravitreally, periocularly, or systemically. Systemic administration will be discussed later in this chapter. Intravitreal injection has been discussed and is quite effective but, as has been mentioned, presents a serious risk to the eye. Periocular drug administration, using subconjunctival, sub-Tenon's, or retrobulbar injection, is

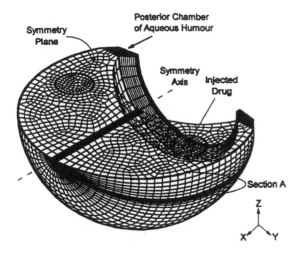

Figure 10 Finite element model of the vitreous body. The injection is hyloid displaced cylindrical. (Reprinted with permission from Friedrich et al. (1997) Finite element modeling of drug distribution in the vitreous humor of the rabbit eye. *Ann. Biomed. Eng.*, 25:306.) (Ref. 84).

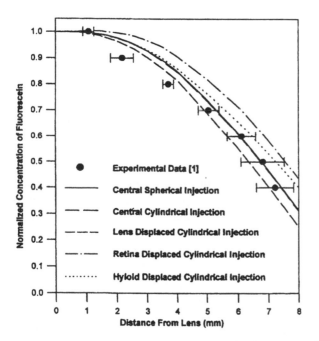

Figure 11 Relationship betwen normalized concentration of fluorescein in the vitreous humor and distance from the lens. (Reprinted with permission from Friedrich et al. (1997) Finite element modeling of drug distribution in the vitreous humor of the rabbit eye. *Ann. Biomed. Eng.*, 25:310.) (Ref. 84).

another and, in many cases, preferred, route for delivering drugs to the posterior segment (59).

1. Subconjunctival Administration

Subconjunctival injection offers the advantage of local drug delivery without the invasiveness of intravitreal injection. This route also allows for the use of drug depots to prolong the duration of drug therapy and avoids much of the toxicity encountered with systemic administration. Drug concentrations in the eye are typically substantially higher following subconjunctival versus systemic administration, while systemic exposure is greatly reduced with subconjunctival dosing. For example, following subconjunctival injection of 6-mercatopurine, mean peak concentrations in aqueous and vitreous were 15 and 10 times those following intravenous administration, while serum levels were about half (85). In another example, rabbits were administered ^{14}C-5-fluorouracil either subconjunctivally or intravenously (86). Peak levels of parent in the serum and urine were similar for the two routes; however, subconjunctival injection resulted in peak aqueous concentrations of 125 and 380 times that after intravenous injectiotn. The localized deliver of hydrocortisone by the subconjunctival route has been demonstrated by McCartney et al. in the rabbit eye (87). Their results showed that hydrocortisone penetrated directly into the eye with minimal spread beyond the site of administration.

Various studies have explored the mechanism by which drugs are absorbed into the eye following subconjunctival administration. Maurice and Mishima point to direct penetration to deeper tissues as the main pathway of entry into the anterior chamber (4). A necessary first condition, however, is the saturation of the underlying sclera with drug. This is followed by diffusion by various possible routes: laterally into corneal stroma and across the endothelium, across trabecular meshwork, through the iris stroma and across its anterior surface, into the ciliary body stroma and into newly generated aqueous humor, and into the vitreous body via the pars plana and across its anterior hyloid membrane (4). In addition to these pathways, depending on the injection volume, regurgitation out the dose site with subsequent spillage onto the cornea can lead to direct transcorneal absorption. For example, Conrad and Robinson investigated the mechanism of subconjunctival drug delivery using pilocarpine nitrate, albino rabbits, and instillation volumes ranging from 60 to 500 μL (88). At high injection volumes (> 200 μL), the primary mechanism for uptake into the aqueous was reflux of the drug solution from the injection site followed by corneal absorption. At lower volumes, the mechanism involved reflux and transconjunctival penetration, permeation of the globe, and systemic absorption followed by redistribution.

2. Periocular Injection (Sub-Tenon's and Retrobulbar)

Sub-Tenon's injection involves delivery of drug, usually as a depot, between the sub-Tenon's capsule and sclera or episclera. This route of administration has the advantage of placing drug in very close proximity to the sclera. Drug can subsequently diffuse through the sclera, which is quite permeable to a wide range of molecular weight compounds (59,89). Because the diffusion of drug from the dose site can be very localized, the preferred location of dose is directly over the target. For example, Freeman et al. performed localization of sub-Tenon's repository injection of corticosteroid (90). Echography showed drug within the sub-Tenon's space over the macula in 11 of 24 cases. The lack of therapeutic response to repository steroids was attributed to placement relative to target.

Except for the observation that bleb retrobulbar injection spreads forward, unlike subconjunctival injection which spreads backward, these two injection routes yield very similar results. Bodker et al. compared ocular tissue levels of dexamethasone 1 and 4 hours after subconjunctival or retrobulbar injection in rabbits (91). In both dosage route groups, concentrations in all three tissues (aqueous, vitreous, retina) were similar 1 hour postdose. After 4 hours, levels in the two groups were again similar except in choroid. Dosed and contralateral undosed eye tissues contained similar levels after 4 hours with the exception of retina, which had lower levels in undosed eye versus dosed. Retrobulbar dosing, however, provided a more sustained drug delivery than with subconjunctival administration.

Retrobulbar (or peribulbar) injection is another option for delivering drug to the posterior segment and the vitreous. Hyndiuk and Reagan determined the penetration and persistence of retrobulbar depot-corticosteroid in monkey ocular tissues (92). High concentrations were found in posterior uvea with persistence of lower concentrations. Steroid tended to concentrate in the optic nerve after retrobulbar but not systemic administration, and no drug was detected in other ocular tissues with the exception of lens and vitreous after 2 and 9 days. Weijten et al. studied the penetration of dexamethasone into the human vitreous and its systemic uptake following peribulbar injection (93). Mean levels in the vitreous peaked at 13 ng/mL at 6–7 hours postdose, and maximal serum level was 60 ng/mL 20–30 minutes postdose.

D. Systemic Administration

Because local drug delivery to the eye generally provides direct access to the site of action and, in most cases, substantially reduces systemic exposure and toxicity, systemic administration of drugs to treat ocular diseases is generally not preferred. Moreover, lower ocular concentrations are usually achieved compared to those following direct ocular dosing. However, for drug delivery to the posterior segment or vitreous body, systemic administration could be the best choice depending on the drug's ability to penetrate the blood-retinal barrier or blood-vitreous barrier and its systemic toxicity profile. For example, in a study by Ueno et al., concentrations of BCNU were measured in aqueous and vitreous of rabbits following intravenous, subconjunctival, and topical ocular administration (94). Distribution was dependent on dose route in that topical, followed by subconjunctival, was best for distribution into the iris, while intravenous, was best for distribution into the choroid-retina. In another example, Liu et al. demonstrated that rifampin penetrated vitreous humor after an intravenous single dose (95).

Compromising the blood-vitreous or -retinal barrier can enhance intraocular absorption following systemic administration. Wilson et al. treated the right eyes of rabbits with triple or single freeze-thaw cryotherapy at one or two locations one day before intravenous carboplatin with or without cyclosporine (96). Cryotherapy increased the intravitreal penetration of carboplatin. In a study by Elliot et al., following intravenous injection of ganciclovir with and without RMP-7, a compound known to increase the permeability of the blood-brain barrier, RMP-7 enhanced retinal uptake through the blood-retinal barrier (97). Interestingly, Palastine and Brubaker demonstrated that systemically administered (intravenous or oral) fluorescein can enter the vitreous through other means beyond an increase in blood-retinal barrier permeability (98).

III. OCULAR METABOLISM

The metabolic capacity of the eye is low compared to that of a primary metabolizing organ such as liver. However, sufficient enzymatic activity is present to cause the breakdown of ophthalmic drugs in the eye. While this biotransformation usually results in loss of efficacy, the development of prodrugs takes advantage of the increased corneal permeability of the prodrug and the subsequent hydrolysis of the prodrug to active compound (16, 99,100). Prodrugs of pilocarpine (101), phenylephrine (102,103), timolol (104), and prostaglandin $F_{2\alpha}$ tromethamine have shown improved corneal penetration.

A variety of esterases responsible for prodrug hydrolysis have been identified in the eye. Lee et al. reported the presence of acetyl-, butyryl-, and carboxylcholinesterases in pigmented eyes (99). Over 75% of cholinesterase activy was due to butyrylcholinesterases in all ocular tissues but corneal epithelium. Their results suggested that esters with chain lengths exceeding four carbons are hydrolyzed principally by butyrylcholinesterase. In a separate study, Lee demonstrated that esterase activity ranked as follows in ocular tissues: iris-ciliary body > cornea > aqueous humor (100). Activities in the pigmented rabbit cornea and iris-ciliary body were greater than in the nonpigmented eye, indicating a higher metabolic capacity in pigmented ocular tissue. Narurkar and Mitra confirmed Lee's ranking of enzymatic hydrolysis activity with aliphatic esters of 5-iodo-2'-deoxyuridine (105). Camber et al. evaluated the permeability and absorption of $PGF_{2\alpha}$ and its methyl and benzyl esters through isolated pig cornea in vitro. Hydrolysis was shown to be due to butyrlcholinesterase in the corneal epithelium (106).

Although esterases have been studied to the largest extent, a number of other enzymes have been identified within the eye. These include catechol-O-methyltransferase, monamine oxidase, steroid 6-betahydroxylase, oxidoreductase, lysosomal enzymes, peptidases, and glucuronide and sulfate transferase (107). In addition, cytochrome P450 enzymatic activity has been observed in ocular tissue (108,109). Campbell et al. demonstrated, using p-aminobenzoate, aminozolamide, and sulfamethazine as substrates that there is significant arylamine acetyltransferase activity in the eye with the highest to lowest ranking compared to a nonocular tissue as liver > iris-ciliary body > corneal epithelium > stroma-endothelum (110). Phenotype (slow versus fast acetylators) had no effect on activity in the eye. Putnam et al. also studied the disposition of aminozolamide in the rabbit eye (111). Their results suggested that the topical IOP-lowering activity of aminozolamide was the result of both metabolite levels in aqueous humor and iris-ciliary body and the 99% + inhibition of carbonic anhydrase. Metabolite levels were highest in cornea and iris-ciliary body, with less in aqueous.

Aldehyde reductase and ketone reductase have also been found in ocular tissues (8). Compounds such as N-oxide, hydroxamic acid, sulfoxide, and nitro drugs are reduced by aldehyde reductase in bovine ciliary body. Using levobunolol as substrate, Lee et al. showed that the rank order of ketone reductase activity was corneal epithelium > iris-ciliary body > conjunctiva > lens. No activity was detected in tears, corneal stroma, sclera, or aqueous humor. Models describing metabolism have been developed for aminozolamide (111) and levobunolol (27).

In general, the iris-ciliary body and corneal epithelium possess the greatest capacity for metabolic activity in the anterior segment. Moreover, activity may be higher in pigmented versus nonpigmented ocular tissue.

IV. OCULAR PHAMACODYNAMICS

Fundamentally, pharmacodynamics is the study of the biological effects of drugs (112). More specifically, it is the study of how the concentration of drug in the biophase (site of action) relates to the magnitude of biological and therapeutic effects produced (113). However, in the evaluation of systemic pharmacodynamics, drug concentrations are typically determined in plasma or serum and not the biophase. As a result, there is not always a direct relationship between measured concentration of drug and biological response. This shortcoming is somewhat overcome with ophthalmic drugs since dose delivery and pharmacokinetic sampling are usually in very close proximity to the biophase. Also, there are several quantifiable ocular responses, which are relatively easy to evaluate in vivo, including miosis, mydriasis, intraocular pressure, corneal sensation, aqueous humor flow, blink rate, tear secretion, and electroretinogram (4).

In conducting human ocular studies, measuring ocular pharmacokinetics in intraocular fluids and tissues is difficult if not impossible. These samples can only be removed at death of the patient or in the case of removal of a diseased eye. As a result, pharmacological response measurements usually replace concentration assays in describing the effect of a drug in the human eye. Unfortunately, responses can vary widely between individuals, presumably because of differences in dose-response relationships and ocular pharmacokinetics (8). Eye pigmentation, wearing of contact lenses, allergies to drug or formulation components, and physiological factors all play a role in causing high variability in response data (8). Nevertheless, pharmacodynamic measurements continue to be applied, and where possible pharmacokinetic data are coupled with pharmacodynamic data.

A mathematical approach developed for miotic or mydriatic response (3,4) is shown in the following equation:

$$R_\ell = \frac{R}{(R_{max} - R)} = qC \tag{6}$$

where R_{max} is the maximal response achieved by a drug with all receptors occupied, q is a proportionality constant, and C is the concentration of drug. Mishima showed that Eq. (6) predicted the miosis of carbachol and pilocarpine on the sphincter muscle of the cat (see Fig. 12) (3).

Based on maximum and minimum pupil diameters of 8.5 and 1 mm, respectively, it can be shown that for a miotic response,

$$R_l = \frac{(D_0 - D)}{(D - 1)} \tag{7}$$

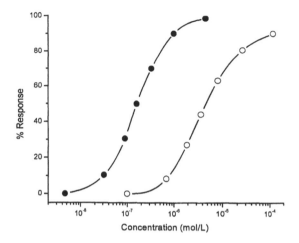

Figure 12 Dose-response relationship from carbachol (●) and pilocarpine (○) in isolated human sphincter muscle strip. (Replotted from Ref. 3.)

and for a mydriasis response,

$$R_I = \frac{(D - D_0)}{(8.5 - D)} \tag{8}$$

where D_0 is the pupil diameter before drug application and D is the pupil diameter following drug administration (9). Figure 13 shows a log-linear plot of the response versus time, from which is derived the following equation:

$$R_I = R_L(e^{-A(t-t_0)} - e^{-B(t-t_0)}) \tag{9}$$

where R_L is the intercept value of R_I, t_0 if the lag time after instillation when response is observed, and A and B are apparent elimination and absorption rate constants (9).

Chien and Schoenwald investigated aqueous humor concentration of phenylephrine and the corresponding mydriatic response in rabbit eyes following topical ocular administration of phenylephrine or a prodrug of phenylephrine (114). Ocular bioavailability of 10% prodrug was eightfold higher than that of the 10% HCl salt. However, mydriatic activity only improved fourfold, demonstrating that the mydriatic response did not accurately reflect drug distribution to the iris. The observed clockwise hysteresis in the response versus concentration plot was suggestive of pharmacological tolerance. An E_{max} model with a Michaelis-Menten relationship between

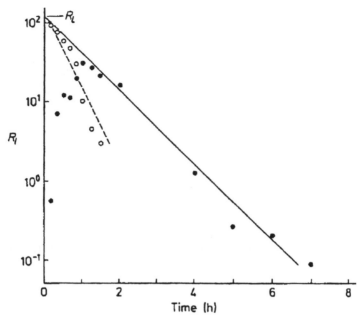

Figure 13 Log-linear plot of pupillary response (miotic or mydriasis) versus time. Dotted line indicates absorption phase after stripping off elimination phase. (Reprinted with permission from Maurice, D. M., and Mishima, S. (1984). Ocular pharmacokinetics. In: *Pharmacology of the Eye*. (M. L. Sears, ed.), Springer-Verlag, Berlin, p. 56.) (Ref. 4).

response and concentration of phenylephrine in the iris was developed and expressed as follows:

$$\Delta E(t) = \frac{\Delta E_{max} \times C_a(t)}{K'_m + C_a(t)} \tag{10}$$

where $\Delta E(t)$ is the difference between pupillary diameter before and after drug instillation at time t, K'_m is the drug concentration in the iris at half maximal mydriatic response (one-half ΔE_{max}), and $C_a(t)$ is the concentration of drug in aqueous humor at time t. In the case of tolerance, K'_m is no longer constant but changes with time and can be calculated for each time interval as:

$$K'_m(t) = \left[\left(\frac{\Delta E_{max}}{\Delta E(t)} \right) - 1 \right] \times C_a(t) \tag{11}$$

A plot of $K'_m(t)$ versus time was linear up to 90 minutes but increased thereafter through 240 minutes postinstillation verifying the development of tolerance (114)

Smolen (115) described a methematical model for pharmacological response from pilocarpine based on its dose-response relationship:

$$I_{\max} = \frac{719.4D}{I + 20.4D} + 0.5D \tag{12}$$

Equation (12) requires the assumptions of nonhysteresis, rapid and reversible binding to the receptor, and first-order kinetics. If these assumptions are met, the equation can be generalized to other drugs.

Smolen and Schoenwald further developed a theoretical basis for the performance of drug-absorption analysis from pharmacological response versus time data following single, multiple, or continuous dosing of drug by any route of administration (116–119). Pharmacological and pharmacokinetic parameters characterizing the mydriatic behavior of tropicamide were derived, and pharmacological response versus time plots yielded two and three-compartment models.

An $E_{\max}$ model, similar to that for miosis, has also been proposed for intraocular pressure (IOP) reduction (9). Mishima reviewed the pharmacodynamics related to IOP lowering (3). By virtue of the complexities of IOP lowering, this response does not necessarily relate directly to drug concentrations as is the case for pupillary response.

Drugs typically have effects other than the measured response. These extraneous actions might include alterations in aqueous humor turnover or blood flow within certain ocular tissues. As a result, nonlinear behavior is likely to be observed, however, as Schoenwald has discussed (8), the difficulty in measuring concentrations in the human eye will likely perpetuate the use of pharmacological responses to evaluate ophthalmic therapies.

V. CONCLUSIONS

Understanding the ocular pharmacokinetic characteristics of a drug is critical to the optimization of its single and multiple dose therapeutic regimens. However, because of the complex nature of ocular absorption, distribution, and elimination, accurately measuring the ocular pharmacokinetics can be difficult. The topical ocular route is preferred for reasons of ease of administration, noninvasiveness, direct drug delivery, and minimization of systemic effects. Even considering the complexities of ocular pharmacokinetics following topical ocular administration, several valid approaches to its study have been developed. Many take into account the competing pathways of absorption, leading to either ocular or systemic exposure. Models in varying detail have also been developed for intravitreal administration. Compared to the kinetics associated with the topical ocular route, vitreal pharmacokinetics is more straightforward in that it avoids convoluted precorneal events. However, due to the nonstirred nature of the vitreous humor, the mathematics can be quite complex due to the inclusion of Fick's law of diffusion. Periocular administration is also dependent to a large extent on diffusion, which can be very localized. Both periocular and systemic administration can be used to deliver drug to the posterior segment, however, the latter is usually the last resort due to the greater risk for systemic drug exposure and toxicity.

Ocular pharmacokinetics, with all its limitations, is an important part of ophthalmic drug development. Coupled with the knowledge of a drug's metabolism and its pharmacodynamics, ocular pharmacokinetics provides invaluable information needed to properly design single and multiple dose regimens. In the future, with the discovery and refinement of animal models and the advent of more sophisticated modeling techniques and computer programs, ocular pharmacokinetics/pharmacodynamics will likely receive even more widespread use.

REFERENCES

1. Burstein, N. L., and Anderson, J. A. (1985). Review: Corneal penetration and ocular bioavailability of drugs. *J. Ocular Pharmacol.*, 1:309.
2. Lee, V. H. L., and Robinson, J. R. (1986). Review: Topical ocular drug delivery: Recent developments and future challenges. *J. Ocular Pharmacol.*, 2:67.
3. Mishima, S. (1981). Clinical pharmacokinetics of the eye. *Invest. Ophthalmol. Vis. Sci.*, 21:504.
4. Maurice, D. M., and Mishima, S. (1984). Ocular pharmacokinetics. In: *Pharmacology of the Eye* (M. L. Sears, ed.). Springer-Verlag, Berlin, pp. 19–116.
5. Schoenwald, R. D. (1990). Ocular drug delivery. Pharmacokinetic considerations. *Clin. Pharmacokinet.*, 18:255.
6. Lang, J. C., and Stiemke, M. M. Biological barriers to ocular delivery. In: *Ocular Therapeutics and Drug Delivery* (I. K. Reddy, ed.). Technomics Publishing, Lancaster, pp. 51–132.
7. Davies, N. M. (2000). Biopharmaceutical consideration in topical ocular drug delivery. *Clin. Exp. Pharmacol. Physiol.*, 27:558.
8. Schoenwald, R. D. (1993). Ocular pharmacokinetics/pharmacodynamics, *Ophthalmic Drug Delivery Systems* (A. K. Mitra, ed.), Marcel Dekker, Inc., New York, pp. 83–110.
9. Worakul, N., and Robinson, J. R. (1997). Ocular pharmacokinetics/pharmacodynamics. *Eur. J. Pharm. Biopharm.*, 44:71.

10. Schoenwald, R. D., and Ward, R. L. (1978). Relationship between steroid permeability across excised rabbit cornea and octanol-water partition coefficients. *J. Pharm. Sci.*, 67:786.
11. Schoenwald, R. D., and Huang, H. S. (1983). Corneal penetration behavior of β-blocking agents I: Physicochemical factors. *J. Pharm. Sci.*, 72:1266.
12. Huang, H. S., Schoenwald, R. D., and Lach, J. L. (1983). Corneal penetration behavior of β-blocking agents II: Assessment of barrier contributions. *J. Pharm. Sci.*, 72:1272.
13. Maren, T. H., Jankowska, L., Sanyal, G., and Edelhauser, H. F. (1983). The transcorneal permeability of sulfonamide carbonic anhydrase inhibitors and their effect on aqueous humor secretion. *Exp. Eye Res.*, 36:457.
14. Cox, W. V., Kupferman, A., and Leibowitz, H. M. (1972). Topically applied steroids in corneal disease. I. The role of inflammation in stromal absorption of dexamethasone. *Arch. Ophthal.*, 88:308.
15. Cox, W. V., Kupferman, A., and Leibowitz, H. M. (1972). Topically applied steroids in corneal disease. II. The role of drug vehicle in stromal absorption of dexamethasone. *Arch. Ophthal.*, 88:549.
16. Chien, D. S., Bundgaard, H., and Lee, V. H. L. (1988). Influence of corneal epithelial integrity on the penetration of timolol prodrugs. *J. Ocular Pharmacol.*, 4:137.
17. Madhu, C., Rix, P. J., Shackleton, M. J., Nguyen, T. G., and Tang-Liu, D. D. S. (1996). Effect of benzalkonium chloride/EDTA on the ocular bioavailability of ketorolac tromethamine following ocular instillation to normal and de-epithelialized corneas of rabbits. *J. Pharm. Sci.*, 85:415.
18. Jani, R., Gan, O., Ali, Y., Rodstrom, R., Hancock, S. (1994). Ion exchange resins for ophthalmic delivery. *J. Ocular Pharmacol.*, 10:57.
19. Gurny, R., Ibrahim, H., Aebi, A., Buri, P., Wilson, C. G., Washington, N., Edman, P., and Camber, O. (1987). Design and evaluation of controlled release systems for the eye. *J. Controlled Release*, 6:367.
20. Ahmed, I., and Patton, T. F. (1985). Importance of the noncorneal absorption route in topical ophthalmic drug delivery. *Invest. Ophthalmol. Vis. Sci.*, 26:584–587.
21. Ahmed, I., and Patton, T. F. (1987). Disposition of timolol and inulin in the rabbit eye following corneal versus non-corneal absorption. *Int. J. Pharmaceutics*, 38:9.
22. Ahmed, I., Gokhale, R. D., Shah, M. V., and Patton, T. F. (1987). Physicochemical determinants of drug diffusion across the conjunctiva, sclera, and cornea. *J. Pharm. Sci.*, 76:583.
23. Chien, D. S., Homsy, J. J., Gluchowske, C., and Tang-Liu, D. D. S. (1990). Corneal and conjunctival/scleral penetration of p-aminoclonidine, AGN 190342, and clonidine in rabbit eyes. *Curr. Eye Res.*, 9:1051.
24. Schoenwald, R. D., Deshpande, G. S., Rethwisch, D. G., and Barfknecht, C. F. (1997). Penetration into the anterior chamber via the conjunctival/scleral pathway. *J. Ocular Pharmacol. Ther.*, 13:41.
25. Romanelli, L., Valeri, P., Morrone, L. A., Pimpinella, G., Graziani, G., and Tita, B. (1994). Ocular absorption and distribution of bendazac after topical administration to rabbits with different vehicles. *Life Sci.*, 54:877.

26. Ling, T. L., and Combs, D. L. (1987). Ocular bioavailability and tissue distribution of [^{14}C]ketorolac tromethamine in rabbits. *J. Pharm. Sci.*, 76:289.

27. Tang-Liu, D. D. S., Liu, S., Neff, J., and Sandri, R. (1987). Disposition of levobunolol after an ophthalmic dose to rabbits. *J. Pharm. Sci.*, 76:780.

28. Patton, T. F., and Robinson, J. R. (1976). Quantitative precorneal disposition of topically applied pilocarpine nitrate in rabbit eyes. *J. Pharm. Sci.*, 65:1295.

29. Chrai, S. S., Patton, T. F., Mehta, A., and Robinson, J. R. (1973). Lacrimal and instilled fluid dynamics in rabbit eyes. *J. Pharm. Sci.*, 62:1112.

30a. Chrai, S. S., Makoid, M. C., Eriksen, S. P., and Robinson, J. R. (1974). Drop size and initial dosing frequency problems of topically applied ophthalmic drugs. *J. Pharm. Sci.*, 63:333.

30b. Keister, J. C., Cooper, E. R., Missel, P. J., Lang, J. C., and Hager, D. F. (1991). Limits on optimizing ocular drug delivery. *J. Pharm. Sci.*, 80:50.

31. Zaki, I., Fitzgerald, P., Hardy, J. G., and Wilson, C. G. (1986). A comparison of the effect of viscosity on the precorneal residence of solutions in rabbit and man. *J. Pharm. Pharmacol.*, 38:463.

32. Patton, T. F., and Robinson, J. R. (1975). Ocular evaluation of polyvinyl alcohol vehicle in rabbits. *J. Pharm. Sci.*, 64:1312.

33. Chrai, S. S., and Robinson, J. R. (1974). Ocular evaluation of methylcellulose vehicle in albino rabbits. *J. Pharm. Sci.*, 63:1218.

34. Edelhauser, H. F., and Maren, T. H. (1988). Permeability of human cornea and sclera to sulfonamide carbonic anhydrase inhibitors. *Arch. Ophthalmol*, 106:1110.

35. Maurice, D. (1995). The effect of the low blink rate in rabbits of topical drug penetration. *J. Ocular Pharmacol. Therap.*, 11:297.

36. Doane, M. G., Jensen, A. D., and Dohlman, C. H. (1978). Penetration routes of topically applied eye medications. *Am. J. Ophthal.*, 85:383.

37. Kaila, T., Huupponen, R., and Salminen, L. (1986). Effects of eyelid closure and nasolacrimal duct occlusion on the systemic absorption of ocular timolol in human subjects. *J. Ocular Pharmacol.*, 2:365.

38. Zimmerman, T. J., Kooner, K. S., Kandarakis, A. S., and Ziegler, L. P. (1984). Improving the therapeutic index of topically applied ocular drugs. *Arch. Ophthalmol.*, 102:551.

39. Linden, C., and Alm, A. (1990). The effect of reduced tear drainage on corneal and aqueous concentrations of topically applied fluorescein. *Acta Ophthal.*, 68:633.

40. Lee, Y.-H., Kompella, U. B., and Lee, V. H.-L. (1993). Systemic absorption pathways of topically applied beta adrenergic antagonists in the pigmented rabbit. *Exp. Eye Res.*, 57:341.

41. Hitoshe, S., Bundgaard, H., and Lee, V. H. L. (1989). Design of prodrugs to selectively reduce systemic timolol absorption on the basis of the differential lipophilic characteristics of the cornea and the conjunctiva. *Invest. Ophthalmol. Vis. Sci.*, 30 (Suppl.):25.

42. Ashton, P., Podder, S. K., and Lee, V. H. L. (1991), V. H. L. (1991). Formulation influence on conjunctival penetration of four beta blockers in

the pigmented rabbit: A comparison with corneal penetration. *Pharm. Res.*, 8:1166.

43. Schoenwald, R. D., and Chien, D. S. (1988). Ocular absorption and disposition of phenylephrine and phenylephrine oxazolidine. *Biopharm. Drug Dispos.*, 9:527.

44. Makoid, M. C., and Robinson, J. R. (1979). Pharmacokinetics of topically applied pilocarpine in the albino rabbit eye. *J. Pharm. Sci.*, 68:435.

45. Huang, H. S., Schoenwald, R. D., and Lach, J. L. (1983). Corneal penetration behavior of β-blocking agents III: In vitro– in vivo correlations. *J. Pharm. Sci.*, 72:1279.

46. Tang-Liu, D. D. S., Liu, S. S., and Weinkam, R. J. (1984). Ocular and systemic bioavailability of ophthalmic flurbiprofen. *J. Pharmacokin. Biopharm.*, 12:611.

47. Ding, S., Chen, C.-C., Salome-Kesslak, R., Tang-Liu, D. D.-S., and Himmelstein, K. J. (1992). Precorneal sampling techniques for ophthalmic gels. *J. Ocular Pharmacol.*, 8:151.

48. Eller, M. G., Schoenwald, R. D., Dixson, J. A., Segarra, T., and Barfknecht, C. F. (1985). Topical carbonic anhydrase inhibitors IV: Relationship between excised corneal permeability and pharmacokinetic factors. *J. Pharm. Sci.*, 74:525.

49. Eller, M. G., Schoenwald, R. D., Dixson, J. A., Segarra, T., and Barfknecht, C. F. (1985). Topical carbonic anhydrase inhibitors III: Optimization model for corneal penetration of ethoxzolamide analogues. *J. Pharm. Sci.*, 74:155.

50. Conrad, J. M., and Robinson, J. R. (1977). Aqueous chamber drug distribution volume measurement in rabbits. *J. Pharm. Sci.*, 66:219.

51. Rittenhouse, K. D., Peiffer, R. L., and Pollack, G. M. (1998). Evaluation of microdialysis sampling of aqueous humor for in vivo models of ocular absorption and disposition. *J. Pharm. Biomed. Anal.*, 16:951.

52. Lindquist, N. G. (1973). Accumulation of drugs on melanin. *Acta Radiol.* 325(Suppl.): 5.

53. Patil, P. N., and Jacobowitz, D. (1974). Unequal accumulation of adrenergic drugs by pigmented and nonpigmented iris. *Am. J. Ophthalmol.*, 78:470.

54. Araie, M., Takase, M., Sadai, Y., Ishii, Y., Yokoyama, Y., and Kitagawa, M. (1982). Beta-adrenergic blockers: ocular penetration and binding to the uveal pigment. *Jpn. J. Ophthalmol.*, 26:248.

55. Lyons, J. S., and Krohn, D. L. (1973). Pilocarpine uptake by pigmented uveal tissue. *Am. J. Ophthalmol.*, 75:885.

56. Chien, D.-S, Richman, J., Zolezio, H., and Tang-Liu, D. (1992). Drug distribution of brimonidine in albino and pigmented rabbit eyes. *Pharm Res.*, 9:S336.

57. Achempoing, A. A., Schackleton, M., and Tang-Liu, D. D-S. (1995). Comparative ocular pharmacokinetics of brimonidine after a single dose application to the eyes of albino and pigmented rabbits. *Drug Metab. Disposition*, 23(7):708.

58. Nagata, A., Mishima, H. K., Kiuchi, Y., Hirota, A., Kurokawa, T., and Ishibashi, S. (1993). Binding of antiglaucomatous drugs to synthetic melanin and their hypotensive effects on pigmented and nonpigmented rabbit eyes. *Jpn. J. Ophthalmol.*, 37:32.

59. Geroski, D. H., and Edelhauser, H. F. (2000). Drug delivery for posterior segment eye disease. *Invest. Ophthalmol. Vis. Sci.*, 41(5):961.

60. Dahlin, D. C., Curtis, M. A., DeSantis, L., Struble, C. B. (2000). Distribution of betaxolol to posterior ocular tissues of the cynomolgus monkey following a 30-day BID topical ocular regimen of Betoptic S. *Invest. Ophthalmol. Vis. Sci.*, 41:S509.

61. Romanelli, L., Morrone, L. A., Guglielmotte, A., Piccinelli, D., and Valeri, P. (1992). Distribution of topically administered drugs to the posterior segment of rabbit eye. *Pharmacol. Res.*, 25(1):39.

62. Schoenwald, R. D., Harris, R. G., Turner, D., Knowles, W., and Chien, D. S. (1987). Ophthalmic bioequivalence of steroid/antibiotic combination formulations. *Biopharm. Drug Dispos.*, 8:527.

63. Tang-Liu, D. D. S., and Burke, P. J. (1988). The effect of azone on ocular levobunolol absorption: Calculating the area under the curve and its standard error using tissue sampling compartments. *Pharm. Res.*, 5:238.

64. Lee, V. H. L. and Robinson, J. R. (1979). Mechanistic and quantitative evaluation of precorneal pilocarpine disposition in albino rabbits. *J. Pharm. Sci.*, 68:673.

65. Gibaldi, M., and Perrier, D. (1982). *Pharmacokinetics*, 2nd ed., Marcel Dekker, New York, pp. 355–384.

66. Himmelstein, K. J., Guvenir, I., and Patton, T. F. (1978). Preliminary pharmacokinetic model of pilocarpine uptake and distribution in the eye. *J. Pharm. Sci.*, 67:603.

67. Chiang, C. H., and Schoenwald, R. D. (1986). Ocular pharmacokinetic models of clonidine-^{3}H hydrochloride. *J. Pharmacokin. Biopharm.*, 14:175.

68. Morlet, N., Graham, G. G., Gatus, B., McLachlan, A. J., Salonikas, C., Naidoo, D., Goldberg, I., and Lam, C. M. (2000). Pharmacokinetics of ciprofloxacin in the human eye: A clinical study and population pharmacokinetic analysis. *Antimicrob. Agents Chemother.*, 44:1674.

69. Gillespie, W. R., Missel, P. J., and Lang, J. C. (1989). Application of system analysis to ocular pharmacokinetics: Prediction of betaxolol concentrations in ocular structures following various modes of administration. *Pharm. Res.*, 6:S224.

70. Sebag, J. (1992). The vitreous, *Adler's Physiology of the Eye: Clinical Applications* (W. M. Hart, Jr., ed.), Mosby Year Book, St. Louis, pp. 305–308.

71. Fatt, I. (1975). Flow and diffusion in the vitreous body of the ey. *Bull. Math. Biol.*, 37:85.

72. Araie, M., and Maurice, D. M. (1991). The loss of fluorescein, fluorescein glucuronide and fluorescein isothiocyanate dextran from the vitreous by the anterior and retinal pathways. *Exp. Eye Res.*, 52:27.

73. Graham, R. O., and Peyman, G. A. (1974). Intravitreal injection of dexamethasone. *Arch. Ophthalmol.*, 92:149.
74. Friedrich, S., Cheng, Y.-L., and Saville, B. (1997). Drug distribution in the vitreous humor of the human eye: The effects of intravitreal injection position and volume. *Curr. Eye Res.*, 16:663.
75. Friedrich, S., Saville, B., and Cheng, Y.-L. (1997). Drug distribution in the vitreous humor of the human eye: the effects of aphakia and changes in retinal permeability and vitreous diffusivity. *J. Ocular Pharmacol. Therap.*, 13:445.
76. Wingard, L. B., Zuravleff, J. J., Doft, B. H., Berk, L., and Rinkoff, J. (1989). Intraocular distribution of intravitreally administered amphotericin B in normal and vitrectomized dyes. *Invest. Ophthalmol. Vis. Sci.*, 30(10)):2184.
77. Ben-Nun, J., Joyce, D. A., Cooper, R. L., Cringle, S. J., and Constable, I. J. (1989). Pharmacokinetics of intravitreal injection. Assessment of a gentamicin model by ocular dialysis. *Invest. Ophthalmol. Vis. Sci.*, 30:1055.
78. Barza, M., Lynch, E., and Baum, J. L. (1993). Pharmacokinetics of newer cephalosporins after subconjunctival and intravitreal injection in rabbits. *Arch. Ophthalmol.*, 111:121.
79. Mochizuki, M. (1980). Transport of indomethacin in the anterior uvea of the albino rabbit. *Jpn J. Ophthalmol*, 24:363.
80. Yoshida, A., Ishiko, S., and Kojima, M. (1992). Outward permeability of the blood-retinal barrier. *Graefe's Arch. Clin. Exp. Ophthalmol.*, 230:78.
81. Barza, M., Kane, A., and Baum, J. (1983). Pharmacokinetics of intravitreal carbenicillin, cefazolin, and gentamicin in rhesus monkeys. *Invest. Ophthalmol. Vis. Sci.*, 24:1602.
82. Ohtori, A., and Tojo, K. (1994). In vivo/in vitro correlation of intravitreal delivery of drugs with the help of computer simulations. *Biol. Pharm. Bull.*, 17:283.
83. Tojo, K. J., and Ohtori, A. (1994). Pharmacokinetic model of intravitreal drug injection. *Math. Biosci.*, 123:59.
84. Friedrich, S., Cheng, Y.-L., and Saville, B. (1997). Finite element modeling of drug distribution in the vitreous humor of the rabbit eye. *Ann. Biomed. Eng.*, 25:303.
85. Gudauskas, G., Kumi, C., Dedhar, C., Bussanich, N., and Rootman, J. (1985). Ocular pharmacokinetics of subconjunctivally versus intravenously administered 6-mercaptopurine. *Can. J. Ophthalmol.*, 20:110.
86. Rootman, J., Ostry, A., and Gudauskas, G. (1984). Pharmacokinetics and metabolism of 5-fluorouracil following subconjunctival versus itnravenous administration. *Can. J. Ophthalmol.*, 19:187.
87. McCartney, H. J., Drysdale, I. O., Gornall, A. G., and Basu, P. K. (1965). An autoradiographic study of penetration of subconjunctivally injected hydrocortisone into the normal and inflamed rabbit eye. *Invest.Ophthalmol.*, 4:297.
88. Conrad, J. M., and Robinson, J. R. (1980). Mechanisms of anterior segment absorption of pilocarpine following subconjunctival injection in albino rabbits. *J. Pharm. Sci.*, 69:875.

89. Maurice, D. M., and Polgar, J. (1977). Diffusion across the sclera. *Exp. Eye Res.*, 25:577.
90. Freeman, W. R., Green, R. L., and Smith, R. E. (1987). Echographic localization of corticosteriods after periocular injection. *Am. J. Ophthalmol.*, 103:281.
91. Bodker, F. S., Ticho, B. H., Feist, R. M., and Lam, T. T. (1993). Intraocular dexamethasone penetration via subconjunctival or retrobulbar injections in rabbits. *Ophthalmic Surg.*, 24:453.
92. Hyndiuk, R. A., and Reagan, M. G. (1968). Radioactive depot-corticosteroid penetration into monkey ocular tissue. I. Retrobulbar and systemic administration. *Arch. Ophthalmol.*, 80:499.
93. Weijten, O., van der Sluijs, F. A., Schoemaker, R. C., Lentjes, E. G. W. M., Cohen, A. F., Romijn, F. P. H. T. M., and van Meurs, J. C. (1997). Peribulbar corticosteroid injection: vitreal and serum concentrations after dexamethasone disodium phosphate injection. *Am. J. Ophthalmol.*, 123:358.
94. Ueno, N., Refojo, M. F., and Liu, L. H. S. (1982). Pharmacokinetics of the antineoplastic agent 1,3-bis(2-chloroethyl)-1-nitrosourea (BCNU) in the aqueous and vitreous of rabbit. *Invest. Ophthalmol. Vis. Sci.*, 23:199.
95. Liu, Q. F., Dharia, N., Mayers, M., and Miller, M. (1995). Rifampin pharmacokinetics in serum and vitreous humor after single dose systemic administration. *Invest. Ophthalmol. Vis. Sci.*, 36:S1018.
96. Wilson, T. W., Chan, H. S. L., Moselhy, G. M., Heydt, D. D., Frey, C. M., and Gallie, B. L. (1996). Penetration of chemotherapy into vitreous is increased by cryotherapy and cyclosporine in rabbits. *Arch. Ophthalmol.*, 114:1390.
97. Elliot, P. J., Bartus, R. T., Mackic, J. B., and Zlokovic, B. V.(1997). Intravenous infusion of RMP-7 increases ocular uptake of ganciclovir. *Pharm. Res.*, 14:80.
98. Palastine, A. G., and Brubaker, R. F. (1981). Pharmacokinetics of fluorescein in the vitreous. *Invest.Ophthalmol. Vis. Sci.*, 21:542.
99. Lee, V. H. L., Chang, S. C., Oshiro, C. M., and Smith, R. E. (1985).Ocular esterase composition in albino and pigmented rabbits: Possible implications in ocular prodrug design and evaluation. *Curr. Eye Res.*, 4:1117.
100. Lee, V. H. L. (1983). Esterase activities in adult rabbit eyes. *J. Pharm. Sci*, 72:239.
101. Bungaard, H., Falch, E., Larsen, C., Mosher, G. L., and Mikkelson, T. J. (1986). Pilocarpine prodrugs II. Synthesis, stability, bioconversion and physicochemical properties of sequentially labile pilocarpine acid diesters. *J. Pharm. Sci.*, 75:775.
102. Chien, D. S., and Schoenwald, R. D. (1986). Improving the ocular absorption of phenylephrine. *Biopharm. Drug Dispos.*, 7:453.
103. Schoenwald, R. D., Folk, V. K., and Piper, J. G. (1987). In vivo comparison of phenylephrine and phenylephrine oxazolidine instilled in the monkey eye. *J. Ocular Pharmacol.*, 3:333.
104. Chang, S-C., Bundgaard, H., Buur, A., and Lee, V. H. L. (1987). Improved corneal penetration of timolol by prodrugs as a means to reduce systemic drug load. *Invest. Ophthalmol. Vis. Sci.*, 28:487.

105. Narurkar, M. M., and Mitra, A. K. (1989). Prodrugs of 5-indo-2′-deoxyuridine for enhanced ocular transport. *Pharm. Res.*, 6:887.
106. Camber, O., Edman, P., and Olsson, L. I. (1986). Permeability of prostaglandin F2α and prostaglandin $F_{2\alpha}$ esters across cornea in vitro. *Int. J. Pharm.*, 29:259.
107. Plazonnet, B., Grove, J., Durr, M., Mazuel, C., Quint, M., and Rozier, A. (1977). Pharmacokinetics and biopharmaceutical aspects of some anti-glaucoma drugs. In: *Ophthalmic Drug Delivery Biopharmaceutical Technological and Clinical Aspects.* Vol. 11 (M. F. Saettone, M. Bucci, and P. Speiser, eds.)., Liviana Press, Springer-Verlag, Berlin, pp. 118–139.
108. Conners, M. S., Stolz, R. A., and Schwarzman, M. L. (1996). Chiral analysis of 12-hydroxyeicosatetraenoic acid formed by calf corneal epithelial microsomes. *J. Ocular Pharmacol. Therap.*, 12:19.
109. Shichi, H., Mahalak, S. M., Sakamoto, S., and Sugiyama. T. (1991). Immunocytochemical study of phenobarbital- and 3-methylcholanthrene-inducible cytochrome P450 isozymes in primary cultures of porcine ciliary epithelium. *Curr. Eye Res*, 10:779.
110. Campbell, D. A., Schoenwald, R. D., Duffel, M. W., and Barfknecht, C. F. (1991). Characterization of arylamine acetyltransferase in the rabbit eye. *Invest. Ophthalmol. Vis. Sci.*, 32:2190.
111. Putman, M. L., Schoenwald, R. D., Duffel, M. W., Barfknecht, C. F., Segarra, T. M., and Campbell, D. A. (1987). Ocular disposition of aminozolamide in the rabbit eye. *Invest. Ophthalmol. Vis. Sci.*, 28:1373.
112. Wagner, J. G. (1975). *Fundamentals of Clinical Pharmacokinetics.* Drug Intelligence Publications, Hamilton, IL, p. 42.
113. Rowland, M., and Tozer, T. N. (1989). *Clinical Pharmacokinetics*, Lea and Febiger, Philadelphia, p. 3.
114. Chien, D. S., and Schoenwald, R. D. (1990). Ocular pharmacokinetics and pharmacodynamics of phenylephrine and phenylephrine oxazolidine in rabbit eyes. *Pharm. Res.*, 7:476.
115. Smolen, V. F. (1981). Noninvasive pharmacodynamic and bioelectrometric methods for elucidating the bioavailability mechanisms of ophthalmic drug preparations. *Prog. Drug Res.*, 25:421.
116. Smolen, V. F., and Schoenwald, R. D. (1971). Drug-absorption analysis from pharmacological data I: Method and confirmation exemplified for the mydriatic drug tropicamide. *J. Pharm. Sci.*, 60:96.
117. Schoenwald, R. D., and Smolen, V. F. (1971). Drug-absorption analysis from pharmacological data II: Transcorneal biophasic availability of tropicamide. *J. Pharm. Sci.*, 60:1039.
118. Smolen, V. F. (1971). Quantitative determination of drug bioavailability and biokinetic behavior from pharmacological data for ophthalmic and oral administrations of a mydriatic drug. *J. Pharm. Sci.*, 60:354.
119. Smolen, V. F., and Schoenwald, R. D. (1974). Drug absorption analysis from pharmacological data III: Influence of polymers and pH on transcorneal biophasic availabiilty and mydriatic response of tropicamide. *J. Pharm. Sci.*, 63:1582.

120. Brazzel, R. K., Wooldridge, C. B., Hackett, R. B.,and McCue, B. A. (1990). Pharmacokinetics of the aldose reductase inhibitor imirestat following topical ocular adminsitration. *Pharm. Res.*, 7:192.

121. Rao, C. S. (1991). *Physicochemical and Biopharmaceutical Evaluation of Ibufenac, Ibuprofen and Their Hydroxyethoxy Analogs in the Rabbit Eye.* Ph.D. thesis, University of Iowa College of Pharmacy, Iowa City.

122. Andermann, G., Guggenbuhl, P., de Burlet, G., and Himber, J. (1989). Pharmacokinetics of falintolol II. Absorption, distribution and elimination from tissues and organs following ocular administration and intravenous injection of falintolol in albino rabbits. *Meth. Find. Exp. Clin. Pharmacol.*, 11:747.

123. Kleinberg, J., Dea, F. J., Anderson, J. A., and Leopold, I. H. (1979). Intraocular penetration of topically applied lincomycin hydrochloride in rabbits. *Arch. Ophthalmol.*, 97:933.

124. Hussain, A., Hirai, S., and Sieg, J. (1980). Ocular absorption of propranolol in rabbits. *J. Pharm. Sci.*, 69:738.

125. Sugrue, M. F., Gautheron, P., Mallorga, P., Nolan, T. E., Graham, S. L., Schwam, H., Shepard, K. L., and Smith, R. L. (1990). L-662,583 is a topically effective ocular hypotensive carbonic anhydrase inhibitor in experimental animals. *Br. J. Pharmacol.*, 99:59.

126. Vuori, M.-L., and Kaila, T. (1995). Plasma kinetics and antagonist activity of topical ocular timolol in elderly patients. *Graef's Arch. Clin. Exp. Ophthalmol.*, 233:131.

127. Valeri, P., Palmery, M., Severini, G., and Piccinelli, D. (1986). Ocular pharmacokinetics of dapiprazole. *Pharmacol. Res. Com.*, 18:1093.

128. Taylor, P. B., Burd, E. M., and Tabbara, K. F. (1987). Corneal and intraocular penetration of topical and subconjunctival fusidic acid. *Br. J. Ophthalmol.*, 71:598.

129. Leibowitz, H. M., Ryan, W. J., Kupferman, A., and DeSantis, L. (1986). Bioavailability and corneal anti-inflammatory effect of topical suprofen. *Invest. Ophthalmol. Vis. Sci.*, 27:628.

130. Hui, H. W., Zeleznick, L., and Robinson, J. R. (1984). Ocular disposition of topically applied histamine, cimetidine, and pyrilamine in the albino rabbit. *Curr. Eye Res.*, 3:321.

131. Sato, H., Fukuda, S., Inatomi, M., Koide, R., Uchida, N., Kanda, Y., Kiuchi, Y., and Ougchi, K. (1996). Pharmacokinetics of norfloxacin and lomefloxacin in domestic rabbit aqueous humour analyzed by microdialysis. *J. Jpn. Ophthalmol. Soc.*, 100:513.

132. Maren, T. H., and Jankowska, L. (1985). Ocular pharmacology of sulfonamides: The cornea as barrier and depot. *Curr. Eye Res.*, 4:399.

133. Grove, J., Gautheron, P., Plazonnet, B., and Sugrue, M. F. (1988). Ocular distribution studies of the topical carbonic anhydrase inhibitors L-643,799 and L-650,719 and related alkyl prodrugs. *J. Ocular Pharmacol.*, 4:279.

134. Anderson, J. A. Chen, C. C., Vita, J. B., and Shackleton, M. (1982). Disposition of topical flurbiprofen in normal and aphakic rabbit eyes. *Arch. Ophthalmol.*, 100:642.

135. Huupponen, R., Kaila, T., Salminen, L., and Urtti, A. (1987). The pharmacokinetics of ocularly applied timolol in rabbits. *Acta Ophthalmol.*, 65:63.

136. Mester, U., Krasemann, C., and Werner, H. (1982). Cefsulodin concentrations in rabbit eyes after intravenous and subconjunctival administration. *Ophthalmic Res.*, 14:129.

137. Vigo, J. F., Rafart, J., Concheiro, A., Martinez, R., and Cordido, M. (1988). Ocular penetration and pharmacokinetics of cefotaxime: An experimental study. *Curr. Eye Res.*, 7:1149.

138. Miller, S. C., Himmelstein, K. J., and Patton, T. F. (1981). A physiologically based pharmacokinetic model for the intraocular distribution of pilocarpine in rabbits. *J. Pharmacokin. Biopharm.*, 9:653.

139. Leeds, J. M., Henry, S.P., Truong, L., Zutshi, A., Levin, A. A., and Kornbrust, D. (1997). Pharmacokinetics of a potential human cytomegalovirus therapeutic, a phosphorothioate oligonucleotide, after intravitreal injection in the rabbit. *Drug Metab. Dispos.*, 25:921.

140. Berthe, P., Baudouin, C., Garraffo, R., Hofmann, P., Taburet, A.-M., and Lapalus, P. (1994). Toxicologic and pharmacokinetic analysis of itnravitreal injections of foscarnet, either alone or in combination with ganciclovir. *Invest. Ophthalmol. Vis. Sci.*, 35:1038.

141. Robertson, J. E., Westra, I., Woltering, E. A., Winthrop, K. L., Barrie, R., O'Dorisio, T. M., and Holmes, D. (1997). Intravitreal injection of octreotide acetate. *J. Ocular Pharmacol. Therap.*, 13:171.

142. Coco, R. M., Lopez, M.I., Pastor, J. C., Vallelado, A. I., Nozal, M. J., and Pampliega, A. (1995). Intravitreal pharmacokinetics of 0.5 and 1 mg of vancomycin in endophthalmic rabbit eyes. *Invest. Ophthalmol. Vis. Sci.*, 36:S613.

143. Barza, M., Kane, A., and Baum, J. (1982). The effects of infection and probenecid on the transport of carbenicillin from the rabbit vitreous humor. *Invest. Ophthalmol. Vis. Sci.*, 22:720.

144. Kwak, H. W. and D'Amico, D. J. (1992). Evaluation of the retinal toxicity and pharmacokinetics of dexamethasone after intravitreal injection. *Arch. Ophthalmol.*, 110:259.

145. Ashton, P., Brown, J. D., Pearson, P. A., Blandford, D. L., Smith, T. J., Anand, R.,Nightingale, S. D., and Sanborn, G. E. (1992). Intravitreal ganciclovir pharmacokinetics in rabbits and man. *J. Ocular Pharmacol.*, 8:343.

4

Ocular Drug Transfer Following Systemic Drug Administration

Nelson L. Jumbe
Albany Medical College, Albany, New York, and Amgen Inc., Thousand Oaks, California, U.S.A.

Michael H. Miller
Albany Medical College, Albany, New York, U.S.A.

I. INTRODUCTION

A discussion of transport models following systemic, intraocular, as well as conventional eyedrop drug administration is important since ocular pharmaceuticals are often administered by more than one route. The primary advantages of direct topical drug administration include targeted drug delivery to the anterior segment of the eye and avoidance of systemic drug toxicity. Many of the disadvantages of eyedrops, such as limited penetration into vitreous and retina, compliance, and the advantages of the use of drug delivery systems, are discussed in other sections of this text.

Intravenous and oral therapy are used in the treatment of generalized systemic disease with ocular involvement (e.g., diabetes mellitus, inflammatory diseases, autoimmune diseases, and sarcoidosis), malignancies such as lymphomas, or when penetration following topical drug administration does not attain therapeutic levels at the site of disease (e.g., vitreous, choroid, or retina). Specific uses of systemic therapy for ocular diseases include photosensitization therapy for the treatment of choroidal neovascularization, cytotoxic agents for the treatment of autoimmune diseases, nonsteroidals and steroids for the treatment of uveitis and scleritis, acetazolamide for macula edema, and antivirals or antibiotics for the prophylaxis or therapy of keratitis, chorioretinitis, and endophthalmitis. Additional applications of systemic therapy include thalidomide for the treatment of proliferative diseases, antioxidants for protection against macular degeneration, and the use of neuroprotective agents in patients with glaucoma.

This chapter primarily deals with the intercompartmental drug translocation (entry and efflux) of antimicrobial agents in the posterior eye. Antimicrobial agents were chosen as the paradigm for systemically administered drugs because the principles governing the intercompartmental drug transfer of antimicrobials are similar for most pharmaceutical agents. Moreover, new methods with enhanced discriminative capabilities used to characterize inter-compartmental drug transfer have primarily characterized the ocular pharmacokinetics and pharmacodynamics of antibiotics, antifungals, and antiviral agents (17,18,52,54,72,73,75).

Systemic, topical, and intraocular administration of antimicrobial agents are all used in the therapy of infectious diseases of the eye. When compared to topical drug administration, the systemic toxicity of antimicrobial agents may be less of an issue since they generally do not alter physiological functions of other organ systems or cause dose-related systemic toxicity. Systemic therapy is used to treat cytomegalovirus (CMV)-retinitis in patients with immunosuppressive diseases such as acquired immunodeficiency syndrome (AIDS) or those on immunosupressive medications such as organ or bone marrow transplant patients. While AIDS patients with CMV-chorioretinitis are often treated with antivirals administered via implanted, long-term drug delivery devices, supplemental systemic therapy is also used to protect the contralateral eye. Recurrent herpes simplex virus (HSV) keratitis can be prevented using oral acyclovir. Finally, while the preferred treatment of deep-seated eye infections such as bacterial and fungalendophthalmitis is direct intraocular (IO) drug administration, the role of systemic therapy remains unclear. In the National Eye Institute (NEI) Endophthalmitis Vitrectomy Study (EVS), systemically administered antibiotics did not improve the outcome in patients with postsurgical, bacterial endophthalmitis (5). However, the drugs used in this trial exhibited poor penetration into noninflamed eyes. As a result, the potential role of adjuvant therapy with systematically administered antimicrobials that show better penetration into the vitreous humor still needs to be addressed. In fact, adjuvant therapy with systemically administered quinolones has been used successfully for the treatment of bacterial endophthalmitis (14,19,58).

While vitrectomy with intravitreal drug administration is the preferred mode of therapy for endophalmitis (23), significant morbidity from this infection persists. Moreover, intraocular drug administration for other ocular infections (e.g., CMV-chorioretinitis) is often associated with serious untoward effects, including endophthalmitis, vitreous hemorrhage, retina detachment, retinal toxicity, cataract formation, and, in the absence of systemic therapy, infection of the contralateral eye. Furthermore, the incidence of opportunistic ocular infections has increased with use of potent immunosuppressive agents in patients with organ transplants, cancer, and autoimmune diseases. While highly active antiretroviral therapy (HAART) for AIDS has decreased the incidence of infections of the eye, viral and fungal infections continue to be seen in patients with HIV diseases. This, in conjunction with the use of more potent immunosuppressive agents in selected patients such as transplant patients, suggest that the use of potent and less toxic systemically administered antimicrobial drugs as adjuncts or alternative therapy of ocular disease has merit in the therapy of deep ocular infections.

A considerable amount of work demonstrating relatedness between drug-specific pharmacodynamic parameters to clinical outcome has been published over the last several years (10,27,30,37,38,50,87). Normally, optimization of the plasma concentration-versus-time profile translates into a similar concentration-versus-time profile for an infection site. However, drugs administered systemically often have poor access to the inside of the eye because of the blood-aqueous and blood-retinal barriers. Thus, ophthalmic drug discovery and intervention therapy development must also deal with the challenge of achieving effective concentrations of these drugs within the eye. The primary focus of this chapter is to review important principles of ocular pharmacokinetics of antimicrobial agents following intravitreal and systemic drug administration and to discuss available strategies for developing effective ocular drug therapies using systemically administered drugs.

II. OVERVIEW OF BLOOD-OCULAR BARRIER TRANSPORT BIOLOGY

The parenteral and oral routes are the principal routes for the systemic delivery of drugs. The most commonly used parenteral routes are intravenous (IV), intramuscular (IM), subcutaneous (SC), and intradermal (ID). The distribution of the drug throughout the body depends on the rates of absorption, distribution, metabolism and excretion from the blood as well as the extent of binding to plasma proteins. The major advantages of intravenous drug administration are rapid and complete absorption and avoidance of first-pass metabolism. However, unlike other parts of the body, specialized barriers regulate drug distribution from the blood into protected compartments like the prostage, eye, and brain. The eye, prostage, and brain are privileged sites in which the concentration-versus-time profile may differ substantially from that observed for the plasma (5). Consequently, understanding of the concentration-versus-time profile of drugs in these sites is of crucial importance.

The blood-brain barrier (BBB), blood–cerebrospinal fluid barrier (BCSFB),and blood-ocular barrier (BOB) share similarities in microscopic structure and function (4–7,22,62). Structurally, the barriers consist of tight endothelial junctions. Functionally, the barriers regulate transfer of sugars, amino acids, organic acids, and ions according to molecular size, protein-binding affinity, lipophilicity, and degree of ionization at the relevant anatomical compartment pH (40,53,59,66–68,80,97). Furthermore, active transport systems and enzymatic degradation contribute to this barrier and regulate the effective penetration of a variety of chemotherapeutic compounds (9,22,53,86). Recent studies have shown that the pharmacokinetics of several antimicrobial agents are similar in both the eye and cerebrospinal fluid (CSF) following systemic drug administration (48,53,61). This observation may have practical as well as theoretical implications since, in the absence of data for site-specific pharmacokinetics, one site may serve as a pharmacokinetic surrogate for the other (48,53,61).

The primary blood supply to the eye is the external ophthalmic artery, a branch of the internal carotid artery. However, because of selective permeability and the presence of "tight" cellular junctions between the endothelial cells lining capillaries, great limitations are placed on which blood components actually reach the intraocular tissue space. The blood-ocular barrier is comprised of three barriers: the corneal epithelial barrier (tear-corneal stroma barrier), retinal capillaries, and the retinal pigmented epithelium (RPE, or blood-retinal barrier). The blood-ocular barrier selectively allows some materials to traverse it, while preventing others from crossing. This anatomical arrangement shields delicate ocular tissue from biochemical fluctuations and toxins in the bloodstream. Although these barriers function as protective mechanisms, they also greatly affect penetration of therapeutic agents into the eye.

Systemically administered drugs gain access into the eye anterior and posterior chambers principally by crossing the blood-aqueous barrier via capillaries perfusing the iris and ciliary body. Once in the posterior chamber, the drugs can diffuse through the lens-iris barrier into the anterior portion of the vitreous body. This barrier is important for two reasons: it can act as an anterior-posterior barrier against infective bacteria, and it imposes limited diffusion of drugs from the anterior chamber to the vitreous humor. The blood-aqueous barrier is composed of the ciliary body, which is posterior to this iris and is far more permissive than the posterior portion of the eye. The iris and ciliary body have fenestrated capillaries, whereas the pigment epithelium and endothelial cell of the retinal capillaries have tight intercellular junctions. These barriers separate drugs equilibrated within the extravascular space of the choroids from entry into the retina and vitreous body.

Drug translocation rates are dependent on the functional anatomy and physiology of the eye as well as pharmacokinetics in the serum. Ocular drug transfer may occur by passive diffusion and active transport. Ultimately, the concentrations of drug achieved in the posterior eye depend upon competing rate constants describing uptake and efflux. Studies showing that the renal and ocular eliminations of fluorescein (20) quinolones, and β-lactam antibiotics in humans and rabbits are blocked by probenecid (52,70,71) and inflammation (4,49,52,85) provide evidence that these barriers have active transport systems that affect drug concentrations in the eye. In vivo and in vitro studies characterizing the rates of renal elimination of zwitterionic quinolones suggest the presence of separate and distinct carrier-mediated systems (44,52). Studies from our laboratory have shown that the elimination rates of four quinolones examined following direct intravitreal injection were prolonged by both probenecid and heat-killed bacteria (52). Unpublished data from our laboratory demonstrated that similarities in drug penetration into the CSF and eye can be explained by the presence of efflux pumps lining these anatomical sites that are targets for probenecid. There is a sidedness to these pumps, which are differentially affected by systemic and intraocular probenecid administration (4,52,62,84,85,102). Furthermore, intracerbroventricular and intravitreal but not systemically administered probenecid block the efflux of quinolone antimicrobials.

III. ALTERATIONS OF THE BLOOD-OCULAR BARRIER IN DISEASED STATE

The blood-ocular barrier shares similar embryological origin, microanatomy, and many physiological functions with the blood-brain barrier. There are many natural (e.g., diabetes, hypertension) or iatrogenic (chemotherapy, retinal photocoagulation) conditions that cause blood-ocular barrier breakdown. Disruption of the tight junctions between the endothelium of the retinal blood vessels (inner blood-retinal barrier) and the tight junctions between adjacent RPE cells (outer blood-retinal barrier) results in breakdown of the BOB and subsequent changes in drug ocular penetration.

Infectious and noninfectious (uveitis and surgery) causes of ocular inflammation represent one category of retinal vascular disorders causing BOB breakdown. Fungi, viruses, and bacteria can be very destructive when they infect the eye. *Candida* endophthalmitis occurs in 5–30% of patients with disseminated *Candida* infections (15). Bacterial endophthalmitis is a severe and often blinding infection of the eye (26,69). Noninfectious inflammation is associated with diseases of immune regulation. Models for non-infectious uveitis include intravitreal antigen injection or heat-killed bacteria (7,33,34,52). Bacterial lipopolysaccharide induces endotoxin-induced uveitis in rabbits, mice, and rats and is a useful tool for investigating ocular inflammation due to immunopathogenic, rather than autoimmune processes (39,94,95).

The integrity of the blood-retinal barrier can be demonstrated both experimentally and clinically by intravenous injection of tracer molecules normally excluded from the retina by the healthy blood-retinal barrier. Horseradish peroxidase (99) and carboxyfluoroscein (20) are the most commonly used tracers). Disruption of the inner or outer blood-retinal barrier is demonstrated by passage of these tracers either between pigment epithelial cells or of retinal blood vessels. Fluorescein isothiocyanate linked to high molecular weight dextrans of varying size can also be used experimentally to evaluate the significance of the molecular weight on differential passage through the disrupted blood-retinal barrier in different pathological conditions (8).

Chemical, mechanical, inflammatory, and infective insults modulate the penetration of drugs into the eye following systemic administration. This is particularly important, especially when the blood-ocular barrier is sufficiently insulted and reduces the integrity of the barrier against normally nonpermeable drugs. As a result, drugs that are normally excluded from the eye may penetrate into the eye due to degenerative effects on junctional barriers. For example, for hydrophilic antimicrobials such as the ciprofloxacin, infection may increase their mean vitreous concentration by more than fivefold (52).

The role of inflammation in drug penetration is particularly informative. Inflammation reduces the elimination rates of intravitreally injected drugs that are not actively exported by the posterior route. For systemically administered quinolones and other antimicrobials, inflammation increases ocular drug accumulation (i.e., penetration) most likely due to increased entry and decreased efflux rates (45,52).

IV. PHYSICOCHEMICAL PROPERTIES GOVERNING DRUG PENETRATION INTO THE EYE

Carrier-independent penetration of antibiotics and other drugs into the eye (11,16,23,63,81), like that at other anatomical sites (16,23,53,63,66), is related to the physicochemical properties of the compound, which include lipophilicity and molecular weight/size and protein binding. The effects of these independent variables on drug penetration into bacteria (96) and into different anatomical compartments have been investigated by several laboratories (35,40,52,66,80,97). Multiple linear regression analysis shows that the logarithm of the penetration of compounds across planar lipid bilayers and tissue membranes correlates with the oil/water partition ratio, the inverse of the square root of the molecular weight (8) and the free fraction of drug (24,53,63). Almost all studies show that the oil/water partition ratio (lipophilicity) is generally the most predictive variable of drug transport into and out of privileged anatomical spaces (Fig. 1).

In relation to ocular drug penetration following systemic administration, only the unbound fraction of drug is in diffusional exchange across the blood-ocular barriers. In principle, protein binding can and should be included in dose determination. Thus, true comparison of drug penetration should be on the basis of the unbound fraction in the plasma, so that binding does not enter as a factor into the ocular kinetics. However, as

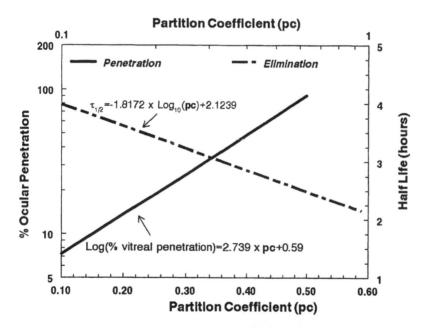

Figure 1 Relationship between the quinolone partition coefficients and levels of drug penetration into the vitreous humor following systemic drug administration, and elimination rate half-lives following direct intravitreal injection. The only statistically significant (when examined univariately; multiple linear regression did not improve model fits) quinolone physicochemical property related to ocular drug translocation was lipophilicity. The partition coefficients for direct and systemic drug administration are shown on the top and bottom abscissas, respectively.

already noted, many factors influence drug entry into protected compartments, and ceftriaxone, which is > 95% protein bound, penetrates into the
CSF better than other, less protein-bound cephalosporins. Since intracameral penetration is inversely related to molecular weight/size, drugs with a
large molecular weight are likely to be excluded from aqueous and vitreous
humors after systemic administration, similar to blood proteins and macromolecules. However, compounds may cross the blood-ocular barriers in
spite of their large molecular size, and the rate of penetration is correlated
with their lipid solubility, as expressed by their oil/water partition ratio.
Unfortunately, the ability to further delineate the relationship between lipo-
phility and molecular size/weight is curtailed due to the limit molecular
weight/size within families of chemotherapeutic compounds.

Independent studies (52,66) have demonstrated the correlation
between lipophilicity and penetration into or elimination from the eye following systemic (17,45,52,73,74) or intravitreal injection (33–35,65) in nonpigmented, uninfected rabbits (42,78). A similar relationship between
lipophilicity, penetration, and efflux occurs in prokaryotes [96].

V.   METHODS FOR IN VIVO ANTRAOCULAR PHARMACOKINETIC MEASUREMENTS

The study of the pharmacokinetics of drugs that penetrate into eye following systemic administration requires assaying ocular specimens obtained at
different time points. In humans these samples are generally obtained by
needle aspiration, often in patients with diseases that alter the BOB. The risk
of iatrogenic complications when perforating the globe with a needle has
restricted human ocular pharmacokinetic studies to a single sample obtained
from patients at the time of intraocular surgery (3). In early studies, the
concern that serial sampling of individual eyes would introduce artifact also
limited animal studies to only one specimen per animal. As a result, single
samples from different individuals are generally pooled to generate single-
subject estimates (1,51,59). This technique is referred to as the naive pooled
data (NPD) approach. A validated animal model from our laboratory
involves sequential sampling of the vitreous humor and CSF in individual
animals to obtain complete concentration-versus-time profiles (52,55,60–
62). In addition, several laboratories have used microdialysis to investigate
drug kinetics in the aqueous and vitreous humors (25,32,41,42,45,46). Both
methods are useful, but it is important to recognize several potential methodological problems that are inherent in both in vivo methods for collecting
ocular drug kinetic data in animals and humans (29,43,60). This section

evaluates these three models and maps out future directions and developments in the art of in vivo intraocular pharmacokinetics measurements.

A. Naïve Pooled Data

Drug penetration into the eye can be estimated by comparing the means of serum and ocular fluid using the mean values of multisubject data sets obtained at sequential time points or at a single sampling time (43,89,90). Determining penetration by either method is imprecise. Two-compartment models best describe ocular kinetics of most systemically administered drugs. The ratios of discrete single pairs of ocular-serum drug concentrations change with time until the subject is well into pseudo-distribution equilibrium. Consequently, obtaining mean penetration ratios from these discrete data will give erroneous estimates of the ability of the drug to penetrate into a specific site, because these ratios would depend largely on the time of collection of the samples. Thus, systemic drug administration is quite different from direct drug administration.

Pharmacokinetics based upon samples obtained sequentially throughout the steady-state dosing interval for a large number of patients should result in reliable pharmacokinetic estimates. Besides difficulties in obtaining serial samples in humans, associated ocular direct-aspiration sampling techniques also include (a) the effects of sampling on BOB and (b) awareness that vitreal aspirates are almost never obtained in the absence of ocular pathology, often with diseases that also alter the BOB. Consequently, comparison of data sets obtained at single time points is also subject to system hysteresis, intersubject variation, and, most noteworthy, parameter estimations generated from fragmentary data. The naive pooled data method prevents the characterization of differences within a population. Therefore, (a) intersubject variation prohibits rigorous determination of pharmacokinetic parameters from small groups of animals (or patients), and (b) parameter estimates from this approach discard the general population information, which reduces the value of the information obtained from these studies (29,60). One way to improve the quality of the data obtained from these models is to study serial drug concentrations in different subjects. Analysis of these data can be evaluated using population models for clinical decision making since exposure-penetration relationships can then be extrapolated to make treatment decisions based on achievable serum steady-state levels.

B. Direct Aspiration

Previous studies have shown that even nontraumatic aspiration of the aqueous humor (a) is associated with BOB breakdown, (b) increased penetration of drugs, and/or (c) decreased aqueous humor flow-dependent drug elimination. In contrast, our laboratory has developed and validated a model that permits repeated vitreous humor paracentesis from the same animal but does not alter the parameters listed above or ocular drug kinetics (60,62). Complete concentration-versus-time curves over the observation period can be obtained using this method. Serial sampling did not alter the pharmacokinetics or terminal elimination rates following direct injection into the vitreous humor (52). Furthermore, serial paracentesis does not alter the BOB or the penetration of the drug into the vitreous from the serum in the majority of the animals (52). BOB breakdown (likely due to trauma to retinal vessels) is easily recognized by measuring albumin concentrations in the vitreous, permitting exclusion of these samples from analysis. The absence of a measurable effect of serial paracentesis on drug pharmacokinetics observed using this method is likely related to both the absence of inflammation and BOB breakdown and the small volume of vitreous humor removed.

Analysis of population pharmacokinetic data using complete concentration-versus-time data following serial aspiration in animals that do not have BOB breakdown is not only theoretically preferable to pooling of data from different subjects (29,56,60,78), but also provides robust kinetic information obtained from a small number of animals. Since pharmacokinetic data are important in the design of clinical trials, this model has fundamental clinical implications for all classes of ocular pharmaceuticals. Furthermore, this model permits the evaluation of the effects of inflammation or surgery on antibiotic penetration after drug elimination following intravitreal injection (52). We have successfully used this model to study (a) similarities between blood-aqueous and blood-cerebrospinal fluid barriers (4,53,61), (b) the relationship between physicochemical properties and ocular drug penetration (52), and (c) determination of mechanisms of active drug transport from the eye and CSF (45). Recent studies characterizing ocular pharmacokinetics of systemically administered ciprofloxacin following a single dose, multiple doses, and continuous infusion to rabbits have shown that microbiological outcome is dependent upon the mean rather than the peak concentrations in the serum (56).

C. Microdialysis

The method of microdialysis provides an important alternative for obtaining intra-ocular pharmacokinetic data (10,32,42,47,100). Complete concentration-versus-time profiles can be obtained in individual animals by perfusing a fine cannula with normal saline at a fixed flow rate. Drug in the surrounding tissue (solute) diffuses down its concentration gradient into the perfusate and is collected for analysis. Details of this method are covered extensively elsewhere in this text.

Microdialysis has proven to be the gold standard of measuring ocular pharmacokinetics following direct intraocular drug injection when drug concentrations are high. Experimental conditions following systemic drug administration are quite different. First, high drug concentrations are not achieved in the eye. Second, and more importantly, the kinetic profile following systemic drug administration follows a rapid distribution phase as drug enters the eye, followed by multiexponential elimination. Therefore, ocular kinetics following systemically administered drug are transient and initially rapidly changing, but change more slowly when the drug is well into pseudo-distribution equilibrium during the elimination phase. This has direct bearing on the methods used for determining probe extraction coefficients. Finally, the lower drug concentrations seen in conjunction with small volumes of dialysate may make the measurement of drug concentrations using conventional HPLC or microbiological assays difficult.

Microdialysis probe calibration is affected by the cannula deadspace, temporal resolution insensitivity, substrate physicochemical properties, and potential BOB breakdown from an indwelling probe. For example, early studies characterizing intravitreal concentrations of aminoglycosides showed time-dependent differences in pharmacokinetic parameters suggesting progressive BOB breakdown. BOB breakdown can be minimized by careful probe placement and/or by allowing the eye to heal completely after probe placement (42). Since BOB is invariable with serial aspirations of the aqueous humor, microdialysis via previously implanted probes in "quiet" eyes is clearly preferable when measuring drug concentrations in the aqueous humor (54,82,83). Both the zero-net flux and retrodialysis methods are used for the determination of probe recovery. The zero-net flux recovery is a steady-state measurement determined at fixed solute concentrations (32,101). Retrodialysis recovery is determined from loss of a drug analog in the solute from the perfusate (32,101). The retrodialysis recovery determination method is most appropriate for in vivo pharmacokinetic studies. However, potential limitations exist in the availability of drug-analog pairs. Microdialysis temporal resolution issues have been greatly reduced by the ability to interface this technique directly with high-performance liquid chromatography – mass spectroscopy (HPLC-MS) for sample analysis. This is possible because collected samples are clean and do not require any preparation before analysis. Moreover, assays with increased sensitivity greatly reduce the sampling time and sample volumes, allow for continuous sampling, and permit faster/slower flow rates, which in turn erase system hysteresis if cannula deadspace noise is removed by integration. Since microdialysis sampling gives an integrated (mean concentration) response over the sampling period, the drug area under the concentration-versus-time curve (AUC) is obtained by pooling the measured concentrations from each sample interval and summing them together (47).

While direct vitreous humor sampling requires paracentesis, a repeated invasive procedure not generally possible in humans, microdialysis provides inroads for ocular pharmacokinetic studies using indwelling probes. Furthermore, our laboratory has shown that the CSF and eye are pharmacokinetic surrogates for systemically administered drugs. Thus, microdialysis measurements in the CSF may provide a practical way to obtain ocular pharmacokinetic data where none is available, and vice versa.

VI. PHARMACOKINETICS AND PHARMACODYNAMICS OF SYSTEMIC DRUG ADMINISTRATION

A. Compartmental Model Analysis

The pharmacokinetic processes of drug absorption, distribution, metabolism, and elimination determine the concentration-versus-time profile in a target organ. Ocular pharmacokinetic models for intraperitoneal (IP), intravenous (IV), and intraocular drug administration are described by three-, two-, or one-compartment models, respectively. These models are not representative of real tissue spaces. Physiologically based models using mass balances and blood-flow limited elimination are least useful for ocular pharmacokinetics because of the nonidentifiable nature of drug transfer by flow, blood diffusional exchange, and anterior-posterior drainage. Compartmental open models are depicted with elimination from the central compartment.

Drugs that distribute rapidly and homogeneously into the plasma and well-perfused, extracellular fluid follow a one-compartment model (and often show first-order kinetics). Drug elimination from the eye generally follows first-order kinetics. One-compartment models best describe monoexponential (log-linear) elimination kinetics (Fig. 2). Two-compartment kinetic models demonstrate identifiable distribution and elimination phases where competing elimination rates govern both the distribution and elimination phases (Fig. 3).

Analysis of concentration-versus-time data optimally co-models plasma samples and ocular samples simultaneously for pharmacokinetic parameter estimation (16). Pharmacokinetic analyses of these data provide apparent volumes of distribution and areas under the concentration-versus-time curve of the serum and peripheral compartments as part of the pharmacokinetic parameter identification procedure. AUCs are determined by numerical integration (or trapezoidal approximation). The calculated

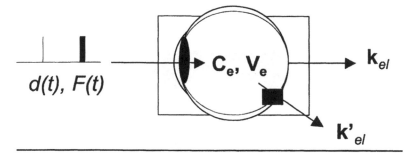

$$d(Amt_e)/dt = F(t) - (k_{el} + k'_{el}) \bullet Amt_e$$

$$C_e = Amt_e/V_e$$

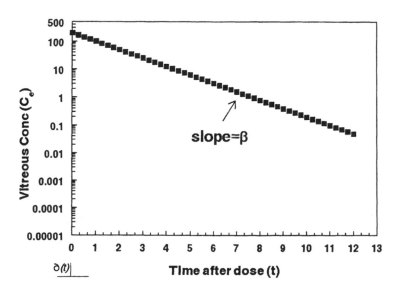

Figure 2 On-compartment open model. The figure depicted shows the pharmaco-kinetic model for changing drug concentrations in the eye, where drug is injected directly into the vitreous either as a bolus [$d(t)$] or rapid prolonged-bolus (infusion) [$F(t)$]. Infusion of drug into the eye is of fixed rate $F(t)$ and known duration. k_{el} is a first order removal rate constant from the eye. k'_{el} is the rate of removal of drug due to active pumping. Amt_e is the drug amount in the eye compartment. Given most achievable concentrations, this behaves in a pseudo-linear fashion. C_e = Concentration in the eye; V_e = volume of distribution of the eye.

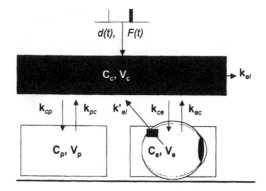

$$d(Amt_c)/dt = F(t) - (k_{ce} + k_{cp} + k_{el}) \bullet Amt_c + k_{ec} \bullet Amt_e + k_{pc} \bullet Amt_p$$

$$d(Amt_e)/dt = k_{ce} \bullet Amt_c - \lfloor k_{ec} + k'_{el} \rfloor \bullet Amt_e$$

$$d(Amt_p)/dt = k_{cp} \bullet Amt_c - k_{pc} \bullet Amt_p$$

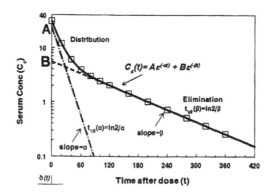

Figure 3 Two-compartment open model. Rates of change in drug concentrations in the eye can alternatively be described by a two-compartment open model, where $c_{e,e,p}$ and $V_{c,e,p}$ represent drug concentrations and apparent volumes of distributions in the central, eye, and peripheral compartments, respectively. F, k'_{el} are as defined previously. k_{cp}, k_{pc}, k_{ce} and k_{ec} are first-order transfer rate constants, and k_{el} is a first-order elimination rate constant. V_e is as previously defined; V_c = volume of central compartment. Amt_c = Drug amount in the central compartment; Amt_p = drug amount in the peripheral compartment; Amt_e = drug amount in the eye compartment.

volumes of distribution do not necessarily correspond to real anatomical tissue space. They are proportionality constants, which relate observed drug concentrations to the amount given. Since ocular compartment volumes are much smaller than the central compartment, the volume of the ocular compartment can be fixed at the physiologically determined mean values to improve identification of the other parameters. The mean drug concentrations after a single dose (or at steady state) are inversely proportional to the AUC. Since the AUC is related to average observed concentrations, the ratio of serum (plasma) AUC to aqueous/vitreous humor AUC provides the most accurate determination of drug penetration into the eye (Fig. 4).

B. Statistical and Population Approaches to Ocular Pharmacokinetics

Optimally, one would like to extend the ocular pharmacokinetics knowledge base to patients. This has been made possible by the recent transfer of adaptive control theory and optimization methods from control systems engineering to the field of pharmaceutical pharmacokinetics/pharmacodynamics (PK/PD). These combined mathematical and statistical tools enable the robust determination of population pharmacokinetic mean parameter values and their dispersions from fragmentary data. There is now software available to support these population-modeling approaches, such as the nonlinear mixed effects modeling (NONMEM) (89), nonparametric expectation maximization (NPEM2) (88), an iterative two-stage (IT2S) population modeling software package (37,38,93) and WinNonMix (Pharsight Corporation, Mountain View, CA). These algorithms have been validated and employed to obtain population pharmacokinetic parameter values from sparse pharmacokinetic data sets (13,29), and comparisons of these packages are available in literature (57,76,77,98).

The utility of these mathematical models can be readily extended to the patient care situation. Most notably, adaptive population models require only a single pair of data where a prior complete kinetic data set exists to begin analysis, no matter how many system parameters are available in the population pharmacokinetic model. Thus, each new data set supplements the population data, which keeps the general population database growing. Most importantly, the more data samples that are obtained for an individual patient, the more patient-specific the model parameter estimation becomes, thereby resulting in customized therapy.

We have used a population modeling approach to characterize ocular pharmacokinetics. We used IT2S population modeling software to characterize and validate this approach following systemic administration of ciprofloxacin in a rabbit model (29). Sequential serum samples were obtained in

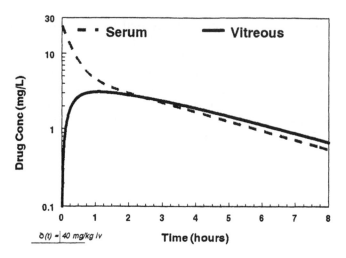

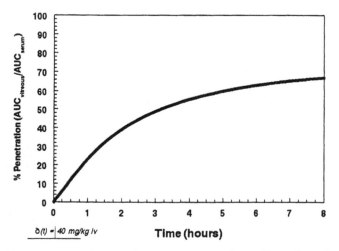

Figure 4 Simulation of mean concentrations of sparfloxacin in the serum and vitreous humor of rabbits following a single intravenous bolus (40 mg/kg) using mean pharmacokinetic parameter estimates from observed data. Penetration was expressed as a cumulative percentage by dividing the area under the concentration versus time curve (AUC) in the vitreous by that in the serum.

different subjects along with a single, sequential vitreous sample from one eye in each subject. We simultaneously also obtained sequential vitreous samples from the contralateral eye of all subjects. Data were analyzed by IT2S to determine the robustness of pharmacokinetic estimates obtained from single data point experiments. Penetration and derived pharmacokinetic constants were equivalent when single or complete ocular data sets were used. This finding suggests that intensive plasma sampling and optimized single sample experimental design holds promise for the analysis or penetration of drugs into privileged spaces, such as the eye and CSF, from which only single samples can be obtained.

C. Pharmacodynamics

Pharmacodynamics characterizes the relationship between drug concentrations (pharmacokinetics) and a quantifiable effect. Modeling this relationship using different dose schedules and determining the effect of derived pharmacodynamic relationships provides a robust approach to optimize therapy. While this approach has primarily focused on antimicrobials, it also can provide useful information for pharmaceutical agents used in the therapy of ocular disease. There has been a long-standing controversy regarding the relative merits of continuous, intermittent, and single dose administration on drug penetration into extravascular foci. It has been argued that the high peak levels achieved by intermittent administration may be more effective than low sustained levels in reaching protected compartments. These questions are best answered via pharmacodynamic analysis. For bacteria and fungi, there are three pharmacodynamic relationships that correlate response to exposure (Fig. 5): the ratios of the area under the concentration-time curve to the MIC (AUC/MIC), the maximal concentration to the MIC (C_{max}/MIC), and the time the drug concentration is above the MIC (time > MIC). The MIC and the 50% inhibitory concentrations (IC_{50}) often closely approximate one another and are often used to signify the same relative effect. These exposure-therapeutic response relationships are used for the selection of the best dose and dose-schedule treatment strategies. To optimize outcome for time dependent drugs, the total daily dose of these compounds is administered in multiple equally divided doses (or as a continuous infusion) over 24 hours. Optimal outcome for peak concentration dependent agents is seen in a single large drug dose per day, while AUC-driven drugs are schedule independent. Pharmacodynamic determinants that link microbial response and antimicrobial exposure have been well characterized in the field of antimicrobial chemotherapy (28,30,31,36–38,79,87). The characterization of the pharmacodynamically linked variables requires the determination of a readily measurable outcome. Once this has been established, separate pharmacokinetic and pharmacodynamic experiments may be designed. Data from these experiments may be analyzed separately, or pharmacokinetic data can be incorporated

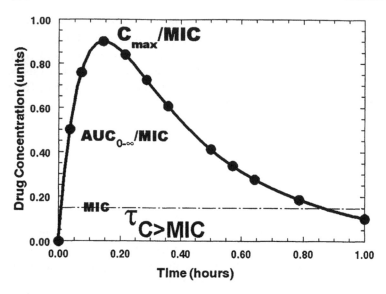

Figure 5 This figures shows the relationship between pharmacokinetic data and the minimum inhibitory concentration (MIC). The relationships that correlate with outcome for antimicrobial agents discussed in the chapter are shown.

into the nonlinear dynamic model analysis. This approach takes advantage of the potential strengths of population modeling outlined above.

Pharmacodynamically based studies comparing the outcome of rabbits with *S. epidermidis* endophthalmitis treated with either ciprofloxacin or trovafloxacin [drugs for which ocular outcome correlates with the AUC/MIC ratio (29) support the utility of PK/PD approaches in optimizing the design of future studies and characterizing the relationship between antimicrobial drug exposure and microbial response for ocular infections (46). Pharmacodynamic modeling may also be useful in determining the optimal mode of systemic drug administration for infectious and noninfectious ocular disease. For example, quinolone antimicrobials show excellent serum and, often, ocular bioavailability following oral administration. Ocular AUCs following systemic drug administration are independent of the schedule of drug administration (single dose, intermittent dose, or continuous infusions) for a given total exposure (56). As a result, for quinolones that show good ocular penetration [e.g., levofloxacin or sparfloxacin, but not ciprofloxacin (47,53)], outcome should be similar following intravenous and oral dosing as long as the AUC/MIC ratios are equivalent. On the other hand, for drugs for which the pharmacodynamically linked parameter is the C_{max}/MIC ratio, intravenously administered agents would be preferred to those given orally.

VII. SUMMARY

Despite the potential benefits of parenteral drug administration as adjunctive or alternative therapy in ocular diseases, there are limited data characterizing ocular pharmacokinetics following systemic drug administration. New population modeling tools for pharmacokinetic data analysis have made it possible to obtain precise and unbiased estimates of the population kinetics for chemotherapeutic agents in a privileged site such as the eye through the use of a complete set of concentration-versus-time profiles as prior estimates plus discreet single serum eye compartment concentration determinations. This approach can be readily extended to the patient care situation to provide optimal information for dose and schedule development and customized patient care management. These methods will prove useful for determining the role of systemically administered drugs in achieving the best outcomes for patients with serious eye disease.

REFERENCES

1. Axelrod JL, Kochman RS. Cefamandole levels in primary aqueous humor in man. Am J Ophthalmol 1978; 85:342–348.
2. Badenoch PR, McDonald PJ, Coster DJ. Effect of inflammation on antibiotic penetration into the anterior segment of the rat eye. Invest Ophthalmol Vis Sci 1986; 27:958–965.
3. Barza M, Kane A, Baum J. Oxacillin for bacterial endophthalmitis: subconjunctival, intravenous, both, or neither? Invest Ophthalmol Vis Sci 1980; 19:1348–1354.
4. Barza M, Kane A, Baum J. The effects of infection and probenecid on the transport of carbenicillin from the rabbit vitreous humor. Invest Ophthalmol Vis Sci 1982; 22:720–726.
5. Barza M, Cuchural G. General principles of antibiotic tissue penetration. J Antimicrob Chemother 1995; 15 (suppl A):59–75.
6. Barza M. Anatomical barriers for antimicrobial agents. Eur J Clin Microbiol Infect Dis 1993; 12 (suppl 1):S31–35.
7. Barza M. Pharmacokinetics of antibiotics in shallow and deep compartments. J Antimicrob Chemother 1993; 31 (suppl D):17–27.
8. Bellhorn MB, Bellhorn RW, Poll DS. Permeability of fluorescein-labelled dextrans in fundus fluorescein angiography of rats and birds. Exp Eye Res 1977; 24:595–605.
9. Bito LZ. A new approach to the medical management of glaucoma, from the bench to the clinic, and beyond: the Proctor Lecture. Invest Ophthalmol Vis Sci 2001; 42:1126–1133.
10. Blaser J, Stone BB, Groner MC, Zinner SH. Comparative study with enoxacin and netilmicin in a pharmacodynamic model to determine importance of ratio

of antibiotic peak concentration to MIC for bactericidal activity and emergence of resistance. Antimicrob Agents Chemother 1987; 31:1054–1060.

11. Bleeker GM, van Haeringen NJ, Glasius E. Urea and the vitreous barrier of the eye. Exp Eyue Res 1968; 7:30–36.

12. Bleeker GM, van Haeringen, NJ, Maas ER, Glasius E. Selective properties of the vitreous barrier. Exp Eye Res 1968; 7:37–46.

13. Bondareva IB, Sokolov AV, Tischenkova IF, Jelliffe RW. Population pharmacokinetic modelling of carbamazepine by using the iterative Bayesian (IT2B) and the nonparametric EM (NPEM) algorithms: implications for dosage. J Clin Pharm Ther 2001; 26:213–223.

14. Brook I, Ledney GD. Quinolone therapy in themanagement of infection after irradiation. Crit Rev Microbiol 1992; 18:235–246.

15. Brooks RG. Prospective study of *Candida* endophthalmitis in hospitalized patients with candidemia. Arch Intern Med 1989; 149:2226–2228.

16. Burns-Bellhorn MS, Bellhorn RW, Benjamin JV. Anterior segment permeability to fluorescein-labeled dextrans in the rat. Invest Ophthalmol Vis Sci 1978; 17:857–862.

17. Cekic O, Batman C, Yasar U, Basci NE, Bozkurt A, Kayaalp SO. Human aqueous and vitreous humour levels of ciprofloxacin following oral and topical administration. Eye 1999; 13:555–558.

18. Cekic O, Batman C, Yasar U, Basci NE, Zilelioglu O, Bozkurt A. Subretinal fluid levels of topical, oral, and combined administered ciprofloxacin in humans. Br J Ophthalmol 2000; 84:1061–1063.

19. Cochereau-Massin I, Bauchet J, Marrakchi-Benjaafar S, Saleh-Mghir A, Faurisson F, Vallos JM, Vallee E, Pocidalo JJ. Efficacy and ocular penetration of sparfloxacin in experimental streptococcal endophthalmitis. Antimicrob Agents Chemother 1993; 37:633–636.

20. Cunha-Vaz JG, Maurice DM. The active transport of fluorescein by the retinal vessels and the retina. J Physiol 1967; 191:467–486.

21. Dacey RG, Sande MA. Effect of probenecid on cerebrospinal fluid concentrations of penicillin and cephalosporin derivatives. Antimicrob Agents Chemother 1974; 6:437–421.

22. Dacey RG, Welsh JE, Scheld WM, Winn HR, Jane JA, Sande MA. Alterations in cerebrospinal fluid outflow resistance in experimental bacterial meningitis. Trans Am Neurol Assoc 1978; 103:142–146.

23. Davidson SI. Post-operative bacterial endophthalmitis. Trans Ophthalmol Soc UK 1985; 104:278–284.

24. Davson H, Segal MB. Effect of cerebrospinal fluid on volume of distribution of extracellular markers. Brain 1969; 92:131–136.

25. de la Pena A, Liu P, Derendorf H. Microdialysis in peripheral tissues. Adv Drug Deliv Re 2000; 15(45):189–216.

26. Driebe WT Jr, Mandelbaum S, Forster RK, Schwartz LK, Culbertson WW. Pseudophakic endophthalmitis. Diagnosis and management. Ophthalmology 1986; 93:442–448.

27. Drusano GL. Role of pharmacokinetics in the otucome of infections. Antimicrob Agents Chemother 1988; 32:289–297.

28. Drusano GL. Pharmacodynamics of antiretroviral chemotherapy. Infect Control Hosp Epidemiol 1993; 14:530–536.

29. Drusano GL, Liu W, Perkins R, Madu A, Madu C, Mayers M, Miller MH. Determination of robust ocular pharmacokinetic parameters in serum and vitreous humor of albino rabbits following systemic administration of ciprofloxacin from sparse data sets by using IT2S, a population pharmacokinetic modeling program. Antimicrob Agents Chemother 1995; 39:1638–1687.

30. Drusano GL, Craig WA. Relevance of pharmacokinetics and pharmacodynamics in the selection of antibiotics for respiratory tract infections. J Chemother 1997; 9 (suppl 3):38–44.

31. Drusano GL. Infection in the intensive care unit: beta-lactamase-mediated resistance among Enterobacteriaceae and optimal antimicrobial dosing. Clin Infect Dis 1998; 27 (suppl 1):S111–116.

32. Elmquist WF, Sawchuk RJ. Application of microdialysis in pharmacokinetic studies. Pharm Res 1997; 14:267–288.

33. Ficker L, Meredith TA, Gardner S, Wilson LA. Cefazolin levels after intravitreal injection. Effects of inflammation and surgery. Invest Ophthalmol Vis Sci 1990; 31:502–505.

34. Ficker LA, Kirkness CM, Steele AD, Rice NS, Gilvarry AM. Intraocular surgery following penetrating keratoplasty: the risks and advantages. Eye 1990; 4:693–697.

35. Fiscella RG, Nguyen TK, Cwik MJ, Phillpotts BA, Friedlander SM, Alter DC, Shapiro MJ, Blair NP, Gieser JP. Aqueous and vitreous penetration of levofloxacin after oral administration. Ophthalmology 1999; 106:2286–2290.

36. Fluckiger U, Segessenmann C, Gerber AU. Integration of pharmacokinetics and pharmacodynamics of imipenem in a human-adapted mouse model. Antimicrob Agents Chemother 1991; 5:1905–1910.

37. Forrest A, Ballow CH, Nix DE, Birmingham MC, Schentag JJ. Development of a population pharmacokinetic model and optimal sampling strategies for intravenous ciprofloxacin. Antimicrob Agents Chemother 1993; 37:1065–1072.

38. Forrest A, Nix DE, Ballow CH, Goss TF, Birmingham MC, Schentag JJ. Pharmacodynamics of intravenous ciprofloxacin in seriously ill patients. Antimicrob Agents Chemother 1993; 37:1073–1081.

39. Forrester JV, McMenamin PG. Immunopathogenic mechanisms in intraocular inflammation. Chem Immunol 1999, 73:159–185.

40. Habgood MD, Begley DJ, Abbott NJ. Determinants of passive drug entry into the central nervous system. Cell Mol Neurobiol 2000; 20:231–253.

41. Hillered L, Persson L. Theory and practice of microdialysis–prospect for future clinical use. Acta Neurochir Suppl (Wien) 1999; 75:3–6.

42. Hughes PM, Krishnamoorthy R, Mitra AK. Vitreous disposition of two acycloguanosine antivirals in the albino and pigmented rabbit models: a novel ocular microdialysis technique. J Ocul Pharmacol Ther 1996; 12:209–224.

43. Jacquez JA. Parameter identifiability is required in pooled data methods. J Pharmacokinet Biopharm 1996; 24(3):301–305.

44. Jaehde U, Sorgel F, Reiter A, Sigl G, Naber KG, Schunack W. Effect of probenecid on the distribution and elimination of ciprofloxacin in humans. Clin Pharmacol Ther 1995; 58:532–541.
45. Jumbe NL, W Liu, Drusano, GL Louie, A Miller MH. Comparison of Quinolone Active Efflux after Systemic, Intra-vitreous or Intra-cerebroventricular Administration. 39th Interscience Conference on Antimicrobial Agents and Chemotherapy, Abstract 1924, 1999, p. 46.
46. Jumbe NL, Drusano GL, Miller MH. Parametric Comparison of Midrodialysis and Direct Vitreous Sampling Techniques at Non Steady State Conditions. 39th Interscience Conference on antimicrobial Agents and Chemotherapy, Abstract 1923, 1999, p. 46.
47. Jumbe NL, W Liu, Kaw P, Drusano G, Louie A, Miller M. Fluoroquinolone-rifampin potentiation in S. epidermidis [SE] endophthalmitis: emergence of rifampin resistance. Abstract 3641–B499, IOVS 40, 1999, p. 5690.
48. Kaw P, Jumbe N, Liu W, Mayers M, Drusano G, Miller M. The penetration of trovafloxacin into the eye and CSF of rabbits. Abstract 469–B429, IOVS 40, 1999, p. 588.
49. Kraff MC, Sanders DR, McGuigan L, Raanan MG. Inhibition of blood-aqueous humor barrier breakdown with diclofenac. A fluorophotometric study. Arch Ophthalmol 1990; 108:380–383.
50. Leggett JE, Fantin B, Ebert S, Totsuka K, Vogelman B, Calame W, Mattie H, Craig WA. Comparative antibiotic dose-effect relations at several dosing intervals in murine pneumonitis and thigh-infection models. J Infect Dis 1989; 159:281–292.
51. Lesar TS, Fiscella RG. Antimicrobial drug delivery to the eye. Drug Intell Clin Pharm 1985; 19:642–654.
52. Liu W, Liu QF, Perkins R, Drusano G, Louie A, Madu A, Mian U, Mayers M, Miller MH. Pharmacokinetics of sparfloxacin in the serum and vitreous humor of rabbits: physicochemical properties that regulate penetration of quinolone antimicrobials. Antimicrob Agents Chemother 1998; 42:1417–1423.
53. Liu W, Jumbe N, Kaw P, Lomastro B, Louie A, Miller M. Comparison of quinolone pharmacokinetics in vitreous humor and CSF following IV drug administration in albino rabbits. Abstract 468–B428, IOVS 40, 1999.
54. Macha S, Mitra AK. Ocular pharmacokinetics in rabbits using a novel dual probe microdialysis technique. Exp Eye Res 2001; 72:289–299.
55. Madu A, Cioffe C, Mian U, Burroughs M, Tuomanen E, Mayers M, Schwartz E, Miller M. Pharmacokinetics of fluconazole in cerebrospinal fluid and serum of rabbits: validation of an animal model used to measure drug concentrations in cerebrospinal fluid. Antimicrob Agents Chemother 1994; 38:2111–2115.
56. Madu AA, Mayers M. Ocular manifestation of systemic infections. Curr Opin Ophthalmol 1996; 7:85–90.

57. Mahmood I, Miller R. comparison of the Bayesian approach and a limited sampling model for the estimation of AUC and C_{max}: a computer simulation analysis. Int J clin Pharmacol Ther 1999; 37:439–445.

58. Marrakchi-Benjaafar S, Cochereau I, Pocidalo JJ, Carbon C. Systemic prophylaxis of experimental staphylococcal endophthalmitis: comparative efficacy of sparfloxacin, pefloxacin, imipenem, vancomycin, and amikacin. J Infect Dis 1995; 172:1312–1316.

59. Maurice DM, Mishima S. Ocular pharmacokinetics. In: Sears ML, ed. Pharmacology of the Eye. Handbook of Experimental Pharmacology. Vol. 69. New York: Springer-Verlag, 1984: 19–116.

60. Mayers M, Rush D, Madu A, Motyl M, Miller MH. Pharmacokinetics of amikacin and chloramphenicol in the aqueous humor of rabbits. Antimicrob Agents Chemother 1991; 35:1791–1798.

61. Mian UK, Mayers M, Garg Y, Liu QF, Newcomer G, Madu C, Liu W, Louie A, Miller MH. Comparison of fluconazole pharmacokinetics in serum, aqueous humor, vitreous humor, and cerebrospinal fluid following a single dose and at steady state. J Ocul Pharmacol Ther 1998; 14:459–471.

62. Miller MH, Madu A, Samathanam G, Rush D, Madu CN, Mathisson K, Mayers M. Fleroxacin pharmacokinetics in aqueous and vitreous humors determined by using complete concentration-versus-time data from individual rabbits. Antimicrob Agents Chemother 1992; 36:32–38.

63. Moog E, Knothe H. [Passage of various tetracyclines into human aqueous humor in dependence on their protein binding in the blood seruem]. Ber Zusammenkunft Dtsch Ophthalmol Ges 1969; 69:536–539.

64. Moog, F, Etzler ME, Grey RD. The differentiation of alkaline phosphatase in the small intestine. Ann NY Acad Sci 1969; 166:447–465.

65. Murray DC, Christopoulou D, Hero M. Intravitreal penetration of teicoplanin. Eye 1999; 13:604–605.

66. Nau R, Sorgel F, Prange HW. Lipophilicity at pH 7.4 and molecular size govern the entry of the free serum fraction of drugs into the cerebrospinal fluid in humans with uninflamed meninges. J Neurol Sci 1994; 122:61–65.

67. Oldendorf WH. Stereospecificity of blood-brain barrier permeability to amino acids. Am J Physiol 1973; 224:967–969.

68. Oldendorf WH, Crane PD, Braun LD, Wade LA, Diamond JM. Blood-brain barrier transport of basic amino acids is selectively inhibited at low pH. J Neurochem. 1983; 40:797–800.

69. Olson JC, Flynn HW Jr, Forster RK, Culbertson WW. Results in the treatment of postoperative endophthalmitis. Ophthalmology 1983; 90:692–699.

70. Ooie T, Suzuki H, Terasaki T, Sugiyama Y. Characterization of the transport properties of a quinolone antibiotic, fleroxacin, in rat choroid plexus. Pharm Res 1996; 13:523–527.

71. Ooie T, Suzuki H, Terasaki T, Sugiyama Y. Kinetics of quinolone antibiotics in rats: efflux from cerebrospinal fluid to the circulation. Pharm Res 1996; 13:1065–1068.

72. Ozdamar A, Aras C, Ozturk R, Karacorlu M, Bahcecioglu H, Ozkan S. Ocular penetration of cefepime following systemic administration in humans. Ophthalmic Surg Lasers 2001; 32:25–29.

73. Ozturk F, Kortunay S, Kurt E, Ilker SS, Basci NE, Bozkurt A. Penetration of topical and oral ciprofloxacin into the aqueous and vitreous humor in inflamed eyes. Retina 1999; 19:218–222.

74. Ozturk F, Kortunay S, Kurt E, Inan UU, Ilker SS, Basci N, Bozkurt A. The effect of long-term use and inflammation on the ocular penetration of topical ofloxacin. Curr Eye Res 1999; 19:461–464.

75. Ozturk F, Kurt E, Inan UU, Kortunay S, Ilker SS, Basci NE, Bozkurt A. The effects of prolonged acute use and inflammation on the ocular penetration of topical ciprofloxacin. Int J Pharm 2000; 25(204): 97–100.

76. Park K, Verotta D, Gupta SK, Sheiner LB. Use of a pharmacokinetic/pharmacodynamic model to design an optimal dose input profile. J Pharmacokinet Biopharm 1998; 26:471–492.

77. Parker TJ, Della Pasqua OE, Loizillon E, Chezaubernard c, Jochemsen R, Danhof M. Pharmacokinetic-pharmacodynamic modelling in the early development phase of anti-psychotics: a comparison of the effects of clozapine, S 16924 and S 18327 in the EEG model in rats. Br J Pharmacol 2001; 132: 151–158.

78. Perkins RJ, Liu W, Drusano G, Madu A, Mayers M, Madu C, Miller MH. Pharmacokinetics of ofloxacin in serum and vitreous humor of albino and pigmented rabbits. Antimicrob Agents chemother 1995; 39:1493–1498.

79. Preston SL, Drusano GL, Berman AL, Fowler CL, Chow AT, Dornseif B, Reichl V, Natarajan J, Corrado M. Pharmacodynamics of levofloxacin: a new paradigm for early clinical trials. JAMA 1998; 279:125–129.

80. Rabkin MD, Bellhorn MB, Bellhorn RW. Selected molecular weight dextrans for in vivo permeability studies of rat retinal vascular disease. Exp Eye Res 1977; 24:607–612.

81. Records RE. The penicillins in ophthalmology. Surv Ophthalmol 1969; 13:207–214.

82. Rittenhouse KD, Peiffer RL Jr, Pollack GM. Evaluation of microdialysis sampling of aqueous humor for in vivo models of ocular absorption and disposition. J Pharm Biomed Anal 1998; 16:951–959.

83. Rittenhouse KD, Peiffer RL Jr, Pollack GM. Microdialysis evaluation of the ocular pharmacokinetics of propranolol in the conscious rabbit. Pharm Res 1999; 16:736–742.

84. Salminen L. Ampicillin penetration into the rabbit eye. Acta Ophthalmol (Copenh) 1978; 56:977–983.

85. Salminen L. Cloxacillin distribution in the rabbit eye after intravenous injection. Acta Ophthalmol (Copenh) 1978; 56:11–19.

86. Sande MA, Sherertz RJ, Zak O, Dacey RG, Bodine JA, Stausbaugh LJ. Factors influencing the penetration of antimicrobial agents into the cerebrospinal fluid of experimental animals. Scand J Infect Dis Suppl 1978; 14:160–163.

87. Schentag JJ, Strenekoski-Nix LC, Nix DE, Forrest A. Pharmacodynamic interactions of antibiotics alone and in combination. Clin Infect Dis 1998; 27:40–46.

88. Schumitzky, A. Nonparametric EM algorithms for estimating prior distributions. Appl Math Comput 1991; 45: 141–157.

89. Sheiner LB, Rosenberg B, Marathe VV. Estimation of population characteristics of pharmacokinetic parameters from routine clinical data. J Pharmacokinet Biopharm 1977; 5:445–479.

90. Sheiner LB, Beal SL. Evaluation of methods for estimating population pharmacokinetics parameters. I. Michaelis-menten model: routine clinical pharmacokinetic data. J Pharmacokinet Biopharm 1980; 8:553–571.

91. Sheiner BL, Beal SL. Evaluation of methods for estimating population pharmacokinetic parameters. II. Biexponential model and experimental pharmacokinetic data. J Pharmacokinet Biopharm 1981; 9:635–651.

92. Sheiner LB, Beal SL. Evaluation of methods for estimating population pharmacokinetic parameters. III. Monoexponential model: routine clinical pharmacokinetic data. J Pharmacokinet Biopharm 1983; 11:303–319.

93. Steimer JL, Mallet A, Golmard JL, Boisvieux JF. Alternative approaches to estimation of population pharmacokinetic parameters: comparison with the nonlinear mixed-effect model. Drug Metab Rev 1984; 15:265–292.

94. Streilein JW, Ksander BR, Taylor AW. Immune deviation in relation to ocular immune privilege. J Immunol 1997; 15(158):3557–3560.

95. Streilein JW. Immunoregulatory mechanisms of the eye. Prog Retin Eye Res 1999; 18:357–370.

96. Tulkens PM. Intracellular distribution and activity of antibiotics. Eur J Clin Microbiol Infect Dis 1991; 10:100 106.

97. van de Waterbeemd H, Camenisch G, folkers G, Chretien JR, Raevsky OA. Estimation of blood-brain barrier crossing of drugs using molecular size and shape, and H-bonding descriptors. J Drug Target 1998; 6:151–165.

98. Vermes A, Math t RA, van der Sijs IH, Dankert J, Guchelaar HJ. Population pharmacokinetics of flucytosine: comparison and validation of three models using STS,NPEM, and NONMEM. Ther Drug Monit 2000; 22:676–687.

99. Vinores SA. Assessment of blood-retinal barrier integrity. Histol Histopathol 1995; 10:141–154.

100. Waga J, Nilsson-Ehle I, Ljungberg B, Skarin A, Stahle L, Ehinger B. Microdialysis for pharmacokinetic studies of ceftazidime in rabbit vitreous. J Ocul Pharmacol Ther 1999; 15:455–463.

101. Wang Y, Wong SL, Sawchuk RJ. Microdialysis calibration using retrodialysis and zero-net flux: application to a study of the distribution of zidovudine to rabbit cerebrospinal fluid and thalamus. Pharm Res 1993; 10:1411–1419.

102. Yoshida A, Ishiko S, Kojima M. Outward permeability of the blood-retain barrier. Graefes Arch Clin Exp Ophthalmol 1992; 230:78–83.

5

Ocular Pharmacokinetics and Pharmacodynamics

Ronald D. Schoenwald
College of Pharmacy, The University of Iowa, Iowa City, Iowa, U.S.A.

I. INTRODUCTION

The study of pharmacokinetic processes—absorption, distribution, and elimination—is fundamental to determining the appropriate dosing regimen for an individual patient administered a drug by systemic routes. Pharmacokinetics has also been indispensable in designing an improved therapeutic agent or the means by which it is delivered. Quite often, pharmacokinetic analyses of systemically useful drugs is approached by dividing the body into a series of compartments that mathematically represent tissue levels of drug over time as a summation of exponentials. The number of compartments that are chosen are equal to and limited by the number of exponentials that can be assigned to the concentration of drug found in a particular body tissue and/or fluid over time.

The compartments are often interpreted physiologically or anatomically to contain tissues and/or organs which are "kinetically homogeneous." The term kinetically homogeneous compartments refers to tissues and/or organs that show similar if not identical kinetics for certain drugs even though the tissues and/or organs within the compartment may be dissimilar physiologically or anatomically. Although the rates within these groups of tissues and/or organs are similar for a particular drug, the extent of drug distribution to each is usually not equal.

The ophthalmic literature contains many reports of drug concentrations measured in eye tissues over time, administered either topically, subconjunctivally, orally, intravenously, or vitreally. The latter route of administration has been of major interest because of the prevalence of cyto-megalovirus retinitis associated with human immunodeficiency virus (HIV). When classical pharmacokinetic approaches (compartmental modeling) have been applied to ophthalmic drugs, a number of limitations have been found to restrict the usefulness of pharmacokinetics in the practice of ophthalmology. Noncompartmental approaches, such as moment analysis, circumvent the difficulty in choosing anappropriate compartmental model, but the assumption of linearity remains, as do various intractable experimental difficulties. Consequently, the majority of the ocular pharmacokinetic reports do not employ a classical approach but focus on whether or not drug reaches target tissues and whether or not the tissue concentrations are within the therapeutic range.

Limitations on the use of classical pharmacokinetic approaches, difficulties in designing and implementing animal studies for the eye, as well as interpretation of the results obtained from animal models are discussed in the following sections.

II. LIMITATIONS ON THE PRACTICAL USE OF CLASSICAL MODELING

At the present time it is not possible to predict optimal dosing regimens in the human eye for different drugs or for the same drug in different dosage forms. The most significant reason for not conducting ocular pharmacokinetic studies in the human eye is the inability to sample tissues or fluids from the intact eye without risking pain and/or injury. Although the rabbit eye is useful in predicting human ocular toxicities (1), the eyes of each species are dissimilar in anatomy and physiology (see Table 1) such that predicting human ocular pharmacokinetics from rabbit data may not be very precise for certain drugs.

As a further complication in predicting human ocular pharmacokinetics based upon animal data, samples from eye tissues cannot be continuously sampled over time. Although a number of tissues can be removed quickly and precisely from the rabbit eye, a different animal is used to determine drug concentration at a single time point, increasing intersubject variability. From this pooling approach a kinetic profile of drug concentration over time is constructed from a number of rabbits, which are sacrificed at each time point. As many as 150–250 rabbit eyes may be required to complete a statistically significant bioequivalence test between two ophthalmic drugs. It is often assumed that a representative pharmacokinetic profile can be constructed from "noncontinuous sampling" if enough time intervals

Table 1 Anatomical and Physiological Differences in the New Zealand Rabbit and Human Eye Pertinent to Ophthalmic Phamacokinetics

Pharmacokinetic factor	Rabbit eye	Human eye
Tear volume	7.5 µL	7.0–30.0 µL[a]
Tear turnover rate	0.6–0.8 µL/min	0.5–2.2 µL/min
Spontaneous blinking rate[b]	4–5 times/min	15 times/min
Nictitating membrane[c]	Present	Absent
pH of tears	[d]	7.14–7.82
Milliosmolarity of tears	[d]	305 mOsm/L
Corneal thickness	0.40 mm	0.52 mm
Corneal diameter	15 mm	12 mm
Aqueous humor volume	[d]	310 µL
Aqueous humor turnover rate	[d]	1.53 µL/min

[a] Range depending on blinking rate and conjunctival sac volume.
[b] Occurs during normal waking hours without apparent external stimuli.
[c] Significance of nictitating membrane is small relative to overall loss rate from precornea area.
[d] Approximately same measurement as human.

and sufficient eyes per time interval are chosen, but this number is not always based on a sound statistical approach.

A. Approaches Designed to Overcome the Pooling of Individual Samples

Because of the use of pooled data obtained from animal eyes, pharmacokinetic profiles of various ocular tissues are limited in their interpretation of the data. Sophisticated models that more adequately explain the data are often too complex and tend to be overly scattered and not as smooth as data obtained in a serial fashion. Therefore, the models have to be oversimplified. As a result of the oversimplification of the modeling and the use of animal eyes instead of human eyes, the value of ocular pharmacokinetic studies are limited to:

1. Validating the minimum effective concentrations in various tissues from different routes of administration
2. Determining the best route of administration for entry into the eye as well as accumulation at the site of action
3. Determining the elimination half-life, which can serve as a guide to selecting dosing regimens for further study

4. Estimating the safety of various drugs by determining their accumulation in tissues of interest, such as the lens or retina

Approaches to extending the application of pharmacokinetics have recently focused on two approaches: serial sampling and microdialysis.

1. Serial Sampling

Serial sampling has not been advocated as a reliable method for obtaining samples from animal eyes because of the possibility of a breakdown of the blood-aqueous barrier, resulting in an alteration of the drug clearance from the eye. Studies by Tang-Liu and coworkers (2,3) established that for a single intracameral injectkion of 5 µL solutions containing flurbiprofen or levobunolol, no significant breakdown of the blood aqueous barrier had occurred since protein concentration was < 1 mg/mL. However, serial sampling is a repetitive process not just a single injection. Miller et al. (4) studied the effect of paracentesis on the pharmacokinetics of fleroxacin following direct intravitreal or systemic drug administration and serially measuring drug levels in serum, aqueous, and vitreous humor. Samples were obtained from aqueous humor with the use of a sterile 30-gauge needle fused to a calibrated 20 µL capillary tube. A volume of 7 µL was removed at each time interval. A 28-gauge needle was used to sample vitrous humor and 20 µL samples were removed. Figure 1 gives the results, for which no statistically significant differences were observed in assigning a correct model for the data, nor were there significant differences in the half-lives for serum, aqueous, and vitreous humor—2.34,3.20, and 3.88 hours, respectively. Similar experiments with similar results were conducted for the pharmacokinetics of amikacin and chloramphenicol in rabbit aqueous humor following anterior chamber injection and serial sampling using 30-gauge needle and removing 7 µL of aqueous (5).

2. Microdialysis Approach

The microdialysis approach was widely used in the analysis of drugs in brain tissue and cerebral spinal fluid with the intention of measuring free drug concentration at the sampling site (6,7). More recently the approach has been adapted for use in the eye, particularly in the measurement of aqueous and vitreal humor concentrations of drug (8–12). Its primary advantage is to measure complete concentration-time profiles in individual animal eyes, reducing the number of animals required, and to more accurately define the pharmacokinetics of ocular drugs.

The procedure consists of surgically placing a probe within the aqueous or vitreous chambers of an anesthetized animal. The microdialysis

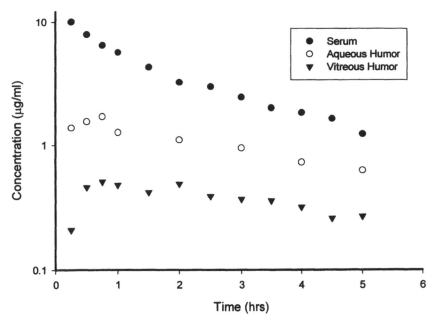

Figure 1 Average concentrations of fleroxacin in serum, aqueous humor and vitreous humor following intravenous administration to 10 rabbits. (Adapted from Ref. 4.)

probe is designed to allow for perfusate to flow into and out of the unit at a fixed rate, usually 2–3.5 μL/min. The base of the probe is constructed with a semipermeable membrane (e.g., a 4 mm polycarbonate membrane with a 20,000 dalton cutoff), which allows drug to diffuse into a perfusate (11). Probe inlet and outlet lines allow for collection of dialysate and analysis of drug over time. It is essential for the percent relative recovery to be determined so that accurate concentrations can be estimated, which may likely vary depending on the membrane used in the probe, the size of the probe and the perfusion rate. For example, reported values for propranolol and two nucleoside antivirals (ganciclovir and acyclovir) were 46 and 15%, respectively (12,13), when probe and perfusion rate varied. Of concern is the insertion of the probe, which appears to result in an increase in protein concentrations in aqueous humor (12), suggesting an alteration of clearance. The use of systemic anesthesia has also been shown to alter the pharmacokinetics of propranolol by increasing the area under the aqueous humor time-concentration plot, possibly by decreasing aqueous humor turnover (12). Nevertheless, results using this technique have reduced the number of animals needed to estimate ocular pharmacokinetic parameter values and have produced curves that are smooth in appearance and, therefore, more reliable in itnerpreting the fitting of models to the results.

III. ADEQUATE CHOICE OF TIME INTERVALS

Studies using pooled data from different rabbits often use as few as 4 or 5 rabbit eyes per time interval or as many as 22, depending on the objective of the study (14–19). A statistical basis for choosing an appropriate number of rabbit eyes in ophthalmic bioavailability studies has been established using areas under the concentration-time curve (AUC) (20,21). The AUC is related to the extent of absorption, which, similar to systemically administered drugs, is most important in determining therapy for chronic medication. The rate of absorption into the eye is less precise a measurement and also less pertinent to chronic therapy.

How many intervals and the length of time between each interval has not always been decided upon using a rational approach. Some general guidelines can be applied based upon the importance of absorption, distribution, and elimination to the kinetic profile. Each kinetic process is practically complete after five half-lives (96.875%); therefore, if the half-life for each kinetic process is known or can be easily arrived at, the theoretical length of time that should be used to generate a concentration × time profile can be estimated (see Fig. 2).

A. Elimination Phase

Elimination of drug from the eye is the least complicated process and can be discussed first. It occurs over the entire concentration-time profile, and as long as it is the slowest of pharmacokinetic processes, the latter log-linear phase of the drug concentration-time profile represents the elimination phase and its slope allows for the calculation of elimination half-life and the time necessary for completion of the process. For example, the half-life for elimination of foscarnet from rabbit vitreous humor is 34 hours (18) after intravitreal injection; therefore, the process is complete in 5 × 34 hours, or 170 hours. Foscarnet can be measured to a sensitivity of 4.5 µg/mL using an electrochemical detector with high-peformance liquid chromatography (HPLC) methodology (22).

In general, at least four or five time intervals should be spaced over the latter log llnear phase following the completion of distribution within the eye. For drugs with a much shorter half-life and a less sensitive assay than foscarnet, a practical limitation to measuring drug in the postdistributive

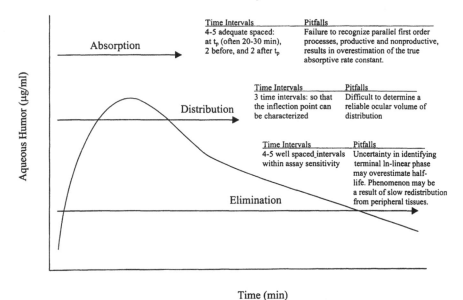

Figure 2 Sampling times and critical problems associated with measuring absorption, distribution, and elimination of an ocularly administered drug.

phase is the sensitivity of the assay, which could limit measuring the decline of the drug over three to five half-lives.

B. Absorption Phase

For many years absorption has been assumed to occur via the cornea; however, recently, scleral routes of administration have been suggested as routes of entry into the eye. Absorption is complex to estimate in the eye since lag time and drainage lengthen and shorten, respectively, the length of time that the absorption process is operative. For example, the first-order absorption rate constant (k_a) for phenylephrine is 4.5×10^{-5} min^{-1}, which gives a half-life of 128.3 hours; however, drainage permits drug to remain at the corneal absorption site for approximately 3–6 minutes only, depending on the volume and viscosity of the instilled solution (16,23–26). Consequently, the absorption process is abruptly terminated from theoretical expectations. The short residence time of drug at the absorption site results in exceptionally poor bioavailability.

Phenylephrine is atypical since it is very hydrophilic and transverses the cornea at a very slow rate. On the other hand, pilocarpine is moderately lipophilic and therefore more rapidly absorbed. Nevertheless, the difference between the theoretically expected time and the actual time during which absorption occurs remains large. For example, Makoid and Robinson (27) reported an accurate k_a of 6.2×10^{-3} min for pilocarpine 15, which gives an absorption half-life of 111.8 minutes and predicts that the process is complete in about 10 hours. However, the drainage rate constant is approximately 100 times larger with an estimated completion of the process in about 6 minues (27). As a result of the very short residence time of drug at the absorption site, the extent of absorption of ophthalmic drugs is about 1–10% (2,14,16,19,28).

The initial time for drug to transverse the cornea, referred to as the lag time, is sufficiently long that most often the time to peak occurs over a much longer time period than the time that a drug solution resides on the cornea (i.e., 3–6 min). The majority of ophthalmic drugs require between 20 and 60 minutes after instillation to reach the time to peak. Therefore, a reasonable time period exists so that up to three to four time intervals can be chosen to characterize the absorption phase. Because of the very low extent of absorption for ophthalmic drugs as well a the large correction needed for the drainage rate, the classical deconvolution techniques (Wagner-Nelson and Loo-Riegelman) (29) cannot be used without severely overestimating the first-order absorption rate consta,t k_a.

The other routes of administration that have been suggested as routes of entry into the eye are penetration across the conjunctiona/sclera (30) and/or absorption via vessels imbedded in the conjunctiva and sclera (e.g., anterior ciliary artery). Vessels embedded in the conjunctiva/sclera only partially empty into sites of action within the eye (i.e., the iris/ciliary body) (31). These routes of entry are in parallel and also contribute to the total value for k_a, the absorption rate constant.

The competing processes, referred to as nonabsorptive processes, have been specifically defined as drainage, conjunctival absorption with ultimate emptying into venous circulation, nictitating membrane absorption, tear turnover, drug-tear protein binding, and drug metabolism (16).

C. Distribution Phase

In an ideal curve, a distribution phase can be identified visually as the concave portion of the log concentration-time curve immediately following the time to peak. The latter log linear phase is the elimination or postdistributive phase (see Fig. 2). The distribution phase, which is expected to be shorter than the elimination phase, cannot be visually identified as easily as absorption and elimination. Depending on the numerical relationship between the microtransfer constants associated with drug disposition, it is possible that the profile representing drug concentration over time cannot be characterized by the proper number of exponentials. Often one less exponential than actually exists, paticularly when $k_{21} > k_a$ and alpha $> k_a$ (32). In addition, the concave portion of the log concentration-time curve may not be apparent because distribution is rapid. On the other hand, when drug concentrations from just after the time to peak to the beginning of the postdistributive phases are concave to the time axis, then the distributive phase is discernible and the concave portion of the profile should be represented by an additional two to four time intervals.

As indicated in Figures 2, 10–12 time intervals will suffice if they are properly chosen to represent absorption, distribution, and elimination. However, if variabiilty is too great, a larger number of eyes could be chosen at each interval to characterize adequately the drug's ocular pharmacokinetics. It is assumed that a smooth representative profile will result if a large enough sample size is chosen and pooling of individual rabbit eyes is used. For bioequivalence, the time to peak (t_p) is a critical concentration to obtain since it represents a maximum concentration. Because of the relatively large and constant nature of the drainage rate for topically administered solutions and suspensions, the t_p only varies from about 20 to 60 minutes for ophthalmic drugs regardless of a drug's physicochemical behavior. As discussed previously, in practice the distribution phase is usually not apparent either because of inherent variabiilty or because the magnitude of the microconstants representing distribution to peripheral tissues prevents observation of the characteristic concavity shown in Figure 2.

D. Other Factors Influencing Choice of Sampling Times

Unfortunately, more subtle factors may be operating to complicate the choice of sampling times and obscure the expected shape of the profile shown in Figure 2. For example, for some drugs, most notably cyclosporine (19,33,34), pilocarpine (35), and verapamil (36), rapid equilibration with aqueous humor is not apparent. As a result, the terminal log-linear elimination phase of the concentration of drug in aqueous humor vs. time is difficult to identify unless time intervals are extended well beyond what is usually considered adequate for ocular studies (i.e., 2–5 hours). For pilocarpine, when drug concentration was measured for 11 hours, a biexponential decline was evident and an elimination half-life of 2.75 hours was observed (27) compared to earlier studies, which estimated the half-life to be about 40–60 minutes. However, the latter log-linear decline of pilocarpine may be due to residual drug slowly redistributing from the lens. Since these levels are low and released slowly, the use of 40–60 minutes is probably better in practical situations. For cyclosporine, the distribution phase was not apparent for 8–10 hours after subconjunctival administration (34). Acheampong et al. (34) observed that cyclosporine in both rabbit and beagle dogs accumulated significantly in the cornea, lens, lacrimal gland, and iris/ciliary body. These tissues acted as reservoirs to prolong retention in the eye likely because of the drug's lipophilic nature and poor water solubility.

Another limiting factor is the sensitivity of the assay. Significant advances have been made in recent years so that it is not necessary to prepare a radioactive tracer for adequate detection of drug in eye tissues. HPLC with ultraviolet, radioactive, or fluorescence detectors, laser scanning confocal Raman spectroscopy, or radioimmunoassay can measure drug concentrations in ocular tissues at levels as low as 1 ng per mL or g of tissue (37–43).

IV. OCULAR PHARMACOKINETIC MODELING

Although there are intractable difficulties in clearly and unambiguously defining pharmacokinetic parameters exclusively for the eye, such as clearance, volume of distribution, as well as rate and extent of absorption, it is also true that ophthalmic drugs are a relatively small commercial market compared to systemically adminstered drugs. Nevertheless, the classical pharmacokinetic approach of expressing the concentration-time curve into a sum of exponentials has been applied to the eye (4,13,14,17,19,28, 36,44–51), but much less extensively than other routes of administration. At the present time, limited application has resulted from these studies in developing new ophthalmic drugs with optimal pharmacokinetic behavior or more specifically in estimating dosing regimens.

Although the classical pharmacokinetic approach has limitations when applied to the eye, in situ or in vitro experiments have been developed that directly measure kinetic phenomena and are more accurate when compared to results obtained from classical compartmental approaches. Very specific techniques have been developed to measure precorneal drug disposition, permeability of various corneal layers, metabolism is various eye tissues (52,53) and to measure fluorescein kinetics, which have led to the understanding of tear, aqueous, and vitreous dynamics (54,55) and have been responsible for the development of very useful clinical applications. These latter approaches are discussed in another chapter.

A. Classical Modeling Approaches

Initially, a classical pharmacokinetic approach is applied to concentration-time curves derived from topical instillation to the eye in much the same manner as data derived from systemically administered drugs. The curve is first expressed by a computer-determined sum of exponentials, which closely fit the experimental data and likewise show no systemic deviation. In the eye, aqueous humor is most often assigned to the central compartment, which is reversibly connected to one or more peripheral compartments and/or a reservoir compartment in the various models (or schemes) that have been derived. This choice is compatible with physiological reality since aqueous humor, which fills the anterior and posterior chambers, is the circulating fluid bathing the peripheral tissues. Drugs instilled topically on the eye primarily reach the first third of the eye, which encompasses these regions. Topically applied ophthalmic drugs do not reach the retina in significant concentrations. Consequently, models can be devised that treat the viscous region as a central compartment particularly when drug is administered intravitreally.

In the eye, the cornea, conjunctiva, lens, iris/ciliary body, choroid, and vitreous are specific tissues that are often lumped together into one or more peripheral compartments. A peripheral compartment can be reversibly connected to a central compartment, but if redistribution into aqueous humor is negligible or nonexistent, peripheral tissues can act as a sink or reservoir compartment. The exit out of the eye is into the blood or circulating fluid of the body.

Figure 3 lists the classical compartmental schemes most commonly applied to ophthalmic drugs following topical application. For many years pilocarpine received the most attention (35,44–47). More recently, publications focusing on classical modeling have decreased, but those that have been published used a varied assortment of drugs for study (5,19,22,36,40,48–51). The most appropriate model seems to depend heavily on the design of the study (i.e., number and length of sampling periods and number of tissues measured for drug content over time), the specificity and sensitivity of the assay, the sophistication of the curve-fitting routine used to analyze the data, and the likelihood that the data can be interpreted by a complex modeling scheme. When aqueous humor or vitreous concentrations of drug are measured over time, either mono- or biexponential equations adequately describe the disposition of drug (5,13,14,22,49–51).

Since it is relatively easy to remove cornea, conjunctiva, lens, iris/ciliary body, and/or choroid tissues along with aqueous humor, the assignment of barriers and peripheral and/or reservoir compartments is not particularly difficult with the exception of the cornea. Although the cornea is clearly a physical barier to drug entry into the anterior chamber, it is actually divided into three significant kinetic barriers: the multilayered lipophilic epithelium, the aqueous-like stroma, and the single-celled lipophilic endothelium. The specific corneal permeability rate for each

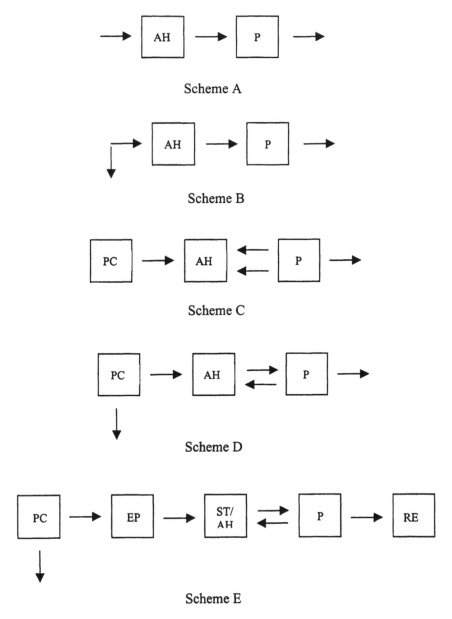

Figure 3 Classic pharmacokinetic schemes used to express compartmentalization for topically applied ophthalmic drugs. PC = precorneal area; EP = corneal epithelium; AH = aqueous humor; P = peripheral or intraocular tissues accessible from aqueous humor; ST/AH = stroma, endothelium and aqueous humor (i.e., kinetic homogeneity), RE = reservoir (i.e., blood and systemic fluids).

drug depends on the drug's partitioning properties and molecular weight relative to the individual properties of each barrier (56–62). The sum of the resistances of each layer represents the apparent corneal permeability rate. However, for pilocarpine a closer study of its kinetics in each barrier by Lee and Robinson (44) indicated that the stroma and endothelium could be more correctly associated with the aqueous humor compartment, and only the corneal epithelium was a barrier for entry of drug into the anterior chamber. Although the endothelium is lipophilic, it is only one cell thick and is apparently not as significant a barrier as the much thicker, more tortuous epithelium with 9 or 10 layers.

This latter division of corneal layers into a single epithelial barrier and the assignment of stroma and endothelium into a compartment along with aqueous humor may be correct not only for pilocarpine, but also for other hydrophilic drugs for which the epithelium is the major significant barrier. Water-soluble drugs of relatively small molecular weight (< 500–900) likely penetrate the epithelium predominantly by paracellular pathways (30,53). Consequently, as long as the drug is soluble, a high topical concentration can be applied tot he cornea to promote a high penetration rate and overcome poor penetrability.

B. Pharmacometric Measurements

Today computer curve-fitting routines are designed for microcomptuers to easily accommodate mathematical treatment of tissue concentrations of drug over time (63). Regardless of the statistical approach employed to arrive at the best representation of the data, it is desirable to characterize and express absorption, distribution, and elimination of drugs. Over the years, attempts that have been made to express pharmacokinetic drug behavior are the fraction absorbed (F), the first-order rate absorption rate constant (k_a) or the time to peak (t_p), the volume of distribution (V_d), and clearance. Clearance is expressed as either excretory (Cl_e), metabolic (Cl_m) or their total, which represents elimination out of the "body" (Cl_t). In the eye, Cl_t becomes ocular clearance, Cl_o. Noncompartmental approaches can be used, for which mean residence times can be calculated to define ocular pharmacokinetics (21,42,51,52). On occasion, no parameter values are given other than half-lives; however, tables are presented summarizing various tissue levels over time (16,34,64). Strictly speaking, classical linear models as well as noncompartmental approaches require that processes follow first-order kinetics and the superposition principle. These assumptions are sometimes not confirmed with ocular pharmacokinetic data, mostly because of intersubject variability, which is often significant enough that reasonable experimentation is not adequate. Difficulties in measuring ocular pharma-cokinetic behavior are discussed in more detail in the following sections.

1. Absorption

As discussed more fully in another chapter, the rate and extent of ophthalmic drug absorption is restricted largely by noncorneal absorption in the precor-neal area and the drainage rate. The latter process, because of its rapidity, limits the ocular contact time for drugs residing at the absorption site to about 3–6 minutes, whereas the rate and extent of penetration across the cornea is restricted by the physicochemical properties of the drug and/or its formulation (14–16,65–69). Drug may also enter the ey by scleral penetration (30,31,53,70–72) or by uptake of drug into the anterior ciliary artery (31).

   a. Fraction Absorbed.   For drugs administered systemically, the frac-tion absorbed is determined by taking the ratio of the area under the plas-ma concentration-time curve or the total amount excreted in the urine for a bolus intravenous dose and an oral dose, respectively. When applied in an analogous manner to the eye, a small volume of drug is injected intra-camerally using a small-bore needle and in a separate group of animals is given topically, each followed by sampling of aqueous humor and measur-ing drug concentration over time (2,3). When given topically, the fraction absorbed for 75 μg and 150 μg ocular doses of flurbiprofen was 10 and 7%, respectively.

   Patton and Robinson (46) estimated the fraction absorbed using a different approach. Topical dosing studies were conducted in both anes-thetized and awake rabbits and with the drainage ducts plugged and unobstructed. Pilocarpine ntirate was measured as the disappearance of drug from the tears of rabbit eyes whose ducts had been plugged and also as appearance of drug in aqueous humor in both experiments. After correct-ing for dilution due to tear production and determining the areas under the tear concentration-time curve (AUC), the fraction absorbed in anesthetized rabbits whose ducts had been plugged was calculated as 0.0187. Equation (1) was used to calculate F:

$$\text{AUC} = \frac{FD}{k_{10}V} \tag{1}$$

In Eq. (1), D is the instilled dose (25 μL), k_{10} is the loss of drug from the precorneal area $(1 \times 10^{-2} \text{ min}^{-1})$, and V is estimated as 0.3 mL. Extrapolating the results to normal rabbits, assuming a volume of distribu-tion approximately equal to the aqueous humor volume, and assuming that negligible drug distributes out of the aqueous humor were approximations required in order to estimate F.

Since drug absorption across the cornea and loss of drug from the precorneal area are parallel loss processes, it was possible to confirm the results of Patton and Robinson (46) by the use of Eq. (2):

$$F = \frac{k_{10}}{k_{10} + k_a} \qquad (2)$$

The fraction absorbed for a 25 μL instilled dose of pilocarpine nitrate in the rabbit eye was estimated to be 1–2% (46,47). Using Eq. (2), Chiang and Schoenwald calculated that for a 30 μL dose of 0.4% clonidine, an F of 1.6% was calculated for the rabbit eye (28).

Ling and Combs (73) compared the areas under the concentration-time curves for ketorolac tromethamine 0.5% administered topically (50 μL) and intracamerally, respectively. The ratio of the areas indicated a fraction absorbed of 3.7%. An identical approach was used by Tang-Liu et al. (3) in determining that 2.5% of the instilled dose of levobunolol was absorbed after a topical dose (50 μL of 0.5%), similar in range to other drugs administered topically.

b. Rate of Absorption. The loss of drug from the precorneal area is a net effect of tear secretion, drainage, and noncorneal and corneal absorption rate processes. When drug concentration in aqueous humor is described biexponentially, the latter, shallower log-linear slope represents elimination out of the eye, whereas the steeper slope is the net effect of the precorneal processes. Because the drainage rate is approximately 100 times more rapid than k_a (44,46), it is correct to assign the more shallow log-linear slope from aqueous humor concentration-time curves as elimination from aqueous humor. Consequently, estimation of the steepest slope and subsequent calculation of k_a can be obtained from nonlinear curve-fitting techniques if the other precorneal processes are known.

Table 2 lists drugs for which k_a has been estimated. These values, when interpreted as half-lives, show how slowly drug is actually absorbed across the cornea. Because of the very rapid loss of drug from the precorneal area, and in particular the drainage rate, it is not surprising to find that only a small fraction of the instilled dose is actually absorbed across the cornea. In addition, the cornea is relatively thick, variable in hydrophilic/lipophilic properties for each layer, and small in surface area. These factors, along with the rapid precorneal loss rate, combine to have a significant effect on the time to peak following topical instillation of drugs to the eye regardless of the drug's physicochemical properties or its elimination rate from internal eye tissues. In general, the time to peak is 20–60 minutes for nearly all ophthalmic drugs when instilled topically to the eye. This has been shown by Makoid and Robinson (27), who determined the ophthalmic pharmaco-

Table 2 Transcorneal First-Order Absorption Rate Constant and
Accompanying Half-Life for Corneal Absorption

Drug	k_a (min^{-1})	$t_{1/2}$(h)	Ref.
Pilocarpine	0.004	2.88	44
Clonidine	0.0014	8.25	28
Ketaprofin	0.0000462	250	52
Phenylephrine	0.00001	1155	120
Ibuprofen	0.00129	9	51
Ibufenac	0.00608	19	51
Ethoxyzolamide	0.0015	7.7	76
Aminozolamide	0.0014	8.25	78
2-Benzothiazolesulfonamide	0.0013	8.88	76
6-Hydroxyethoxy-2-benzothiazolesulfonamide	0.0042	5.37	76
N-Methylacetazolamide	0.00126	9.17	121
Acetazolamide	0.00153	75.5	121

kinetics of pilocarpine following topical application to the rabbit eye. From
their work an equation was developed for t_p:

$$t_p = \frac{\ln(k_{na}/k_a)}{K_{na} - K_a} \tag{3}$$

In Eq. (3), k_{na} and k_a are the nonabsorptive loss rate constant and the
transcorneal absorption rate constant, respectively. Equation (3) assumes
that k_{na} is much larger than uptake into the epithelium of the cornea
from the precorneal area. This assumption can be applied to most, if
not all, ophthalmic drugs, since k_{na} is approximately twofold larger
than k_a.

On occasion, a drug cannot be given systemically by a bolus intravenous dose, and therefore equations have been developed so that a slow
intravenous infusion could be used instead (74,75). Eller et al. (76) developed a topical infusion technique for estimating the ophthalmic pharmacokinetics of drugs, which was based upon noncompartmental methods. The
procedure consisted of maintaining a constant concentration of drug on the
cornea through the use of a plastic cylinder secured over the sclera, which
allowed only the cornea to be exposed to drug solution (see Table 3). A
volume of 0.7 mL is maintained over the cornea of an anesthetized rabbit
until steady-state ocular concentrations are reached. Rabbits are sacrificed
at various time intervals, ocular tissues aer excised, and then assayed for
drug content. This topical infusion approach permits an estimate of k_a the
apparent volume of distribution at steady state (V_{ss}), and ocular clearance

Table 3 Topical Infusion Method Depicting Well[a] and Equations[b]

Ocular well used for topical infusion	Equations used for topical infusion method

$$k_a = \frac{V_A(dC_a/dt)_t}{C_W V_W} \tag{3a}$$

$$Cl_0 = \frac{K_0 T}{AUC} \tag{3b}$$

$$V_{SS} = \frac{K_0 T \, AUMC}{(AUC)^2} - \frac{K_0 T^2}{2AUC} \tag{3c}$$

$$K_0 = (dC_a/dt)_t V_A \tag{3d}$$

[a] Well is a fixed over cornea of anesthetized rabbit; drug solution is maintained at a constant concentration for 90–160 minutes until steady-state concentrations of drug are reached in the aqueous humor.

[b] K_a = first-order transcorneal rate constant; V_a = volume of the anterior chamber; $(dC_a/dt)_I$ = initial rate of appearance of drug in aqueous humor minus lag time; Cl_0 = ocular clearance ($\mu L/min$); K_0 = constant rate of input into anterior chamber; AUC and AUMC = areas (to infinity) under the aqueous humor concentration × time curve and concentration × time-time curve, respectively; C_W = constant concentration maintained on the cornea over time (90–160 min); V_W = volume of drug solution maintained in well.

(Cl_o). Figure 4 shows a semilogarithmic plot of the aqueous humor concentration of ibufenac and ibuprofen following topical infusion of 0.3% maintained on the cornea for 120 minutes (51). Table 3 lists the equations and pharmacokinetic parameter values for drugs for which this procedure has been used.

2. Distribution

The volume of distribution represents a proportionality constant to relate concentration to amount or dose and also as a relative measure of tissue accumulation. It is the most difficult pharmacokinetic process to measure primarily because the amuont of drug in the eye at any time is not known. Aqueous humor is the circulating fluid of the eye, and in order to measure V_d accurately, an instantaneous input (i.e., intracameral injection) or an injection at a known rate must be introduced. Estimates of apparent volumes of distribution are lacking for ocular drugs. Table 4 lists values estimated either from an intracameral injection (see figure 5) or from topical

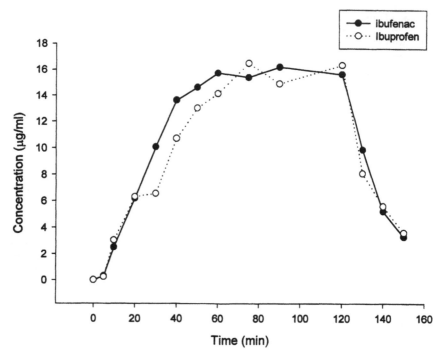

Figure 4 Average aqueous humor concentrations of ibufenac and ibuprofen following topical infusion of a 300 μg/mL solution to anesthetized rabbit eyes ($n = 6$) for 120 minutes. (Adapted from Ref. 51.)

infusion. Estimating the volume of distribution for amikacin and for chloramphenicol yielded values of 2.67 and 3.33 mL (5), which are about 8.5- and 10.5-fold larger than aqueous humor volume. Although these values are the largest summarized in Table 4, they are relatively small relative to aqueous humor volume. For systemically administered drugs, for which serum or plasma is measured, V_d can easily be 100 times larger than plasma volume, the latter of which is about 4.3% of body weight.

Nevertheless, tissues in the anterior and posterior chamber are adjacent to circulating aqueous humor and therefore readily available for transfer of drug. Also, protein concentration in aqueous humor is about 10% of proteins in plasma, so that it is not likely that tissue distribution is prevented because of binding to components in aqueous humor. Consequently, it is surprising that V_d is so small. Although accurate determinations of V_d are necessary for estimates of optimal multiple dosing regimens, few are available, mainly because of the pharmacometric difficulties in obtaining such measurements.

Table 4 Volumes of Distribution (V_d) for Drugs of Ophthalmic Interest

Drug	V_d (mL)	Method	Ref.
Pilocarpine	0.58	EXT[a]	47
Clonidine	0.53	SS[b]	28
Phenylephrine	0.42	SS	120
Flubiprofen	0.62	EXT	2
Ibufenac	0.21	EXT	51
Ibuprofen	0.53	EXT	51
Ketanserin	0.97	EXT	52
Amikacin	2.67	EXT	5
Chloramphenicol	3.33	EXT	5
Levobunolol	1.65	EXT	3
Dihydrolevobunolol	1.68	EXT	3
Phenylephrine	0.42	SS	120
Ketorolac tromethamine	1.93	EXT	73
Ethoxzolamide	0.28	SS	57
Aminozolamide	0.53	SS	78
2-Benzothiazolesulfonamide	0.24	SS	76
6-Hydroxyethoxy-2-benzothiazolesulfonamide	0.33	SS	76
N-Methylacetaxolamide	0.42	SS	121
Acetazolamide	0.47	SS	121

[a] EXT = extrapolated method; determined by extrapolating log-linear elimination phase t_0 C at t_0 and dividing into the intracameral dose.

[b] SS = steady-state method; determined by maintaining a constant concentration of drug on the cornea of an anesthetized rabbit and measuring aqueous humor concentrations of drug over time during infusion and postinfusion. See Table 3 for equatiaon for V_{SS}.

The pharmacokinetic parameter, V_d, also provides a general assessment of distribution. However, it does not differentiate between sites that are active and those that are either devoid of activity of potentially responsible for side effects. In lieu of making these measurements, it is not difficult to measure eye tissue concentrations over time, which provides a direct indication of whether or not drug distributes to the active site. In contrast to the paucity of pharmacokinetic measurements for ophthalmic drugs, tissue concentrations of drug have been widely reported for many years. With recent improvements in assay methodology, tissue profiles over time are routinely measured for aqeous humor and cornea, but less frequently for lens, iris/ciliary body, conjunctiva, choroid, lacrimal gland, and/or retina.

In the interest of therapy, it is of importance to determine the percent of the dose that reaches a particular tissue and to determine if the concentrations that are reached meet and/or exceed the minimum therapeutic

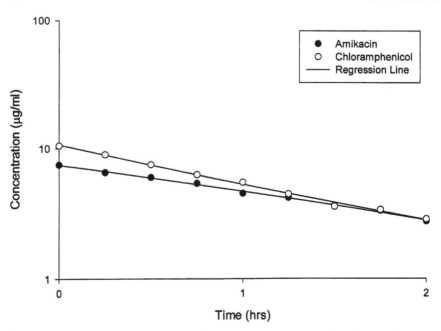

Figure 5 Average ($n = 5$) aqueous humor concentrations of amikacin (2 μg/μL) and chloramphenicol (5 μg/μL) following direct injection of into the anterior chamber of the rabbit eye (10 μL). (Adapted from Ref. 5.)

range. For example, in a recent study by Morlet et al. (77), ciprofloxacin, which is active against a wide variety of bacteria, was given orally in doses of 750 or 1500 mg prior to eye surgery and then assayed for levels in blood, aqueous, and vitreous humor during surgery. Population pharmacokinetics was applied to the data, and the mean half-lives for loss of ciprofloxacin were determined for aqueous and vitreous humor, which were found to be 3.5 and 5.3 hours, respectively. At steady state, the concentrations of drug in aqueous and viterous were 23 and 17% of serum levels, respectively. The authors concluded that the use of oral ciprofloxacin would be below the minimum inhibitory concentration (MIC) of 0.5 μg/mL in treating bacterial endophthalmitis or for use for perioperative prophylaxis.

It is reasonable to expect that if drug is instilled topically to the eye and no unusual tissue affinity occurs for a particular drug, the order of decrasing tissue concentrations are as follows: cornea > conjunctiva > aqueous humor > iris/ciliary body > lens, vitreous, and/or choroid/retina. Many studies (37,51,52,67,78,80,81) show that iris/ciliary body concentrations are higher than aqueous humor concentrations, even though the dose is instilled topically to the cornea. A number of reasons have been suggested to account for this phenomenon. For example, the drug may distribute extensively to iris/ciliary body, but drug may equilibrate rapidly with aqueous humor so that the elimination rate during distribution equilibrium is the same as elimination from aqueous humor. If this explanation is correct, the iris/ciliary body would have a large capacity for drug but not exhibit an unusually high binding affinity. It is also conceivable that the binding affinity as well as its capacity is very high so that the elimination rate from iris/ciliary body and aqueous are not the same but drug remains in the former tissue much longer.

This latter observation was observed by Putnam et al. (78) for aminozolamide, a topically active carbonic anhydrase inhibitor (CAI), which showed a relatively slow elimination for drug as well as metabolite, 6-acetamido-2-benzothiazolesulfonamide, from iris/ciliary body compared to aqueous humor following topical administration to the rabbit eye. In another example, a derivative of methazolamide, 5-acetoxyacetylimino-4-methyl-Δ^2-1,3,4,-thiadiazoline-2-sulfonamide, is an ester prodrug that lowered intraocular pressure in albino New Zealand rabbits but was found to be active in pigmented Dutch Belt rabbits (79). From various studies it was concluded that melanin binding in the iris, and to some extent metabolism occurring only in the Dutch Belt rabbits, were valid explanations.

Alternatively, support for the possibility of high concentrations of drug in the iris-ciliary body after topical application come from the likelihood that drugs reach iris-ciliary body by scleral absorption (i.e., paracellular penetration) and/or uptake by vessels imbedded in the conjunctiva that deposit drug. Certain drugs, when applied topically to the eye, may be preferentially absorbed by the sclera, as opposed to the cornea, and enter the iris/ciliary body without first entering the aqueous humor. In a study by Ahmed et al. (71), corneal and scleral penetration were determined for propranolol, timolol, nadalol, penbutolol, sucrose, and inulin. The results of the study showed that the outer layer of the sclera provides much less resistance to penetrabiilty for hydrophilic drugs than the corneal epithelium. Hämäläinen et al. (30) estimated that the conjunctival and scleral tissues were 15–25 times more permeable than the cornea and that conjunctival permeability was less affected by molecular size than the cornea. In addition, the total paracellular space of the conjunctiva was estimated to be 230 times greater than that in the cornea. For lipophilic drugs, such as propranolol, timolol, and penbutolol, the difference in penetrability between the tissues has been estimated to be similar. In a study by Schoenwald and Zhu (52), ketanserin and its metabolite, ketanserinol, were infused topically to anesthetized rabbits for 120 minutes. Drug was instilled either within the well and, therefore, in direct contact with the cornea, or outside the well, excluding the cornea but allowing drug to come in contact with conjunctiva (see Fig. 3). The results showed that iris–ciliary body concentrations were three and two times higher for ketanserin and ketanserinol when applied exclusively to the sclera as opposed to the cornea (52).

In a similar study by Chien et al. (79), various anterior chamber tissue levels were measured over time for clonidine, p-aminoclonidine, and a 6-quinoxalinyl derivative of chlonidine (AGN 190342) using the infusion method. Whenever drug was maintained on conjunctiva or cornea for a period of 60 minutes, tissue concentration followed a clear trend. the order of highest to lowest concentration of drug following conjunctival contact was conjunctiva > cornea > ciliary body > aqueous humor. When drug solution was in contact with cornea only, the order was cornea > aqueous humor > ciliary body > conjunctiva. From the results of recent studies (30,31,79–82), various pathways of ocular absorption have been proposed, as summarized in Figure 6.

Although many anterior and, to a lesser extent, posterior tissues have been measured for drug concentration over time following topical or systemic administration, little definitive information exists regarding the ability of tissues to accumulate drug through either partitioning or binding of drug. Of critical importance is the iris/ciliary body, which is the biophasic location for many pharmacological responses acting on the eye. Also of interest is the lens, since drug accumulation may be responsible for inducing cataract formation. Both of these tissues are easily removed and often treated as a kinetically homogeneous tissue, but drug concentrations within these tissues are likely to be quite variable in concentration since these tissues are not anatomically homogenous.

For example, iris tissue in the rabbit eye is porous and highly vascular with a large surface area in direct contact with aqueous humor; consequently, distribution equilibrium between iris and aqueous humor should occur rapidly. Also, as the iris becomes darker, the capacity for pigmented iris to bind to catecholamines increases. This was also observed for carbonic anhydrase inhibitors (CAIs) (82). Dark-eyed individuals have a delayed onset and a reduced but prolonged response to catecholamines, presumably due to the reservoir effect that the pigmented iris has on ocular disposition of catecholamines. Latanoprost, an isopropyl ester of prostglandin $F_{2\alpha}$, can darken the iris in susceptible individuals due to increased pigmentation of the anterior surface of the iris (83). In contrast to iris tissue, the ciliary body epithelial layer of the pars plicata, containing a high concentration of carbonic anhydrase and presumed to be the active site for CAIs, is not easily reached via topical instillation (84), requiring a lipophilic drug substance to readily penetrate cellular membranes. Although the separation of these tissues from one another would provide useful information, it is usually not done because of the difficulty in separating one tissue entirely from the other.

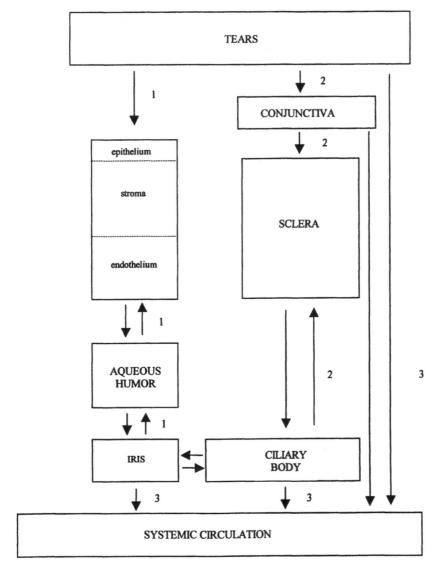

Figure 6 Probable ocular penetration routes for topically applied drugs: (1) transcorneal pathways; (2) noncorneal pathways; (3) systemic pathways.

The entire lens is also easy to remove during kinetic studies; nevertheless, the lens should not be treated as a kinetically homogeneous tissue. Maurice and Mishima (85) reported that fluorescein, a water-soluble dye, spreads laterally and rapidly in the outer layers of the lens but does not diffuse readily into the lens nucleus. The initial barrier for entry into the lens is the epithelium, which is a single layer of cells lying just below the anterior lens capsule. Internal to the epithelial layer are densely packed lens fibers and the nucleus. Because it consists of hard, condensed cellular material, the nucleus possesses high tortuosity and low porosity. With age, old fibers are not disposed of but become compressed centrally to form a larger, less elastic nucleus. Consequently, drugs are not expected to readily penetrate the lens interior. Ahmed et al. (86) came to this conclusion from a study of the diffusion of timolol through the lens fibers of rabbit lens. A pharmacokinetic model for drug entering aqueous humor and distributing into the lens included the capsule and its epithelium as a compartment adjacent to aqueous, but excluded the lens interior since drug did not reach significant levels in this region. It was concluded that unless a steady state of drug is present and maintained through repetitive dosing, significant accumulation would not occur. Drug elimination from the eye is too rapid to allow for significant concentrations to accumulate into the interior of the lens from a few doses.

3. Elimination

Drug is eliminated from the anterior chamber, at least in part, by aqueous humor turnover, which in the rabbit eye is 1.5% of the volume of the anterior chamber per minute or expressed as a half-life, 46.2 minutes (87). Although clearance is of greatest interest for drugs used systemically, half-life representing loss from aqueous humor is the most common pharmacokinetic parameter measured following topical administration to the eye. Table 5 lists half-lives for drugs of ophthalmic interest. Surprisingly, nearly all the drugs fall within a range of 0.6–3 hours, which is less than when these same drugs are studied systemically. Either there are few tissue-binding sites in the eye to allow for drugs to resist clearance, or the pathways by which drugs are eliminated are very efficient. The latter may be the most likely explanation, since aqueous humor volume is relatively large compared to ocular tissue volume.

Elimination can also be expressed as a clearance, and if the anterior chamber of the rabbit contains about 0.311 mL, an average aqueous humor clearance due to bulk flow becomes 4.67 µL/min based upon Eq. (4). Ocular clearances (Cl_o) can be calculated from the following equations:

$$Cl_o = K_e V_d \tag{4}$$

$$Cl_o = \frac{K_o T}{\text{AUC}_{\text{INF}}} \tag{5}$$

$$Cl_o = \frac{D_{\text{IC}}}{\text{AUC}_{\text{INF}}} \tag{6}$$

where K_c represents the first-order elimination rate constant out of aqueous humor, V_d is the apparent volume of distribution for the eye, K_o is the constant rate input into the anterior chamber, T is the time for the constant rate input, D_{IC} is an intracameral dose, and AUC_{INF} is the area (to infinity) under the aqueous humor concentration-time curve.

Each equation above depends on assumption that require experimentation to be carefully planned. In Eq. (4), K_e can be easily obtained. It is calculated from the latter linear slope of the logarithm of drug concentration in aqueous humor measured over time or obtained from any other tissue concentration in distribution equililbrium with aqueous humor. The V_d term in Eq. (3) has been correctly determined for the eye by either of two methods. One method, the topical infusion technique (28,37,52,76), has been discussed previously and is the basis for Eq. (5), also shown in Figure 4. The other method for determining V_d is based upon measuring drug concentration in aqueous humor over time following an intracameral injection of a very small volume (5 μL) of drug solution. Whenever an intracameral injection is made, there is concern that drug elimination can be altered because of a breakdown of the blood-aqueous barrier. However, Mayers, Miller, and coworkers (4,5,88,89), as well as Tang-Liu and coworkers (2,3), have established that for intracameral injections of 5 μL solutions containing various drugs, no significant breakdown of the blood-aqueous barrier had occurred since protein concentration was < 1 mg/mL. Equation (6), sometimes referred to as a "dose-area" determination, was used by Tang-Liu et al. (2,3) to calculate V_d for flurbiprofen and levobunolol.

Table 6 contains Cl_o values for those drugs for which accurate determinations have been made. Values range from 13 to 28.7 mL/min, which are 2.8-6.1 times higher than aqueous humor clearance, suggesting pathways of elimination other than aqueous turnover. The two most likely alternate routes of elimination are metabolism and systemic uptake by the vascular tissues of the anterior uvea. However, accumulation and retention by the lens (over the time course of the experiment), as well as back diffusion into the cornea and tears followed by subsequent drainage, are all minor routes that are not likely to significantly contribute to ocular clearance values.

C. Metabolic Models

Although the eye is not a primary drug-metabolizing organ, a knowledge of metabolic pathways in the eye has become increasingly important in order to optimize drug action and therapeutic effect. Esterases have been studied most extensively (90–93), no doubt because of their importance in the development of prodrugs for use in the eye. Prodrugs that have shown a significant improvement in corneal penetrability are phenylephrine (94,95),

Table 5 Aqueous Humor Half-Lives[a] of Drugs Administered to
the Rabbit Eye Either Topically, Intracamerally, or
Subconjunctivally

Drug	Half-life (h)	Ref.
Cyclosporine	24.9	19
Dapiprazole	5.8	122
Imirestat	4.75	123
6-Mercaptopurine	4.6	124
Falintolol	3.0	123
Fusidic acid	2.8	125
Suprofen	2.6	126
Dorzolamide	2.4	144
Histamine	2.2	128
Cimetidine	2.2	127
Ketorolac tromethamine	2.1	73
Benzolamide	2.0	128
Ceftazidime	2.0	129
Gentamicin	1.9	130
L-Alphamethyldopa[b]	1.8	131
1-643,799[c]	1.8	132
Diclofenac	1.7	133
Diclofenac[d]	5.0	38
Diclofenac[e]	1.0	38
Diclofenac[f]	0.2	38
Flurbiprofen	1.7	134
Fluorometholone acetate	1.5	20
Cefamandole	1.5	135
Thiamphenicol	1.5	49
Phenylephrine	1.4	120
D-Alphamethyldopa[b]	1.4	131
Amikacin	1.4	5
Timolol	1.2	136
Timolol	0.84	137
Timolol	0.2	40
Lincomycin	1.2	138
6-Amino-2-benzothiazolesulfonamide	1.15	78
L-662,583[g]	1.11	139
Acetbutolol	1.1	137
Cefsulodin	1.0	140
Fluorouracil	1.0	141
Chloramphenicol	1.0	5
Dihydrolevobunolol	0.98	3
N-Methylacetazolamide	0.98	121
6-Hydroxyethoxy-2-benzothiazolesulfonamide	0.97	76

Table 5 Continued

Drug	Half-life (h)	Ref.
Propranolol	0.96	10
Propranol	1.2	12
6-Acetamido-2-benzothiazolesulfonamide	0.93	78
L-650,719[h]	0.81	132
Ketanserrin	0.86	64
Saperconazole	0.86	52
Tobramycin	0.75	20
Trifluoromethazolamide	0.78	128
Pilocarpine	0.72	142
Methazolamide	0.58	128
Cefotaxime	0.57	143
Bufuralol	0.50	137
Levobunolol	0.67	3
Ethoxzolamide	0.63	76
Ethoxzolamide	0.23	128
Pyrilamine	0.61	127
Verapamil	0.55	36
Clonidine	0.49	28
Acetazolamide	0.35	121
Tilisolol	0.35	40
Ibuprofen	0.31	51
2-Benzothiazolesulfonamide	0.29	76
Ibufenac	0.28	51

[a] Concentrations from the last two to four times intervals were used in calculating $t_{1/2}$ values.
[b] A small dose dependency was observed (statistically NS); IV dose = 10 mg/kg.
[c] 6-Hydroxybenzol[b]thiophene-2-sulfonamide.
[d] Normal rabbit eyes were used.
[e] Keratitis model.
[f] Uveitis model.
[g] 6-Hydroxybenzol[b]thiophene-2-sulfonamide.
[h] 6-Hydroxy-2-benzothiazidesulfonamide.

timolol (96), pilocarpine (97,98), and idoxuridine (99). Two sterioisomers, both isopropyl ester prodrugs of prostaglandin $F_{2\alpha}$, latanoprost, and unoprostone, have approved been recently for clinical use (83). Acetyl-, butyryl-, and carboxylesterases have been identified in the pigmented rabbit eye (90) and are responsible for rapid conversion of ester prodrugs to the active drug species.

Bodor and coworkers (100–105) have applied knowledge of metabolic pathways in the eye to alter a drug's elimination pathway. New

Table 6 Ocular Clearances $(Cl_0)^a$ for Drugs of Ophthalmic
Interest

Drug	Cl_0 (μL/min)	Ref.
Pilocarpine	13.0	35
Clonidine	14.9	28
Ketanserin	13.6	52
Phenylephrine	14.6	120
Flurbiprofen	14.4	2
Levobunolol	28.7	3
Dihydrolevobunolol	19.7	3
Propranolol	0.86	12
Phenylephrine	14.6	120
Ketorolac tromethamine	11.0	73
Ibufenac	18.7	51
Ibuprofen	8.4	51
Ethoxolamide	9.0	76
2-Benzothiazolesulfonamide	1.15	76
6-Hydroxyethoxy-2-benzothiazolesulfonamide	3.0	76
N-Methylacetazolamide	1.56	121
Acetazolamide	5.27	121

$^a Cl_0$ calculated from Eq. 4–6 in text.

drugs, referred to as "soft drugs," are designed for rapid metabolism and subsequent conversion to an active species before being eliminated from the eye. For example, an adamantylethyl of metaprolol has shown a prolonged and greater reduction of IOP and also a reduced potential to cause tachycardia when compared to timolol in the rabbit eye (103). In another example, timolol maleate was oxidized to a keto analog and coupled with either hydroxylamine or methoxyamine. The resulting drug candidates, timolone oxime and timolone methoxime, showed greater reduction of IOP than timolol in rabbits administered the drugs topically and did not show cardiovascular effects when administered intravenously to rabbits or rats (104).

Many enzyme systems have been identified within ocular tissues. As summarized by Plazonnet et al. (15), these are catechol-O-methyltransferase, monoamine oxidase, steroid 6-betahydroxylase, oxidoreductase, lysosomal enzymes, peptidases, glucuronide and sulfate transferase, and glutathione-conjugating enzymes. Arylamine acetyltransaferase activity was demonstrated by Campbell et al. (106) in an anterior chamber tissues using p-aminobenzoate, aminozolamide, and sulfamethazine as substrates. The rank order of arylamine acetyltransferase activity regardless of substrate was liver > iris/ciliary process > corneal epithelium > stroma/endothelium. Although fast- and slow-acetylating rabbits, classified with respect to their rate of hepatic acetylation, metabolized aminozolamide at different rates in liver tissue, no differences between phenotypes were observed for aminozolamide either in ocular disposition or in decline of IOP following topical instillation.

The distribution of ketone reductase activity in anterior chamber tissues was determined by Lee et al. (107) in order to explain the metabolism of levobunolol to dihydrolevobunolol. The rank order of activity was corneal epithelium > iris/ciliary body > conjunctiva > lens. No activity was detected in the tears, corneal stroma, sclera, or aqueous humor. Bovine ciliary body apparently contains aldehyde oxidase, which is responsible for the reduction of a number of compounds: N-oxide, hydroxamic acid, and sulfoxide and nitro compounds (108).

Metabolic models have been devised for ketanserin (52) and levobunolol (3) (Fig. 7). It is important to study ocular metabolism so that drug disposition is better understood and also in anticipation of a new drug candidate. For example, an endogenous corneal epithelial arachidonic acid metabolite formed by the cytochrome P450 system and a potent inhibitor of Na^+-K^+-ATPase was found to significantly lower IOP in the rabbit eye (109).

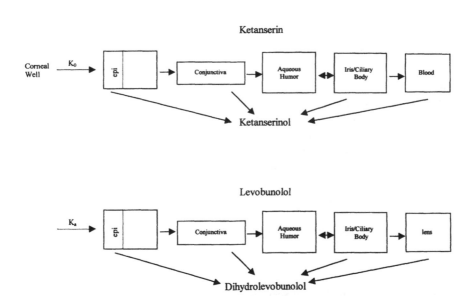

Figure 7 Metabolic schemes devised for ketanserin and levobunolol following absorption in the eye. (Adapted from Refs. 3 and 52.)

In general, the iris/ciliary body and the epithelium of the cornea appear to be anterior chamber tissues with the greatest capacity for metabolism.

V. PHARMACODYNAMICS

Because ophthalmic drugs are relatively potent and because of the difficulty in routinely measuring ophthalmic pharmacokinetics, the measurement of pharmacological responses in the animal or human eye has become a convenient and necessary aid in anticipating the clinical effect of an ophthalmic drug. The principal shortcoming to the use of pharmacological measurements either for optimizing therapy or for use as an aid in the development of new ophthalmic drugs is that the same dose often produces a different intensity of effect in different individuals. This variability occurs because of differences in dose-response relationships as well as differences in ocular pharmacokinetic behavior between individuals. Other factors that contribute to variability are eye pigmentation, whether or not an individual wears contact lenses, allergies to drugs or preservatives, and a number of physiological factors, which also determine intrasubject variation, such as eye discomfort leading to induced tearing, changes in blood pressure, hormonal concentrations, genetic differences, and/or changes in autonomic tone.

Although many ophthalmic pharmacological responses, such as miosis, mydriasis, IOP, flicker fusion, tear secretion, and aqueous turnover, can be easily measured over time, variability has been a major reason for the lack of a mathematical model. Pilocarpine and other muscarinic agonists that constrict the pupil have been studied extensively with respect to their miotic response. The response of an isolated strip of human sphincter muscle to carbachol and pilocarpine follows a typical sigmoidal-shaped dose or concentration-response relationship (110). Figure 8 is a recent representation of a concentration-response curve for S(+)flurbiprofen to COX-1 and COX-2 inhibition activity in homogenate human iris, with the latter treated with lippolysaccharide (111). Mishima (111) showed that this response, which represents one molecule binding competitively to a single muscarinic receptor, can be described as follows:

$$\frac{R}{R_{max} - R} = qC \tag{7}$$

In Eq. (7), R_{max} is the largest response that can be achieved by drug when all receptors are occupied, C is the drug concentration present in the incubation media, and q is a proportionality constant, which is equal to 1 if a single

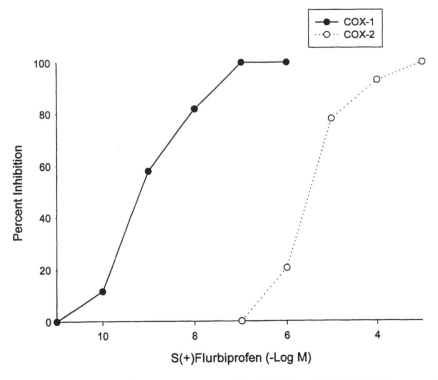

Figure 8 Concentration-response curves for inhibitin of the COX-1 (untreated) and COX-2 (treated with lipopolysaccharide) activity in human eye homogenate ($n = 4$–6). (Adapted from Ref. 112.)

molecule binds to a single receptor. Maurice and Mishima (85) further reported that Eq. (7) also correctly characterized the miosis of carbachol on the sphincter muscle of the cat, mydriasis of isoproterenol on bovine and rabbit sphincter muscle, mydriasis of 1-epinephrine and atropine on guinea pig iris, and mydriasis of epinephrine and acetylcholine on cat iris.

Gabrielsson and Weiner (113) analyzed the miotic response in the cat eye over time after application of three different doses of latanoprost. A simple one-compartment model was assumed with a first-order input into the eye with the biophase (site of the miotic response) associated with the central compartment. The concentration in the biophase was assumed to act directly on the response according to the sigmoid E_{max} model equation:

$$E(t) = E_0 + \frac{E_{max} C^n}{EC_{50}^n + C^n} \tag{8}$$

In Eq. (8), E_0 is the baseline value for the pupil size, E_{max} is the maximum effect, C is the concentration of drug in the biophase estimated from a kinetic model equation, EC_{50} is the concentration in the biophase at half-maximal effect, and n is the sigmoidicity factor.

Smolen and coworkers (114–118) developed a mathematical model for which pharmacological response intensities were transformed into biophasic drug levels for tropicamide, tridihexethylchloride, carbachol, and pilocarpine. The transformation was accomplished with the use of a precisely determined dose-response curve. The method requires a graded response that can be measured over time and expressed according to:

$$I = \frac{K_1 Q'_B}{1 + K_2 Q'_B} + P Q'_B \qquad (9)$$

where I is the intensity of response at any time and $Q'B$ is the concentration of drug in the biophase at the same time of measurement (normalized for dose: $Q'_B = Q_B/D$) and K_1, K_2, and P are constants derived from the fitting procedure.

Figure 9 shows the kinetics of the expected biophasic concentration of a drug after fitting miosis vs. time data to a kinetic model. After calculating the expected biophasic drug concentrations to Eq. (8) or (9), the response

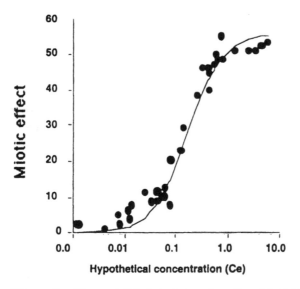

Figure 9 Observed (filled circles) and predicted (solid line) kinetics of a drug in the effect compartment following topical administration of three different doses. (Adapted from Ref. 113.)

intensities (I) or effect (E) can be fit to the concentration of drug estimated to be in the biophase. Figure 9 represents a fit to Eq. (8) for S(+)flurbipofen inhibition of prostaglandin E_2 to the COX-1 and COX-2 isoenzymes (113).

Use of Eq. (9) requires that the following assumptions are valid: (1) the same biophasic concentration of drug produces the same intensity of response (i.e., nonhysteresis), (2) binding to the receptor site is rapid and reversible, and (3) the pharmacokinetic processes are first order and therefore do not differ with dose. Application of this approach permits the optimization of a delivery system for an ophthalmic drug, insight into a drug's kinetics of response, and determination of a product's "biophasic bioavailability." The later term refers to the drug's absorption and disposition to the ocular site of action (114).

A mydriatic tolerance of the pupil response has been interpreted for phenylephrine from the application of the classic pharmacodynamic E_{max} model (119):

$$K_M = \left(\frac{\Delta E_{max}}{\Delta E(t)} - 1\right) C_a(t) \tag{10}$$

where K'_m is the drug concentration in aqueous humor required to produce one half of the maximal mydriatic response of phenylephrine ($1/2\ E_{max}$), $E(t)$ is the change in the mydriatic response from baseline at any time, and $Ca(t)$ is the concentration of drug in aqueous humor at the same time of measurement of E. In Eq. (10), K'_m is linearly related to $Ca(t)$ for a drug that does not develop tolerance, but if mydriatic tolerance is developed following topical instillation, the value of K'_m will vary with time. Chien and Schoenwald (119) measured the aqueous humor concentration of phenylephrine and its corresponding mydriatic response over time in the rabbit eye following a 10 uL topical instillation of phenylephrine HCl viscous solution (10%). A clockwise hysteresis effect of mydriasis vs. $C_a(t)$ is shown in Figure 10, which illustrates the development of tolerance over time. At the 240-minute time interval, the phenylephrine was twofold higher than that measured at the 20-minute time interval. However, at these two time intervals, the mydriatic response was similar. K'_m was linear up to 90 minutes, but steadily increased beyond 90 minutes through 240 minutes postinstillation.

Nonlinear pharmacokinetic behavior may be more common than has been observed since many ophthalmic drugs are known to alter physiological processes. Drugs that affect aqueous humor turnover or blood flow within the iris/ciliary body would be expected to show some degree of nonlinear pharmacokinetic behavior. Nevertheless, the inability to routinely measure concentrations of drug in the human eye provides a strong incentive to continue exploring the use of pharmacological response intensities to

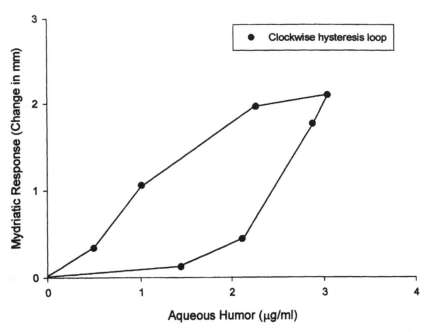

Figure 10 Average mydriasis measurement vs. aqueous humor concentrations of phenylephrine (clockwise hysteresis loop) following a 10 μL topical instillation of 10% phenylephrine HCl viscous solution. (Adapted from Ref. 119.)

either optimize therapy or povide a screning tool for use in developing new ophthalmic agents.

VI. CONCLUSION

It is important that the ocular pharmacokinetic behavior for drugs of ophthalmic interest be determined. Without a detailed knowledge of these processes, we must rely on the screening of new ophthalmic drugs intended for systemic use. For many years, drugs originally intended for systemic use and screened for use in the eye have provided good leads but were not optimized for ophthalmic potency or structurally altered to be devoid of systemic side effects when instilled topically to the eye. More recently, dipivefrin, latanoprost, unoprostone, dorzolamide, and brinzolamide were developed exclusively for the eye. A knowledge of ocular pharmacokinetic behavior is critical for optimizing therapeutic regimens following single and, particularly, multiple doses. It is not for lack of interest that prevents study of the ocular pharmacokinetic behavior of drugs, but because of the technical problems that have yet to be solved, the application of pharmacokinetics to the design of dosing regimens remains a goal. Specifically, a reliable method for serially measuring drug levels in aqueous humor without injury, pain, or risk of infection is yet to be developed for widespread use in the human eye.

At the present time, pharmacokinetic determinations in the human eye can only be made in subjects undergoing eye surgery. The patient is given the ophthalmic drug prior to entering surgery, and a sample of aqueous humor (or other tissue) is removed when it does not interfere with the surgery. In these experiments the time interval may not be measured accurately, and each patient's sample represents only one time interval. Consequently, a number of patient determinations at different time intervals must be averaged.

In lieu of human measuerments, an animal model is needed that is readily available and can accurately predict human ocular pharmacokinetics. The ideal animal model, whether a rabbit or monkey eye, should allow for accurate predictions in the human eye so that dosing regimens can be predicted. The pharmacokinetic measurements should be capable of assessing absorption (rate and extent), distribution, and elimination in volunteers and, in particular, patients. The model may be mathematically based but useful without extensive training and/or requiring specialized computer programs for its use. It should also allow for accurate predictions even though the drug itself may alter its own pharmacokinetic or pharmacodynamic processes over time, which may also complicate pharmacokinetic modeling since nonlinearity requires a unique set of assumptions for each drug. No doubt as these limitations are solved, the application of pharmacokinetics will become as extensively studied and applied to the human eye as it is now to drugs administered systemically. In the interim, it is useful to study various routes of administration and to measure tissue levels of drug for the purpose of determining if the minimum effective concentration is reached.

REFERENCES

1. McDonald, T. O., and Shadduck, J. A. (1977). *Eye Irritation. Determatoxicology and Pahrmacology* (H. Maibach and F. N. Marzulli, eds.). J. Wiley & Sons, New York, pp. 139–191.
2. Tang-Liu, D. D. S., Liu, S. S., and Weinkam R. J. (1984). Ocular and systemic bioavailability of ophthalmic flurbiprofen. *J. Pharmacokin. Biopharm.*, 12:611.

3. Tang-Liu, D. D. S., Liu, S. S., Neff, J., and Sandri, R. (1987). Disposition of levobunolol after an ophthalmic dose to rabbits. *J. Pharm. Sci.*, 76:780.

4. Miller, M. M., Madu, A., Samathanam, G., Rush, D., Madu, C. N., Mathisson, K., and Mayers, M. (1992). Flexoxacin pharmacokinetics in aqueous and vitreous humors determined by using complete concentration-time data from individual rabbits. *Antimicrob. Agents Chemother.*, 36:32.

5. Mayers, M., Rush, D., Madu, A., Motyl, M., and Miller, M. H. (1991). Pharmacokinetics of amikacin and chloramphenicol in the aqueous humor of rabbits. *Antimicrob. Agents Chemother.*, 35:1791.

6. Bito, L., Davson, H., Murray, L. M., and Snider, N. (1966). The concentration of free amino acids and other electrolytes in cerebrospinal fluid, in vivo dialysate of brain, and blood plasma of dog. *J. Neurochemistry* 13:1056.

7. Wang, Y., Wong, S. L., and Sawchuk, R. J. (1993). Microdialysis calibration using retrodialysis and zero-net flux: application to a study of the distribution of zidovudine to rabbit cerebrospinal fluid and thalamus. *Pharm. Res.*, 10:1411.

8. Sato, H., Fukuda, S., Inatomi, M., Koide, R., Uchida, N., Kanda, Y., Kiuchi, Y., and Oguchi, K. (1995). Pharmacokinetics of norfloxacin and lomefloxacin in domestic rabbit aqueous humor analyzed by microdialysis. *J. Jpn. Ophthalmol.*, 7:513.

9. Ohtori, R., Sato, H., Fukuda, S., Ueda, T., Koide, R., Kanda, Y., Kiuchi, Y., and Oguchi, K. (1998). Pharmacokinetics of topical beta-adrenergic antagonists in rabbit aqueous humor evaluated with the microdialysis method. *Exp. Eye Res.*, 66:487.

10. Rittenhouse, K. D., Peiffer, R. L., and Pollack, G. M. (1999). Microdialysis evaluation of the ocular pharmacokinetics of propanolol in the conscious rabbit. *Pharm. Res.*, 16:736.

11. Ben-Nun, J., Cooper, R. L., Cringle, S. J., and Constable, I.J. (1988). A new technique for in vivo intraocular pharmacokinetic measurements. *Arch. Ophthalmol*, 106:254.

12. Rittenhouse, K. D., Peiffer Jr., R. L., and Pollack, G.M. (1998). Evaluation of microdialysis sampling of aqueous humor for in vivo models of ocular absorption and disposition. *J. Pharm. Biomed. Anal.*, 16:951.

13. Hughes, P. M., Krishnamoorthy, R., and Mitra, A. (19xx.) Vitreous disposition of two acycloguanosine antivirals in the albino and pigmented rabbit models: a novel ocular microdialysis technique. *J. Ocul. Pharmacol. Ther.*, 12:209.

14. Schoenwald, R. D. (1990). Ocular drug delivery. Pharmcokinetic considerations. *Clin. Pharmacokinet.*, 18:255.

15. Plazonnet, B., Grove, J., Durr, M., Mazuel, C., Quint, M., and Rozier, A. (1977). Pharmacokinetics and biopharmaceutical aspects of some anti-glaucoma drugs. In *Ophthalmic drug Delivery Biopharmaceutical Technological and Clinical Aspects* (M. F. Saettone, M. Bucci, and P. Speiser, eds.). Springer-Verlag, Berlin, pp. 118–139.

16. Lee, V. H. L., and Robinson, J. R. (1986). Review: topical ocular drug delivery: recent developments and future challenges. *J. Ocular Pharmacol.* 267.

17. O'Day, D. M., Head, W. S., Foulds, G., Robinson, R. D., Williams, T. E., and Ferraina, R. A. (1994). Ocular pharmacokinetics of orally administered azithromycin in rabbits. *J. Ocul. Pharmacol.*, 10:633.

18. Berthe, P., Baudouin, C., Garraffo, R., Hofmann, P., Taburet, A.-M., and Lapalus P. (1994). Toxicologic and pharmacokinetic analysis of intravitreal injections of foscarnet, either alone or in combination with ganciclovir. *Invest. Ophthalmol. Vis. Sci.*, 35:1038.

19. Oh, C., Saville, B. A., Cheng, Y.-L., and Rootman, D. S. (1995). A compartmental model for ocular pharmacokinetics of cyclosporine in rabbits. *Pharm. Res.*, 12:433.

20. Schoenwald, R. D., Harris, R. G., Turner, D., Knowles, W. and Chien, D. S. (1987). Ophthalmic bioequivalence of steroid/antibiotic combination formulations. *Biopharm. Drug Disposit.*, 8:527.

21. Tang-Liu, D. D. S., and Burke S. S. (1988). The effect of azone on ocular levobunolol absorption: calculating the area under the curve and its standard error using tissue sampling compartments. *Pharm. Res.*, 5:238.

22. Pettersson, K. J., and Nordgren, T. (1989). Determination of phosphonoformate (foscarnet) in biological fluids by ion pair reversed-phase liquid chromatography. *J. Chromatogr.*, 488:447.

23. Chrai, S. S., Makoid, M. C., Eriksen, S. P., and Robinson, J. R. (1974). Drop size and initial dosing frequency problems of topically applied ophthalmic drugs. *J. Pharm. Sci.*, 63:333.

24. Chrai, S. S., and Robinson, J. R. (1974). Ocular evaluation of methylcellulose vehicle in albino rabbits. *J. Pharm. Sci.*, 63:1218.

25. Chrai, S. S., Patton, T. F., Mehta, A. and Robinson, J. R. (1973). Lacrimal and instilled fluid dynamics in rabbit eyes. *J. Pharm. Sci.*, 62:1112.

26. Burstein, N. L., and Anderson, J. A. (1985). Corneal penetration and ocular bioavailability of drugs. *J. Ocular Pharmacol.*, 1:309.

27. Makoid, M. C., and Robinson, J. R. (1979). Pharmacokinetics of topically applied pilocarpine in the albino rabbit eye. *J. Pharm. Sci.*, 68:435.

28. Chiang C. H., and Schoenwald, R. D. (1986). Ocular pharmacokinetic models of clonidine-^{3}H hydrochloride. *J. Pharmacokin. Biopharm.*, 14:175.

29. Gibaldi, M., and Perrier, D. (1982). *Pharmacokinetics*, 2nd ed. Marcel Dekker, New York, pp. 145–166.

30. Hämäläinen, K.M., Kananen, K., Auriola, S., Kontturi, K., and Urtti, A. (1997). Characterization of paracellular and aqueous penetration routes in cornea, conjunctiva, and sclera. *Invest. Ophthalmol. Vis. Sci.*, 38:627.

31. Schoenwald, R. D., Deshpande, G. S., Rethwisch, D. G., and Barfknecht, C. F. (1997). Penetration into the anterior chamber via the conjunctival/scleral pathway. *J. Ocular Pharm. Ther.*, 13:41.

32. Wagner, J. G. (1975). *Fundamentals of Clinical Pharmacokinetics*. Drug Intelligence Publications, Hamilton, IL, pp. 102–106.

33. Kalsi, G. S., Gudauskas, G., Bussanich, N., Freeman, D. J., and Rootman, J. (1991). Ocular pharmacokinetics of subconjunctivally administered cyclosporine in the rabbit. *Can. J. Ophthalmol.*, 26:200.

34. Acheampong, A. A., Shackleton, M., Tang-Liu, D. D.-S., Ding, S., Stern, M. E., and Decker, R. (1998). Distribution of cyclosporin A in ocular tissues after topical administration to albino rabbits and beagle dogs. *Curr. Eye Res.*, 18:91.

35. Miller, S. C., Himmelstein, K. J., and Patton, T. F. (1981). A physiologically based pharmacokinetic model for the intraocular distribution of pilocarpine in rabbits. *J. Pharmacokin. Biopharm.*, 9:653.

36. Ettl, A., Hofmann, U., Daxer, A., Dietrich, H., Schmid, E., and Eichelbaum, M., (1998). Ocular pharmacokinetics of verapamil in rabbits. *Naunyn-Schmiedeberg's Arch. Pharmacol.*, 357:331.

37. Schoenwald, R. D., Gadiraju, R. R., and Barfknecht, C. F. (1997). Serotonin antagonists for use as antiglaucoma agents and their ocular penetration. *Eur. J. Pharm. Biopharm.*, 43:273.

38. Palmero, M., Bellot, J. L., Alcoriza, N., and García-Cabanes, C. (1997). The ocular pharmacokinetics of topical dicloenac is affected by ocular inflammation. *Ophthalmic Res.*, 31:309.

39. Bauer, N.J. C., Motamedi, N., Wicksted, J. P., March, W. F., Webers, C. A. B., and Hendrikse, F. (1999). Non-invasive assessment of ocular pharmacokinetics using confocal raman spectroscopy. *J. Ocular Pharmacol. Ther.*, 15:123.

40. Yamamura, K., Sasaki, H., Nakashima, M., Ichikawa, M., Mukai, T., Nishida, K., and Nakamura, J. (1999). Characterization of ocular pharmacokinetics of beta-blockers using a diffusion model after instillation. *Pharm. Res.*, 16:1595.

41. Sasaki, H., Yamamura, K., Mukai, T., Nishida, K., Nakamura, J., Nakashima, M., and Ichikawa, M. (1999). Characterization of ocular pharmacokinetics of tilisolol after instillation into anesthetized rabbits. *Biol. Pharm. Bull.*, 22:1253.

42. Velpandian, T., Gupta, S. K., Gupta, Y. K., Agarwal, H. C., and Biswas, N. R. (1999). Comparative studies on topical lomefloxacin and ciprofloxacin on ocular kinetic and experimental corneal ulcer. *J. Ocular Pharmacol. Ther.*, 15:505.

43. Desai, S. (1993). Ocular pharmacokinetics of tobramycin. *Int. Ophthalmol.*, 17:201.

44. Lee, V. H. L., and Robinson, J. R. (1979). Mechanistic and quantitative evaluation of precorneal pilocarpine disposition in albino rabbits. *J. Pharm. Sci.*, 68:673.

45. Himmelstein, K. J., Guvenir, I., and Patton, T. P. (1978). Preliminary pharmacokinetic model of pilocarpine uptake and distribution in the eye. *J. Pharm. Sci.*, 67:603.

46. Patton, T. F., and Robinson, J. R. (1976). Quantitative precorneal disposition of topically applied pilocarpine ntirate in rabbit eyes. *J. Pharm. Sci.*, 65:1295.

47. Conrad, J. M., and Robinson, J. R. (1977). Aqueous chamber drug distribution volume measurements in rabbits. *J. Pharm. Sci.*, 66:219.

48. Kitaura, T, Tsukiai, S., Arai, S., Miyake, K., Kimura, M., and Fukuchi, H. (1998). Ocular pharmacokinetics of latamoxef and cefaclor in humans. Penetration into aqueous humor. *J. Pharmacobio-Dyn.*, 12:60.

49. Aldana, I., Fos, D., Peñas, E. G., Gazzaniga, A., Gianesello, V., Monti, N. C., Figini, P. G., Zato, M. A., Bruseghini, L., and Esteras, A. (1992). Ocular pharmacokinetics of thiamphenicol in rabbits. *Asneim. Forsch. Drug Res.*, 42:1236.

50. Ben-Nun, J., Joyce, D. A., Cooper, R. L., Cringle, S. J., and Constable, I. J. (1989). Pharmacokinetics of intravitreal injection. 30:1055.

51. Rao, C. S., Schoenwald, R. D., Barfknecht, C. F., and Laban S. L. (1992). Biopharmaceutical evaluation of ibufenac, ibuprofen, and their hydroxyethoxy analogs in the rabbit eye. *J. Pharmcokin. Biopharm.*, 230:357.

52. Schoenwald, R. D., and Zhu, J. (2000). The ocular pharmacokinetics of ketanserin and its metabolite, ketansreinol, in albino rabbits. *J. Ocular Pharmacol. Ther.*, 16:479.

53. Huang, A. J. W., Tseng S. C. G., and Kenyon, K. R. (1989). Paracellular permeability of corneal and conjunctival epithelia. *Invest. Ophthalmol. Vis. Sci.*, 30:684.

54. Occhipinti, J. R., Mosier, M. A., LaMotte, J., and Monji G. T. (1988). Fluorophotometric measurement of human tear turnover rate. *Curr. Eye Res.*, 7:995.

55. Palestine, A. G., and Brubaker, R. F. (1981). Pharmacokinetics of fluorescein in the vitreous. *Invest. Ophthalmol. Vis. Sci.*, 21:542.

56. Igarashi, H., Sato, Y., Hamada, S., and Kawasaki, T. (1984). Studies on rabbit corneal permeability of local anesthetics. *Jpn. J. Pharmacol.*, 34:429.

57. Schoenwald, R. D., and Huang, H. S. (1983). Corneal penetration behavior of beta-blocking agents I: Physicochemical factors. *J. Pharm. Sci.*, 72:1266.

58. Huang, H. S., Schoenwald, R. D., and Lach, J. L. (1983). Corneal penetration behavior of beta-blocking agents II: Assessment of barrier contributions. *J. Pharm. Sci.*, 72:1272.

59. Chiang, C. H., Huang, H. S., and Schoenwald, R. D. (1986). Corneal permeability of adrenergic agents potentially useful in glaucoma. *J. Taiwan Pharm. Assoc.*, 38:67.

60. Grass, G. M., and Robinson, J. R. (1988). Mechanisms of corneal drug penetration II: Ultrastructural analysis of potential pathways for drug movement. *J. Pharm. Sci.*, 77:15.

61. Camber, O., Edman, P., and Olsson, L. I. (1986). Permeability of Prostaglandin F_{2alpha} and prostaglandin F_{2alpha} and prostaglandin F_{2alpha} esters across cornea in vitro. *Int. J. Pharm.*, 29:259.

62. Corbo D. C., Liu, J. C., and Chien, Y. W. (1990). Characterization of the barrier properties of mucosal membranes. *J. Pharm. Sci.*, 79:202.

63. Gibaldi, M., and Perrier, D. (1982). *Pharmacokinetics*, 3nd ed. Marcel Dekker, New York, pp. 475–477.

64. O'Day, D, Head, W. S., Robinson, R. D., Williams, T. E., and Wolff, R. (1992). Ocular pharmacokinetics of saperconazole in rabbits. *Arch. Ophthalmol.*, 110:550.

65. Baeyens, V., and Gurney, R., (1997). Chemical and physical parameters of tears relevant for the design of the ocular drug delivery formulations. *Pharm. Acta Helvetica*, 72:191.

66. Le Bourlais, C., Acar, L., Zia, H., Sado, P. A., Needham, T.,and Leverage, R. (1998). Ophthalmic drug delivery systems—recent advances. *Prog. Ret. Eye Res.*, 17:33.

67. Tang-Liu, D. D.-S., and Sandri, R. (1989). Ocular biodistribution of clonidine after topical application with ophthalmic rods or solution. *J. Ocular Pharmacol.*, 5:133.

68. Ito,Y., Cai, H., Koizumi, Y., Hori, R., Terao, M., Kimura, T., Takagi, S., and Tomohiro, M. (2000). Effects of lipid composition on the transcorneal penetration of liposomes containing disulfiram, a potential anti-cataract agent, in the rabbit. *Biol. Pharm. Bull.*, 23:327.

69. Zane, P. A., Brindle, S. D., Gause, D. O., O'Buck, A. J., Raghavan, P. R., and Tripp, S. L. (1990). Physiological factors associated with binding and retention of compounds in ocular melanin or rats: correlations using data from whole body autoradiography and molecular modeling for multiple linear regression analyses. *Pharm. Res.*, 9:935.

70. Kahn, M., Barney, N. P., Briggs, R. M., Bloch, K. J., and Allansmith, M. R., (1990). Penetrating the conjunctival barrier. *Invest. Ophthalmol. Vis. Sci.*, 31:258.

71. Ahmed, I., Gokhale, R. D., Shah, M. V., and Patton, T. F. (1987). Physicochemical determinants of drug diffusion across the conjunctiva, sclera, and cornea. *J. Pharm. Sci.*, 76:583.

72. Maurice, D. (1997). Characterization of paracellular penetration routes. *Invest. Ophthalmol. Vis. Sci.*, 38:2177.

73. Ling, T. L., and Combs, D. L. (1987). Ocular bioavailability and tissue distribution of [^{14}C]ketorolac tromethamine in rabbits. *J. Pharm. Sci.*, 76:289.

74. Wagner, J. G. (1993). *Pharmacokinetics for the Pharmaceutical Scientist.* Technomic Publishing Co., Lancaster, PA, pp. 27–33.

75. Gibaldi, M., and Perrier, D. (1982). *Pharmacokinetics*, 2nd ed. Marcel Dekker, New York, pp. 409–417.

76. Eller, M. G., Schoenwald, R. D., Dixson, J. A., Segarra, T., and Barfknecht, C. F. (1985). Topical carbonic anhydrase inhibitors IV: relationship between excised corneal permeability and pharmacokinetic factors. *J. Pharm. Sci.*, 74:525.

77. Morlet, N., Graham, G. G., Gatus, B., McLachlan A. J., Salonikas, C., Naidoo, D., Goldberg, I., and Lam, C. M. (2000). Pharmacokinetics of ciprofloxacin in the human eye; a clinical study and population pharmacokinetic analysis. *Antimicrob. Agents Chemother.*, 44:1674.

78. Putnam, M. L., Schoenwald, R. D., Duffel, M. W., Barfknecht, C. F., Segarra, T. M., and Campbell, D. A. (1987). Ocular disposition of aminozolamide in the rabbit eye. *Invest. Ophthalmol. Vis. Sci.*, 28:1373.

79. Chien, D. S., Homsy, J. J., Gluchowski, C., and Tang-liu, D. D. S. (1990). Corneal and conjunctival/scleral penetration of p-aminoclonidine, AGN 190342, and clonidine. *Curr. Eye Res.*, 9:1051.

80. Schoenwald, R. D., Tandon, V., Wurster, D. E., and Barfknecht, C. F. (1998). Significance of melanin binding and metabolism in the activity of 5-acetoxyacetylimino-4-methyl-Δ^2-1,3,4-thiadiazoline-2-sulfonamide. *Eur. J. Pharm. Biopharm.*, 46:39.

81. Hitoshi, S., Bundgaard, H., and Lee, V.H. L. (1989). Design of prodrugs to selectively reduce timolol absorption on the basis of the differential lipophilic characteristics of the cornea and the conjunctiva. *Invest. Ophthalmol. Vis. Sci.*, 30(Suppl.):25.

82. Edelhauser, H. F., and Maren, t. H. (1988). Permeability of human cornea and sclera to sulfonamide carbonic anhydrase inhibitors. *Arch. Ophthalmol.*, 106:110.

83. Camras, C. B., Bito, L. Z., and Toris, C. B. (19xx). Prostaglandins and prostaglandiin analogues. In *Textbook of Ocular Pharmacology* (T. J. Zimmerman, K. S. Kooner, M. Sharir, and R. D. Fechtner, eds.). Lippincott-Raven Publishers, Philadelphia, pp. 315–328.

84. Friedland, B. R., and Muther, T. F. (1978). Autoradiographic localization of carbonic anhydrase in the ciliary body. *Invest. Ophthalmol. Vis. Sci.*, (suppl.):162.

85. Maurice, D. M., and Mishima, S. (1984). Ocular pharmacokinetics. In *Pharmacology of the Eye* (M. L. Sears, ed.). Springer-Verlag, Berlin, pp. 19–116.

86. Ahmed, I. Francoeur, M. L., Thombre, A. G., and Patton, T. F. (1989). The kinetics of timolol in the rabbit lens: implications for ocular drug delivery. *Pharm. Res.*, 6:772.

87. Maurice, D. (1987). Kinetics of topically applied ophthalmic drugs. In *Ophthalmic Drug Delivery: Biopharmaceutical, Technological and Clinical Aspects* (M. F. Saettone, M. Bucci, and P. Speiser, eds.). Springer-Verlag, Berlin, pp. 19–26.

88. Liu, W., Liu, Q. F., Perkins, R., Drusano, G., Louie, A., Madu, A., Mian, U., Mayers, M., and Miller, M. H. (1998). Pharmacokinetics of sparfloxacin in the serum and vitreous humor of rabbits: physicochemical properties that regulate penetration of quinolone antimicrobials. *Antimicrob. Agents Chemother.*, 42:1417.

89. Perkins, R. J., W. Liu, Drusano, G., Madu, M., Mayers, M., Madu, and Miller, M. H. (1995). Pharmacokinetics of ofloxacin in serum and vitreous humor of albino and pigmented rabbits. *Antimicrob. Agents Chemother.*, 39:1493.

90. Lee, V.H. L., Chang, S. C., Oshiro, C. M., and Smith, R. E. (1985). Ocular esterase composition in albino and pigmented rabbits: possible implications in ocular prodrug design and evaluation. *Curr. Eye Res.*, 4:1117.

91. Chien, D. S., Bundgaard, H., and Lee, V. H. L. (1988). Influence of corneal epithelial integrity on the penetration of timolol prodrugs. *J. Ocular Pharmacol.*, 4:137.

92. Lee, V. H. L., Morimoto, K. M., and Stratford, Jr., R. E. (1982). Esterase distribution in the rabbit cornea and its implications in ocular drug bioavailability. *Biopharm. Drug Disposit.*, 3:291.

93. Lee, V. H. (1983). Esterase activities in adult rabbit eyes. *J. Pharm. Sci.*, 72:239.

94. Chien, D. S., and Schoenwald, R. D. (1986). Improving the ocular absorption of phenylephrine. *Biopharm. Drug Disposit.*, 7:45.

95. Schoenwald, R. D., Folk, J. C., Kumar, V., and Piper, J. G. (1987). In vivo comparison of phenylephrine and phenylephrine oxazolidine instilled in the monkey eye. *J. Ocular Pharmacol.*, 3:333.

96. Chang, S. C., Bundgaard, H., Buur, A., and Lee, V. H. L. (1987). Improved corneal penetration of timolol by prodrugs as a means to reduce systemic drug load. *Invest. Ophthalmol. Vis. Sci.*, 28:487.

97. Bundgaard, H., Falch, E., Larsen, C., and Mikkelson, T. (1986). Pilocarpine prodrugs I. Synthesis, physicochemical properties and kinetics of lactonization of pilocarpic acid esters. *J. Pharm. Sci.*, 75:36.

98. Bundgaard, H., Falch, E., Larsen, C., Mosher, G. L., and Mikkelson, T. (1986). Pilocarpine prodrugs II. Synthesis, stbility, bioconversion, and physicochemical properties of sequentially labile pilocarpine acid diesters. *J. Pharm. Sci.*, 75:775.

99. Narukar, M. M., and Mitra A. K. (1989). Prodrugs of 5-iodo-2'-deoxyuridine for enhanced ocular transport. *Pharm. Res.*, 6:887.

100. Bodor, N., and Buchwald, P. (2000). Soft drug design: general principles and recent applications. *Med. Res. Rev.*, 20:58.

101. Buchwald, A., Browne, C. E., Wu, W. M., and Bodor, N. (2000). Soft cannabinoid analogues as potential anti-glaucoma agents. *Pharmazie*, 55:196.

102. Farag, H. H., Wu, W. M., Barros, M. D., Somogyi, G., Prokai,L., and Bodor, N. (1997). *Drug Des. Disc.*, 15:117.

103. Bodor, N., El-Koussi, A., Kano, M., and Khalifa, M. M. (1988). Soft drugs. 7. Soft β-blockers for systemic and ophthalmic use. *J. Med. Chem.*, 31:1651.

104. Bodor, N., Farag, H. H., Somogyi, G., Wu, W.M., and Prokai, L. (1997). Ocular-specific delivery of timolol by sequential bioactivation of its oxime and methoxime analogs. *J. Ocular Pharmacol. Ther.*, 13:389.

105. Kumar, G. N., Hammer, R. H., Wu, W. M., and Bodor, N. S. (1993). Mydriatic activity and transcorneal penetration of phenylsuccinic soft analogs of methscopolamine as short acting mydriatics. *Curr. Eye. Res.*, 12:501.

106. Campbell, D. A., Schoenwald, R. D., Duffel, M. W., and Barfknecht, C. F. (1991). Characterization of arylamine acetyltransferase in the rabbit eye. *Invest. Ophthalmol. Vis. Sci.*, 32:2190.

107. Lee, V. H. L., Chien, D. S., and Sasaki, H. (1988). Ocular ketone reductase distribution and its role in the metabolism of ocular applied levobunolol in the pigmented rabbit. *J. Pharmacol. Exp. Ther.*, 246:871.

108. Shimada, S., Mishima, H., Kitamura, S., and Tatsumi, K. (1987). Nicotinamide N-oxide reductase activity in bovine and rabbit eyes. *Invest. Ophthalmol. Vis. Sci.*, 28:1204.

109. Masferrer, J. L., Dunn, M. W., and Schwartzman, M. L. (1990). 12(R)-Hydroxyeicosatetraenoic acid, an endogenous corneal arachidonate metabolite, lower intraocular pressure in rabbits. *Invest. Ophthamol. Vis. Sci.*, 31:535.

110. O'Hara, K. (1977). Effects of cholinergic agonists on isolated iris sphincter muscles: a pharmacodynamic study. *Jpn. J. Ophthalmol.*, 21:516.

111. Mishima, S. (1981). Clinical pharmacokinetics of the eye. *Invest. Ophthalmol. Vis. Sci.*, 21:504.

112. Van Haeringen, N. J., Van Sorge, A. A., and Carballosa Coré-Bodelier, V. M. W. (2000). Constitutive cyclooxygenase-1 and induced cyclooxygenase-2 in isolated human iris inhibited by S(+) flurbiprofen. *J. Ocular Pharmacol. Ther.*, 16:353.

113. Gabrielsson, J., and Weiner, D. (1997). Dose-response-time analysis I. In *Pharmacokinetic and Pharmacodynamic Data Analysis Concepts and Applications*, 2nd ed. Swedish Pharmaceutical Society, Swedish Pharmaceutical Press, Stockholm, Sweden, pp. 717–723.

114. Smolen, V. F., and Schoenwald, R. D. (1971). Drug absorption analysis from pharmacological data I. The method and its confirmation exemplified for a mydriatic drug, tropicamide. *J. Pharm. Sci.* 60:96.

115. Schoenwald, R. D., and Smolen, V. F. (1971). Drug absorption analysis from pharmacological data. II Transcorneal biophasic availability of tropicamide. *J. Pharm. Sci.*, 60:1039.

116. Smolen, V. F., and Schoenwald, R. D. (1974). Drug absorption analysis from pharmacological data. III. Influence of polymers and pH on transcorneal biophasic availability and myriatic response of tropicamide. *J. Pharm. Sci.*, 63:1582.

117. Smolen, V. F. (1972). Applications of a pharmacological method of drug absorption analysis to the study of the bioavailability characteristics of mydriatic drugs. *Can. J. Pharm. Sci.*, 7:7.

118. Smolen, V. F. (1975). Drug bioelectrometric study of the mechanisms of carbachol interactions with the cornea and its relation to miotic activity. *J. Pharm. Sci.*, 64:526.

119. Chien, D. S., and Schoenwald, R. D. (1990). Ocular pharmacokinetics and pharmacodynamics of phenylephrine and phenylephrine oxazolidine in rabbit eyes. *Pharm. Res.*, 7:476.

120. Schoenwald, R. D., and Chien D. S. (1988). Ocular absorption and disposition of phenylephrine and phenylephrine oxazolidine. *Biopharm. Drug Disposit.*, 9:527.

121. Eng. I. S. (1986). Ph.D. thesis, University of Iowa College of Pharmacy.

122. Valeri, P., Palmery, M., Severini, G., Piccinelli, D, and Catanese, B. (1986). Ocular pharmacokinetics of dapiprazole. *Pharmacol. Res. Comm.*, 18:1093.

123. Brazzell, R. K., Wooldridge, C. B., Hackett, R. B., and McCue B. A. (1990). Pharmacokinetics of the aldose reductase inhibitor inhibitor imirestat following topical ocular administration. *Pharm. Res.*, 7:192.

124. Gudauskas, G., Kumi, C., Dedhar, C., Bussanich, N., and Rootman, J. (1985). Ocular pharmacokinetics of subconjunctivally versus intravenously administered 6-mercaptopurine. *Can. J. Ophthalmol.*, 20:110.
125. Taylor P. B., Burd, E. M., and Tabbara, K. (1987). Corneal and intraocular penetration of topical and subconjunctival fusidic acid. *Bri. J. Ophthalmol.*, 71:598.
126. Kleinberg, J., Dea, F. J., Anderson, J. A., and Leopold I. H. (19xx). Intraocular penetration of topically applied lincomycin hydrochloride in rabbits, Arch. Ophthalmol, 97:933.
127. Hui, H. W., Zeleznick, L., and Robinson J. R. (1984). Ocular disposition of topically applied histamine, cimetidine and pyrilamine in the albino rabbit. *Curr. Eye Res.*, 3:321.
128. Maren T. H., and Jankowska, L. (1985). Ocular pharmacology of sulfonamides: the cornea as barrier and depot. *Curr. Eye Res.*, 4:399.
129. Walstad, R. A., Hellum K. Blika S., Dale L. G., Fredriksen, T., Myhre, K. I., and Spencer, G. R. (1983). Pharmacokinetics and tissue penetration of ceftazidime: studies on lymph, aqueous humor, skin blister, cerebrospinal and pleural fluid. *J. Antimicrob. Chemother.*, 12 (Suppl. A):275.
130. Barza, M., Kane, A., and Baum, J. L. (1979). Intraocular levels of cefamandole compared with cefazolin after subconjunctival injection in rabbits. *Invest. Ophthalmol. Vis. Sci.*, 18:250.
131. Auclair, E., Laude, D., Wainer, I. W., Chaouloff, F., and Elghozi, J. L. (1988). Comparative pharmacokinetics of D- and L-alphamethyldopa in plasma, aqueous humor, and cerebrospinal fluid in rabbits. *Fundam. Clin. Pharmacol.*, 2:283.
132. Grove, J., Gautheron, P., Plazonnet, B., and Sugrue, M. F. (1988). Ocular distribution studies of the topical carbonic anhydrase inhibitors L-643,799 and L-650,719 and related alkyl prodrugs. *J. Ocular Pharmacol.*, 4:279.
133. Agata, M., Tanaka, M., Nakajima, A., Fujii, A., Kuboyama, N., Tamura, T., and Araie, M. (1984). Ocular penetration of topical diclofenac sodium, a nonsteroidal anti-inflammatory drug, in rabbit eye. *Nippon Ganka Gakkai Zashi*, 88:991.
134. Anderson, J. A., Chen, C. C., Vita, J. B., and Shackleton, M. (1982). Disposition of topical flurbiprofen in normal and aphakic rabbit eyes. *Arch. Ophthalmol.*, 100:642.
135. Barza, M., and McCue, M. (1983). Pharmacokinetics of aztreonam in rabbit eyes. *Invest. Ophthalmol. Vis. Sci.*, 24:468.
136. Huuopponen, R., Kaila, T., Salminen, L., and Urtti, A. (1987). The pharmacokinetics of ocularly applied timolol in rabbits. *Acta Ophthalmol.*, 65:63.
137. Huang, H. S., Schoenwald, R. d., and Lach, J. L. (1983). Corneal penetration behavior of beta-blocking agents III: in vitro-in vivo correlations. *J. Pharm. Sci.*, 72:1279.
138. Leibowitz, H. M., Ryan, W. J., Kupferman, A., and DeSantis, L. (1986). Bioavailability and corneal anti-inflammatory effect of topical suprofen. *Invest. Ophthalmol. Vis. Sci.*, 27:628.

139. Sugrue, M. F., Gautheron, P., Mallorga, T. E., Nolan, S. L., Graham, H., Schwam, H., Shepard, K. L., and Smith R. L. (1990). L-662,583 is topically effective ocular hypotensive carbonic anhydrase inhibitor in experimental animals. *Br. J. Pharmacol.*, 99:59.

140. Mester, U., Krasemann, C., and Werner, H. (1982). Cefsulodine concentrations in rabbit eyes after intravenous and subconjunctival administration. *Ophthalmol. Res.*, 14:129.

141. Rootman, J., Ostry, A., and Gudauskas, G. (1984). Pharmacokinetics and metabolism of 5-fluorouracil following subconjunctival versus intravenous administration. *Can. J. Ophthalmol.*, 19:187.

142. Lee, v. H.L., and Robinson, J. R. (1982). Disposition of pilocarpine in the pigmented rabbit eye. *Int. J. Pharm.*, 11:155.

143. Vigo, J. F., Rafart, J., Concheiro, A., Martinez, R., and Cordido, M. (1988). Ocular penetration and pharmacokinetics of cefotaxime: an experimental study. *Curr. Eye Res.*, 7:1149.

144. Sugrue, M. F. (1996). The preclinical pharmacology of dorzolamide hydrochloride, a topical carbonic anhydrase inhibitor. *J. Ocular Pharmacol. Ther.*, 12:363.

6
Mathematical Modeling of Drug Distribution in the Vitreous Humor

Stuart Friedrich, Bradley Saville, and Yu-Ling Cheng
University of Toronto, Toronto, Canada

I. INTRODUCTION

A. Vitreous Physiology

The vitreous humor is a viscous fluid occupying the space between the lens and retina of the eye. A number of diseases that can affect the vitreous or the surrounding retina can be treated by administration of various therapeutic drugs. Due to physiological barriers within the eye that prevent drug in the systemic circulation from entering the vitreous, the most common method of treating diseases affecting the vitreous or retina is a direct intravitreal injection of drug (1). Many of the drugs used to treat vitreous and retinal disorders have a narrow concentration range in which they are effective, and they may be toxic at higher concentrations (2–6). Therefore, knowledge of the drug distribution following intravitreal administration is important if the disease is to be properly treated and damage to tissues by high concentrations of drug is to be avoided.

There are three main tissues that bound the vitreous humor: the retina, lens, and hyaloid membrane. The retina covers the posterior portion of the interior of the globe and is immediately adjacent to the vitreous. In a rabbit eye, the retina is supplied with nutrients via the choroid, the tissue layer directly outside the retina. The choroid has a vast network of capillaries, while the retina is avascular. The retina is made up of several cellular layers, some of which form the blood-retinal barrier that prevents extraneous compounds from entering the vitreous from the bloodstream. The vitreous to blood permeability of the blood-retinal barrier depends on the physicochemical properties of the drug. Some drugs cannot penetrate the barrier, while others may be actively transported between the vitreous and the blood. The lens forms the majority of the anterior boundary of the vitreous humor. The lens is composed of highly compacted cellular material and is therefore highly impermeable to most drugs. The hyaloid membrane is composed of loosely packed collagen fibers and spans the gap between the lens and the ciliary body. Although the hyaloid membrane forms a boundary between the stagnant vitreous and the flowing aqueous humor, it does not form a limiting barrier to the transport of low molecular weight compounds. The aqueous humor is continuously produced by the ciliary body and drained from the anterior chamber of the aqueous humor after it passes between the iris and the lens. Therefore, once drug passes through the hyaloid membrane from the vitreous it is eliminated by the flow of aqueous humor.

B. Properties of Intravitreal Injected Drug Solutions

The distribution of a drug solution within the vitreous immediately following intravitreal injection may be dependent on several factors. Needle gauge, needle length, penetration angle of the needle, speed of the injection, rheology of the injected solution, and rheology of the vitreous could all affect how the drug solution is initially distributed in the vitreous. The shape that the drug solution assumes immediately after injection may range from globular to irregular shapes that vary in the extent of fingering. Such variations in shapes would influence the diffusional surface area and hence drug distribution within the vitreous (7).

C. Experimental Measurements of Drug Distribution in the Vitreous and Retinal Permeability

Due to the difficulty in measuring solute concentrations within the vitreous, there has only been one published report that shows experimentally measured concentration profiles of model compounds across an entire cross section of the rabbit vitreous (8). The compounds used in the study were fluorescein, fluorescein glucuronide, and fluorescein isothiocyanate. The main elimination route for fluorescein is across the retina; conversely, fluorescein glucuronide has a very low retinal permeability and is eliminated mainly across the hyaloid membrane. As a result of their contrasting elimination characteristics, the experimental fluorescein and fluorescein glucuronide concentration profiles observed by Araie and Maurice (8) are ideal for comparing to concentration profiles calculated by a mathematical model as a test of the model's robustness.

The in vitro permeability of an excised rabbit retina to fluorescein and fluorescein glucuronide has been measured by Koyano et al. (9). Retinal permeabilities can also be determined by fitting vitreous concentrations calculated by a mathematical model to experimental data, such as the data observed by Araie and Maurice (8). Therefore, the in vitro retinal permeability found by Koyano et al. can be compared to model calculated retinal permeabilities as a method of model validation.

II. EARLY MATHEMATICAL MODELS OF THE VITREOUS HUMOR

Several models have been developed to simulate the distribution and elimination of drugs from the vitreous (8,10–13). A number of other models have been used to determine the retinal permeability from the blood to the vitreous (14–19). In each of the former models, a simplified geometry and set of boundary and initial conditions were used so that the mathematical expression of the model would be easier to develop and solve. Some of these simplifications affect the generality of the model and may affect model calculations and estimates of the retinal permeability.

A. Araie and Maurice Model

Araie and Maurice (8) used the simplest approach to model distribution and elimination in the vitreous by representing the vitreous as a sphere with the entire outer surface representing the retina (Fig. 1). The predicted concentration profile within the vitreous will be the same for any cross section that passes through the center of the sphere, with the highest concentration in the center and the lowest concentration next to the outer surface. In a rabbit eye, the center of curvature of the retina is immediately next to the lens, on the symmetry axis of the vitreous. Qualitatively, the concentration profile calculated by a spherical model will be correct for the posterior hemisphere of the vitreous, which is behind the center of curvature of the retina. In a spherical geometry model like the Araie and Maurice model, the concentration profile in the anterior hemisphere will be the same as in the posterior hemisphere, since the two hemispheres are the same. Therefore, the concentration profile calculated by a spherical model for the portion of the vitreous that is in front of the center of curvature of the retina will not accurately reflect the actual profile that would be present in vivo. A spherical model also assumes that there is no flux across the plane that passes through the center of curvature of the retina and is perpendicular to the symmetry

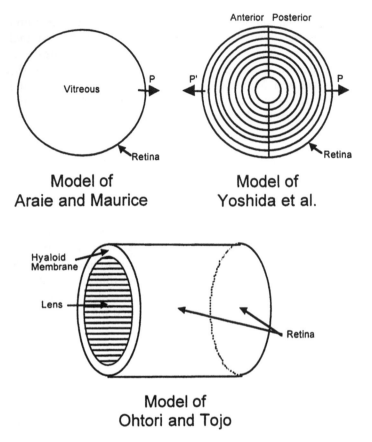

Figure 1 Comparison of models developed by Araie and Maurice (8), Yoshida et al. (12,13), and Ohtori and Tojo (10,11).

axis. For this assumption to be true, the loss across the portion of the retina located behind its center of curvature must equal the sum of the loss across the hyaloid membrane plus the loss across the portion of the retina in front of the center of curvature of the retina. This condition will only be true for a particular retinal permeability.

B. Yoshida Model

Yoshida et al. (12,13) extended the model used by Araie and Maurice by dividing the vitreous into an anterior and posterior hemisphere (Fig. 1). Each hemisphere was further subdivided into eight compartmental shells, and a separate permeability was used for the outer surface of each hemisphere. Within each concentric compartmental shell, the concentration calculated by the model would be uniform since each compartment was assumed to be perfectly mixed. Yoshida's model is a more accurate representation of the true vitreous than a spherical model, since a separate permeability is calculated for the outer surface of the anterior and posterior hemispheres. However, if this model is used to estimate retinal permeabilities using vitreous concentration data, an accurate estimate of the retinal permeability will only be obtained for compounds that are primarily eliminated across the retina. As discussed in further detail (in Sec. 3.2), compounds that are eliminated mainly across the hyaloid membrane will have concentration contours within the vitreous which are perpendicular to the retina, and, therefore, the concentric compartmental shells will not accurately calculate the correct concentration profile. The profile calculated by a model that uses concentric compartmental shells will always have concentration contours that are parallel to the retina since the concentration within each compartmental shell must be uniform. Furthermore, the concentric shell compartmental model will always predict a uniform vitreal concentration over the entire inner surface of the retina; the model will be unable to account for conditions that result in nonuniform concentrations adjacent to the retina (such as displaced or irregular injections or diseases that cause the retinal permeability to vary over the retinal surface).

C. Ohtori and Tojo Model

The geometry and boundary conditions of the vitreous were more accurately modeled by Ohtori and Tojo (10,11). The model was cylindrical in shape with one end of the cylinder and the curved surface representing the retina, and the opposite end of the cylinder divided into an outer section representing the hyaloid membrane and an inner section representing the lens (Fig. 1). This model design allowed the use of different permeability values for the boundaries representing the lens, hyaloid membrane, and retina. The main advantage of this model is a more accurate representation of drug loss from the anterior portion of the vitreous. The boundary conditions representing the lens and hyaloid membrane are different than for the retina, thereby allowing more accurate calculated concentrations within the region of the vitreous close to these boundaries. The main limitations of this model are the use of a cylinder to approximate the spherical shape of the vitreous and the inability to study complex and nonsymmetric initial conditions.

III. FINITE ELEMENT MODEL BASED ON RABBIT EYE

Modelling drug distribution and elimination in the vitreous is particularly suitable to finite element analysis, which allows the complex geometry and boundary conditions of the vitreous to be more accurately incorporated into the model. Finite element analysis also allows complex initial conditions to be studied.

A finite element model has been developed (20), and the model was initially based on the physiological dimensions of a rabbit eye, using the cross sections of the eye shown by Araie and Maurice as a guide (8). The rabbit eye was initially chosen rather than the human eye due to the availability of data for confirmation of model calculations.

A. Model Development

A detailed description of the model equations and solution methods are presented elsewhere (20). The tissues included in the model were the vitreous, retina, posterior surface of the lens, and the posterior chamber of the aqueous humor (Fig. 2). Mass transport by both convection and diffusion was accounted for in the aqueous humor. Due to the viscous nature of the vitreous, especially in the rabbit eye, only diffusive mass transport was considered in the vitreous.

The only unknown variables in the model were the initial distribution of drug solution in the vitreous following injection (initial condition) and the retinal permeability. The initial distribution of the injected drug solution is a variable that could affect the elimination of drug from the vitreous. Therefore, rather than simulating only a central injection, four extreme initial conditions were considered. These conditions covered a range of possible positions where the injected drug solution may have been placed in the in vivo experiments performed by Araie and Maurice (8): (a) a central injection, (b) an injection placed next to the lens on the symmetry axis, (c) an injection placed next to the retina on the symmetry axis, and (d) an injection placed close to the hyaloid membrane (Fig. 3). The model simulated the shape of the injected solution as a sphere in cases 1–3 and a cylinder of equal height and diameter for case 4. In reality, a drug solution injected into the vitreous will not take the shape of a perfect sphere or a cylinder. Complex and poorly characterized shapes that depend on drug solution and vitreous properties as well as the injection procedure may be observed (7). These complex shapes would be difficult to incorporate in the finite element model, so for the purpose of studying the effect of injection position, a simpler shape was selected. The concentration profiles produced by the model using each initial condition were fit to the concentration profiles observed by Araie and Maurice (8), resulting in four

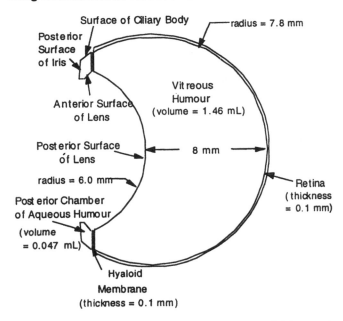

Figure 2 Cross section view of the model. In addition to the vitreous, the model includes the posterior aqueous compartment and the surrounding retina layer. The aqueous compartment was included to properly account for drug loss across the hyaloid membrane.

possible values of retinal permeability that best fit the experimental profiles. By simulating extreme injection positions, the range of retinal permeabilities calculated by the model should include the actual retinal permeability. If the actual injection position used by Araie and Maurice was precisely known, a single retinal permeability could be calculated using the model.

B. Comparison of Model Calculated and Experimental Data

Figures 4 and 5 show the model calculated concentration profiles for fluorescein at 15 hours and for fluorescein glucuronide at 24 hours, respectively, after a spherical central injection (A), and a cylindrical injection displaced towards the hyaloid membrane (B). The concentration profiles for the injection displaced towards the lens and the injection displaced towards the retina were qualitatively similar to the concentration profile produced by the central injection.

Qualitatively, the contour profiles calculated using the model are similar to those found experimentally by Araie and Maurice (8). In Figure 4, the

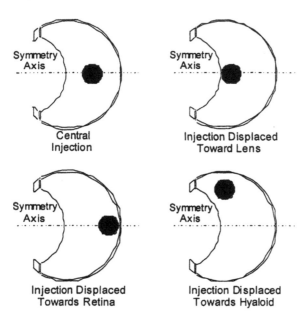

Figure 3 Injection positions studied using the model. Four extreme and distinct injection positions were studied to determine the sensitivity of the model calculated retinal permeability to the initial location of the injected drug.

concentration contour lines are parallel to the retina as expected, since the flux of fluorescein across the retina was the dominant elimination mechanism. For each injection position along the symmetry axis, the maximum model calculated concentrations were next to the lens, on the symmetry axis as shown in Figure 4A. In the case where fluorescein was injected closer to the hyaloid membrane (Fig. 4B), the maximum model calculated concentration was next to the lens; however, it is displaced slightly, closer to the site of the injection.

In Figure 5, the model calculated concentration contour lines are perpendicular to the retina since fluorescein glucuronide is eliminated mainly across the hyaloid membrane. Araie and Maurice (8) found that the concentration of fluorescein glucuronide in the vitreous was approximately the same next to the retina and next to the lens on the symmetry axis of the vitreous at 24 hours. However, the model calculated that the concentration next to the retina (12.1 µg mL^{-1}) was slightly higher than the concentration next to the lens (10.4 µg mL^{-1}) for all injection positions. For the hyaloid-displaced injection, the maximum concentration was shifted slightly towards the injection site, similar to that noted for the hyaloid-displaced

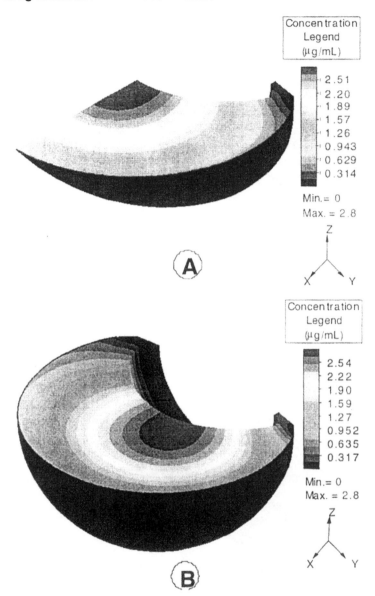

Figure 4 Model calculated concentration profile for fluorescein at 15 hours for a spherical central injection (A) and a hyaloid-displaced injection (B). The dominant elimination route for fluorescein is across the retina; therefore, the concentration contour lines are parallel to the retina surface. The concentration profile for the lens-displaced injection and the retina-displaced injection were qualitatively similar to the central injection.

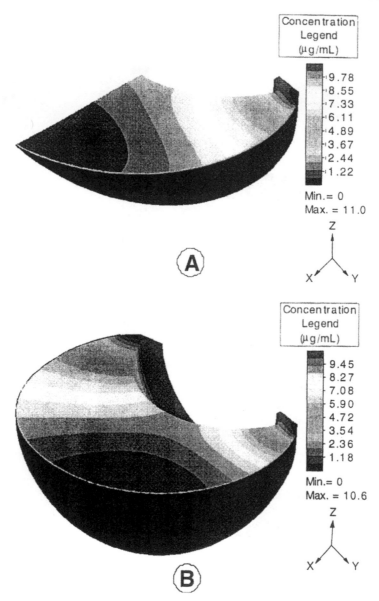

Figure 5 Model calculated concentration profile for fluorescein glucuronide at 24 hours for a spherical central injection (A) and a hyaloid-displaced injection (B). Fluorescein glucuronide has a very low retinal permeability; therefore, the concentration contour lines are perpendicular to the retina. The concentration profile for the lens-displaced injection and the retina-displaced injection were qualitatively similar to the central injection.

injection of fluorescein. If the hyaloid membrane was the only elimination route, theory would suggest that the maximum concentration would be next to the retina on the symmetry axis, since this is the point where a drug molecule must travel furthest to be eliminated.

In Figure 6, the model calculated concentration gradients of fluorescein between the lens and the retina along the symmetry axis are compared with the experimental data of Araie and Maurice (8). In each case, the concentrations have been normalized with respect to the concentration found next to the lens. Considering that the concentration gradients were calculated by fitting only the experimental concentration measured 1 mm adjacent to the

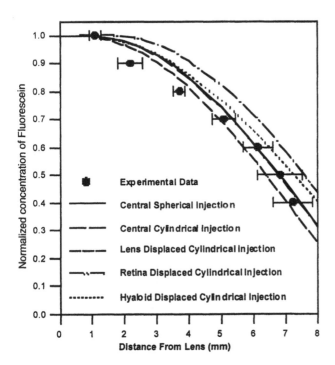

Figure 6 Concentration gradient between the lens and retina 15 hours after an intravitreal injection of fluorescein. Concentrations have been normalized with respect to the concentration next to the lens. The experimental bars represent the minimum and maximum distance from the center of curvature of the retina that each specific experimental concentration contour line was observed (8). The model calculated profiles were produced using the retinal permeabilities shown in Table 1. The retinal permeabilities were calculated by fitting only the experimental concentration observed 1 mm adjacent to the lens measured at 15 hours. However, the model was able to accurately fit the entire profile.

lens, the fact that the model-calculated concentration gradients follow the experimentally observed gradient provides strong validation of the model and its inherent assumptions. Of particular note is that even 15 hours after the intravitreal injection, significant variations in the concentration profiles were observed when different injection locations were considered. At earlier times after the injection, the concentration variations would be much larger, which suggests that injection position is an important variable that must be controlled when performing animal experiments and in clinical treatment.

For each of the simulated injection positions, Table 1 shows the model calculated retinal permeabilities of fluorescein and fluorescein glucuronide that were determined by fitting the experimental data and compares them to values calculated by other published models and found in vitro by Koyano (9) using an excised rabbit retina. As mentioned earlier, the retinal permeability for a compound is a constant. The different values obtained from the various simulations occurred because the retinal permeability was the only parameter with an unknown value that could be adjusted to fit the experimental data. Since the injection position affects the concentration gradients in the vitreous, different estimates for retinal permeabilities were obtained. The estimated fluorescein retinal permeabilities were much lower when the injection was displaced towards the retina or the hyaloid membrane. In the former case, fluorescein was placed closer to the retina, producing a higher initial concentration gradient of fluorescein across the retina than obtained from a central injection. Since the concentration gradient is higher, a lower

Table 1 Comparison of Finite Element Model Calculated Retinal Permeabilities and Other Published Values

Position of injection and other published values	Retinal permeability (cm/s)	
	Fluorescein	Fluorescein glucuronide
Central Injection	2.88×10^{-5}	6.41×10^{-7}
Injection Displaced Towards Lens	3.50×10^{-5}	3.89×10^{-7}
Injection Displaced Towards Retina	2.03×10^{-5}	7.62×10^{-7}
Injection Displaced Towards Hyaloid Membrane	1.94×10^{-5}	0
Araie and Maurice (8)	2.33×10^{-5}	NC
Koyano et al. (9)	$0.6–1.8 \times 10^{-5}$	6.3×10^{-6}
Yoshida et al. (12,13)[a]	1.27×10^{-5}	1.5×10^{-6}

[a] These data were collected using monkey eyes but were included for comparison.
NC = Not calculated.

retinal permeability is required to fit the experimental data. In the latter case, the injection position is closer to both the retina and the hyaloid membrane than with a central injection. Retinal penetration is the dominant elimination mechanism for fluorescein; however, when the injection is placed closer to the hyaloid membrane, more fluorescein will be eliminated across the hyaloid membrane than if the injection was placed in the center of the vitreous. The combination of a greater loss across the hyaloid membrane and a higher initial concentration gradient across the retinal results in a lower retinal permeability required to fit the experimental data. Displacement of the injection towards the lens led to the highest estimate of the retinal permeability, because this injection position places fluorescein furthest from the retina compared to the other three injection positions.

A retinal permeability of zero was obtained when the injection of fluorescein glucuronide was displaced towards the hyaloid membrane. A low retinal permeability was expected since penetration across the hyaloid membrane is the main elimination route for fluorescein glucuronide, and an injection placed closer to the hyaloid membrane will increase the amount of fluorescein glucuronide eliminated across the hyaloid membrane. Therefore, a lower retinal permeability will be required to fit the experimental data. Since fluorescein glucuronide is known to penetrate the retina at least to a small degree and the model has estimated a retinal permeability of zero, it is reasonable to conclude that the extreme position of the hyaloid-displaced injection is significantly different than the actual experimental injection position, leading to an error in the estimation of the retinal permeability. This result was also due to the low sensitivity of the fluorescein glucuronide concentration at 24 hours to the retinal permeability. For the other three injection positions, as the injection site was moved further from the hyaloid membrane, the net elimination across the hyaloid was reduced. To compensate, the simulated amount of drug transferred across the retina must increase, and, therefore, the estimated retinal permeability increases as the injection site was placed further from the hyaloid membrane.

The retinal permeability of fluorescein calculated by the models of Araie and Maurice (8) and Yoshida et al. (12,13) and found in vitro by Koyano (9) are close to the range of retinal permeabilities calculated by the finite element model. Since the fluorescein retinal permeability calculated by Araie and Maurice (8) with their spherical model agrees with the retinal permeability calculated with the finite element model, the fluorescein permeability value is coincidentally the value that is required to balance the anterior and posterior losses. The retinal permeability calculated with a spherical model for any compound that does not have an actual retinal permeability similar to fluorescein will be in error.

Yoshida et al. (12,13) used their model to calculate the retinal permeability of fluorescein and fluorescein glucuronide in monkey eyes. Therefore, any differences between the retinal permeability calculated by their model and the finite element model could be due to differences between the models and also due to differences between the physiology of the rabbit and monkey retina. However, a comparison of the two models on a theoretical basis can still be made. Yoshida et al. (12,13) divided the vitreous into an anterior and posterior hemisphere. Each hemisphere was further subdivided into eight compartmental shells, and a separate permeability was used for the outer surface of each hemisphere. Within each concentric compartmental shell, the concentration calculated by the model would be uniform since each compartment was assumed to be perfectly mixed. As noted experimentally by Araie and Maurice (8), and with the finite element model, the concentration contours of fluorescein form concentric rings that are parallel to the retina in the rabbit eye. The concentration contours in a monkey eye would be similar, due to the high permeability of fluorescein through the monkey retina. The concentration contours calculated using Yoshida's model (12,13) for the posterior portion of the vitreous, therefore, would be qualitatively correct. Since the anterior portion of Yoshida's model (12,13) is also defined by concentric compartmental shells and the concentration contours in the region close to the hyaloid membrane are not parallel to the retina, the concentration profile calculated for the anterior portion of the vitreous would be incorrect. Yoshida's model (12,13) is a more accurate representation of the true vitreous than a spherical model, since a separate permeability is calculated for the outer surface of the anterior and posterior hemispheres. However, an accurate estimate of the retinal permeability will only be obtained for compounds that are primarily eliminated across the retina. Compounds that are eliminated mainly across the hyaloid membrane will have concentration contours perpendicular to the retina, and, therefore, the concentric compartmental shells will not accurately calculate the correct concentration profile. The profile calculated by a model that uses concentric compartmental shells will always have concentration contours that are parallel to the retina since the concentration within each compartmental shell must be uniform. Furthermore, since the concentration in the vitreous (adjacent to the retina) calculated by a concentric shell compartmental model will be always uniform over the entire inner surface of the retina, the model will be unable to account for conditions that result in nonuniform concentrations adjacent to the retina (such as displaced or irregular injections or diseases that have a local effect on retinal permeability).

Although the retinal permeability of fluorescein found in vitro by Koyano et al. (9) is similar to the values found using the finite element model, their retinal permeability of fluorescein glucuronide is significantly different from the value found using the finite element model. To test the value that was found by Koyano et al. (9), a simulation was performed with the finite element model using their permeability value and a central injection of fluorescein glucuronide with the same injected concentration used by Araie and Maurice (8). As mentioned previously, the concentration contour lines of fluorescein glucuronide were found to be perpendicular to the retina at 24 hours, experimentally by Araie and Maurice (8), and by the finite element model for any of the injection positions. However, when the retinal permeability value found by Koyano et al. (9) was used in the model, the concentration contour lines at 24 hours were found to be parallel to the retina, similar to the profiles for fluorescein. If the profiles found experimentally by Araie and Maurice (8) are assumed to be correct, then it must be concluded that the retinal permeability values found in vitro by Koyano et al. (9) are not accurate. This may be due to the difficulty of excising a retina from the eye and maintaining its viability while permeation experiments are performed.

IV. USING FINITE ELEMENT MODELING TO INVESTIGATE CLINICAL CONDITIONS

A. Modification of Finite Element Model to Anatomy and Physiology of Human Eye

To determine the implications of changing conditions which may affect drug distribution in the vitreous in a more clinically relevant setting, the finite element model can be modified to match the geometry of the human eye (21) (Fig. 7). The most significant differences between the posterior segment of a rabbit and human eye are the size of the lens and the volume of the vitreous humor. In a human eye, the lens occupies a smaller portion of the vitreous than in the rabbit eye. The volume of the vitreous humor in the human eye is approximately 4 mL, and the volume of the rabbit vitreous is approximately 1.5 mL. Another difference between the human and rabbit eye is the flow dynamics in the posterior aqueous humor chamber. The volumetric flow rate of aqueous humor is similar in human and rabbit eyes; however, the cross-sectional area for flow is approximately four times larger in human eyes, resulting in a lower flow velocity in human eyes. Similar to the rabbit eye model, fluorescein and fluorescein glucuronide were used as test compounds to study the effects of injection position and volume in the human eye model. In humans, the exact retinal permeabilities of fluorescein and fluorescein glucuronide are not known, so the values used were 2.6×10^{-5} cm/s and 4.5×10^{-7} cm/s, respectively, which are the average of the values that were found using the rabbit eye finite element model. For the purpose

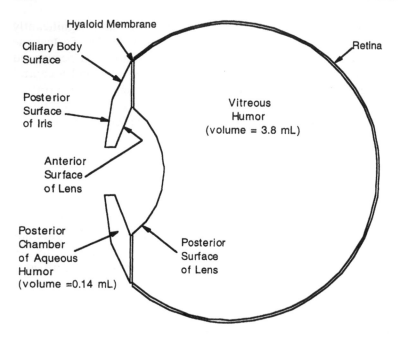

Figure 7 Cross-section view of human eye model. The model was based on the physiological dimensions of the human eye. The posterior chamber of the aqueous humor was included to account for the loss of drug from the vitreous across the hyaloid membrane. Transport of drug by convection and diffusion was accounted for in the posterior chamber of the aqueous humor, and only diffusive transport was accounted for in the vitreous humor.

of examining the effects of changing intravitreal injection variables, the accuracy of the retinal permeability is not of prime importance. The retinal permeability value will impact the quantitative results of each injection variable case studied, but qualitative intercase comparisons using a constant retinal permeability will be valid.

B. Effects of Injection Position and Volume on Drug Distribution in the Vitreous

1. Injection Conditions Studied

The actual position and shape of an intravitreal injection will most likely not be the same as any of the initial conditions that are described in Sec. III.A; however, the model results indicated the variability that can occur when the injection is not placed in the same position each time. Not only is knowledge of the actual injection position and shape required to calculate the correct retinal permeability, it is also very important for calculating the correct concentrations within the vitreous. Different injection positions and shapes will produce different concentrations within the vitreous, and, therefore, the efficacy of the treatment produced by the drug will change. Although other authors have suggested that the location of an intravitreal injection is significant with respect to drug toxicity (16), a detailed study has not been performed due to the difficulty of experimentally measuring drug distribution within the vitreous.

Similar to the rabbit eye finite element model, four extreme injection positions were studied using the human eye finite element model: (a) a central injection, (b) an injection displaced towards the lens, (c) an injection displaced towards the retina, and (d) an injection displaced towards the hyaloid membrane. The most common intravitreal injection volume in human patients is 100 µL; however, different volumes may be used for clinical trials and in animal studies (8,12,13). The two injection volumes compared using the model were 15 and 100 µL. The mass injected in each case was the same (30 µg), resulting in drug solution concentrations of 2000 and 300 µg/mL for the 15 and 100 µL injections, respectively. In each of the 100 µL injection cases, the distance between the outer boundary of the injected drug and the adjacent tissue surface was the same as for the corresponding 15 µL injection. Therefore, the overall displacements of the 100 µL injections from the central injection were not as large as the displacements of the 15 µL injections due to the larger diameter sphere that was used to represent the 100 µL injection.

At any time following an intravitreal injection, there may be significant concentration gradients within the vitreous due to the localized initial distribution and the fact that in the finite element model, mass transfer within the vitreous occurs by diffusion alone. Changing the variables of an intravitreal injection dramatically affects the concentration gradients and local concentrations. Therefore, the concentrations within the vitreous were monitored at three different sites (Fig. 8): (a) adjacent to the lens on the symmetry axis, (b) adjacent to the retina on the symmetry axis, and (c) adjacent to the hyaloid membrane. For the case where the injection was placed close to the hyaloid membrane, the concentration was also monitored at the opposite side of the vitreous adjacent to the hyaloid membrane.

2. Results of Changing Injection Conditions

Figures 9 and 10 show the model calculated concentrations in the vitreous adjacent to the retina on the symmetry axis of the vitreous following 15 µL injections of fluorescein or fluorescein glucuronide, respectively, at the four different vitreous locations. Tables 2 and 3 contain the peak concentrations

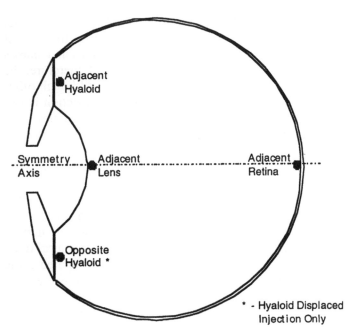

Figure 8 Sites within vitreous where concentrations were monitored using the finite element model. In addition to studying the effects of injection position and volume on mean concentrations within the vitreous, concentrations were also monitored at several distinct points within the vitreous. The variation of drug concentrations within the vitreous will be revealed using this method of analysis.

and area-under-the-curve (AUC) values for all the vitreous sites and injection locations of fluorescein and fluorescein glucuronide.

In general, the data illustrate that injecting fluorescein or fluorescein glucuronide at different locations within the vitreous may produce significantly different local concentrations and concentration profiles. The peak concentrations that were calculated by the model depended on the location of the injection relative to the site where the concentration was monitored. The largest variations in the peak concentrations of fluorescein were observed at the vitreous site adjacent to the retina, where the retina-displaced injection produced a peak concentration over three orders of magnitude higher than that obtained from the hyaloid-displaced injection (Table 2). At the vitreous site adjacent to the hyaloid membrane, the peak concentration of fluorescein produced by the hyaloid-displaced injection was also over three orders of magnitude higher than the concentration produced by the retina-displaced injection. Peak concentrations of fluorescein at the vitr-

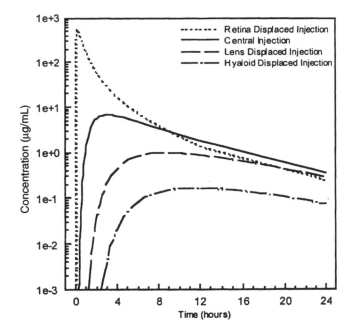

Figure 9 Concentration of fluorescein at the vitreous site adjacent to the retina following 15 μL injections at four different vitreous locations. Peak concentrations of fluorescein at this vitreous site varied by up to three orders of magnitude, depending on the initial injection position. Similar variations were noted for the other sites within the vitreous where the concentrations were monitored.

eous site adjacent to the lens varied by up to two orders of magnitude, depending on the location of the injection (Table 2). Similar variations were also noted for fluorescein glucuronide; peak concentrations produced by the different injection sites varied by up to two orders of magnitude at the different vitreous sites (Table 3).

It is also important to note that there were significant variations in the model calculated peak concentrations at each vitreous site produced by an individual injection location. For example, for the hyaloid-displaced injection, the peak concentration next to the injection (adjacent hyaloid) was over three orders of magnitude higher than the peak concentration next to the hyaloid membrane opposite the injection location (Table 3). Furthermore, the time to reach the maximum fluorescein concentration varied from approximately 6 minutes to 12 hours, depending upon the proximity of the monitoring site to the injection site. Similarly, the time to reach the peak concentration of fluorescein glucuronide ranged from approximately 10 minutes to 24 hours. The variations observed for the AUC-time curve followed

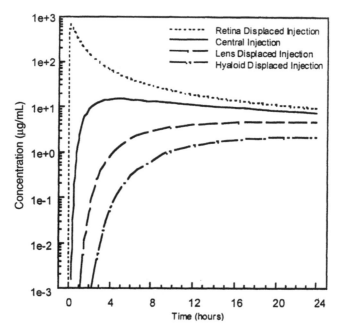

Figure 10 Concentration of fluorescein glucuronide at the vitreous site adjacent to the retina following 15 μL injections at four different vitreous locations. Peak concentrations of fluorescein glucuronide varied by up to three orders of magnitude at this site within the vitreous, depending on the initial position of the injection. Similar variations in concentrations were noted for the other sites within the vitreous.

trends similar to those observed for the peak concentration values. For fluorescein, AUC values for a specific vitreous site varied by over two orders of magnitude, depending on the location of the injection. AUC values for fluorescein glucuronide for a specific vitreous site also varied by over an order of magnitude. The AUC represents the cumulative exposure of a particular tissue to a drug over time and may therefore be related to the efficacy and/or toxicity of a drug at a particular site.

The data in Table 3 also further emphasize the importance of the injection location. After 24 hours there is one-quarter the amount of fluorescein left in the vitreous following the 15 μL hyaloid-displaced injection compared to after the 15 μL central injection. Similarily, there is one-third the amount of fluorescein glucuronide left in the vitreous following the 15 μL hyaloid-displaced injection compared to after the 15 μL retina-displaced injection. For the larger 100 μL injections, the difference between the amount of drug remaining at 24 hours for the different injection locations

Table 2 Peak Concentrations and Area Under Curve Values at Various Vitreous Sites Following 15 μL Intravitreal Injections of Fluorescein at Four Different Vitreous Locations

| | | Vitreous site where concentration was monitored | | | |
		Adjacent retina	Adjacent lens	Adjacent hyaloid	Adjacent opposite hyaloid
	Injection location				
Peak	Central	6.77 (3.2)	9.53 (3.8)	0.673 (6.9)	
concentration	Lens-displaced	0.989 (7.9)	628 (0.13)	2.97 (2.8)	
(μg/mL)	Retina-displaced	563 (0.10)	1.52 (9.9)	0.154 (11)	
	Hyaloid-displaced	0.166 (12)	5.73 (3.3)	210 (0.10)	0.084 (9.3)
AUC	Central	56.7	104	8.72	
(μg h/mL)	Lens-displaced	13.9	800	23.6	
0–24 h	Retina-displaced	548	22.4	2.22	
	Hyaloid-displaced	2.44	49.6	217	1.22

Values in parentheses indicate the time (hours) to reach the peak concentrations.

Table 3 Peak Concentrations and Area Under Curve Values at Various Vitreous Sites Following 15 μL Intravitreal Injections of Fluorescein at Four Different Vitreous Locations

| | | Vitreous site where concentration was monitored | | | |
		Adjacent retina	Adjacent lens	Adjacent hyaloid	Adjacent opposite hyaloid
	Injection location				
Peak	Central	14.6 (4.6)	9.54 (3.8)	0.904 (11)	
concentration	Lens-displaced	4.68 (21)	628 (0.13)	3.04 (3.1)	
(μg/mL)	Retina-displaced	680 (0.14)	4.14 (21)	0.742 (24)	
	Hyaloid-displaced	2.15 (24)	6.38 (3.4)	210 (0.10)	0.188 (22)
AUC	Central	244	138	17.3	
(μg h/mL)	Lens-displaced	77.1	843	32.7	
0–24 h	Retina-displaced	1290	66.6	10.4	
	Hyaloid-displaced	28.6	79.9	260	3.15

Values in parentheses indicate the time (hours) to reach the peak concentrations.

Table 4 Mean Vitreous Concentrations of Fluorescein and Fluorescein Glucuronide 24 Hours After 30 μg Injections

		Intravitreal injection volume	
	Injection location	15 μL	100 μL
Mean concentration of	Central	0.603	0.527
fluorescein in vitreous	Lens-displaced	0.564	0.535
(μg/mL)	Retina-displaced	0.339	0.361
	Hyaloid-displaced	0.159	0.214
Mean concentration of	Central	5.16	5.11
fluorescein glucuronide	Lens-displaced	3.73	4.09
in vitreous (μg/mL)	Retina-displaced	5.71	5.60
	Hyaloid-displaced	1.87	2.49

is not as large; however, variations of up to a factor of 2.5 are still observed. As the injection volume increases, the effect of injection position would be dampened, with the upper limit of injection volume being a single injection that completely replaces the whole vitreous.

Table 4 lists the mean model calculated concentrations of fluorescein and fluorescein glucuronide in the vitreous as a function of the injection position, following either a 15 or a 100 μL injection. As mentioned earlier, the simulated mass of drug injected in each case was the same (30 μg). As indicated by the lower values of the mean fluorescein concentration at 24 hours, elimination of fluorescein was faster for the 100 μL central and lens-displaced injections than for the 15μL injections. However, when the fluorescein was injected closer to the retina or hyaloid membrane, elimination was higher for the 15 μL injections. These results are consistent with the fact that fluorescein is primarily eliminated across the retina. When the 15 μL injection is placed next to the retina, the flux of drug across the retina immediately after the injection is faster than for the 100 μL injection, due to the higher concentration within the 15 μL injection. This is illustrated by Figure 11, which shows the concentration of fluorescein adjacent to the retina on the symmetry axis of the vitreous following both the 15 and 100 μL retina-displaced injections. For the central and lens-displaced injections of fluorescein, elimination was higher for the 100 μL injection than for the 15 μL injection. In these cases, the 100 μL injection produces a higher concentration at the surface of the retina than the 15 μL injection, resulting in a higher rate of elimination. For injections of fluorescein glucuronide, the same trends were observed. Since fluorescein glucuronide is eliminated

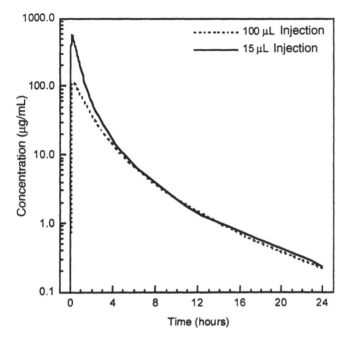

Figure 11 Concentration of fluorescein at the vitreous site adjacent to the retina following a 15 or 100 μL injection adjacent the retina on symmetry axis of vitreous. The mass of fluorescein injected in each case was identical, resulting in higher peak concentrations adjacent to the retina following the 15 μL injection case and, therefore, a higher initial loss of fluorescein across the retina.

mainly across the hyaloid membrane, the 15 μL injections placed closer to the hyaloid membrane (hyaloid-displaced and lens-displaced) resulted in lower mean concentrations at 24 hours than the 100 μL injections at the same locations, due to a higher initial rate of elimination across the hyaloid membrane. Figure 12 shows the concentration adjacent to the hyaloid membrane for the 15 and 100 μL hyaloid-displaced injections of fluorescein glucuronide. Similar to fluorescein, when the injection of fluorescein glucuronide was not placed next to its elimination surface (central and retina-displaced), higher elimination is produced by the 100 μL injection.

3. Clinical Implications of Changes in Injection Conditions

From a clinical perspective, the results of changes in injection conditions are very significant. Retinal damage from excessive drug concentrations is observed periodically following an intravitreal injection. The results of this

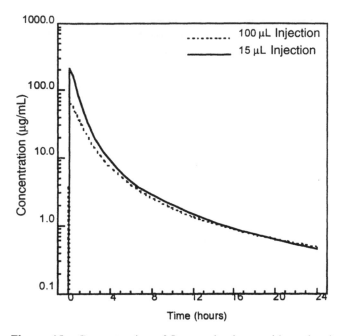

Figure 12 Concentration of fluorescein glucuronide at the vitreous site adjacent to the hyaloid membrane following a 15 or 100 μL injection adjacent to the hyaloid membrane. The mass of fluorescein glucuronide injected in each case was identical, resulting in a higher peak concentration, adjacent to the hyaloid membrane following the 15 μL injection case and, therefore, a higher initial loss of fluorescein across the hyaloid membrane.

modeling work show that enormous variations in local concentrations can arise due to variations in injection positions, suggesting that small deviations from a central injection position may contribute to retinal damage. For treatment of infectious diseases, a specific minimum inhibitory level of drug must be maintained for a specified length of time to eradicate the infectious agent. Due to the potentially devastating effects of a vitreoretinal infection, the antibiotics are used at the highest possible nontoxic doses (22); however, these studies indicate that a nontoxic dose injected at one location of the vitreous may be toxic if injected in a different location. Furthermore, the time interval the antibiotic drug remains above its therapeutic concentration at a specific site in the vitreous is dependent on the injection location.

The results are also relevant to early clinical trials or experiments with animal models, when the efficacy of new drugs is tested. Significant variability in the results may occur if care is not taken to ensure that the conditions of the intravitreal injections are kept constant. Although the injection positions that were examined in this study are extremes within the anatomy of the eye, a variation of only 5–8 mm from a central injection will produce these extremes. Slight changes in the injection conditions can easily produce these variations. Knowledge of concentration variations that are present at different sites within the vitreous will facilitate the optimization of administration techniques for diseases that affect the posterior segment of the eye.

C. Effects of Aphakia and Changes in Retinal Permeability and Vitreous Diffusivity on Drug Distribution in the Vitreous

Posterior segment infections that result in endophthalmitis most often occur as a complication following cataract extraction, anterior segment procedures, and traumatic eye injuries (23–25). Vitreoproliferative disease, a disorder in which there is uncontrolled proliferation of nonneoplastic cells, accounts for the majority of failures following retinal detachment surgery (26). A common result of both of these diseases states is inflammation of the retina, which results in a breakdown of the blood-retinal barrier (27). Long-term diabetes is also known to result in a breakdown of the blood-retinal barrier (28). The permeability of the retina will be affected as a result of these disorders and will depend on the extent to which the blood-retinal barrier has been compromised. The retinal permeability of compounds normally unable to cross the blood-retinal barrier will be increased; however, the retinal permeability of compounds that are normally actively transported across the retina may actually decrease due to a disruption in the active transport processes. Another transport parameter that may change indirectly with changes in the pathophysiology of the eye is the diffusivity of drugs in the vitreous. Changes in drug diffusivity will be most significant when drugs of different molecular weight are used to treat different pathological conditions. The developed human eye finite element model was used to estimate how the pathophysiology of the posterior eye segment affects the distribution and elimination of drug from the vitreous (29). In particular, the effect of three conditions were examined: changes in the diffusivity of drugs in the vitreous, changes in retinal permeability, and, since it is common to inject drugs into aphakic eyes, the presence or absence of the lens.

1. Range of Vitreous Diffusivity and Retinal Permeability Values Considered

In order to cover a large number of drugs with a wide range of physicochemical properties, retinal permeabilities between 1×10^{-7} and 1×10^{-4}

cm/s were considered. Retinal permeabilities have been estimated for only a small number of compounds, including fluorescein (2.6×10^{-5} cm/s), fluorescein glucuronide (4.5×10^{-7} cm/s), and dexamethasone sodium m-sulfobenzoate (4.9×10^{-5} cm/s) (1,9,15–17,30). All of the reported values fall within the range of permeabilities that were studied.

The vitreous is composed of water and low concentrations of collagen and hyaluronic acid. As the vitreous ages, the concentration of collagen and hyaluronic acid increases; however, even when elevated, the concentrations are still relatively low, at 0.13 mg/mL and 0.4 mg/mL, respectively (31). It has long been accepted that the diffusivity of solutes in the vitreous is unrestricted (32). An empirical relationship developed by Davis (33) can be used to determine if the concentration of collagen and hyaluronic acid would affect drug diffusivity in the vitreous. The diffusivity of a substance in a hydrogel can be estimated relative to its free aqueous diffusivity using the following equation:

$$\frac{D_P}{D_o} = \exp\left[-\left(5 + 10^{-4}(M_w)\right)C_p\right]$$

where D_P and D_o represent the hydrogen (vitreous) diffusivity and the diffusivity in a polymer-free aqueous solution, respectively, M_W represent the molecular weight of the diffusing species, and C_P represents the concentration of polymer (collagen and hyaluronic acid) in the hydrogel in units of grams of polymer per gram of hydrogel. Using the sum of the maximum concentration of collagen and hyaluronic acid (5.3×10^{-4} g/g) as C_P and the molecular weight of fluorescein (330 Da) gives a D_P to D_o ratio of 0.997. This value indicates that the diffusivity of a small molecule like fluorescein in the vitreous is virtually identical to the diffusivity of fluorescein in a polymer-free aqueous solution. Even if a molecular weight of 100,000 Da is used, the ratio of D_P to D_o is still 0.992, indicating that for virtually all drugs of interest, the diffusivity in a free aqueous solution is an accurate representation of vitreous diffusivity. This conclusion will hold for any molecule that does not have some form of binding interaction with collagen and hyaluronic acid. The diffusivity of molecules that do not interact with hyaluronic acid and collagen is simply a function of the molecular weight of the diffusing species. The molecular weight of drugs administered to the vitreous fall within a range of approximately 100–10,000. Davis (33) estimated the diffusivity of Na^{125}I (125 Da), [^{3}H]prostaglandin $F_{2\alpha}$ (354 Da), and ^{125}I-labeled bovine serum albumin (67,000 Da) in water. Although these compounds would not be administered therapeutically to the vitreous, their diffusivities represent a reasonable range of values for testing the sensitivity of drug distribution and elimination using the model. Therefore, the diffusivities used in the model simulations are 2.4×10^{-5} cm^2/s (125 Da), 5.6×10^{-6} cm^2/s (354 Da), and 5.4×10^{-7} cm^2/s (67,000 Da).

The effects of changing the retinal permeability or vitreous diffusivity were studied using the phakic eye model. When the sensitivity to the vitreous diffusivity was studied, the retinal permeability was held constant at 5×10^{-5} cm/s. Likewise, when the sensitivity to the retinal permeability was studied, the vitreous diffusivity was held constant at 5.6×10^{-6} cm²/s. When the effects of changing the vitreous diffusivity and retinal permeability were studied in the phakic eye model, only a central injection was considered to reduce the number of variables that were changed.

2. Modifications to Finite Element Model to Simulate Aphakic Eyes

Although cataract extractions previously involved removal of the entire lens, it is more common today to leave the posterior lens capsule intact in order to reduce postoperative complications such as vitreous changes and retinal detachment (34). To study elimination in an aphakic eye, the human phakic eye model was modified so that the curved barrier formed by the lens (Fig. 7) was replaced by the posterior capsule of the lens (Fig. 13). All of the other tissues of the aphakic eye model were assumed to be in the same

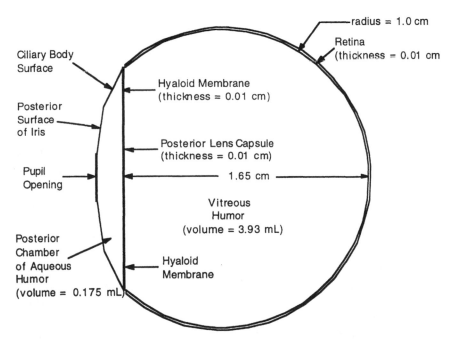

Figure 13 Cross-section view of aphakic human eye model.

configuration as in the phakic eye model. The values noted earlier for the retinal permeability of fluorescein and fluorescein glucuronide were also used in the aphakic model to study the effects of removing the lens on the elimination of compounds that have either a high or a low retinal permeability. The diffusivity of fluorescein and fluorescein glucuronide used for the vitreous and hyaloid membrane was 6.0×10^{-6} cm^2/s, which is the same as the diffusivity in free solution (35). Kaiser and Maurice (30) studied the diffusion of fluorescein in the lens and concluded that the mass transfer barrier formed by the posterior capsule of the lens was the same as an equal thickness of vitreous. The drug diffusivity used within the posterior lens capsule, therefore, was also 6.0×10^{-6} cm^2/s.

3. Results of Changes in Vitreous Diffusivity and Retinal Permeability

The effects of changing the retinal permeability and vitreous diffusivity are summarized in Table 5. The results agree with what would be expected based on mass transfer principles. The effect of vitreous diffusivity was examined with the retinal permeability set to an intermediate value of 5.0×10^{-5} cm/s, such that both the hyaloid membrane and the retina are expected to be important elimination routes. Decreasing the drug diffusivity through the vitreous increases the time required for drug molecules to travel from the injection site to an elimination boundary. Accordingly, the mean concentrations in the vitreous, calculated at 4, 12, and 24 hours after injection, increased as the drug diffusivity was reduced. Furthermore, the rate of drug elimination, which is inversely related to the drug's elimination half-life, decreased significantly as the drug diffusivity was reduced. (*Note*: The half-life noted in these studies is not the terminal phase half-life normally quoted for a drug's pharmacokinetic properties, but rather the time required for the average concentration in the vitreous to drop by a factor of two immediately following injection.) At the lowest diffusivity considered (5.4×10^{-7} cm^2/s), the mean intravitreal concentration at 24 hours was only 7.5% lower than the concentration at 4 hours. In contrast, at the highest diffusivity examined (2.36×10^{-5} cm^2/s), the mean vitreal concentration decreased by more than 99% between 4 and 24 hours. Consequently, drug diffusivity can have a drastic effect upon drug distribution and elimination.

Table 5 shows the peak concentrations in the vitreous adjacent the lens were only slightly affected by changes to the drug diffusivity. However, the time at which the peak concentration occurred increased as the drug diffusivity decreased because the average time required for a drug molecule to reach the lens increased. In the regions adjacent to the retina and hyaloid membrane, the peak concentrations increased as the drug diffusivity

Table 5 Sensitivity of Half-Life, Mean Vitreous Concentration, and Peak Vitreous Concentration to Drug Diffusivity and Retinal Permeability

D_{vit} (cm^2/s) $\times 10^{-7}$	P_{retina} (cm/s) $\times 10^{-7}$	$t_{1/2}$ (hr)[a]	C_{mean} in vitreous (μg/mL)			C_{peak} in vitreous (μg/mL)		
			4 h	12 h	24 h	Adjacent lens	Adjacent retina	Adjacent hyaloid
5.4	500	63.9	7.97	7.93	7.37	9.51 (38.6)	0.591 (26.5)	0.366 (61.7)
56	500	7.64	6.49	2.22	0.435	9.54 (3.89)	4.36 (2.97)	0.621 (7.03)
236	500	2.69	2.54	0.264	0.0169	9.48 (0.897)	9.26 (0.897)	0.775 (1.75)
56	1.0	44.4	7.88	7.0	5.69	9.54 (3.89)	14.8 (5.44)	0.915 (11.3)
56	10	31.1	7.80	6.53	4.79	9.54 (3.89)	14.1 (4.67)	0.876 (11.3)
56	100	12.3	7.30	4.07	1.54	9.54 (3.89)	9.86 (3.89)	0.742 (7.78)
56	1000	6.94	6.21	1.90	0.323	9.53 (3.89)	2.59 (2.66)	0.587 (6.25)

All values were obtained using a central injection into the vitreous.
Values in parentheses indicate the time (hours) to reach the peak concentration.
[a] The half-life noted in these studies is not the terminal phase half-life, but rather the time required for the average concentration in the vitreous to drop by a factor of 2 immediately following injection.

increased, and the time to reach the peak concentration decreased as the drug diffusivity increased. When the vitreous diffusivity is high, the retina limits the rate of elimination. Therefore, the drug rapidly diffuses to the retina, but cannot be rapidly transferred across the retina, leading to a high concentration adjacent to the retina. When the diffusivity is low, the retina is no longer a rate-limiting barrier, and molecules are eliminated almost as soon as they reach the retina surface, and the concentration adjacent to the retina is low. The diffusivity within the hyaloid membrane is equal to the diffusivity within the vitreous, and, therefore, the hyaloid membrane is never a rate-limiting transport barrier. The observation that peak concentrations adjacent to the hyaloid membrane decrease as the vitreous diffusivity decreases is due to the proximity of the hyaloid membrane to the retina.

Changing the retinal permeability had similar effects on the mean and peak concentrations within the vitreous (Table 5). The effect of retinal permeability was examined with the vitreous diffusivity held constant at an intermediate value (5.6×10^{-6} cm^2/s). Increasing the retinal permeability increases the rate of elimination; consequently, the mean concentration in the vitreous at 4, 12, and 24 hours decreases as the retinal permeability increases. The increase in elimination rate is also apparent by the fact that the half-life dramatically decreases as the permeability increases. At the lowest retinal permeability considered (1.0×10^{-7} cm/s), the mean concentration in the vitreous at 24 hours was approximately 27% lower than at 4 hours. In contrast, when the retinal permeability was 1.0×10^{-4} cm/s, the mean vitreal concentration at 24 hours was 95% lower than the concentration at 4 hours.

Peak concentrations and peak times in the vitreous adjacent to the lens were virtually unaffected by changes to the retinal permeability. The largest changes in the peak concentrations were noted adjacent to the retina, where changing the retinal permeability by four orders of magnitude caused a sixfold variation in peak concentrations. As the retinal permeability increases, it is less likely to be a rate-limiting barrier. Therefore, where the permeability is high, drugs are eliminated faster, leading to a lower concentration adjacent to the retina.

Figure 14 contains a plot of the half-life of a drug within the vitreous as a function of either its vitreous diffusivity or its retina permeability.

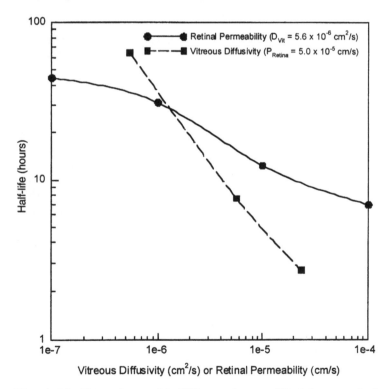

Figure 14 Dependence of half-life on vitreous diffusivity or retinal permeability. Note the half-life noted in these studies is not the terminal phase half-life, but rather the time required for the average concentration in the vitreous to drop by a factor of two immediately following injection.

Similar relationships between retinal permeability, vitreous diffusivity, molecular weight, and half-life have been shown by Maurice (32,36). Within the range studied, half-life is inversely dependent on the vitreous diffusivity and retinal permeability. The half-life has a greater dependence on the vitreous diffusivity than on the retinal permeability, although neither relationship is linear. As the retinal permeability either decreases towards zero or increases to a high value, the half-life approaches either a high or a low limit, respectively. This is consistent with expectations because all drug is eliminated across the hyaloid membrane when the retinal permeability is zero. Therefore, the half-life will be dependent on the rate at which drug reaches the hyaloid membrane, which is determined by the drug diffusivity through the vitreous. Likewise, when the retinal permeability is high, the rate of elimination will be limited by the rate of diffusion across the vitreous. Although the range of drug diffusivities considered is not large enough to show the effect of extreme values of diffusivity on half-life, it is expected that as the vitreous diffusivity decreases, the half-life should increase without bound. However, as the vitreous diffusivity increases, drug elimination would occur primarily through the hyaloid membrane into the aqueous humor and ultimately through the aqueous/blood barrier. Since diffusivity in the aqueous humor should be at the same as in the vitreous and hyaloid, the flowing aqueous humor should not represent a limiting mass transfer barrier. Although the finite element model did not account for the aqueous/blood barrier, the properties of this barrier would dictate the lower limit of vitreous half-life when vitreous diffusivity increases to large values.

Most drugs administered intravitreally have molecular weights ranging from 300 to 500 Da; therefore, Figure 14 (for a vitreous diffusivity of 5.6×10^{-6} cm^2/s, 354 Da) will be representative of most drugs. However, for smaller or larger compounds, the quantitative relationship between half-life and the permeability will be different, as will the limiting values. Nevertheless, the same qualitative relationship should still be observed, regardless of the vitreous diffusivity. Consequently, Figure 14 permits qualitative comparisons between the elimination of different drugs (molecular weight affects diffusivity). Furthermore, Figure 14 demonstrates the importance of dose adjustment if a drug is administered into an eye compromised by retinal inflammation or other disease that alter the permeability of the blood-retinal barrier.

4. Results of Aphakia on Drug Distribution in the Vitreous

Figure 15 shows the model calculated concentration profile of fluorescein on half of a cross section of the vitreous 24 hours after a central intravitreal injection in the phakic and aphakic eye models. The concentration contours

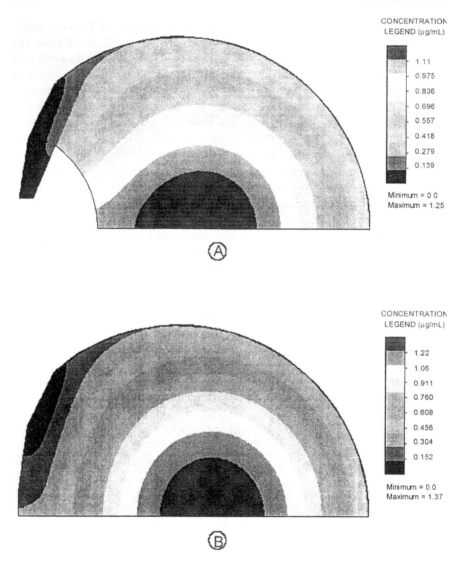

Figure 15 Model calculated concentration profile of fluorescein on half of a cross-section of the vitreous 24 hours after a central intravitreal injection in the phakic eye model (A) and the aphakic eye model (B).

are parallel to the retina, as expected, since fluorescein is eliminated mainly across the retina. Table 6 lists the half-lives, mean concentrations, and peak concentrations of fluorescein within the vitreous as a function of injection position for both the phakic eye model or the aphakic eye model. Different

Table 6 Half-Life and Peak and Mean Vitreous Concentrations of Fluorescein Calculated Using the Aphakic and Phakic Eye Models Following Intravitreal Injections at Different Locations

Injection location	$t_{1/2}$ (h)[a]	C_{mean} in vitreous (µg/mL)			C_{peak} in vitreous (µg/mL)		
		4 h	12 h	24 h	Adjacent lens	Adjacent retina	Adjacent hyaloid
Phakic							
Central	8.36	6.61	2.61	0.60	9.53 (3.78)	6.77 (3.17)	0.673 (6.89)
Lens Displaced	8.08	6.49	2.49	0.564	628 (0.128)	0.989 (7.94)	2.97 (2.83)
Retina Displaced	3.54	3.79	1.27	0.339	1.52 (9.89)	563 (0.119)	0.154 (11.1)
Hyaloid Displaced	1.39	2.11	0.695	0.158	5.73 (3.28)	0.166 (12.1)	210 (0.104) 0.084[b] (9.31)[b]
Aphakic							
Central	8.38	6.61	2.47	0.646	3.34 (4.33)	4.13 (4.33)	0.873 (5.22)
Lens Displaced	3.54	3.72	1.26	0.312	328 (0.093)	0.430 (10.3)	3.58 (2.01)
Retina Displaced	3.75	3.84	1.35	0.303	0.421 (11.2)	563 (0.131)	0.144 (11.2)
Hyaloid Displaced	2.29	2.41	0.626	0.146	3.98 (2.03)	0.163 (12.9)	238 (0.137) 0.102[b] (8.44)[b]

Values in parentheses indicate the time (hours) to reach the peak concentrations.

[a] The half-life noted in these studies is not the terminal phase half-life, but rather the time required for the average concentration in the vitreous to drop by a factor of 2 immediately following injection. The terminal phase half-life would not be expected to change with changes in injection position since the terminal phase occurs after a pseudo equilibrium has been achieved in the vitreous. After this point only vitreous diffusivity and retinal permeability would govern the rate of elimination.

[b] Peak concentration in vitreous adjacent hyaloid opposite the location of the intravitreal injection.

trends were noted when comparing the half-life of fluorescein in the phakic versus aphakic eye model. In both cases, the longest half-life was found for a central injection and the shortest half-life was found for a hyaloid-displaced injection. The half-life for the lens-displaced injection, however, was much lower in the aphakic eye model than in the phakic eye model. Placing the injected drug closer to the lens capsule in the aphakic eye model would initially produce a rapid loss of drug to the posterior chamber of the aqueous humor. However, in the phakic eye model, since there is no loss across the lens, injecting the drug closer to the lens has little effect. The initial drug loss across the lens capsule in the aphakic eye model is confirmed by comparing, in the aphakic and phakic eye models, the ratio between the mean concentrations at 4 and 24 hours for the central and lens-displaced injections. In the aphakic eye model, the mean concentration 4 hours following a central injection is 1.75 times greater than the mean concentration from a lens-displaced injection; this ratio increases slightly at 24 hours. In the phakic eye model, however, this ratio is only approximately 1.02, despite the fact that the mean concentration in the vitreous is the same for the phakic and aphakic eye models 4 hours following a central injection. The higher ratio in the aphakic eye model is therefore due to increased transport across the lens capsule, much of which occurs within the first 4 hours following an injection.

The mean vitreous concentrations in the phakic and aphakic eye models differ by less than 10% following central, retinal-displaced, and hyaloid-displaced injections, regardless of the sample time considered. However, the peak concentrations of fluorescein adjacent to the lens and retina were higher in the phakic eye model than in aphakic eye model for all the injection positions. Adjacent to the lens, the peak concentrations were higher in the phakic eye model because there is no loss across the lens. Adjacent to the retina, the peak fluorescein concentrations were only significantly higher in the phakic eye model for the central and lens-displaced injections. This is due to increased loss across the lens capsule in the aphakic eye model and the fact that the distance between the injection site and the recording site is slightly larger in the aphakic eye model than in the phakic eye model. The peak concentrations adjacent to the hyaloid membrane were higher in the aphakic eye model than in the phakic eye model for the central and lens-displaced injections. This is due to the fact that, in the aphakic eye model, the injection sites are slightly closer to the site adjacent to the hyaloid where the concentrations were recorded.

Figure 16 shows the model calculated concentration profile of fluorescein glucuronide in half of a cross section of the vitreous 36 hours after a central injection in the phakic and aphakic eye models. In this case, since fluorescein glucuronide has a low retinal permeability and is eliminated primarily across the hyaloid membrane, the concentration contours are perpendicular to the surface of the retina. Table 7 lists the half-lives, mean concentrations, and peak concentrations of fluorescein glucuronide within the vitreous as a function of injection position for both the phakic

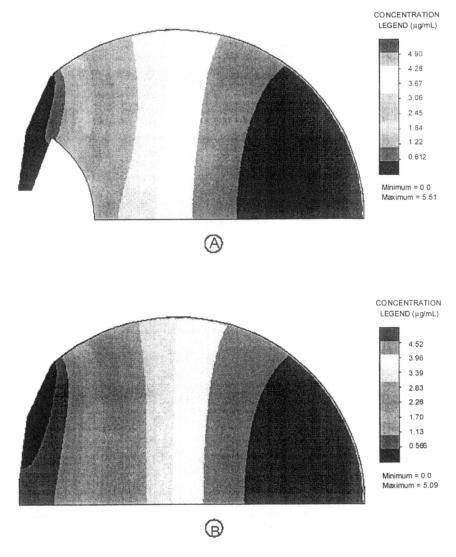

Figure 16 Model calculated concentration profile of fluorescein glucuronide on half of a crosssection of the vitreous 24 hours after a central intravitreal injection in the phakic eye model (A) and the aphakic eye model (B).

and aphakic eye models. It should be noted that the different half-lives reported in Table 6 or Table 7, with respect to injection position, are due to differences in elimination rates immediately following the injection that depend upon the injection position.

Table 7 Half-Life and Peak and Mean Vitreous Concentrations of Fluorescein Calculated Using the Aphakic and Phakic Eye Models Following Intravitreal Injections at Different Locations

Injection location	$t_{1/2}$ (h)[a]	C_{mean} in vitreous (µg/mL) 4 h	12 h	24 h	C_{peak} in vitreous (µg/mL) Adjacent lens	Adjacent retina	Adjacent hyaloid
Phakic							
Central	35.4	7.73	6.71	5.16	9.54 (3.77)	14.6 (4.61)	0.904 (11.0)
Lens Displaced	21.5	6.99	5.15	3.74	628 (0.128)	4.68 (21.0)	3.04 (3.11)
Retina Displaced	40.4	7.73	7.13	5.71	4.14 (21.0)	680 (0.138)	0.742 (24.0)
Hyaloid Displaced	3.33	3.76	2.62	1.87	6.38 (3.4)	2.15 (24.0)	210 (0.104) 0.188[b] (22.2)[b]
Aphakic							
Central	30.4	7.45	6.13	4.60	3.36 (4.78)	10.0 (6.53)	1.02 (6.53)
Lens Displaced	4.08	4.01	2.60	1.83	328 (0.093)	2.21 (21.7)	3.60 (2.01)
Retina Displaced	38.1	7.59	6.97	5.49	1.39 (21.6)	678 (0.130)	0.702 (21.6)
Hyaloid Displaced	3.97	3.96	2.46	1.71	4.23 (2.11)	2.0 (24.0)	238 (0.137) 0.180[b] (19.6)[b]

Values in parentheses indicate the time (hours) to reach the peak concentrations.

[a] The half-life noted in these studies is not the terminal phase half-life, but rather the time required for the average concentration in the vitreous to drop by a factor of 2 immediately following injection. The terminal phase half-life would not be expected to change with changes in injection position since the terminal phase occurs after a pseudo equilibrium has been achieved in the vitreous. After this point only vitreous diffusivity and retinal permeability would govern the rate of elimination.

[b] Peak concentration in vitreous adjacent hyaloid opposite the location of the intravitreal injection.

The rate of elimination from the vitreous at longer times (in the terminal phase) should be independent of the injection position. In general, the half-life of fluorescein glucuronide is higher than that for fluorescein. However, the elimination behavior observed with the phakic model and the aphakic model is different for fluorescein and fluorescein glucuronide. These differences are due to the fact that fluorescein glucuronide is eliminated mainly across the hyaloid membrane, rather than across the retina. In both the aphakic model and the phakic model, the highest half-life occurred for the retina-displaced injection and the lowest half-life occurred for the hyaloid-displaced injection, which is consistent with the fact that the hyaloid is the main elimination pathway. Similar to fluorescein, the half-life following a lens-displaced injection was much lower in the aphakic model than in the phakic model due to transport of drug across the lens capsule in the aphakic eye model. Mean intravitreal concentrations of fluorescein glucuronide at 12 and 24 hours are lower in the aphakic model for all the injection locations considered.

A comparison of peak concentrations (Table 7) shows that fluorescein glucuronide concentrations adjacent to the lens and retina were consistently lower in the aphakic eye model. However, concentrations adjacent to the hyaloid membrane were typically higher following injection in the aphakic eye model. Similar trends are observed for the peak fluorescein concentrations (Table 6). The aphakic model calculated lower peak concentrations near the retina and lens, for all the injection positions, but calculated higher concentrations near the hyaloid membrane. Thus, this comparison of elimination in the aphakic and phakic eye models has indicated that not only does the presence of the lens affect elimination, but the difference in elimination from an aphakic eye and a phakic eye is highly dependent on the injection location and the retinal permeability of the drug. If the drug has a low retinal permeability, then the half-life of the drug in an aphakic eye is highly dependent on the distance between the injection location and the lens capsule.

V. SUMMARY

Finite element modeling has been shown to be a useful tool to study drug distribution within the vitreous humor, with fewer limitations than previously developed mathematical models. Using a finite element model of the vitreous, the site of an intravitreal injection was shown to have a substantial effect on drug distribution and elimination in the vitreous. The retinal permeability of fluorescein and fluorescein glucuronide in rabbit eyes calculated by the model ranged from 1.94 to 3.5×10^{-5} and 0 to 7.62×10^{-7} cm/s, respectively, depending on the assumed site of the injection. The actual physiological retinal permeability will be a constant that is expected to lie within these ranges. If the exact initial location and distribution of the drug following injection were known, a single retinal permeability value could be calculated using the model.

By using a finite element model that matched the geometry and physiology of the human eye, it was shown that variations in intravitreal injection conditions can produce radically different levels of drug exposure in different sites within the vitreous. Variations in the injection location resulted in peak concentrations that varied by over three orders of magnitude. These variations are very important to consider if toxicity to the retina and other tissues is to be avoided. The mean calculated vitreous concentration 24 hours after an intravitreal injection varied by up to a factor of 3.8, depending on the initial location of the injected drug. Changing the volume of the injection from 15 to 100 µL dampened the effects of the initial injection location; however, mean concentrations at 24 hours still varied by up to a factor of 2.5.

Using finite element modeling, it has also been shown that the rate of drug elimination from the vitreous is highly dependent on diffusivity through the vitreous and retinal permeability. For a constant retinal permeability of 5.0×10^{-5} cm/s, increasing the vitreous diffusivity from 5.4×10^{-7} to 2.4×10^{-5} cm^2/s decreased the calculated half-life from 64 hours to 2.7 hours. For a constant drug diffusivity of 5.6×10^{-6} cm^2/s, increasing the retinal permeability from 1.0×10^{-7} to 1.0×10^{-4} cm/s decreased the calculated half-life of drug from 44 to 7 hours. Therefore, the drug diffusivity and retinal permeability are key factors that affected elimination from the vitreous and must be considered when selecting drugs and doses, particularly if the blood-retinal barrier has been compromised. Drug elimination was higher in an aphakic eye model than in a phakic eye model, especially for drugs with a low retinal permeability and if the injection was close to the lens capsule.

In the modeling work presented in this chapter, injection solutions have been assumed to be spherical or cylindrical in shape. It is known, however, that the distribution or shape of a drug solution within the vitreous immediately following intravitreal injection may vary depending on factors such as needle gauge and length, injection speed, solution viscosity, and vitreous rheology. Such variations in shape would influence the diffusional surface area and hence drug distribution within the vitreous. An attempt has been made to quantitate the effect of shape by using the extent of fingering as a quantitative indicator of shape irregularity and simulating intravitreal drug distribution using various shapes as the initial condition (7). Although such simulations provide some insight into the effect of shape, given the spurious nature of injections, it is difficult to relate the results to any given injection.

Another limitation of the models discussed in this chapter is that transport of drug in the vitreous was assumed to occur only by diffusion. Vitreous liquefaction as a result of age or disease may result in pockets of liquefied vitreous where there may be convective transport of drug. This convection would dampen both the concentration gradients calculated by the model and the effects of using different intravitreal injection conditions. However, knowledge of exactly where liquefaction occurs or how much convection occurs in liquefied pockets was not available at the time the modeling was performed. When better knowledge of vitreous liquefaction becomes available, this could be incorporated into the models.

REFERENCES

1. Lee, V. H. L., Pince, K. J., Frambach, D. A., et al. Drug delivery to the posterior segment. In: *Retina*, T. E. Ogden and A. P. Schachat, eds. St. Louis: C. V. Mosby, 1989, pp. 483–498.
2. Forster, R. K., Abbott, R. L., and Gelender, H. Management of infectious endophthalmitis. *Ophthalmology* 87:313–319, 1980.
3. Pflugfelder, S. C., Hernandez, E., Fliesler, S. J., Alvarez, J., Pflugfelder, M. E., and Forster, R. K. Intravitreal vancomycin. Retinal toxicity, clearance, and interaction with gentamicin. *Arch. Ophth.* 105:831–837, 1987.
4. Stainer, G. A., Peyman, G. A., Meisels, H., and Fishman, G. Toxicity of selected antibiotics in vitreous replacement fluid. *Ann. Ophth.* 9:615–618, 1977.
5. Tabatabay, C. A., D'Amico, D. J., Hanninen, L. A., and Kenyon, K. R. Experimental drusen formation induced by intravitreal aminoglycoside injection. *Arch. Ophth.* 105:826–830, 1987.
6. Talamo, J. H., D'Amico, D. J., Hanninen, L. A., and Kenyon, K. R., and Shanks, E. T. The influence of aphakia and vitrectomy on experimental retinal toxicity of aminoglycoside antibiotics. *Am. J. Ophth.* 100:840–847, 1985.
7. Lin, H.-H. Finite element modelling of drug transport processes after an initravitreal injection. MASc. thesis, University of Toronto, 1997.
8. Araie, M., and Maurice, D. M. The loss of fluorescein, fluorescein glucuronide and fluorescein isothiocyanate dextran from the vitreous by the anterior and retinal pathways. *Exp. Eye Res.* 52:27–39, 1991.
9. Koyano, S., Araie, M., and Eguchi, S. Movement of fluorescein and its glucuronide across retinal pigment epithelium-choroid. *Invest. Ophth. Vis. Sci.* 34:531–538, 1993.
10. Ohtori, A., and Tojo, K. In vivo/in vitro correlation of intravitreal delivery of drugs with the help of computer simulation. *Biol. Pharm. Bull.* 17:283–290, 1994.
11. Tojo, K., and Ohtori, A. Pharmacokinetic model of intravitreal drug injection. *Math. Biosci.* 123:359–375, 1994.

12. Yoshida, A., Ishiko, S., and Kojima, M. Outward permeability of the blood-retinal barrier. *Graef. Arch. Clin. Exp. Ophth.* 230:78–83, 1992.
13. Yoshida, A., Kojima, M., Ishiko, S., et al. Inward and outward permeability of the blood-retinal barrier. In: *Ocular Fluorophotometry and the Future*, J. Cunha-Vaz and E. Leite, eds. Amsterdam: P Kugler & Ghedini Pub., 1989, pp. 89–97.
14. Hosaka, A. Permeability of the blood-retinal barrier in myopia. An analysis employing vitreous fluorophotometry and computer simulation. *Acta Ophth. Suppl.* 185:95–99, 1988.
15. Larsen, J., Lund-Andersen, H., and Krogsaa, B. Transient transport across the blood-retina barrier. *Bull. Math. Bio.* 45:749–758, 1983.
16. Lund-Andersen, H., Krogsaa, B., la Cour, M., and Larsen, J. Quantitative vitreous fluorophotometry applying a mathematical model of the eye. *Invest. Ophth. Vis. Sci.* 26:698–710, 1985.
17. Lund-Andersen, H., Krogsaa, B., and Larsen, J. Calculation of the permeability of the blood-retinal barrier to fluorescein. *Graef. Arch. Clin. Exp. Ophth.* 222:173–176, 1985.
18. Oguru, Y., Tsukahara, Y., Saito, I., and Kondo, T. Estimation of the permeability of the blood-retinal barrier in normal individuals. *Invest. Ophth. Vis. Sci.* 26:969–976, 1985.
19. Palestine, A. G., and Brubaker, R. F. Pharmacokinetics of fluorescein in the vitreous. *Invest. Ophth. Vis. Sci.* 21:542–549, 1981.
20. Friedrich, S. W., Cheng, Y.-L., and Saville, B. A. Finite element modelling of drug distribution in the vitreous humour of the rabbit eye. *Ann. Biomed. Eng.* 25(2):303–314, 1997.
21. Friedrich, S. W., Saville, B. A., and Cheng, Y.-L. Drug distribution in the vitreous humor of the human eye: the effects of intravitreal injection position and volume. *Curr. Eye Res.* 16(7):663–669, 1997.
22. Baum, J. Therapy for ocular bacterial infection. *Trans. Ophthalmol. Soc. U.K.* 10:569–577, 1986.
23. Kattan, H. M., Flynn, H. W., Pflugfelder, S. C., et al. Nosocomial endophthalmitis survey. Current incidence of infection after intraocular surgery. *Ophthalmology* 98:227–228, 1991.
24. Peyman, G. A., and Schulman, J. A. Intravitreal drug therapy. In: *Intravitreal Surgery*. Norwalk: Appleton-Century-Crofts, pp. 407–455.
25. Speaker, M. G., and Menikoff, J. A. Postoperative endophthalmitis: pathogenesis, prophylaxis, and management. *Int. Ophthalmol. Clin.* 33:51–79, 1993.
26. The Retina Society Terminology Committee. The classification of retinal detachment with proliferative vitreoretinopathy. *Ophthalmology* 90:121–125, 1983.
27. Goldberg, M. F. Diseases affecting the inner blood-retinal barrier. In: *The Blood-Retinal Barriers*, Cunha-Vaz, J. G., eds. New York: Plenum Press, 1979, pp. 309–363.
28. Frank, R. N. The mechanism of blood-retinal barrier breakdown in diabetes. *Arch. Ophthalmol.* 103:1303–1304, 1985.

29. Friedrich, S. W., Saville, B. A., and Cheng, Y.-L. Drug distribution in the vitreous humour of the human eye: the effects of aphakia and changes in retinal permeability and vitreous diffusivity. *J. Ocular Pharm. Therap.* 13(5);445–459, 1997.

30. Kaiser, R., and Maurice, D. M. The diffusion of fluorescein in the lens. *Exp. Eye Res.* 3:156–165, 1964.

31. Sebag, J. Aging of the vitreous. *Eye* 1:254–262, 1987.

32. Maurice, D. M., and Mishima, S. Ocular pharmacokinetics. In: *Pharmacology of the Eye.* Vol. 69, *Handbook of Experimental Pharmacology*, Sears, M. L., ed. New York: Springer-Verlag, 1984, p. 72.

33. Davis, B. K. Diffusion in polymer gel implants. *Proc. Natl. Acad. Sci. USA* 71:3120–3123, 1974.

34. Blinkhorst, C. Corneal and retinal complications after cataract extraction. The mechanical aspect of endophthalmodonesis. *Ophthalmology* 87:609–617, 1980.

35. Algvere, P. V., Hallnas, K., Dafgard, E., et al. Panretinal photocoagulation aggravates experimental proliferative vitreoretinopathy. *Graef. Arch. Clin. Exp. Ophthalmol.* 228:461–466, 1990.

36. Tsukahara, Y., and Maurice, D. M., Local pressure effects on vitreous kinetics. *Exp. Eye Res.* 60:563–574, 1995.

7

Anterior Segment Microdialysis

Kay D. Rittenhouse
Pfizer Inc., San Diego, California, U.S.A.

I. INTRODUCTION

Preservation of sight is the major objective of many scientific studies. Topically administered drugs effectively treat many important ocular diseases. Short-term efficacy endpoints are sometimes difficult to assess following these treatment approaches. Hence, it is important to determine whether therapeutically relevant concentrations reach the site of action, as in other regions of the body. The anterior chamber of the eye is a relatively straightforward region for sampling. Anatomically accessible by paracentesis procedures, it is possible to obtain a single sample for measurement of drug concentrations. However, challenges are encountered when time-course or steady-state data are collected. Repeat sampling of this region is not possible by conventional methods in general. Traditionally, rabbits or other mammal species have been used for the assessment of intraocular concentrations of topically administered drugs. In order to obtain time-course data in aqueous humor, many animals are required, with each time point requiring multiple individual aqueous humor samples following sacrifice. These procedures present a number of challenges to be managed.

The anterior segment is an interesting and important ocular region for exploration with research tools such as microdialysis. More than 20 papers describing microdialysis approaches for assessment of ocular drug delivery and endogenous substrate characterization have been published, which include both vitreous and aqueous humor sampling.

223

II. PHYSIOLOGICAL CONSIDERATIONS OF THE ANTERIOR SEGMENT

Aqueous humor, the watery solvent produced by the ciliary body in the posterior chamber, is, in part, an ultrafiltrate of plasma (1). However, a number of the electrolytes are present in higher concentration in aqueous humor than in blood, providing evidence of active secretory and metabolic components to aqueous formation. For example, ascorbate and lactate are 20-fold and 2-fold higher in concentration in aqueous relative to plasma, respectively (2). Aqueous humor serves a nutritive role for avascularized ocular tissues such as the cornea, trabecular meshwork, and lens (2).

A. Aqueous Humor Formation and Turnover

1. Inflow Dynamics

Blood, presented at the ciliary body arterioles at relatively high hydrostatic pressure ($\sim$ 30 mmHg) (3–5), is converted into aqueous humor through complex and not completely characterized ways. The protein concentration in aqueous humor is less than 1% of that present in plasma (1). Plasma proteins are prevented from entry into aqueous humor by the tight junctions located at the nonpigmented ciliary epithelium, a component of the so-called blood-aqueous barrier, analogous to the blood-brain barrier (1). Active secretion of electrolytes such as sodium, deposited at the intercellular clefts of the tight junction regions of the nonpigmented ciliary epithelium, provide for a concentration gradient favoring fluid flow from the ciliary processes to the posterior chamber (6). A number of active secretory pathways have been identified (7,8) with specific active transport systems such as Na^+/K^+-ATPase and others providing a major contribution. The formed aqueous humor flows into the posterior chamber, down a pressure gradient, and is transported via convective bulk flow through the pupil into the anterior chamber, where the pressure is $\sim$ 16 mmHg (6).

2. Outflow Dynamics

Return of aqueous humor to the systemic circulation is facilitated by the lower pressure of the episcleral venous system ($\sim$ 9 mmHg) relative to the anterior chamber ($\sim$ 16 mmHg), as aqueous percolates through the trabecular meshwork and collects into the canal of Schlemm (1). A second pressure-independent pathway, called the uveoscleral route, provides an important contribution to aqueous outflow in humans. In contrast, rabbits have virtually no aqueous outflow by this route (9). Resistance to flow, or aqueous humor outflow facility, is used to describe the passive resistance of the trabecular meshwork to the passage of aqueous humor (10,11). The pressure-independent flow pathway behaves like a constant-rate pump; however, no metabolically dependent process has been identified as a driving force for pressure-independent flow (11). The uveoscleral pathway is described as the slow entry of aqueous humor through the face of the ciliary body just posterior to the scleral spur, with movement by bulk flow through the tissue and absorption into the uveal vessels or into periocular orbital tissues (10). There is considerable discussion concerning whether or not a significant energy-dependent component of the outflow pathway exists (10). The cells of the trabecular meshwork have phagocytic activity (12–14), which may contribute to increased facility of outflow. Trabecular meshwork outflow is biologically active, providing biochemical modulation of a passive physical process (10).

The relationship between inflow and outflow provides a means for estimating the intraocular pressure (IOP). This relationship is described as:

$$\text{IOP} = \frac{F - U}{C} + Pv$$

where F is aqueous humor formation, or flow, U is pressure-insensitive flow, C is the facility of inflow or pressure sensitive flow, and Pv is the episcleral venous pressure (2).

III. AQUEOUS HUMOR DYNAMIC IMPACT ON ANTERIOR SEGMENT DRUG DISPOSITION

The pharmacokinetics of drugs in aqueous humor is complex. Aqueous turnover, as well as availability of unbound substrate (i.e., tissue binding), complicate the assessment of ocular clearance. Anterior chamber volume in rabbit and humans is estimated to be ∼ 250–300 μL. Aqueous humor turnover is ∼ 1% of anterior chamber volume (∼ 2.5 μL/min) (15). In the anterior chamber environment, volume and clearance are not independent in the sense that drug clearance is a function of aqueous turnover and turnover rate is a function, in part, of anterior chamber volume (16). The nature of aqueous humor turnover and the pharmacodynamics of drugs that affect aqueous formation can also complicate the characterization of drug disposition. As drug is absorbed and exerts the pharmacological effect resulting in decreased aqueous humor formation, for example, the resulting aqueous concentrations are elevated relative to that of substrates that would not exert this effect (17). Tissue binding and drug lipophilicity, for example, provide input into the dispositional characteristics of the drug. Systemic effects can also influence the ocular disposition of drugs. Analgesia may result in decreased aqueous humor turnover (17), which in turn results in elevated aqueous humor drug concentrations.

IV. MICRODIALYSIS SAMPLING OF AQUEOUS HUMOR

A. Important Problems in the Anterior Chamber

1. Anterior Segment Pharmacokinetics

The ocular pharmacokinetics of ophthalmic drugs has been evaluated for many years by paracentesis sampling of anterior chamber aqueous. Lee et al. (18) examined the systemic disposition of a series of beta-adrenergic antagonists following topical administration to the pigmented rabbit (18) in order to establish the relationship between the physicochemical drug properties and absorption pathways. The efficiency of nasolacrimal punctum occlusion for minimization of systemic exposure and increased local absorption also was examined. Ross et al. (19) reported a propranolol aqueous humor C_{max} of $\sim$ 5000–5500 ng/mL ($\sim$ 10–11 ng/mL/μg, dose normalized) in anesthetized rabbits with paracentesis sampling. Others have examined the aqueous humor disposition of propranolol and other beta-adrenergic antagonists using this sampling technique (19–21). Disadvantages to this approach include the large number of animals required for evaluation and that paracentesis sampling is usually a terminal procedure.

Rabbits are the species of choice for most ocular pharmacokinetic experiments, although work in the cat, dog, and primate has been reported (22,23). The rabbit eye is similar to the human eye in size and aqueous humor volume. The rabbit eye has a thinner corneal thickness (0.35 mm vs. 0.52 mm in humans) (9), slower blink reflex (9), a nictitating membrane (absent in humans) (24), and virtually no uveoscleral outflow pathway (9).

2. Approaches to the Assessment of Modulation of Aqueous Humor Inflow and Outflow

In order to study pharmacodynamics of drugs that affect aqueous humor formation and turnover, a number of techniques have been developed. Approaches such as fluorophotometry have been used (25,26). In essence, fluorophotometry is a noninvasive technique that uses sophisticated instrumentation for the evaluation of the anterior chamber time course of topically or systemically administered fluorescing compounds such as fluorescein or fluorescein conjugates; the dilution of a topically or systemically administered dye in aqueous is measured without direct assay of aqueous humor contents. This procedure is advantageous for use in the clinical setting due to its lack of invasive sampling. Measurement of fluorescein in the eye using fluorophotometry is a somewhat complex procedure with a number of possible sources of error (25). Tonography, also a noninvasive approach, can be used to assess aqueous humor formation indirectly. Briefly, tonography tests the ability of the eye to recover from the elevation of IOP induced by a tonometer. Such recovery primarily occurs through increased outflow of aqueous humor (27). Tonography depends on the assumption that aqueous humor formation is insensitive to moderate changes in IOP; the facility of trabecular meshwork outflow is estimated. This method neglects the pseudofacility component. With this approach, it is difficult to separate out the different contributions to facility (27). Constant pressure perfusion techniques have been used to estimate outflow facility (28–30). A phenomenon described as a "washing-out" effect is commonly observed with the use of this method; the perfusion results in the clearing of macromolecules (30) usually present at the trabecular meshwork that partially occlude these outflow channels (10). Inaccuracy in flow estimates can result since time dependent changes in facility are observed (29). An invasive approach used by Miichi and Nagataki (31) to estimate aqueous humor formation involves the assessment of the time course of "dilution" of a nondiffusable compound or dye, which is perfused at a constant rate into aqueous humor. Perturbation of the rate of dilution of the dye can be estimated via a change in the time course of the dye following administration of the pharmacological agent. The time-course data are approximated mathematically employing nonlinear least-squares regression analysis in order to obtain aqueous humor flow parameters perturbed by drugs that affect inflow. This method offers some attractive features in the quantitation of the physiological effect. However, the technical procedures are quite involved, with numerous intrusions simultaneously to the same eye (31–36).

B. Principles of Microdialysis: Probe Design and Recovery

Microdialysis offers a novel means for obtaining samples of biological fluids while providing a relatively clean matrix, which may require little or no sample preparation prior to analysis. However, microdialysis, in general, does not provide meaningful information concerning endogenous or exogenous compounds implicitly. Microdialysis is a means of collecting the sample for further analysis. The dialysate must be analyzed by other conventional analysis techniques. Such analytical techniques used in conjunction with microdialysis include high-performance liquid chromatography (HPLC) (37,38), capillary electrophoresis (39,40), UV-visible spectrophotometry (41), and liquid scintillation spectroscopy (42).

1. Principles of Dialysis

Dialysis involves the separation of two compartments containing differing concentrations of a solute in solution by a semi-permeable membrane. This membrane allows passage of solutes of sufficiently small size from one compartment to the other along a concentration gradient. Theoretically, the solute concentration in both compartments will establish equilibrium such that there is no net flux of solute; the concentration of solute not bound to nonpermeable macromolecules then will be equal in both compartments. The solute diffusion rate, as described by Fick's law, is a function of membrane surface area, thickness, concentration gradient, compartment volume, and ligand diffusion coefficient (43).

Tissue and plasma proteins often bind drugs and other low molecular weight compounds. Hypothesis regarding mechanisms of binding include the generally held view that a reaction occurs between two oppositely charged ions (essentially salt formation). Negatively charged drugs bind to the positively charged amino acid groups, such as histidine or lysine, of plasma proteins. Additional contributions to binding phenomena include hydrophobic interactions (44). Nonpolar functional groups of drug and protein or tissue interact via van der Waals forces.

Pharmacodynamic effects of drugs are considered to be a function of the unbound concentration in plasma (45). For this reason, it is important to determine the unbound (i.e., therapeutically relevant) concentration of pharmacological agents. Dialysis techniques are well suited to make these determinations. In the anterior chamber, low concentrations of proteins are encountered (4). However, under conditions of compromised blood-aqueous barrier, an increased influx of proteins from plasma may result in elevated aqueous protein concentrations (46). Under these conditions, the assessment of unbound concentrations in aqueous humor may become more important in the establishment of the pharmacodynamics arising from intraocular exposures to the substrate in question.

Microdialysis is a dynamic process. Perfusion medium is perfused through the probe. Analyte concentrations in perfusate and in the surrounding medium are not in equilibrium (41). This introduces a number of technical problems that must be overcome in creative ways. Microdialysis is a relatively sophisticated tool. There are a number of challenges to appropriate use of this technique. Although nonspecific binding to the microdialysis membrane is minimized as compared to other dialysis methods, plastic tubing is used to deliver perfusate to the probe and to deliver the dialysate from the probe to the collection vessel. Nonspecific binding to the tubing is possible (47). This situation can be exacerbated when coupling microdialysis directly to other instrumentation since longer tubing usually is required. In experiments examining plasma protein binding of drug in vivo, microdialysis requires sufficient time to achieve stable concentrations. This process requires more time (than ultrafiltration, for example), and recovery of substrate across the membrane can be time- and temperature-dependent.

2. Microdialysis Probe Design Issues

The unique and dynamic environment of the anterior chamber provides features amenable to microdialysis sampling. Continuous flow of aqueous humor about the probe tip prevents the creation of microenvironments near the probe membrane. This is an important advantage for microdialysis use in this organ as opposed to placement in other extracellular spaces. Special problems that develop for specific placement into the anterior chamber include fibrin formation (17), which must be circumvented in order to prevent reduced recovery of substrate in probe effluent. Additionally, due to possible disruption of the blood-aqueous barrier, protein influx may alter the drug disposition of highly protein-bound substrates (17).

Specific advantages to microdialysis use for anterior chamber sampling are:

1. There is no extraction of internal aqueous humor fluids; IOP is not adjusted artificially since aqueous humor volume is not altered by influx of fluids.
2. Microdialysis sampling of both pharmacological agent and endogenous substrate is performed simultaneously.
3. Although this method involves some intrusion via surgical placement of the microdialysis probe into the anterior chamber, a more quantitative approach to the estimation of aqueous humor formation rates and pharmacokinetic experimentation is possible than with many conventional noninvasive approaches.

Fukada et al. (48–50) used a linear probe design that involved both entry and exit ports through the anterior chamber, a similar approach to that taken by Macha and Mitra (51,52). For their work in conscious animals, Rittenhouse et al. (19,53,54) modified a concentric microdialysis probe design according to the scheme presented in Figure 1, incorporating a 90° bend in the probe shaft for each of anchoring the probe to the sclera of the rabbit eye. In Figure 2, a photograph of an intact rabbit eye with a microdialysis probe in the anterior chamber is presented.

3. Microdialysis Probe Recovery

A major concern in using microdialysis as a tool for the determination of unbound drug concentrations in the in vivo as well as in vitro settings is the

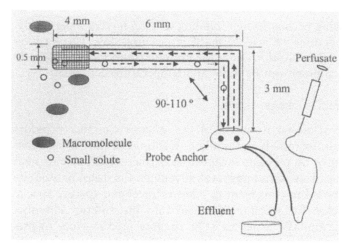

Figure 1 Custom-designed microdialysis probe for posterior or anterior chamber placement into the rabbit eye.

assessment of recovery. Recovery may be defined as the proportion of solute extracted from the medium surrounding the probe (55). Recovery is dependent on the following parameters: dialysis membrane length, perfusion flow rate, diffusion rate of the solute through the compartment (the usual rate-limiting step in the process), and membrane properties (47). Recovery can

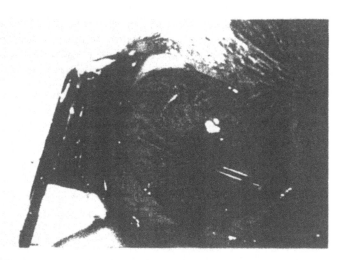

Figure 2 Rabbit eye with a microdialysis probe in the anterior chamber (magnification ~ 4×).

also be time- and temperature-dependent. Typical recovery values observed in the literature range from a low of ~ 10 up to 100%. By maximizing the dialysis membrane length, significant increases in recovery can be realized. Decreases in perfusion flow rate also increase the relative recovery (although they also decrease the available sample volume). The recovery of solute can be difficult to ascertain. Ideally, probe perfusate composition should closely match the environment of the medium in which it is placed. The probe also can create a microenvironment near the probe surface, which may be different than the medium more distant from the membrane (47). Several different types of recoveries are evaluated in microdialysis studies; these include relative recovery (or concentration recovery) and absolute recovery (mass recovery). Relative recovery is the fraction of solute obtained in the dialysate relative to the actual concentration in the medium in which the probe is placed. Absolute recovery is the total amount of solute collected over a specified time period. A number of approaches are used to estimate the recovery of a solute by the microdialysis probe, including water recovery, no-net-flux (or difference method), perfusion rate, and relative loss (55,56).

The water-recovery method is of limited use for in vivo settings because drug diffusion characteristics are usually different in artificial aqueous physiological buffers or solutions than in the dynamic in vivo environment. Where a solid in vitro–to–in vivo correlation is established, the water-recovery method has utility. For this method, the microdialysis probe is placed in a reservoir (usually stirred) containing a known concentration of solute. The perfusion medium, an aqueous solution of similar composition to the medium in which it is placed but without solute, is delivered through the probe at a constant rate. Dialysate is collected and the amount of solute determined via appropriate analytical methods. The ratio of the dialysate concentration of the known concentration of the medium in which the probe is placed is the relative recovery. This method is known to underestimate the concentration in the medium sampled (55).

The point of no-net-flux or difference method is used for in vitro and in vivo studies. By varying the concentration of solute in the perfusion medium and fixing the solute concentration in the surrounding medium, the dialysate solute concentration is assessed. The direction of the concentration gradient of solute depends on whether the concentration in the perfusion medium is higher or lower than the concentration in the surrounding medium (55). A plot of the perfusate solute concentration versus the difference in concentration between perfusate and dialysate is constructed; the x-intercept identifies the concentration at which no net flux of solute occurs (55). In theory, this value will be the concentration of the surrounding medium. This method is very time-consuming.

The perfusion rate method is based on the principle that recovery is dependent on the rate of perfusate transit through the probe. With an increase in perfusate transit, there is a corresponding decrease in relative recovery. Conversely, the lower the perfusion rate, the higher the relative recovery. For the perfusion rate method, the initial surrounding medium contains no solute and the probe is perfused with a fixed concentration of solute (55). This method is the most exhaustive in that several different surrounding media concentrations must be assessed separately, each at different perfusion rates (in vitro). A typical experiment might evaluate four different concentrations for the medium at three different perfusion rates each over an extended period. Frequently regression models are employed to provide the best estimates of probe performance. Typically for in vivo determinations, the lowest possible perfusion rate (e.g., 0.1 μL/min) is selected. This maximizes the relative recovery to nearly 100% in some cases. At such low flow rates, longer collection times are required to obtain sufficient sample for further analysis.

The relative loss method is similar to the water-recovery method, but is operated in reverse. Rather than placing a known concentration of solute in the medium surrounding the probe, the solute concentration of the perfusate is fixed. The surrounding medium, which in most situations contains small quantities of solute (i.e., sink conditions), then provides a negative concentration gradient of the solute. The net loss of solute reflects the relative loss of solute to medium. This method, which is based on the premise that recovery is the same in both directions across the membrane (47), is by far the simplest to use in the in vivo setting and provides a reliable estimate of recovery. Relative loss is the ratio of the difference in perfusate to dialysate solute concentrations to the perfusate concentration (56). This method is often referred to as retrodialysis recovery. Under nonsink conditions of the surrounding medium, an internal standard is sometimes employed.

C. Anterior Versus Posterior Chamber Sampling

Anterior chamber aqueous microdialysis sampling approaches have been explored by a number of researchers (16,17,48–54). Challenges that were managed using this approach include sensitivity of the eye to immunoprotective cascades following manipulation (17) and the requirement of the protection of visual function, also a major concern for any procedures proposed for observation of ocular pathophysiology or ocular pharmacokinetic/pharmacodynamic experimentation.

In published reports as early as the 1940s, researchers attempted to obtain information regarding aqueous endogenous substrate concentrations in the posterior versus the anterior chambers. Becker (57) and Kinsey and

Palmer (58,59) examined posterior chamber versus anterior chamber aqueous humor ascorbate concentrations. Rittenhouse et al. (53) used a microdialysis approach to estimate posterior versus anterior chamber ascorbate aqueous concentrations; the probe tip was introduced into the anterior chamber and directed through the pupil towards the posterior chamber. The posterior chamber is a much smaller region (~ 55 μL Vs ~ 250 μL for the anterior chamber) and provides additional challenges due to size constraints.

V. CASE STUDIES OF MICRODIALYSIS USE IN THE ANTERIOR SEGMENT

A. Ocular Pharmacokinetics

Recently, drug disposition in the anterior segment has been explored using microdialysis. Fukuda et al. (48–50) were the first to examine the utility of microdialysis sampling of anterior chamber aqueous humor. In their studies, linear probes inserted into the temporal cornea through the anterior chamber and exteriorized out of the nasal cornea were used to examine intraocular disposition of fluoroquinolones following oral or topical administration of ofloxacin, norfloxacin, or lomefloxacin in the anesthetized rabbit (48,49). Fukada et al. (48) characterized the ocular pharmacokinetics (C_{max}, T_{max}, $T_{1/2}$) of ofloxacin. Sato et al. [of the same laboratory as Fukada (49)] were able to conclude that lomefloxacin penctrated into aqueous sooner and was eliminated faster than norfloxacin. In later experiments, Ohtori et al. [of the same laboratory as above (50)] examined the ocular pharmacokinetics of timolol and carteolol in rabbits shortly after recovery from anesthesia. A 5 mm cellulose membrane (50 kDa) linear probe of fused silica (0.2 mm o.d., 23 g tubing) was used. In vitro recoveries of 16–20% for norfloxacin/lomefloxacin and ~ 17–22% for timolol and carteolol were reported. Pigmented rabbits (1.5–3.0 kg) were studied. The surgery involved stitching the nictitating membrane in order to immobilize the eye followed by the insertion of a 23 gauge needle attached to one end of the probe in the temporal cornea and passing the needle through anterior chamber and out of nasal side. The exteriorized tubing was glued at the puncture sites with epoxy resin. The polyethylene tubing was taped to the face of the rabbit.

Rittenhouse et al. (16) developed an animal model for the evaluation of microdialysis sampling of aqueous humor to assess the ocular absorption and disposition of beta-adrenergic antagonist drugs. For this study using anesthetized dogs ($n = 3$) and rabbits ($n = 3$), microdialysis probes (10 mm CMA/20) were implanted in the anterior chamber. Immediately following probe implantation (~ 30 min), a single dose of [^{3}H]DL-propranolol was administered topically or intracamerally in order to estimate intraocular bioavailability of [^{3}H]DL-propranolol. [^{3}H]DL-Propranolol collected from probe effluent was assayed by liquid scintillation spectroscopy. The results of this study indicated a 10-fold higher intraocular exposure to propranolol in the rabbit relative to the dog (F_{AH} ~ 0.55 vs. ~ 0.056). Time to peak was longer in the dog relative to the rabbit (~ 87 vs. ~ 54 min), and the terminal rate constant for the dog was ~ twofold higher than the rabbit (~ 0.0189 vs. ~ 0.00983). Propranol recoveries of ~ 32–45% were reported. The results obtained in this initial examination of propranolol disposition in aqueous humor using microdialysis were highly variable. In general, aqueous humor protein concentrations would have minimal influence on ocular exposure (3) due to the low concentrations present. However, since propranolol is a highly protein-bound substrate (45), Rittenhouse et al. (17) examined the possibility that time-dependent protein binding might have been a contributing factor to variability in parameter estimates, due to surgical insult from probe implantation and subsequent increased influx of proteins into aqueous humor. In addition, anesthesia is a known contributor to alterations in the pharmacokinetics and pharmacodynamics of drugs (60). Thus, development of relevant experimental techniques for use in conscious animals was imperative.

Following redesign of the microdialysis probes for anterior or posterior chamber placement (4 mm, CMA/20 with 90° bend) (Fig. 1) in the conscious rabbit, studies were conducted with propranolol (17) to estimate the intraocular exposure (AUC_{AH}), time to peak (T_{max}), and aqueous humor peak concentrations (C_{max}) following a > 5-day recovery. This minimum recovery period was established by following the time course of ocular wound healing and anterior segment resorption of fibrin, a phenomenon that could result in reduced substrate recovery via microdialysis aqueous humor sampling. Briefly, the surgical probe implantation procedure for New Zealand white rabbits (2.3–50 kg) proceeded as follows: A limbal-based conjunctival flap was created superior nasally or temporally ~ 3 mm from the limbus. A 10–12 mm conjunctival pocket was prepared, and the probe inlet/outlets were exteriorized to the top of head. A 20 gauge needle was inserted ~ 2–3 mm from limbus into the anterior chamber and removed. The microdialysis probe was then placed into the opening and the anchor of probe sutured to the sclera and covered with conjunctiva. Propranolol ocular pharmacokinetic parameter estimates obtained from a previous study (16) were compared to those obtained in the present study (17). It was observed that reduced dose-normalized AUC_{AH} and C_{max} were obtained in the previous study relative to the present study (~ 1.9-fold relative to anesthetized results with >5-day recovery period). It was hypothesized that time-dependent aqueous humor protein concentrations may have been present immediately postsurgery, but that protein concentrations returned to basal levels given a sufficient recovery period. Increased aqueous humor protein concentrations have been reported in vivo shortly after cannulation of the eye (46). In order to examine this possible explanation for the apparent decrease in dose-normalized AUC_{AH} observed in the previous study (16), the time course of aqueous humor protein concentrations after microdialysis probe implantation in the anterior chamber was examined in 16 rabbits (17). Immediately following probe implantation, aqueous humor protein concentrations were comparable to control. At 30 minutes postimplantation, aqueous humor protein concentrations were maximal ($\sim$ 30 mg/mL) and were maintained for up to 90 minutes. Aqueous humor protein concentrations were half-maximal at 150 minutes. A simulation approach was used to examine the hypothesis that altered protein concentrations were responsible for differences in propranolol exposure between the two experiments. Results of the simulations indicated that time-dependent binding of propranolol in aqueous humor was probably the major contributor to the reduced aqueous humor intraocular exposure to propranolol observed in rabbits with a minimal recovery period postimplantation (2.4-fold for simulation results vs. $\sim$ 1.9-fold difference observed in vivo). Another salient observation in this study was the appreciable difference between the ocular pharmacokinetics of propranolol in the conscious versus the anesthetized rabbit. Dose-normalized AUC_{AH} was $\sim$eight-fold lower in conscious rabbits as compared to anesthetized rabbits. Propranolol dose-normalized C_{max} values for the conscious rabbits were appreciably lower than those reported in the literature for conscious animal experimentation (20,21). A careful examination of this question resulted in the hypothesis that traditional sampling procedures (euthanasia of conscious rabbits following topical administration of drug, with paracentesis sampling of aqueous humor as the last step) may result in artifactually higher intra-ocular exposures to topically administered xenobiotics. This work provided a framework for examination of ocular pharmacokinetics in a more physiologically relevant model.

Although a number of researchers have examined the blood-to-aqueous transport of ascorbate in ciliary body tissue and cell culture in vitro (61–68), the transport kinetics information derived from these studies, in most instances, does not correlate to in vivo determinations. In vivo investigations have been limited due to difficulties inherent in studies of ascorbate transport kinetics; K_m, the blood concentration of ascorbate at half-maximal transport, is reputed to be at or below physiological blood concentrations (58,63). Rittenhouse et al. (53), following the development of an analytical procedure for assay of ascorbate in blood and aqueous humor, examined the transport kinetics of ascorbate using the recently developed conscious animal model with microdialysis sampling of aqueous humor.

Microdialysis probes were placed in the anterior chamber of one eye and the posterior chamber of the fellow eye (53). Basal blood–to–aqueous transport of ^{14}C-ascorbate was established by the examination of aqueous humor ascorbate corrected for specific activity. Following a 30-day recovery period, the rabbits ($n = 4$) were placed in restraining devices, the marginal ear veins of respective ears were cannulated, and ascorbate was administered via an i.v. bolus loading dose followed by maintenance incremental infusions in order to characterize the linear-to-nonlinear kinetic profile in blood to aqueous humor transport. Blood and probe effluent were analyzed via UV spectrophotometry at 265 nm. A nonlinear least-squares regression analysis assessment of the transport kinetics of ascorbate was performed. Contrary to previous reports (58,63), ascorbate blood concentrations, which were increased in a stepwise fashion (an overall ~twofold increase), did not result in saturable ascorbate uptake into aqueous (blood concentrations from ~ 14 to ~ 21 to ~ 30 mg/L). Nonlinear least-squares regression analysis of a model that incorporated nonsaturable uptake into aqueous with first-order translocation from the posterior to the anterior chamber and first-order efflux from the anterior chamber, with an incorporated lag time of ~ 1 hour, appeared to describe the data best. The model fits to the serum, anterior, and posterior aqueous ascorbate concentration-time data are presented in Figure 3. Physiologically relevant parameter estimates were obtained with this approach. The analysis provided indications that reduced aqueous humor turnover occurred in this group of rabbits (translocation rate constants were ~ 0.005 min^{-1} as compared to 0.01 min^{-1} in intact animals). The parameter estimates were also in agreement with the model independent ascorbate ocular clearance determinations (~ 39 µL/min or ~ 0.003 min^{-1}, when divided by the estimated aqueous humor volume of 200 µL) (53). It is possible that the apparent transport of ascorbate was perturbed by surgery. Surgical trauma can result in increased peroxide generation as a result of the inflammatory cascade (69). There are no reports of studies evaluating basal ascorbate transport as a function of the degree of intraocular inflammation. It also is possible that time-dependent changes to ascorbate blood to aqueous transport were observed. In order to examine this possibility, the relationship between aqueous humor ascorbate concentrations and time post–probe implantation was examined (Fig. 4) (17,53,54). At 0 minutes, physiologically relevant ascorbate aqueous humor concentrations are observed (~ 1.4 mM). An appreciable decrease ($\sim 50\%$) was observed from day 1 to day 12. Hence, recovery periods were lengthened for subsequent experiments in order to examine ascorbate transport kinetics (> 30 days). However, from

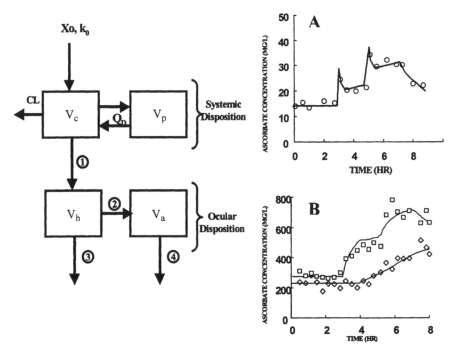

Figure 3 Four-compartment model and associated ascorbate disposition in serum (A) and aqueous humor (B). Lines represent fit of the kinetic model to the data. (Adapted from Ref. 53.)

the data presented in Figure 5, it appeared that as early as ~ 21 days, ascorbate aqueous humor concentrations returned to physiologically relevant concentrations (~ 1.3 mM). The relationship between basal blood to aqueous transport and time postsurgery is presented in Figure 5. Basal transport rates comparable to the expected value (~ 27 μg/hr) were observed for rabbits following a minimum of 21 days of recovery. These data were examined retrospectively (53,54).

Macha and Mitra (51,52) explored an innovative approach in ocular microdialysis experimentation. A dual microdialysis probe experimental design provided the unique opportunity to examine intraocular drug disposition in both vitreous and aqueous humors simultaneously. Using this approach, the pharmacokinetics of systemically versus intravitreously administered fluorescein (51) was examined in the anesthetized rabbit. Concentric probes (CMA/20 with 0.5 × 10 mm, polycarbonate membrane and 14 mm shaft) were used for vitreous sampling. Linear probes (MD-2000, 0.32 × 10 mm, polyacrylonitrile membrane and 0.22 mm tubing)

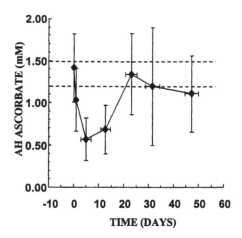

Figure 4 Relationship between aqueous humor ascorbate concentrations and recovery period in rabbits with intraocular microdialysis probes placed into the anterior or posterior chamber of the eye. Area between dashed lines represents reported steady-state aqueous humor ascorbate concentrations.

were used for aqueous sampling. For the implantation of the probe in the vitreous, a 22 gauge needle was inserted into the eye about 3 mm below the corneal-scleral limbus through the pars plana. The needle was then removed and the probe adjusted such that the membrane was in the mid-

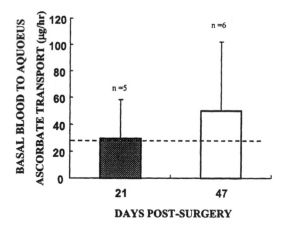

Figure 5 Relationship between basal ascorbate blood aqueous transport versus recovery period in rabbits with intraocular microdialysis probes in the anterior and posterior chambers. Dashed line represents theoretical basal transport. (Bars represent ± SD).

vitreous region as ascertained by microscopic examination. The linear probe was implanted in the aqueous humor using a 25 gauge needle. The needle was inserted across the cornea just above the corneal scleral limbus so that it traversed through the center of the anterior chamber to the other end of the cornea. The sample-collecting end of the linear probe was inserted into the bevel edge end of the needle. The needle was then retracted, leaving the probe with the membrane in the middle of the anterior chamber. The outlets of both probes were then fixed. The rabbits were maintained under general anesthesia throughout the experiment. A permeability index was calculated by taking the ratio of the area under the aqueous or vitreous fluorescein concentration curve relative to plasma following intravenous administration. This assessment provided experimental documentation of the pathway for fluorescein entry into the eye primarily via the ciliary body; the aqueous permeability index was ~fivefold higher than vitreous. The plasma, aqueous, and vitreous disposition of fluorescein is presented in Figure 6.

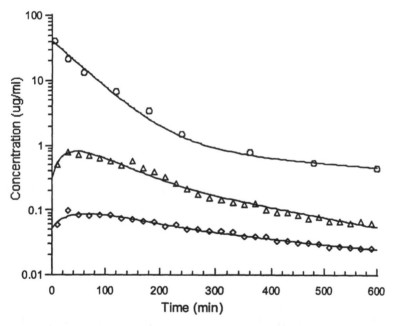

Figure 6 Concentration-time profiles of plasma, anterior chamber, and vitreous fluorescein after systemic administration (10 mg/kg): (○) plasma concentrations; (△) aqueous concentration; (◇) vitreous concentration. The line drawn represents the nonlinear least-squares regression fit of the model to the concentration-time data. (Ref. 52.)

B. Ocular Pharmacology and Pharmacodynamic Experimentation

A second study using the dual–probe approach—simultaneous sampling of aqueous and vitreous humor using microdialysis—was conducted (52) for the examination of cephalosporin ocular pharmacokinetics and the pharmacodynamics of inhibitory drugs on the intraocular disposition of cephalosporins. New Zealand albino rabbits (2–2.5 kg) were kept under anesthesia throughout the experiment. The concentric and linear microdialysis probes were implanted into the vitreous and aqueous chambers, respectively, as described above (51). Microdialysate samples were collected every 20 minutes over a period of 10 h. The animals were allowed to stabilize for 2 hours prior to initiation of each experiment. The ocular pharmacokinetics of cephalosporins were investigated following intravitreal administration of 500 µg dose of cephalexin, cephazolin, and cephalothin, respectively. In vivo inhibition experiments were conducted by coadministration of one of two dipeptides, gly-pro or gly-sar, with a 50 µg dose of cephalexin or cefazolin. The dipeptides were administered by a bolus injection into the vitreous 30 minutes prior to administration of the drugs, as well as by continuous perfusion through the vitreous probes to maintain the study state dipeptide concentrations throughout the experiment. The intravitreal elimination half-lives of cephalexin, cefazolin, and cephalothin after intravitreal administration were found to be 185.38 ± 27 $.25$ min, 111.40 ± 17.17 min, and 146.68 ± 47.52 min, respectively. Higher aqueous cephalexin concentrations were observed in comparison to cefazolin concentrations. With respect to the pharmacokinetic parameters of cephalexin in the presence of gly-pro, increased AUC (~3-fold), decreased clearance (~ 3-fold), and increased terminal elimination half-life (~ 3.5-fold) was observed. The cephalexin intravitreal concentration time course with or without inhibitor is presented in Figure 7. For cefazolin, no change in the pharmacokinetic parameters was observed except for an ~fourfold increase in terminal elimination half-life in the presence of gly-pro. Gly-sar had no significant effect on the pharmacokinetics of either drug.

An important first step toward the ultimate endpoint, the assessment of the pharmacodynamics of beta-adrenergic antagonists, involved characterization of the disposition of the proposed endogenous marker for aqueous humor turnover, ascorbate, discussed in the previous section (53). The utility of this approach was examined initially in the pioneering work of Becker (57,70,71,72) for the pharmacodynamics of a systemically administered carbonic anhydrase inhibitor (CAI), acetazolamide. CAIs decrease IOP via reduction in aqueous humor production (73). Ascorbate concentra-

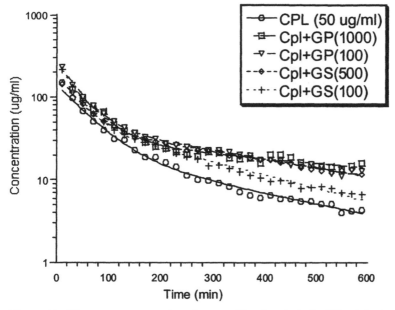

Figure 7 Vitreous concentration-time profile of cephalexin (50 μg) in the presence of inhibitors after intravitreal administration. (Ref. 51.)

tions in aqueous humor were observed to increase following acetazolamide administration (70). This observation provided the impetus for examining ascorbate as an endogenous substrate for the assessment of aqueous humor production inhibition.

Examination of the pharmacodynamics of aqueous humor production by beta-adrenergic antagonists was performed with a novel approach, microdialysis sampling of aqueous humor ascorbate. The time course for ascorbate in aqueous humor was used in order to determine the relative changes in aqueous humor flow as a result of beta-blocker pharmacodynamics. The volume dilution technique (31,32) involves assessment of the time course of an exogenously administered dye in aqueous humor following pharmacodynamic modulation of aqueous humor production (Fig. 8A), as described previously. Due to the intrusiveness of the procedure, studies of this nature are possible only in anesthetized animals. Rittenhouse et al. (54) selected an approach that would permit examination in a conscious animal model and would minimize the number of exogenous substrates required for this examination. By using an endogenous substrate, ascorbate, a less intrusive method for the examination of in vivo aqueous humor turnover, was developed (Fig. 8B).

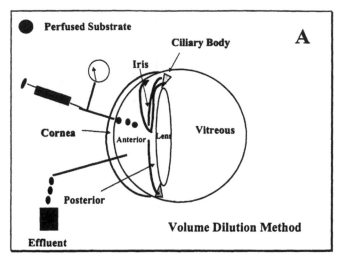

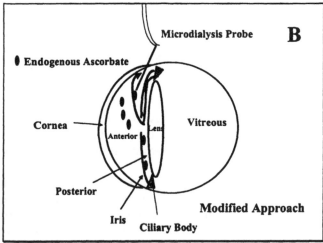

Figure 8   Schematic of volume dilution method (A) and modified volume dilution method: microdialysis probe placement (B).

Following anterior chamber placement of microdialysis probes into each eye of six rabbits and a >14-day recovery period, each rabbit received a tracer i.v. bolus of ^{14}C-ascorbate (53). Basal ascorbate blood to aqueous transport, R_o, and ascorbate ocular clearance, CL_{AH} were estimated. After a 1-hour washout, each rabbit received a series of three doses of ^{3}H-propranolol (750–3000 μg, 16.5 μCi/mg) every 60 minutes into the lower cul-de-sac of each eye. Microdialysis probe effluent was analyzed for ascorbate with a spectrophotometric assay (53,54), and the time course of aqueous humor ascorbate was determined (Fig. 9) (54). Nonlinear least-squares regression analysis of the ascorbate time-course in aqueous humor was performed in order to estimate the altered CL_{AH} following propranolol perturbation of aqueous humor production. The relative difference in the basal CL_{AH} and the CL_{AH} determined subsequent to propranolol administration was calculated. The major assumption for this approach was that this difference in CL_{AH} could be attributed solely to inhibition of aqueous humor production. A $\sim 47\%$ reduction in flow was observed

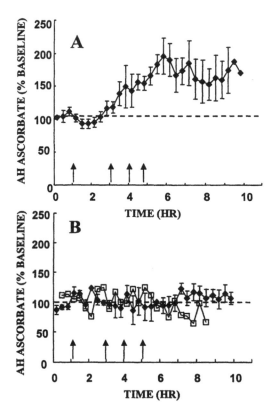

Figure 9 Ascorbate aqueous humor concentrations following three doses of topically administered propranolol: (A) AH ascorbate as % baseline (bars indicate ± SE; $n = 3$) versus time profile for the 1500 µg dose (◆); (B) AH ascorbate as % baseline (bars indicate ± SE; $n = 3$ versus time profiles for the 750 µg (◆) and for the 3000 µg (□) doses. Arrows represent time for administration of ^{14}C-ascorbate i.v. dose and the hourly propranolol topical doses. (From Ref. 57.)

following topical administration of propranolol (1500 μg). No modulation in the ascorbate aqueous humor time-course was observed for the 750 and 3000 μg groups. The model fit to three individual ascorbate aqueous concentration–time data is presented in Figure 10. Examination of iris-ciliary body tissue concentrations of ascorbate and propranolol provided evidence that a spectrum of intraocular responses to propranolol was observed in this experiment. It appeared that the 750 μg dose provided aqueous humor

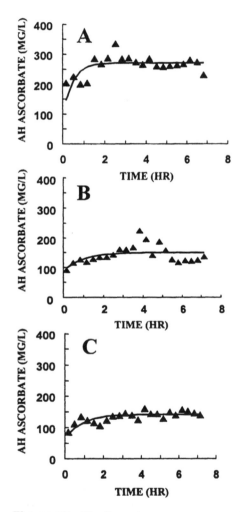

Figure 10   Nonlinear least-squares regression fit of aqueous humor ascorbate concentration versus time profiles following three 1500 μg doses of topically administered propranolol in three individual rabbits. (From Ref. 54.)

propranolol concentrations below those that could inhibit aqueous humor production. Reduction in aqueous humor production was observed for the 1500 µg group, while the simultaneous inhibition of ascorbate ciliary tissue accumulation and aqueous humor formation resulting in no change in the ascorbate aqueous humor time course was observed for the 3000 µg group (54). Anterior segment microdialysis provided an excellent approach to examine complex ocular physiology and pharmacology.

VI. FUTURE CHALLENGES, MILESTONES, AND OPPORTUNITIES

The anterior segment microdialysis technique has provided the framework for novel approaches to the examination of the mechanisms involved in ophthalmic drug ocular pharmacokinetics and the pharmacodynamics of aqueous humor formation and modulation. Anesthetized and conscious animal models, in some cases involving the long-term placement of microdialysis probes into the anterior segment (i.e., anterior and posterior chambers), were established, which have provided a substantial advance in experimental approaches to ocular pharmacokinetic/pharmacodynamic experimentation. Reduction in the number of animals required for these studies ($n = 48$ reduced to $n = 3 - 6$) provides a clear market advantage via reduction in costs and in animal-sparing research approaches. Animal experimentation with probe placement in the anterior segment, pioneered by Sato et al. (49), Fukada et al. (48), and Ohtori et al. (50), up to papers describing conscious animal experimental with microdialysis probes in the anterior chamber for 5 to > 30 days (17,53,54), demonstrate the rapid development and increased utility of the microdialysis approach in the study of ocular drug delivery and disposition. Unique applications of the microdialysis approach in the examination of drug ocular disposition such as a dual probe implantation technique involving simultaneous examination of aqueous and vitreous drug disposition have been performed (51,52). The importance and broad-based applicability of the microdialysis sampling approach for the examination of ocular pharmacokinetics and dynamics of ophthalmics is of large impact. Reuse of animals is possible because of the long-term tolerability of the animals to probe implantation. A series of substrates could be examined using the same subject to assess phenomenon such as tolerance development. Possible reduction in inter-subject responses to ophthalmic drugs is possible via this approach. This approach also provided the framework for a detailed examination of in vivo basal blood to aqueous transport of ascorbate, a labile substrate of utmost importance to intraocular health and homeostasis. Moreover, the pharmacodynamics of beta-adrenergic antagonist–associated modulation of both aqueous humor formation and ascorbate ciliary accumulation was examined in detail using anterior segment microdialysis. Pharmacokinetic modeling was facilitated with this technique; by using alterations in the ascorbate aqueous humor time-course as a means of estimating aqueous humor flow, the modulatory effects of a model substrate, propranolol, on aqueous humor turnover, was examined.

REFERENCES

1. Morrison, J. C., and Freddo, T. F. (1996). Anatomy, microcirculation, and ultrastructure of the ciliary body. In *The Glaucomas*, 2nd ed., Ritch, R., Sields, M. B., Krupin, T., eds. C. V. Mosby Publishers, St. Louis, pp. 125–138.
2. Krupin, T., and Civan, M. M. (1996). Physiologic basic of aqueous humor formation. In *The Glaucomas*, 2nd ed., Ritch, R., Sields, M. B., Krupin, T., eds. C. V. Mosby Publishers, St. Louis, pp. 252–253.
3. Cole, D. F. (1974). Comparative aspects of intraocular fluids. In *The Eye: Comparative Physiology*, H. Dason, L. T. Graham, eds. Academic Press, New York.
4. Cole, D. F. (1977). Secretion of the aqueuos humor. *Exp. Eye Res.* 25 (suppl):161.
5. Bill, A. (1973). The role of ciliary body blood flow and ultrafiltration in aqueous humor formation. *Exp. Eye Res.* 16:287.
6. Freddo, T. F. (1989). Ocular anatomy and physiology related to aqueous production and outflow. In *The Glaucomas*, Ritch, R., Sields, M. B., Krupin, T., eds. C. V. Mosby Publishing Co., St. Louis, pp. 23–46.
7. Sears, M. L. and Kondo, K. (1986). Drugs effects upon aqueous production. *Trans. Ophthalmol. Soc. U.K.* 105:171–179.
8. Krupin, T., and Nichols, P. F. (1984). In *Glaucoma: Applied Pharmacology in Medical Treatment*. Drance, S. E., and Neufeld, A. H., eds. Grune and Stratton, New York, pp. 71–85.
9. Maurice, D. M., and Mishma, S. (1984). Ocular pharmacokinetics. In *Handbook Experimental Pharmacology*, Sears, M. L., ed. Springer-Verlag, New York, p. 32.
10. Kaufman, P. L. (1996). Pressure-dependent outflow. In *The Glaucomas*, 2nd ed., Ritch, R., Sields, M. B., Krupin, T., eds. C. V. Mosby Publishing Co., St. Louis, pp. 307–311.
11. Hart, W. M. (1992). Intraocular pressure. In *Adler's Physiology of the Eye, Clinical Application*, 9th ed., Hart, W. M. ed., Mosby Year Book, St Louis, pp. 248–267.
12. Johnson, D. H., Richardson, T. M., and Epstein, D. L. (1989). Trabecular meshwork recovery after phagocytic challenge. *Curr. Eye Res.* 8:1121–1130.

13. Epstein, D. L., Freddo, T. F., Anderson, P. J., Patterson, M. M., and Bassett-Chu, S. (1986). Experimental obstruction to aqueous outflow by pigment particles in living monkeys. *Invest. Ophthalmol. Vis. Sci.* 27:387–395.

14. Crean, E. V., Tyson, S. L., and Richardson, T. M. (1986). Establishment of calf trabecular meshwork cell cultures. *Exp. Eye Res.* 43:503–517.

15. Brubaker, R. F. (1991). Flow of aqueous humor in humans. *Invest. Ophthalmol. Vis. Sci.* 32:3145–3166.

16. Rittenhouse, K. D., Peiffer, Jr., R. L. and Pollack, G. M., (1998). Evaluation of microdialysis for in vivo models of ocular absorption and disposition. *J. Pharm. Biomed. Anal.* 16:951–959.

17. Rittenhouse, K. D., Peiffer, Jr., R. L. and Pollack, G. M. (1999). Microdialysis evaluation of the ocular pharmacokinetics of propranolol in the conscious rabbit. *Pharm. Res.* 16:736–742.

18. Lee, Y. H., Kompella, U. B., and Lee, V. H. L. (1993). Systemic absorption pathways of topically applied adrenergic antagonists in the pigmented rabbit. *Exp. Eye Res.* 57:341–349.

19. Ross, F. E., Innemee, H. C., and van Zwieten, P. A. (1980). Ocular penetration of beta-adrenergic blocking agents. An experimental study with atenolol, metoprolol, timolol and propranolol. *Docum. Ophthalmol.* 48:291–301.

20. Hussain, A., Hirai, S., and Sieg, J. (1980). Ocular absorption of propranolol in rabbits. *J. Pharm. Sci.* 69:738–739.

21. Schmitt, C., Lotti, V. J., and Le Douarec, J. C. (1981). Penetration of five beta-adrenergic antagonist into the rabbit eye after ocular instillation. *Albrecht Graefes Arch. Klin. Ophthalmol.* 217:167–174.

22. Ben-Nun, J., Joyce, D. A., Cooper, R. L., and Cringle, I. J. (1989). Pharmacokinetics of intravitreal injection. *Invest. Ophthalmol. Vis. Sci.* 30:1055–1061.

23. Urtii, A. (1993). Animal pharmacokinetics studies. In *Ophthalmic Drug Delivery Systems*, Mitra, A. K., ed. Marcel Dekker, New York, pp. 83–108.

24. Prince, J. H. (1964). *The Rabbit in Eye Research.* Charles C Thomas, Springfield IL.

25. Brubaker, R. F. (1996). Measurement of aqueous flow by fluorophotometry. In *The Glaucomas*, 2nd ed., Ritch, R., Sields, M. B., Krupin, T., eds. Mosby Publishing Co., St. Louis, pp. 447–453.

26. Jones, R. F., and Maurice, D. M. (1966). New methods of measuring the rate of aqueous flow in man with fluorescein. *Exp. Eye Res.*, 5:208–220.

27. Dueker, D. (1996). Tonography. In *The Glaucomas*, 2nd ed., Ritch, R., Sields, M. B., and Krupin, T., eds. Mosby Publishing Co., St. Louis, pp. 399–401.

28. Peiffer, R. L. Jr., Gelatt, K. N., and Gum, G. G. (1976). Determination of the facility of aqueous humor outflow in the dog, comparing in vivo and in vitro tonographic and constant pressure perfusion techniques. *Am. J. Vet. Res.* 12:1473–1477.

29. Peiffer, R. L. Jr., Gum, G. G., Grimson, R. C., and Gelatt, K. N. (1980). Aqueous humor outflow in beagles with inherited glaucoma: constant pressure perfusion. *Am. J. Vet. Res.* 41:1808–1813.

30. Johnson, M., Chen, A., Epstein, D. L., and Kamm, R. D. (1991). The pressure and volume dependence of the rate of wash-out in the bovine eye. *Curr. Eye Res.* 10:373–375.

31. Miichi, H., and Nagataki, S. (1982). Effects of cholinergic drugs and adrenergic drugs on aqueous humor formation in the rabbit eye. *Jpn. J. Ophthalmol.* 26:425–436.

32. Miichi, H., and Nagataki, S. (1983). Effects of pilocarpine, salbutamol, and timolol on aqueous humor formation in cynomolgus monkeys. *Invest. Ophthalmol. Vis. Sci.* 24:1269–1275.

33. Green, K., and Padgett, D. (1979). Effect of various drugs on pseudofacility and aqueous humor formation in the rabbit eye. *Exp. Eye Res.* 28:239–246.

34. Green, K., and Elija, D. (1981). Drug effects on aqueous humor formation and pseudofacility in normal rabbit eyes. *Exp. Eye Res.* 33:239–245.

35. Liu, H. K., Chiou, G. C., and Garg, L. C. (1980). Ocular hypotensive effects of timolol in cat eyes. *Arch. Ophthalmol.* 98:1467–1469.

36. Oppelt, W. W. (1967). Measurement of aqueous humor formation rates by posterior-anterior chamber perfusion with inulin: normal values and the effect of carbonic anhydrase inhibition. *Invest. Ophthalmol.* 6:76–83.

37. Evrard, P. A., Deridder G., and Verbeeck, R. K. (1996). Intravenous microdialysis in the mouse and the rat: Development and pharmacokinetic application of a new probe. *Pharm. Res.* 13:12–17.

38. Deguchi Y., Terasaki, T., Yamada, H., and Tsuji, A. (1992). An application of microdialysis to drug tissue distribution study: in vivo evidence for free-ligand hypothesis and tissue binding of Beta-Lactam antibiotics in interstitial fluids. *J. Pharmacobiol. Dyn.* 15:79–89.

39. Hogan, B., and Lunte, S. (1994). On-line coupling of in vivo microdialysis sampling with CE. *Anal. Chem.* 66:596–602.

40. Tellez, S., Forges, N., and Roussin, A. (1992). Coupling of microdialysis with CE: a new approach to the study of drug transfer between two compartments of the body in freely moving rats. *J. Chromatography* 581:257–266.

41. Eisenberg, E. J., and Eichoff, W. M. (1993). A method for estimation of extracellular concentration of compounds by microdialysis using urea as a endogenous recovery marker in vitro validation. *JPM* 30:27–31.

42. Dubey, R. K., McAllister C. B., Inoue, M., and Wilkinson, G. R. (1989). Plasma binding and transport of diazepam across the BBB. No evidence for in vivo enhanced dissociation. *J. Clin. Invest.* 84:1155–1159.

43. Sebille, B., Zini, R., Madjar, C. V., Thuaud, N., and Tillement, J. P. (1990). Review: separation procedures used to reveal and follow drug protein binding. *J. Chromatography* 531:51–77.

44. Rietbrock, N., and Woodcock, B., eds. (1981). Progress in drug protein binding: proceedings of lectures presented at a symposium in Frankfurt am Main, April 1980. *Methods in Clinical Pharmacology*, Vieweg, Braunschweig/Wiesbaden.

45. Rowland, M., and Tozer, T. N. (1995). *Clinical Pharmacokinetics: Concepts and Applications*, 3rd ed. Williams and Wilkins, Media, PA.

46. Kulkarni, P. S., and Srinvasan, B. D. (1987). Nonsteroidal anti-inflammatory drugs in ocular inflammatory conditions. In *Nonsteroidal Anti-inflammatory Drugs*, A. J. Lewis, D. E. Furst, eds., Marcel Dekker, New York.

47. Robinson, T. E., and Justice J. B., Jr. eds. (1991). *Microdialysis in the Neurosciences*. Elsevier Science Publishers, Amsterdam.

48. Fukuda, M., Mikitani, M., Ueda, T., Inatomi, M., Koide, Y., Kurata, T., et al. (1995). Application of microdialysis on analysis of pharmacokinetics in domestic rabbits aqueous humor. *J. Jpn. Ophthalmol. Soc.* 99:400–405.

49. Sato, H., Fukuda, S., Inatomi, M., Koide, R., Uchida, N., Kanda, Y., Kiuchi, Y., and Oguchi, K. (1996). Pharmacokinetics of norfloxacin and lomefloxacin in domestic rabbit aqueous humor analyzed by microdialysis. *J. Jpn. Ophthalmol. Soc.* 100:513–519.

50. Ohtori, R., Sato, H., Fukuda, S., Ueda, T., Koide, R., Kanda, Y., Kiuchi, Y., and Oguchi, K. (1988). Pharmacokinetics of topical beta-adrenergic antagonists in rabbit aqueuos humor evaluated with the microdialysis method. *Exp. Eye Res.* 66:487–494.

51. Macha, S., Mitra, A. K. (2001). Ocular pharmacokinetics of cephalosporin using microdialysis. *J. Ocul. Pharmacol Ther.* 17:485–498.

52. Macha S., Mitra A. K. (2001). Ocular pharmacokinetics in rabbits using a novel dual probe microdialysis technique. *Exp. Eye Res.*, 72:289–299.

53. Rittenhouse, K. D., Peiffer, R. L., Jr. and Pollack, G. M. (2000). Assessment of ascorbate ocular disposition in the conscious rabbit: an approach using the microdialysis technique. *Curr. Eye Res.* 20:351–360.

54. Rittenhouse, K. D., and Pollack, G. M. (2000). Pharmacodynamics of beta-blocker modulation of aqueous humor. *Exp. Eye Res.* 70:429–439.

55. Stahle, L., Segersvard, S., and Ungerstedt, U. (1991). A comparison between three methods for estimation of extracellular concentrations of exogenous and endogenous compounds by microdialysis. *J. Pharmacol. Methods* 25:41–52.

56. Scheller, D., and Kolb, J. (1991). The internal reference technique in microdialysis: a practical approach to monitoring dialysis efficiency and to calculating tissue concentration from dialysate samples. *J. Neurosci. Methods* 40:31–38.

57. Becker, B. (1955). The effects of the carbonic anhydrase inhibitor, acetazolamide, on the composition of aqueous humor. *Am. J. Ophthalmol.* 40:129–136.

58. Kinsey, V. E. (1947). Transfer of ascorbic acid and related compounds across the blood-aqueous barrier. *Am. J. Ophthalmol.* 30:1262–1266.

59. Kinsey, V. E. and Palmer, E. (1955). Posterior and anterior chamber aqueous humor formation. *AMA Arch. Ophthalmol.* 53:330.

60. Ausinsch, B., Rayborn, R. L., Munsen, E. S., and Levy, N. S. (1976) Ketamine and IOP in children. *Anesthesia Analgesia* 55:773–775.

61. Delamere, N. A., Coca-Prados, M., and Shelinder, A. (1993). Studies on regulation of the ascorbic acid transporter in a cell line derived from rabbit non-pigmented ciliary epithelium. *Biochem. Biophys. Acta* 1149:102–108.

62. Candia, O. A., Shi, X. P., and Chu, T. C. (1991). Ascorbate-stimulated active Na^+ transport in rabbit ciliary epithelium. *Curr. Eye Res.* 10:197–203.

63. Becker, B. (1967). Ascorbate transport in guinea pig eyes. *Invest. Ophthalmol.* 51:410–415.
64. Socci, R. R., and Delamere, N. A. (1988). Characteristics of ascorbate transport in the rabbit iris-ciliary body. *Exp. Eye Res.* 46:853–861.
65. Chu, T., and Candia, O. A. (1988). Active transport of ascorbate across the isolated rabbit ciliary epithelium. *Invest. Ophthalmol Vis. Sci.* 29:594–599.
66. Helbig, H., Korbmacher, C., Wohlfarth, J., Berweck, S., Kuhner, D., and Wiederholt, M. (1989). Electrogenic Na^+-ascorbate cotransport in cultured bovine pigmented ciliary epithelial cells. *Am. J. Physiol.* 256:C44–C49.
67. Mead, A., Sears, J. and Sears, M. (1996). Transepithelial transport of ascorbic acid by the isolated intact ciliary epithelial bilayer of the rabbit eye. *J. Ocular Pharmacol. Ther.* 12:253–258.
68. Hou, Y., Pierce, W. M., Jr., and Delamere, N. A. (1998). The influence of ascorbic acid on active sodium transport in cultured rabbit nonpigmented ciliary epithelium. *Invest. Ophthalmol. Vis. Sci.* 39:143–149.
69. Slater, T. F. (1972). *Free Radical Mechanisms in Tissue Injury.* Pion Publishing, London.
70. Becker, B. (1956). The effects of acetazolamide on ascorbic acid turnover. *Am. J. Ophthalmol.* 41:522–529.
71. Becker, B. (1957). Chemical composition of human aqueous humor. *AMA Arch. Ophthalmol.* 57:793–799.
72. Becker, B. (1959). Carbonic anhydrase and the formation of aqueous humor. *Am. J. Ophthalmol.* 47:342–359.
73. Hurvitz, M., Kaufman, P. L., Robin, A. L., Weinreb, R. N., Crawford, K., and Balke, S. (1991). New developments in the drug treatment of glaucoma. *Drugs* 41(4):514–532.

8
Posterior Segment Microdialysis

Sreeraj Macha* and Ashim K. Mitra
University of Missouri–Kansas City, Kansas City, Missouri, U.S.A.

I. INTRODUCTION

The eye is a specialized sensory organ that is relatively secluded from systemic access by the blood-retinal, blood-aqueous, and blood-vitreous barriers (1). Ocular infections can involve the lids, orbits and ocular adnexia, anterior segment (cornea and conjunctiva), or the eye interior, i.e., retina-choroid. While often benign and self-limiting, certain infections can involve delicate structures of the eye and destroy visual function (2). Postoperative endophthalmitis, which is bacterial in origin, is one of the most important complications following intraocular surgery. It is a sight-threatening condition and occurs with an incidence of 0.05–0.33% (1,3). Unfortunately, the outcome of clinical diagnosed postoperative endophthalmitis is far from satisfactory. More than 50% of all such cases suffer irreparable visual loss, despite presently available antimicrobial agents (4). Human cytomegalovirus retinitis is another most common cause of visual loss among patients suffering from acquired immunodeficiency syndrome (AIDS), occurring in about 30–40% of patients (5–8).

Management of these ocular diseases demands immediate diagnosis and treatment to maximize recovery of vision. Because of blood-ocular barriers, therapeutic intravitreal concentrations of drugs cannot be readily achieved by periocular or parenteral administration (9–11). Although standard therapy consists of both intravitreal and parenteral delivery, recent clinical evidence suggests that intravitreal administration alone is as effective in restoring vision as the combined therapy (3). Experimental pharmacoki-

---

* *Current affiliation*: Boehringer Ingelheim Inc., Ridgefield, Connecticut, U.S.A.

netic studies have repeatedly confirmed the need to administer drugs intra-vitreally because systemic or subconjunctival therapy does not deliver ade-quate concentrations of the drug into the vitreous body (9).

The major constraint on the development and assessment of posterior segment pharmacokinetics of drugs is the inaccessibility of the vitreous for continuous serial sampling. Imprecise or nonexistent pharmacokinetic infor-mation on vitreous drug disposition has prevented the delineation of the fundamental mechanisms of vitreal clearance and retinal uptake of drugs (12). More often, ocular pharmacokinetics are determined by obtaining single sample of the ocular fluids from individual animals (13–15) or by direct serial sampling (16,17).

Microdialysis has gained wide recognition as a valuable tool for sam-pling the extracellular space of the living tissue. It has become a standard technique in the field of neurochemistry, as well as in sampling other tissues and fluids including liver, kidney, skin, tumor, bile, and blood (18–21). Recently, microdialysis has been employed for sampling the vitreous (10,22–27) and aqueous humors (28) in rabbits. The present chapter deals with the methodological aspects to the use of this technique to study ocular pharmacokinetics. This chapter also presents a brief overview of the vitreal microdialysis studies reported recently.

II. ANATOMY OF THE POSTERIOR SEGMENT

The posterior segment of the eye is comprised of lens, sclera, choroid, vitr-eous, and retina. Vitreous is a clear gel composed almost entirely of water (99%) and collagen fibrils. Vitreous humor occupies a volume of 4 mL and comprises about 80% of the internal volume of the human eye. Its pH is about 7.5, and the water turnover rate in vitreous is reported to be about 10–15 minutes. It is separated from the lens and posterior chamber by the anterior vitreous membrane (anterior hyaloid membrane), which is anchored by ligaments to the retina. Vitreous chamber has three important anatomical adhesions: (a) ligamentum hyaloideo-capsulare, a pseudomem-brane consisting of collagen tissue, (b) circular attachment around the optic disc, and (c) the vitreous base, which is annular and lies against posterior surface of the ciliary body and pars plana. Vitreous in humans can be divided into two zones: the cortical zone and the medullary zone. Cortical vitreous is closest to the retina and is gel-like, mainly composed of collagen fibrils and hyaluronic acid. Medullary zone mainly consists of interstitial substance and tissue. Special cells called hyalocytes are dispersed in the outer parts of the cortical vitreous, particularly in the vicinity of pars plana.

Vitreous shows a fibrillar structure, which can be differentiated into two types: Coarse branching fibers originate at the base of the vitreous and disappear behind the equator after having divided into two or three fibrils. They are arranged in the cortex of the vitreous in two or more planes and are approximately 30 μm long. Fine parallel fibers are brittle with a diameter of 3 μm and are more closely joined. They divide behind the equator.

Retina, a transparent tissue, is the innermost coating of the eye that lines the posterior two thirds of the eyeball. It is firmly attached to the ciliary body at its anterior termination (ora serrata) and at the margins of the optic nerve. It consists of two major functional parts: the neural layer and the pigment epithelium. Pigment epithelium cells are connected by tight junctions and form a tight barrier between the choroid and retina. It selectively transfers nutrients to the retina from the choroid. There also exists a fluid pump mechanism in the direction of the choroid through the pigment epithelium.

Choroid is a highly vascularized tissue present between the retina and sclera. It forms the posterior part of the uvea, the anterior part consisting of the iris and ciliary body. Choroid mainly consists of three parts: (a) a vessel layer, consisting of veins and arteries; (b) a choriocapillary layer, consisting of a very fine and dense network of fenestrated capillaries, which is very permeable to plasma proteins and colloids; and (c) Bruch's membrane, which is in direct contact with the retinal pigment epithelium.

Sclera is the outermost layer of the eye, which is mainly protective in function. It is about 0.5–1.0 mm thick, consisting mainly of collagen bundles and elastic fibers.

III. OCULAR BARRIERS TO VARIOUS ROUTES OF ADMINISTRATION

Drug delivery to the posterior segment of the eye is of high clinical significance in treating various ocular disorders, i.e., endophthalmitis, viral retinitis, proliferative vitreoretinopathy, uveitis, etc. The problem of administering potent drugs to the posterior segment of the eye, which is a relatively closed and well-defined compartment, may be approached in different ways. The most common and patient-acceptable route is the topical instillation of drugs. Many studies have shown that approximately 5% or less of the topically applied dose is absorbed across the cornea, which forms the major barrier to drug penetration to anterior segment tissues. Amounts of drug absorbed into the posterior segment of the eye will only be a minute fraction of the amounts achieved in the anterior segment. The main constraints afforded by the eye upon topical delivery are the protective mechanisms, which include solution drainage, lacrimation, diversion of exogenous chemicals into the systemic circulation via conjunctiva, and a highly selective corneal barrier to exclude these compounds from the eye (29). In addition, there is a finite limit to the size of the dose that can be applied and tolerated by the cul-de-sac (usually 7–10 µL) and the contact time of the drug with the absorptive surfaces of the eye. The drugs usually disappear in about 5–10 minutes in rabbits and 1–2 minutes in humans following topical instillation (30,31) and at an even faster rate at the pH where most of the ophthalmic drugs are formulated (32).

Intraocular drug concentrations achieved after systemic administration depend primarily on the ocular blood circulation. With most drugs, very low intraocular concentrations were achieved after systemic administration, due mainly to the presence of blood-aqueous barrier, which restricts substances from entering into the aqueous humor, and blood-retinal barrier, which prevents the drugs entering into the vitreous chamber (33–37). Higher levels are generally found in the aqueous humor compared to vitreous, as the blood-aqueous barrier is known to be leakier than the blood-retinal barrier.

Subconjunctival administration of drugs can also generate elevated intraocular concentrations compared to topical and systemic administration, with minimal systemic adverse effects. The aqueous and vitreous concentrations of various drugs have been determined after subconjunctival administration (38–41). Even in this case the intraocular concentrations achieved were found to be only a fraction of the dose administered, as conjunctival epithelium constitutes a relatively tight barrier. The sclera does not offer a very tight barrier to the penetration of even relatively large molecular weight drugs (42).

The only possible way to achieve therapeutic concentrations in the posterior segment of the eye was found to be the intravitreal administration (43–51). This route of administration has become the recommended therapy for the treatment of endophthalmitis and cytomegalovirus retinitis. Drugs injected into the vitreous may be eliminated by two routes. Drugs eliminated by diffusion into the posterior chamber with subsequent removal by normal egress of fluid from the anterior chamber (52,53) generally exhibit half-lives within a range of 20–30 hours (53). The second route is through the retina via penetration of the blood-retinal barrier (52,53). Drugs eliminated by this route usually exhibit half-lives in the range of 5–10 hour (53).

IV. CONVENTIONAL TECHNIQUES TO STUDY OCULAR PHARMACOKINETICS

Delineation of ocular pharmacokinetics is complicated due to the complex nature of the retina and the presence of blood-ocular barriers. In addition, the small volume of the intraocular fluids aggravates the problem. Limited volumes of the aqueous and vitreous humors does not allow multiple and continuous sampling. Most of the studies were carried out with an objective to decide a dosage regimen that can provide therapeutic concentrations of drugs in the eye. These studies were conducted in human subjects by collecting vitreous and/or aqueous humor samples prior to surgery (such as cataract, paracentesis, vitrectomy, etc.) after administration of the drug by the route of interest (48). This method allows for collection of only one sample per subject at a specific time period. The data obtained can be interpreted only to determine whether the therapeutic concentrations of the drug have been achieved with the dose administered.

Ocular pharmacokinetic studies have been carried mainly in rabbits, the ocular physiology of which is most similar to the human eyes. Initially, the studies were carried out by collecting single samples from each animal at a specified time point (13,14). The pooling of the data from individual rabbits requires at least 100 animals for each profile (12,13). Moreover, it introduces a significant amount of intersubject variability.

Serial sampling technique has been developed to obtain more reliable data with a significantly reduced number of animals, compared to the single sample approach, needed for the estimation of pharmacokinetic parameters (15–17). Miller et al. (15) have developed and validated on animal model by measuring the protein concentrations of the intraocular fluids for serial sampling of the aqueous and/or vitreous humors in New Zealand albino rabbits. Animals were anesthetized and vitreous samples of about 20 µL were collected using a 28 gauge needle inserted into the vitreous chamber, 4 mm below the limbus. For serial sampling of the aqueous humor a 30 gauge needle fused to a calibrated 25 µL capillary tube was gently inserted into the anterior chamber near the limbus, and approximately 7 µL of aqueous humor was withdrawn.

V. MICRODIALYSIS

The in vivo microdialysis technique has gained significant importance in the field of the neurochemistry and neurophysiology. This technique has been successfully adapted to sample various tissues and fluids such as skin, liver, kidney, blood, etc. Recently, microdialysis has found important applications in the fields of pharmacokinetics, (especially in the area of drug distribution and metabolism) and pharmacodynamics. It has also been used to study the in vitro protein and melanin binding of drugs (54).

Microdialysis is based on the principle of diffusion. It involves perfusion of a probe, containing a semipermeable membrane, implanted in a tissue under nonequilibrium conditions. The driving force for the diffusion of drugs across the semipermeable membrane is the concentration gradient. Endogenous compounds (harmones, neurotransmitters, etc.) and exogenous compounds (drugs and metabolites) diffuse into the probe, whereas compounds added to the perfusate diffuse out into the tissue. Therefore, the technique can be used not only to monitor the extracellular concentrations of the analyte, but also to deliver drugs to a specific tissue region (55,56).

Microdialysis offers a number of advantages: (a) it permits continuous monitoring of the tissue concentration of a drug with limited interference with the normal physiology; (b) no fluid is introduced nor is any withdrawn from the tissue, which is particularly important in sampling tissues/organs with limited volume; (c) concentration versus time profiles can be obtained from individual animals; (d) the method provides protein free samples, thus eliminating clean up procedures and ex vivo enzymatic degradation; (e) the samples can be analyzed by any analytical technique, which contributes to the selectivity and sensitivity of the method. Its disadvantages include a need to determine the recovery of the probe (which is still controversial), the diluting effect of dialysis, which requires sensitive analytical methods to measure small concentrations, and the invasive nature of the probe implantation.

A. Probe Design and Selection

A variety of probes have been employed to study posterior segment pharmacokinetics. Probes are selected mainly on the basis of the drug under investigation, surgical accessibility, type, and length. A vertical probe with a concentric design, either as such or with modification, is most commonly used, both in fixed and repeated models, by reinsertion via a guide cannula. The molecular mass cut-off range of the commercially available probes is 5–50 kDa, and selection of a particular probe is based on the molecular weight of the drug and/or metabolites being studied. The probe membrane type is one more important factor to be considered in microdialysis. Tao and Hjorth (57) demonstrated the difference in the recoveries of three different probe types: GF (regenerated cellulose cuprophan), CMA (polycarbonate ether), and HOSPAL (polyacrilonitril/sodium methallylsulfonate copolymer). GF and CMA probes exhibited maximal recovery immediately after the introduction of 5-HT in the artificial CSF, whereas it took about 2 hours for the HOSPAL probe. Landolt et al. (58) have shown that the CMA probe recovery of cysteine and glutathione varied with concentration.

Ben-Nun et al. (10) used a sampling catheter for simultaneous sampling of the vitreous of both eyes for short-term experiments. Waga et al. (25,59,60) designed a new probe consisting of soft protecting tube (outer diameter 0.6 mm) with a long opening toward one side and a dialysis membrane mounted inside for long-term implantation in the vitreous chamber. The dialysis membrane consisted of a tube of polycarbonate-polyether copolymer, with an outer diameter of 520 μm and an inner diameter of 400 μm. In the later experiments the commercially available vertical probe (CMA 20), with a stiff plastic shaft, was used. The shaft length was set to 9 mm and was bent 60–90°. Probes with a molecular weight cut-off of 20 and 100 kDA were selected for small and large molecules, respectively. Stempels et al. (23) used CMA probe with a shaft diameter of 0.6 mm, length 3 mm, semipermeable membrane diameter of 0.52 mm, and a cut-off value of 20 kDa.

Probe recovery is directly proportional to the dialysis membrane surface area (61–63). By increasing the area, low drug concentrations can be detected with reasonably high perfusion flow rates while maintaining an adequate time resolution. To obtain optimal recovery, Macha and Mitra (26,27) selected a commercially available CMA probe with a membrane length of 10 mm, shaft 14 mm, and a cut-off value of 20 kDa.

Recovery is shown to be independent of the extracellular analyte concentration (61–63). A concentration gradient across the dialysis membrane changes in unison with the extracellular analyte concentration, thus maintaining a constant recovery.

B. Composition and Temperature of the Perfusate Solution

Intraocular fluid homeostasis is maintained by the highly perfused retina and iris-ciliary body. A perfusion fluid isosmotic with the plasma is preferred, as it has direct access to the vitreous humor. Previous studies have revealed that perfusion with anisosmotic fluid changes the dialysate concentration of taurine in brain (64–66) and muscle (64) microdialysis. In addition, problems arise when a compound already present in the perfusion medium is also measured using dialysis.

In vitro recovery is dependent on the temperature of the standard solution. Wages et al. (67) have shown that the in vitro recovery of 3,4-dihydroxyphenylacetic acid increased by approximately 30% when the solution temperature was raised from 23 to 37°C. Therefore, the in vitro probe calibration is always carried out at a constant temperature usually the physiological temperature.

C. Perfusion Flow Rate

Recovery has been shown to improve with a decrease in the perfusion flow rate. It is fairly high at the beginning but rapidly decelerates after 30–60 minutes of perfusion. The high dialysate concentrations immediately after probe implantation may be due to the traumatic tissue response and also due to the steep concentration gradient across the dialysis membrane when the probe is first inserted into the medium. Although this may play an important role, it is usually neglected as the similar time-dependent decrease in recovery is observed in aqueous solutions (68,69).

D. Recovery

Dialysate concentration of an analyte of interest is only a measure of its concentration in the extracellular space. The ratio between the concentration of a substance in the outflow solution following microdialysis of a tissue or a biological fluid and the undisturbed concentration of the same substance in the solution outside the probe is defined as "recovery," expressed either as a ratio or as a percentage (70).

Recovery factor of the probes is an important parameter in determining the extracellular concentrations of the drug. In vitro recovery was found to be not only simple and time consuming, but also very appropriate for ocular microdialysis. In case of in vitro recovery technique, the recovery of a drug is usually determined by placing the probe in a standard solution. The probe is continuously perfused at a constant flow rate with saline containing no analyte. Samples are collected during fixed time intervals. The recovery of the substance of interest is calculated as follows:

$$\text{Recovery}_{\text{in vitro}} = \frac{C_{\text{out}}}{C_i} \tag{1}$$

where C_{out} is the concentration in the outflow solution and C_i is the concentration in the medium.

The dialysate substances concentrations are transformed into tissue concentrations as follows:

$$\overline{C}_i = \frac{\overline{C}_{\text{out}}}{\text{Recovery}_{\text{in vitro}}} \tag{2}$$

where $\overline{C}_i$ is the substance concentration in the tissue and $\overline{C}_{\text{out}}$ is the concentration of the dialysate.

Several other techniques have been used to assess probe recovery in vivo, especially for tissue microdialysis. Jacobsen et al. (71) calculated the extracellular concentrations by varying the perfusion flow during an in vivo experiment, measuring the change in the analyte concentration exiting the probe, and then extrapolating to zero flow rate. This method is called as flow-rate or stop-flow method. Lonnroth et al. (72) developed a method where in vivo recovery is estimated by perfusing the probes with varying concentrations of the test analyte and then calculating the equilibrium concentration, i.e., the concentration at which the analyte in the perfusate does not change during the perfusion because it has the same concentration inside the probe as in the extracellular fluid. This is called as the concentration difference method or zero-net flux method. The two in vivo methods require that the drug concentration in the tissue remains constant during the experiment. Probe recovery has also been calculated using a reference substance in the perfusate (73). The method is based on the fact that recovery across the membrane is same in both directions. The percentage loss of the reference substance from the perfusate is used to calculate the concentration of the compound of interest in the tissues.

Although the recovery of a drug as determined in saline solution was used to calculate the drug concentrations in the extracellular space in ocular microdialysis, several studies have been carried out to determine the effect of extracellular milieu on probe recovery. In the case of brain microdialysis, in order to account for factors that may affect mass transport from brain ECF to membrane, in vivo recovery techniques have gained more popularity. In addition, complex solutions like agar gel or red blood cell media have been used to simulate the brain ECF conditions (74). However, these systems have limitations, since it is unlikely that a relatively simple solution like agar gel accurately reflects the complexity of the in vivo physiology. Vitreal microdialysis appears to be less complicated in terms of assessment of the actual vitreal drug concentration compared to other tissues/organs. Vitreous humor consists of almost 99% water. As a result, diffusion of drugs in the vitreous humor has been shown to be similar to that in water. As the microdialysis probe is surrounded by the vitreous humor without any direct contact with the tissue, in vitro recovery appears to be a good approximation of in vivo recovery.

The readers are referred to a review article by de Lange et al. (56) for a detailed description of microdialysis recovery methods.

E. Surgical Trauma and Blood-Retinal Barrier Integrity

Probe-induced inflammation at the site of implantation and subsequent healing is of major concern in in vivo microdialysis. Such physiological changes may affect the intraocular pharmacokinetics significantly. The inflammatory response of the eye mainly depends on the precision of the surgical procedure; therefore, proper precautions should be taken during probe implantation. The time interval between the surgery and the onset of an experiment must be carefully determined, allowing the animal to completely recover.

Stempels et al. (23) reported that the scleral ports (internal diameter of 0.6 mm), implanted 2–3 mm from the limbus, were well tolerated during the observation period. A transient flare or minimal cell count was observed during the first few days following implantation at or near the entry port, but it was not considered to be due to intolerance. Endophthalmitis, the most common inflammatory response of the eye, and uveitis were not observed for up to 6 months following probe implantation. Endophthalmitis was detected in 4 of the 23 insertions (17%) in which probes were reused without sterilization; uveitis was not observed when dialysis was conducted with new probes or probes treated with 25% ethanol.

According to Waga et al. (59) the probes were well tolerated for up to 30 days. Topical antibiotics effectively controlled the purulent discharge observed in few cases. Clinical observations and histopathological analysis demonstrated that the probes were well tolerated in majority of the cases. The inserted probe did not elicit any vitreous reactions and the retina in the posterior fundus remained normal. In a few cases when the probe touched the lens due to improper implantation, cataract formation was noticed.

Macha and Mitra (26) selected intraocular pressure (IOP) to determine the effect of microdialysis probe implantation in the anterior and vitreous chambers. The baseline IOP prior to any probe implantation was 10.6 ± 1.9 mmHg. A sharp fall in the IOP was observed immediately after the implantation of the dialysis probes. IOP reverted $(10.9 \pm 1.4 \text{ mmHg})$ to the basal level within 2 hours after the implantation and remained constant throughout the duration of an experiment. The steady IOP after 2 hours following probe implantation suggests that there was no long-term effect of probe implantation on the aqueous humor dynamics.

Blood-aqueous and blood-retinal barriers restrict the passage of serum proteins into the aqueous and vitreous humors. Elevated protein levels and high enzymic activities in the ocular fluids indicate either a breakdown of the respective barrier or a leakage from the injured ocular tissue. Paracentesis (75) and vitrectomy (76) cause breakdown of the blood-ocular barriers, thereby producing elevated protein levels in the intraocular fluids. Integrity of the blood ocular barriers must be maintained following probe implantation, and this issue has been addressed in detail by Macha and Mitra (26). A change in the total protein concentration in the aqueous and vitreous humors was measured. Vitreal protein concentrations measured at 2 $(0.5619 \pm 0.3085 \text{ mg/mL})$ and 12 hours $(0.2696 \pm 0.0897 \text{ mg/mL})$ after the probe implantation was not significantly different from the basal concentration $(0.3045 \pm 0.1712 \text{ mg/mL}$ at 2 hours and 0.2087 ± 0.1050 mg/mL). Although the aqueous humor total protein concentration was higher at 2 hours $(1.6971 \pm 0.3766 \text{ mg/mL})$ compared to the control $(0.3895 \pm 0.1183 \text{ mg/mL})$, the basal level was reached during the course of the experiment (0.7986 ± 0.3460 mg/mL in the probe implanted and 0.5876 ± 0.2336 mg/mL in the control eye at 12 hr). A transient rise observed in case of aqueous humor protein level was assumed to be mainly due to the trauma caused during probe implantation.

The blood-ocular barriers maintain the homeostasis of the intraocular environment by restricting the movement of compounds from the systemic circulation to the retinal tissue and vitreous cavity. Several reports discussed the measurement of blood-ocular barrier integrity with the aid of posterior vitreous fluorophotometry (PVF) using fluorescein. Penetration of the dye depends on its concentration in the blood as well as its permeability across the blood-ocular barriers. Macha and Mitra (26) evaluated the blood-ocular barrier integrity by studying the fluorescein kinetics after probe implantation. The rate constant for fluorescein penetration into the anterior chamber was found to be significantly higher than into the vitreous, indicating that tighter barrier surrounds the vitreous compartment compared to the anterior chamber. Integrity of the blood-retinal and blood-aqueous barriers was ascertained by determining the permeability index (PI). PI of the anterior (9.48%) and the vitreous chamber (1.99%) determined using ocular microdialysis was found to be similar to the values reported using PVF (77).

VI. INTRAOCULAR PHARMACOKINETICS USING MICRODIALYSIS

Gunnarson et al. (22) first utilized in vivo dialysis technique to sample the vitreous chamber. Studies were carried out to measure endogenous amino acids in the preretinal vitreous space. The effects of high potassium and nipecotic acid, a potent gamma-aminobutyric acid (GABA) inhibitor, on amino acid concentrations were measured. A dialysis probe was implanted in the vitreous of the eye of albino rabbits (Fig. 1). The integrity of the blood-retinal barrier was demonstrated by measuring the concentrations of ^{3}HOH and [^{14}C] | mannitol in the vitreous effluent following intracarotid injections. ^{3}HOH was detected in the vitreous within a few minutes, whereas [^{14}C]mannitol was mostly excluded. Among the amino acids, glutamine had a concentration similar to that in the plasma and cerebrospinal fluid (CSF). Vitreous concentration of all amino acids was lower than in plasma, the majority being below 50% of the plasma concentrations. The taurine level was approximately 70% that of plasma. A comparison with CSF shows that all amino acids except for glutamine and phosphoethanolamine (PEA) are present at higher concentrations in vitreous. Taurine was significantly elevated (fourfold) in the vitreous, as are valine and alanine. Perfusion with 125

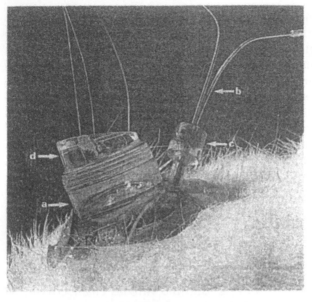

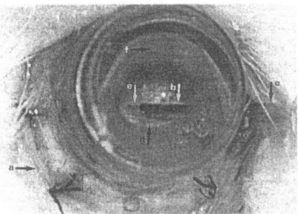

Figure 1 (Top) The positioner device for the dialysis probe on the rabbit eye. The Perspex cylinder (a) is sewn to the sclera. The probe (b) is placed in the guide channel (c). The prismatic lens (d) used for biomicroscopy is in contact with the cornea. (Bottom) The biomicroscopic view of the fundus and the inserted dialysis loop (e). The iris (f) and the retina (g) can also be observed through the lens.

mM KCl-containing media for 30 minutes, 4 hours after probe implantation raised the taurine content by sixfold and PEA content by twofold. Other amino acids remained unchanged (Fig. 2). Perfusion with 60 mM nipecotic acid increased GABA concentration by 60 times and taurine levels by almost 10 times, while other amino acids remained fairly constant (Fig. 3).

Ben-Nun et al. (10) evaluated the intraocular pharmacokinetics of gentamicin after intravitreal administration. The experiments were carried out for a short duration in domestic cats weighing 2.5–5 kg. The animals were anesthetized and the pupils were dilated with tropicamide 0.5% and phenylephrine 10%. Lateral canthotomy was performed in both eyes and the area of the upper part of the sclera was exposed. The superior rectus muscle was divided and cotton wool was inserted into the gap between the posterior sclera and the superior margin of the orbit to stop bleeding. The cotton wool was fixed with a drop of cyanoacrylate glue. A rubber disk (5 mm in diameter and 1 mm thick) was glued to the sclera over the pars plana region in the superotemporal quadrant of each eye. A 1 mm diameter hole was made through the rubber disks and a 20 gauge needle was then passed through each hole into the eye. A sampling catheter for ocular dialysis was

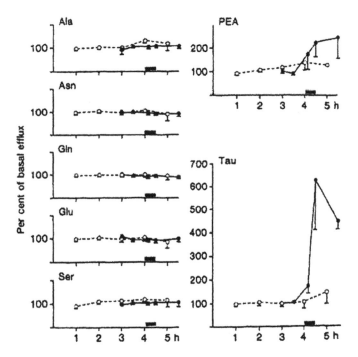

Figure 2 Change of amino acid concentration with time. (○) Amino acid level on perfusion with Krebs-Ringer buffer. (●) Level on perfusion with high potassium.

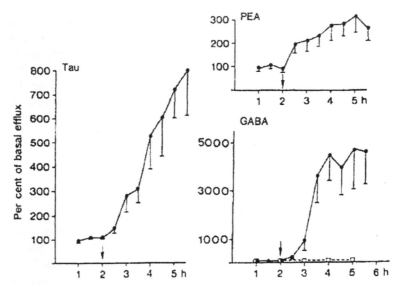

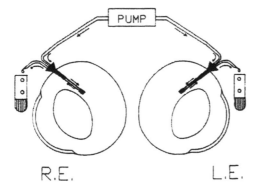

Figure 3 Change of concentration of taurine, phosphoethanolamine, and GABA in response to 60 mM nipecotic acid. The change from Krebs-Ringer buffer to nipecotic acid perfusion media is indicated by an arrow on the time axis.

passed into the sclerotomy site in each eye and glued by a drop of cyanoacrylate glue, followed by a drop of rapid setting epoxy adhesive. The catheters were connected in parallel to a double barrel Harvard pump and perfused at a rate of 3.5 μL/min (Fig. 4). Gentamicin was administered at a site away from the sampling site. The experiments were carried in two groups of cats: normal and bacterial endophthalmitis (*Staphylococcus*

Figure 4 Diagram representing the bilateral simultaneous sampling of vitreous humor by ocular dialysis.

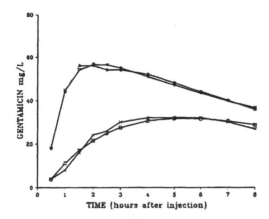

Figure 5 Plots of vitreal gentamicin concentrations fitted with the pharmacokinetic model sampled over 8 hours from the time of injection. The top curve represents the gentamicin concentrations in control eye and the bottom curve the concentrations in the eye with endophthalmitis.

aureus)-induced eyes. Perfusate was collected over 30-minute periods for 3 hours and then hourly to 8 hours. Concentration-time data fitted into a one-compartment model that incorporated the diffusion of drug within the vitreous and its elimination from the vitreous (Fig. 5). The elimination rate constants were greater in infected eyes (0.107 hr^{-1}) than in controls (0.055 hr^{-1}), which might be due to increased permeability of the blood-retinal barrier. Aqueous humor gentamicin concentrations in control eyes were three to six times those in the infected eyes at the end of the experiment.

Waga et al. (59) developed the ocular microdialysis technique for long-term pharmacokinetic studies in rabbits (Fig. 6). A probe (CMA 20) with a

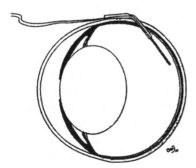

Figure 6 Diagrammatic representation of the microdialysis probe in the rabbit eye.

membrane length of 4 mm and the shaft bent at 60–90° was used. Adult pigmented rabbits were anesthetized with Hypnorm vet®, and a small opening was made in the sclera by conjunctival dissection, about one quarter of the circumference around the limbus. The beginning was at the nasal end of the superior rectus muscle, and the end was at the temporal side, before the lateral rectus. Sling sutures at the superior rectus and a U-shaped suture was made intrasclerally temporal to the rectus superior muscle. The tip of the U was pulled out and a loop was formed. At the loop the sclera was punctured with a 0.9 mm cannula, the probe was inserted, and the sutures were fixed. The tubes of the probe were led under the skin out between the ears. Ceftazidime was injected intramuscularly (1 mg/kg) (Fig. 7) or intravitreally (1 mg) (Fig. 8) in two groups: normal and the inflammation-induced eyes. The penetration of ceftazidime into the vitreous was higher (42%) in inflamed than in normal eyes (20%), suggesting an interference with the blood-retinal barrier. The vitreal half-life of ceftazidime after intravitreal administration was 8.1 hours and 11.7 hours in normal and inflamed eyes, respectively.

Microdialysis was also used to administer drugs into the vitreous chamber. Waga and Ehinger (78) investigated the ability of ^{125}I-labeled NGF to cross a previously implanted probe. The probes were perfused for different time periods with a solution containing NGF. With an inlet NGF concentration of 8×10^{-11} M, the vitreous concentrations were found to be 0.08×10^{-12}, 0.87×10^{-12}, and 0.86×10^{-12} M when the solution was perfused for 1, 4, and 6 hours, respectively. When 9×10^{-10} and 7.6×10^{-9} M concentrations of NGF were perfused for 4 hours, the vitreous concentrations were 012×10^{-11} and 3.8×10^{-11} M, respectively. The same model was used to delivery ganciclovir into the rabbit vitreous (60). Ganciclovir concentration in the vitreous after microdialysis infusion of 120 μl 3.4×10^{-4} M solution was $10.5 \times 10^{-7} \pm 0.99$ M. Microdialysis probe was also used to administer 5-fluorouracil, benzyl penicillin, daunomycin, and dexamethasone into the vitreal space of rabbits (25). The vitreal concentrations achieved after perfusion were 5×10^{-5} M, 2 μM, 1.2 μM, and 1.2×10^{-7} M, respectively.

Stempels et al. (23) developed a removable ocular microdialysis system using scleral port for the first time for measuring the vitreous levels of biogenic amines. This model allowed long-term experiments using microdialysis. Dutch pigmented rabbits were equipped with a scleral entry port (internal diameter 0.6 mm) with a removal closing plug. The scleral port was sutured bilaterally about 2–3 mm from the limbus in the temporal superior quadrant and covered with conjunctiva. The light-adapted rabbits were intubated and maintained under halothane anesthesia with spontaneous breathing. The pupils were dilated with one drop of homatropine 1%.

(a)

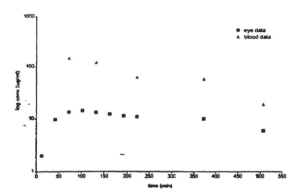

(b)

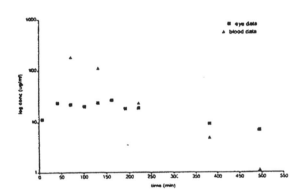

Figure 7 Vitreous and blood concentration of ceftazidime after an intramuscular injection of 1 mg/kg in (a) healthy rabbit eye and (b) mildly inflamed eye.

The conjunctiva was reopened, the closing plug was removed and a microdialysis probe, with a shaft diameter of 0.6 mm and a cut-off value of 20 kDa, was inserted into the midvitreous. The position of the probe tip was confirmed by direct illumination through the pupil. The perfusion fluid used was Ringer's solution with a Ca^{2+} concentration of 0.75 mM. The perfusion fluid was pumped at a flow rate of 2 μL/min, and the samples were collected every 20 minutes. Using this model, the concentration dihydroxyphenyl acetic acid was found to be three times higher than in the bovine vitreous. No significant difference was observed between simultaneously taken left

(a)

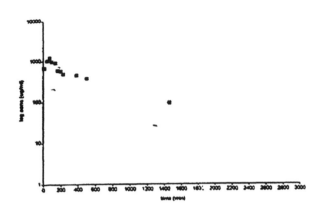

(b)

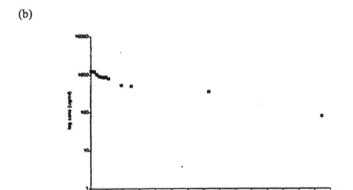

Figure 8   Vitreous concentration of ceftazidime after an intravitreal injection of 1 mg ceftazidime in (a) healthy eye and (b) mildly inflamed eye.

and right eye samples nor between days 1, 7, 11, and 14 for dopamine, dihydroxyphenyl acetic acid (Fig. 9) and noradrenaline. This study proved that ocular microdialysis could be carried out over several hours and repeatedly in the same animal.

Macha and Mitra (27) have used the technique to study the ocular pharmacokinetics of cephalosporins after intravitreal administration and also investigated the presence of peptide transporters on the retina. New

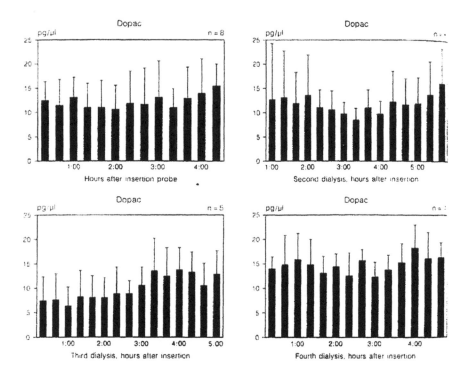

Figure 9 Concentrations of dihydroxyphenyl acetic acid in the dialysates of rabbit vitreous on days 1, 7, 11, and 14.

Zealand albino male rabbits, weighing 2–2.5 kg, were kept under anesthesia throughout the experiment. A concentric microdialysis probe was implanted into the midvitreous chamber using a 22 gauge needle about 3 mm below the limbus through the pars plana. Another linear microdialysis probe was implanted across the cornea in the aqueous humor using a 25 gauge needle (Fig. 10). The probes were perfused with isotonic phosphate buffer saline (pH 7.4) at a flow rate of 2 µL/min and the samples were collected every 20 minutes over a period of 10 hours. Animals were allowed to stabilize for 2 hours prior to initiation of a study. Ocular pharmacokinetics of cephalosporins were investigated following intravitreal administration of 500 µg of cephalexin, cephazolin, and cephalothin. Inhibition experiments were carried in vivo using two dipeptides, gly-pro and gly-sar. The dipeptides were administered by a bolus injection intravitreally 30 minutes prior to the administration of cephalosporins, followed by continuous perfusion through the vitreous probe to maintain the

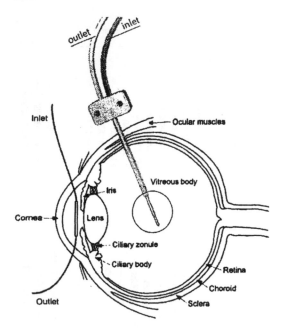

Figure 10 Diagrammatic representation of the microdialysis probes implanted in the anterior chamber and vitreous of the eye.

steady-state dipeptide concentration during an experiment. Vitreal elimination half-lives of cephalexin, cefazolin, and cephalothin after intravitreal administration were found to be 185.38 ± 27.25 min, 111.40 ± 17.17 min, and 146.68 ± 47.52 min, respectively. Cephalexin (224.39 ± 84.56 µg.min/mL) was found to generate higher concentrations in the aqueous humor compared to cefazolin (85.37 ± 45.11 µg.min/mL). The pharmacokinetic parameters of cephalexin in the presence of gly-pro, i.e., AUC (44452.06 ± 3326.55 µg.min/mL), clearance (0.0013 ± 0.0004 mL/min), and terminal elimination half-life (825.12 ± 499.95 min), were found to be significantly different from that of the control (14612.83 ± 4036.47 µg.min/mL, 0.0036 ± 0.0011 mL/min, and 187.96 ± 65.12 min, respectively) (Fig. 11). In the case of cefazolin, the control parameters (30199.06 ± 8819.07 µg.min/mL, 0.0018 ± 0.0006 mL/min, and 229.53 ± 3 7.31 min, respectively) were found to be similar, except the terminal elimination half-life, to those in the presence of gly-pro (26648.31 ± 4156.56 µg.min/mL, 0.0019 ± 0.0003 mL/min, and 881.03 ± 469.67 min, respectively) (Fig. 12). Gly-sar was found to have no significant effect on the pharmacokinetics of both drugs. These studies indicated the involvement

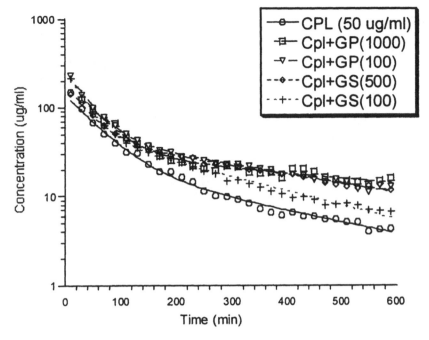

Figure 11 Vitreous concentration-time profile of cephalexin (50 µg) in the presence of inhibitors after intravitreal administration. The line drawn represents the non-linear least-squares regression fit of the model to the concentration-time data.

of a peptide carrier in the transport of cephalosporins across the retina. Although gly-pro inhibited the elimination of cephalexin from the vitreous, the effect of the α-amino group on the specificity of cephalosporins towards peptide carriers was not clearly established.

Furthermore, Macha and Mitra have utilized the microdialysis technique to delineate the ocular pharmacokinetics of ganciclovir (GCV) and its ester prodrugs (acetate, propionate, butyrate, and valerate). The prodrugs generated sustained therapeutic concentrations of GCV over a prolonged period of time after intravitreal administration. Drugs were administered (0.2 µmol) intravitreally and the samples were collected every 20 minutes over a period of 10 hours. The representative anterior and vitreous chamber concentration-time profiles of GCV following intravitreal administration are shown in Figure 13. The vitreal terminal phase elimination half-life ($t_{1/2}$ β) of GCV was found to be 426 ± 109 minutes. The proportion of GCV eliminating through the anterior chamber pathway was about 1%. The representative vitreous concentration-time profile

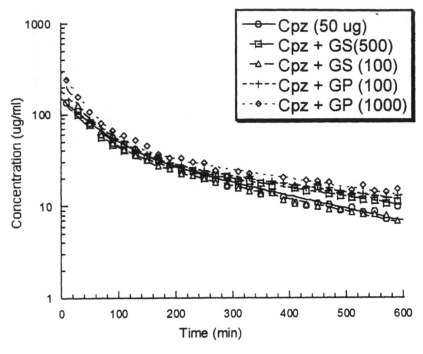

Figure 12 Vitreous concentration-time profile of cefazolin (50 μg) in the presence of inhibitors after intravitreal administration. The line drawn represents the nonlinear least-squares regression fit of the model to the concentration-time data.

of the GCV butyrate is depicted in Figure 14. The hydrolysis rate and clearance of the prodrugs increased with the ascending ester chain length. Vitreal elimination half-lives ($t_{1/2}k_{10}$) of GCV, monoacetate, monopropionate, monobutyrate, and valerate esters of GCV were 170 ± 37, 117 ± 50, 122 ± 13, 55 ± 26, and 107 ± 14 minutes, respectively. A parabolic relationship was observed between the vitreal elimination rate constant (k_{10}) and the ester chain length. The C_{max} for the regenerated GCV after the prodrug administration was found to be 2.75 ± 0.431, 6.66 ± 0.570, 8.03 ± 1.19, and 8.26 ± 1.76 μg for acetate, propionate, butyrate, and valerate esters, respectively. The mean residence time of the regenerated GCV after prodrug administration was found to be three to four times the value obtained after GCV injection. The low proportions of aqueous levels of GCV indicate the retinal pathway as the major route of elimination. These studies have shown that the ester prodrugs generated therapeutic concentrations of GCV in vivo and the MRT of GCV could be enhanced three-to-fourfold through prodrug modification.

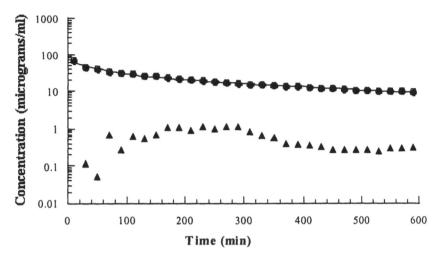

Figure 13 Concentration-time profile of GCV (50.0 µg) following intravitreal administration: (●) vitreal and (▲) anterior chamber concentrations. The line drawn represents the nonlinear least-squares regression fit of the model to the concentration-time data.

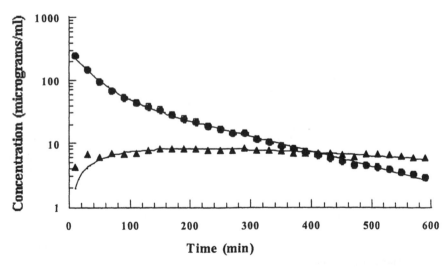

Figure 14 Concentration-time profile of GCV monobutyrate (63.3 µg) following intravitreal administration: (●) vitreal GCV monobutyrate and (▲) vitreal GCV concentrations. The line drawn represents the nonlinear least-squares regression fit of the model to the concentration-time data.

VII. CONCLUSIONS

Microdialysis has been shown to be a very useful tool to study ocular pharmacokinetics. The major strengths of the technique appear to be its simplicity and its ability to monitor drug and metabolite concentration and deliver the drugs. Despite its increasing popularity, microdialysis is still far from being a routine method in eye research. Until now, much work has gone into adapting and improving the technology involved. Future studies need to be focused on the methodological problems and limitations that could lead to erroneous data interpretation and conflicting results.

ACKNOWLEDGMENTS

Supported by NIH grants R01 EY09171-08 and R01 EY10659-07.

REFERENCES

1. G. Raviola. (1977). The structural basis of the blood-ocular barriers. *Exp. Eye Res.* 25:27–63.
2. S. P. Donahue, J. M. Khoury, and R. P. Kowalski. (1996). Common ocular infections. A prescriber's guide. *Drugs* 52:526–540.
3. P. R. Pavan, E. E. Oteiza, B. A. Hughes, and A. Avni. (1994). Exogenous endophthalmitis initially treated without systemic antibiotics. *Ophthalmology* 101:1289–1297.
4. L. IH. (1984). Anti-infective agents. In: *Pharmacology of the Eye*. M. Sears, ed. New York: Springer-Verlag, pp. 385–446.
5. B. D. Kuppermann, J. G. Petty, D. D. Richman, W. C. Mathews, S. C. Fullerton, L. S. Rickman, and W. R. Freeman. (1993). Correlation between CD4+ counts and prevalence of cytomegalovirus retinitis and human immunodeficiency virus-related noninfectious retinal vasculopathy in patients with acquired immunodeficiency syndrome. *Am. J. Ophthalmol.* 115:575–582.
6. J. G. Gross, S. A. Bozzette, W. C. Mathews, S. A. Spector, I. S. Abramson, J. A. McCutchan, T. Mendez, D. Munguia, and W. R. Freeman. (1990). Longitudinal study of cytomegalovirus retinitis in acquired immune deficiency syndrome. *Ophthalmology* 97:681–686.
7. D. A. Jabs, C. Enger, and J. G. Bartlett. (1989). Cytomegalovirus retinitis and acquired immunodeficiency syndrome. *Arch. Ophthalmol.* 107:75–80.
8. D. A. Jabs. (1992). Treatment of cytomegalovirus retinitis—1992. *Arch. Ophthalmol.* 110:185–187.

9. M. J. Daily, G. A. Peyman, G. Fishman. (1973). Intravitreal injection of methicillin for treatment of endophthalmitis. *Am. J. Ophthalmol.* 76:343–350.

10. J. Ben-Nun, D. A. Joyce, R. L. Cooper, S. J. Cringle, and I. J. Constable. (1989). Pharmacokinetics of intravitreal injection. Assessment of a gentamicin model by ocular dialysis. *Invest. Ophthalmol. Vis. Sci.* 30:1055–1061.

11. A. G. Palestine, M. A. Polis, M. D. DeSmet, B. F. Baird, J. Falloon, J. A. Kovacs, R. T. Davey, J. J. Zurlo, K. M. Zunich, M. Davis, et al. (1991). A randomized controlled trial of foscarnet in the treatment of cytomegalovirus retinitis in patients with AIDS. *Ann. Intern. Med.* 115:665–673.

12. L. B. Sheiner, B. Rosenberg, and V. V. Marathe. (1977). Estimation of population characteristics of pharmacokinetic parameters from routine clinical data. *J. Pharmacokinet. Biopharm.* 5:445–479.

13. G. L. Drusano, W. Liu, R. Perkins, A. Madu, C. Madu, M. Mayers, and M. H. Miller. (1995). Determination of robust ocular pharmacokinetic parameters in serum and vitreous humor of albino rabbits following systemic administration of ciprofloxacin from sparse data sets by using IT2S, a population pharmacokinetic modeling program. *Antimicrob. Agents Chemother.* 39:1683–1687.

14. M. Mayers, D. Rush, A. Madu, M. Motyl, and M. H. Miller. (1991). Pharmacokinetics of amikacin and chloramphenicol in the aqueous humor of rabbits. *Antimicrob. Agents Chemother.* 35:1791–1798.

15. M. H. Miller, A. Madu, G. Samathanam, D. Rush, C. N. Madu, K. Mathisson, and M. Mayers. (1992). Fleroxacin pharmacokinetics in aqueous and vitreous humors determined by using complete concentration-time data from individual rabbits. *Antimicrob. Agents Chemother.* 36:32–38.

16. R. J. Perkins, W. Liu, G. Drusano, A. Madu, M. Mayers, C. Madu, and M. H. Miller. (1995). Pharmacokinetics of ofloxacin in serum and vitreous humor of albino and pigmented rabbits. *Antimicrob. Agents Chemother.* 39:1493–1498.

17. W. Liu, Q. F. Liu, R. Perkins, G. Drusano, A. Louie, A. Madu, U. Mian, M. Mayers, and M. H. Miller. (1998). Pharmacokinetics of sparfloxacin in the serum and vitreous humor of rabbits: physicochemical properties that regulate penetration of quinolone antimicrobials. *Antimicrob. Agents Chemother.* 42:1417–1423.

18. L. Bito, H. Davson, E. Levin, M. Murray, and N. Snider. (1966). The concentrations of free amino acids and other electrolytes in cerebrospinal fluid in vivo dialysate of brain, and blood plasma of the dog. *J. Neurochem.* 13:1057–1067.

19. M. Telting-Diaz, D. O. Scott, and C. E. Lunte. (1992). Intravenous microdialysis sampling in awake, freely-moving rats. *Anal. Chem.* 64:806–810.

20. J. E. Robinson. (1995). Microdialysis: a novel tool for research in the reproductive system. *Biol. Reprod.* 52:237–245.

21. D. G. Maggs, W. P. Borg, and R. S. Sherwin. (1997). Microdialysis techniques in the study of brain and skeletal muscle. *Diabetologia* 40(Suppl. 2):S75–82. (1987).

22. G. Gunnarson, A. K. Jakobsson, A. Hamberger, and J. Sjostrand. (1987). Free amino acids in the pre-retinal vitreous space. Effect of high potassium and nipecotic acid. *Exp. Eye Res.* 44:235–244.

23. N. Stempels, M. J. Tassignon, and S. Sarre. (1993). A removable ocular microdialysis system for measuring vitreous biogenic amines. *Graefes Arch. Clin. Exp. Ophthalmol.* 231:651–655.

24. P. M. Hughes, R. Krishnamoorthy, and A. K. Mitra. (1996). Vitreous disposition of two acycloguanosine antivirals in the albino and pigmented rabbit models: a novel ocular microdialysis technique. *J. Ocul. Pharmacol. Ther.* 12:209–224.

25. J. Waga and B. Ehinger. (1997). Intravitreal concentrations of some drugs administered with microdialysis. *Acta Ophthalmol. Scand.* 75:36–40.

26. S. Macha and A. K. Mitra. (2001). Ocular pharmacokinetics in rabbits using a novel dual probe microdialysis technique. *Exp. Eye Res.* 72:289–299.

27. S. Machal and A. K. Mtira. Ocular pharmacokinetics of cephalosporins using microdialysis. *J. Ocul. Pharmacol. Ther.* (in press).

28. K. D. Rittenhouse, R. L. Peiffer, Jr., and G. M. Pollack. (1999). Microdialysis evaluation of the ocular pharmacokinetics of propranolol in the conscious rabbit. *Pharm. Res.* 16:736–742.

29. V. H. Lee and J. R. Robinson. (1986). Topical ocular drug delivery: recent developments and future challenges. *J. Ocul. Pharmacol.* 2:67–108.

30. S. S. Chrai, M. C. Makoid, S. P. Eriksen, and J. R. Robinson. (1973). Drop size and initial dosing frequency problems of topically applied ophthalmic drugs. *J. Pharm. Sci.* 63:333–338.

31. S. S. Chrai, T. F. Patton, A. Mehta, and J. R. Robinson. (1973). Lacrimal and instilled fluid dynamics in rabbit eyes. *J. Pharm. Sci.* 62:1112–1121.

32. A. K. Mitra and T. J. Mikkelson. (1988). Mechanism of transcorneal permeation of pilocarpine. *J. Pharm. Sci.* 77:771–775.

33. R. Abel, Jr., G. L. Boyle, M. Furman, and I. H. Leopold. (1974). Intraocular penetration of cefazolin sodium in rabbits. *Am. J. Ophthalmol.* 78:779–787.

34. S. J. Faigenbaum, G. L. Boyle, A. S. Prywes, R. Abel, Jr., and I. H. Leopold. (1976). Intraocular penetrating of amoxicillin. *Am. J. Ophthalmol.* 82:598–603.

35. B. M. Faris and M. M. Uwaydah. (1974). Intraocular penetration of semi-synthetic penicillins: methicillin, cloxacillin, ampicillin, and carbenicillin studies in experimental animals with a review of the literature. *Arch. Ophthalmol.* 92:501–505.

36. G. A. Peyman, D. R. May, P. I. Homer, and R. T. Kasbeer. (1977). Penetration of gentamicin into the aphakic eye. *Ann. Ophthalmol.* 9:871–880.

37. L. Salminen. (1978). Ampicillin penetration into the rabbit eye. *Acta Ophthalmol. (Copenh.)* 56:977–983.

38. M. Barza, A. Kane, and J. L. Baum. (1979). Intraocular levels of cefamandole compared with cefazolin after subconjunctival injection in rabbits. *Invest. Ophthalmol. Vis. Sci.* 18:250–255.

39. M. Barza, A. Kane, and J. Baum. (1980). Oxacillin for bacterial endophthalmitis: subconjunctival, intravenous, both or neither? *Invest. Ophthalmol. Vis. Sci.* 19:1348–1354.

40. W. M. Jay, R. K. Shockley, A. M. Aziz, M. Z. Aziz, and J. P. Rissing. (1984). Ocular pharmacokinetics of ceftriaxone following subconjunctival injection in rabbits. *Arch. Ophthalmol.* 102:430–432.

41. F. P. Furgiuele, J. P. Smith, and J. G. Baron. (1978). Tobramycin levels in human eyes. *Am. J. Ophthalmol.* 85:121–123.

42. D. M. Maurice, and S. Mishima. (1984). Ocular pharmacokinetics. In: *Pharmacology of the Eye II.* M. L. Sears, ed. New York: Springer-Verlag, p. 19.

43. M. Barza, A. Kane, and J. Baum. (1983). Pharmacokinetics of intravitreal carbenicillin, cefazolin, and gentamicin in rhesus monkeys. *Invest. Ophthalmol. Vis. Sci.* 24:1602–1606.

44. V. N. Reddy, B. Chakrapani, and C. P. Lim. (1977). Blood-vitreous barrier to amino acids. *Exp. Eye Res.* 25:543–545.

45. A. G. Schenk and G. A. Peyman. (1974). Lincomycin by direct intravitreal injection in the treatment of experimental bacterial endophthalmitis. *Albrecht Von Graefes Arch. Klin. Exp. Ophthalmol.* 190: 281–291.

46. S. C. Pflugfelder, E. Hernandez, S. J. Fliesler, J. Alvarez, M. E. Pflugfelder, and R. K. Forster. (1987). Intravitreal vancomycin. Retinal toxicity, clearance, and interaction with gentamicin. *Arch. Ophthalmol.* 105:831–837.

47. F. M. Ussery, 3rd, S. R. Gibson, R. H. Conklin, D. F. Piot, E. W. Stool, and A. J. Conklin. (1988). Intravitreal ganciclovir in the treatment of AIDS-associated cytomegalovirus retinitis. *Ophthalmology*, 95:640–648.

48. K. Henry, H. Cantrill, C. Fletcher, B. J. Chinnock, and H. H. Balfour, Jr. (1987). Use of intravitreal ganciclovir (dihydroxy propoxymethyl guanine) for cytomegalovirus retinitis in a patient with AIDS. *Am. J. Ophthalmol.* 103:17–23.

49. G. A. Peyman, D. R. May, E. S. Ericson, and D. Apple. (1974) Intraocular injection of gentamicin. Toxic effects of clearance. *Arch. Ophthalmol.* 92:42–47.

50. R. K. Shockley, W. M. Jay, T. R. Friberg, A. M. Aziz, J. P. Rissing, and M. Z. Aziz. (1984). Intravitreal ceftriaxone in a rabbit model. Dose- and time-dependent toxic effects and pharmacokinetic analysis. *Arch. Ophthalmol.* 102:1236–1238.

51. A. G. Schenk, G. A. Peyman, and J. T. Paque. (1974). The intravitreal use of carbenicillin (Geopen) for treatment of pseudomonas endophthalmitis. *Acta Ophthalmol.* 52:707–717.

52. S. K. Gardner. (1987). Ocular drug penetration and pharmacokinetic principles. In: *Clinical Ophthalmic Pharmacology.* D. W. Lamberts and D. E. Potter, eds.

53. T. S. Lesar and R. G. Fiscella. (1985). Antimicrobial drug delivery to the eye. *Drug Intell. Clin. Pharm.* 19:642–654.

54. J. D. Wright, F. D. Boudinot, and M. R. Ujhelyi. (1996). Measurement and analysis of unbound drug concentrations. *Clin. Pharmacokinet.* 30:445–462.

55. U. Ungerstedt. (1991). Microdialysis—principles and applications for studies in animals and man. *J. Intern. Med.* 230:365–373.

56. E. C. de Lange, M. Danhof, A. G. de Boer, and D. D. Breimer. (1997). Methodological considerations of intracerebral microdialysis in pharmacokinetic studies on drug transport across the blood-brain barrier. *Brain Res. Brain Res. Rev.* 25:27–49.

57. R. Tao and S. Hjorth. (1992). Differences in the in vitro and in vivo 5-hydroxytryptamine extraction performance among three common microdialysis membranes. *J. Neurochem.* 59:1778–1785.

58. J. Landolt, H. Langemann, T. H. Lutz, and O. Gratzl. (1991). Non-linear recovery of cysteine and glutathione in microdialysis. In: H. Rollema, et al., eds. Meppel, Netherlands: Krips Repro, pp. 63–65.

59. J. Waga, I. Nilsson-Ehle, B. Ljungberg, A. Skarin, L. Stahle, and B. Ehinger. (1999). Microdialysis for pharmacokinetic studies of ceftazidime in rabbit vitreous. *J. Ocul. Pharmacol. Ther.* 15:455–463.

60. J. Waga. (2000). Ganciclovir delivery through an intravitreal microdialysis probe in rabbit. *Acta Ophthalmol. Scand.* 78:369–371.

61. A. Hamberger, C. H. Berthold, B. Karlsson, A. Lehmann, and B. Nystrom. (1983). Extracellular GABA, glutamate and glutamine in vivo perfusion dialysis of the rabbit hyppocampus. In: *Glutamine, Glutamate and GABA in the Central Nervous System.* New York: Alan R. Liss Inc., pp. 473–492.

62. M. Sandberg and S. Lindstrom. (1993). Amino acids in the dorsal lateral geniculate nucleus of the cat—collection in vivo. *J. Neurosci. Methods.* 9:64–74.

63. U. Tossman and U. Ungerstedt. (1986). Microdialysis in the study of extracellular levels of amino acids in the rat brain. *Acta Physiol. Scand.* 128:9–14.

64. A. Lehmann. (1989). Effects of microdialysis-perfusion with anisoosmotic media on extracellular amino acids in the rat hippocampus and skeletal muscle. *J. Neurochem.* 53:525–535.

65. J. M. Solis, A. S. Herranz, O. Herreras, J. Lerma, and R. Martin del Rio. (1988). Does taurine act as an osmoregulatory substance in the rat brain? *Neurosci. Lett.* 91:53–58.

66. J. V. Wade, J. P. Olson, F. E. Samson, S. R. Nelson, T. L. Pazdernik. (1988). A possible role for taurine in osmoregulation within the brain. *J. Neurochem.* 51:740–745.

67. S. A. Wages, W. H. Church, and J. B. Justice, Jr. (1986). Sampling considerations for on-line microbore liquid chromatography of brain dialysate. *Anal. Chem.* 58:1649–1656.

68. J. M. Delgado, J. Lerma, R. Martin del Rio, and J. M. Solis. (1984). Dialytrode technology and local profiles of amino acids in the awake cat brain. *J. Neurochem.* 42:1218–1228.

69. G. Amberg, and N. Lindefors. (1989). Intracerebral microdialysis: II. Mathematical studies of diffusion kinetics. *J. Pharmacol. Methods* 22:157–183.

70. T. Zetterstrom, L. Vernet, U. Ungerstedt, U. Tossman, B. Jonzon, and B. B. Fredholm. (1982). Purine levels in the intact rat brain. Studies with an implanted perfused hollow fibre. *Neurosci. Lett.* 29:111–115.

71. I. Jacobson, M. Sandberg, and A. Hamberger (1985). Mass transfer in brain dialysis devices—a new method for the estimation of extracellular amino acids concentration. *J. Neurosci. Methods* 15:263–268.

72. P. Lonnroth, P. A. Jansson, and U. Smith. (1987). A microdialysis method allowing characterization of intercellular water space in humans. *Am. J. Physiol.* 253:E228–231.

73. D. Scheller and J. Kolb. (1991). The internal reference technique in microdialysis: a practical approach to monitoring dialysis efficiency and to calculating tissue concentration from dialysate samples. *J. Neurosci. Methods* 40:31–38.

74. H. Benveniste, A. J. Hansen, and N. S. Ottosen. (1989). Determination of brain interstitial concentrations by microdialysis. *J. Neurochem.* 52:1741–1750.

75. G. Raviola. (1974). Effects of paracentesis on the blood-aqueous barrier: an electron microscope study on Macaca mulatta using horseradish peroxidase as a tracer. *Invest. Ophthalmol.* 13:828–858.

76. F. P. Killey, H. F. Edelhauser, and T. A. Aaberg. (1980). Intraocular fluid dynamics. Measurements following vitrectomy and intraocular sulfur hexafluoride administration. *Arch. Ophthalmol* 98:1448–1452.

77. L. L. Knudsen, T. Olsen, and F. Nielsen-Kudsk (1988). Anterior chamber fluorescein kinetics compared with vitreous kinetics in normal subjects. *Acta Ophthalmol. Scand.* 76:561–567.

78. J. Wagar and B. Ehinger. (2000). NGF administered by microdialysis into rabbit vitreous. *Acta Ophthalmol. Scand.* 78:154–155.

9
Ocular Penetration Enhancers

Thomas Wai-Yip Lee and Joseph R. Robinson
School of Pharmacy, University of Wisconsin-Madison, Madison, Wisconsin, U.S.A.

I. INTRODUCTION

Drug delivery to the eye is not an easy assignment. The cornea, being a very important component in the visual pathway, is well protected by a number of very effective defense mechanisms, e.g., blinking, high tear secretion rate flushing its surface, induced lacrimation and tear protein production in response to foreign substances, etc. These protective mechanisms provide a challenge for pharmaceutical scientists to design drug delivery systems that can deliver therapeutic agents in sufficient concentrations to target sites.

After topical instillation of an eye drop, the drug is subject to a number of very efficient elimination mechanisms such as drainage, binding to proteins, normal tear turnover, induced tear production, and nonproductive absorption via the conjunctiva. Typically, drug absorption is virtually complete in 90 seconds due to the rapid removal of drug from the precorneal area. To make matters worse, the cornea is poorly permeable to both hydrophilic and hydrophobic compounds. As a result, only approximately 10% or less of the topically applied dose can be absorbed into the anterior segment of the eye.

Basically, the two major barriers encountered in ocular drug delivery are (a) short residence time in the precorneal area and (b) poor permeability of the cornea.

Various efforts have been made to prolong the drug solution residence time via vehicle modification (1,2), bioadhesives (3), inserts (4), etc. Another approach to improve ocular bioavailability, which is less well understood, is penetration enhancement. Penetration enhancement can be achieved via prodrugs, penetration enhancers, etc. Prodrugs will be covered elsewhere in this book. The main focus of this chapter will be on the use of penetration enhancers to improve ocular drug delivery. Fundamental aspects of ocular penetration enhancers will be covered, and recent advances will be presented as well.

II. KINETIC BASIS OF THE NEED FOR PENETRATION ENHANCEMENT

The simplest model for ocular pharmacokinetics is shown in Figure 1 (5). It is well known that for most drugs the true absorption rate constant is much smaller than the elimination rate constant. This will normally give rise to a flip-flop model. However, when the parallel elimination pathway is introduced (Fig. 2) (5), the apparent absorption rate constant is defined as:

Apparent $k_{abs} = k_{abs} + k_{loss,pp}$

Thus, the model is not a flip-flop model and drug concentration can be described as

$$C = (FD/V_d)[k/(k - K)](e^{-Kt} - e^{-kt}) \tag{1}$$

where F is the fraction of dose absorbed, D is the dose, k and K are absorption and elimination rate constants, respectively, and V_d is the apparent volume of distribution. Obviously, $K = k_{elim}$, $k = k_{abs} + k_{loss,pp}$.

For many drugs, $k_{loss,pp}$ is of the order of 0.5–0.7 min^{-1}, being several orders of magnitude larger than k_{abs}, which is typically of the order of 0.001 min^{-1}. As a result, the peak time, which is controlled by $k_{loss,pp}$ and k_{abs}, is similar (20–40 min) for a wide range of compounds since $k_{loss,pp}$, which is mainly due to drainage, induced lacrimation, etc., predominates over k_{abs} in controlling the peak time.

In order to improve the bioavailability ($F = k_{abs}/[k_{abs} + k_{loss,pp}]$) significantly, it is essential to increase k_{abs} by one or two order of magnitudes or reduce $k_{loss,pp}$ to a similar extent.

Several approaches have attempted to reduce the magnitude of $k_{loss,pp}$. However, it has its limit. Keister et al. (6) showed that reducing the dose volume from 25 µL to zero brings only a fourfold improvement in bioavailability for a poorly permeable compound. However, it is practically impos-

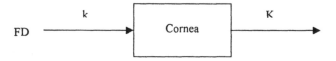

Figure 1 A one-compartment model for ocular absorption.

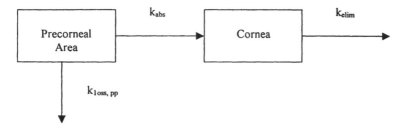

Figure 2 A two-compartmental model for ocular absorption.

sible to have zero dosing volume. Therefore, small dose volumes will give an improvement in bioavailability that is less than fourfold. Similarly, theoretical calculations showed that use of bioadhesives does not necessarily give any benefit if the cornea is poorly permeable to that compound (7). These calculations are as follows: steady-state, at which the rates of delivery and elimination are equal, is approached after about five drug half-lives, and the amount of the drug in a particular ocular compartment can be expressed as

$$dA/dt = R - KA$$

where A is the amount of the drug (in mg), R is the rate of drug input, and K is the elimination rate constant. At steady state, $dA/dt = 0$, leading to

$$A_{SS} = R/K = M_p t_{1/2}/0.693T$$

where M_p is the mass penetrating and $t_{1/2}$ is the half-life of the drug. It is clearly shown that prolonging the contact time (T) via the use of bioadhesives will lower A_{SS} provided that M_p and $t_{1/2}$ are kept constant. For drugs where permeability is not a problem, the use of bioadhesives is beneficial since the therapeutic drug level can be sustained. On the contrary, for a poorly permeable compound, the use of adhesives may lower A_{SS} below the therapeutic level. In order to bring A_{SS} back to a therapeutic level, M_p has to be increased. This requires the use of penetration enhancers.

Methods of penetration enhancement such as prodrugs, ion pairing, etc. are beyond the scope of this chapter and will not be discussed. The main focus of this chapter will be ocular penetration enhancers.

III. TRANSPORT CHARACTERISTICS OF EPITHELIAL TISSUES

The normal expected mechanisms of corneal penetration is shown in Table 1 (8). Transport across epithelia occurs via two pathways: transcellular and paracellular. The former involves cell/tissue partitioning/diffusion, channel

Table 1 Expected Mechanisms of Corneal Penetration

Drug type	Apparent rate-limiting membrane	Mechanisms
Water soluble	Epithelium	Low o/w partition into epithelium
		Slow diffusion through epithelium
		High partition rate + rapid diffusion through stroma/ endothelium
		Via leaky channels
		Solute movement may be intercellular and/or transcellular
Water and oil soluble	Epithelium-stroma	Both mechanisms operate
Oil soluble	Stroma	High o/w partition into epithelium
		Rapid diffusion through epithelium
Ionizable	Epithelium + stroma or leaky channel	Mechanism not solely dependent upon partition coefficient

Source: Adapted from Ref. 8.

diffusion, and carrier-mediated transport. In contrast, the latter represents diffusive and convective transport occurring through intercellular spaces and tight junctions. Due to its aqueous nature, hydrophilic solutes would preferably adopt the paracellular pathway. However, there are three forms of junctional complexes that form between cells which hinder transport of hydrophilic molecules, namely, tight junctions (zonula occludens), intermediate junctions (belt desmosome or zonula adherens), and spot desmosomes (macula adherens) (Fig. 3) (9). Among them, the tight junction is the uppermost and tightest, and it gives the greatest resistance for hydrophilic molecules to go between cells. The barrier property of the tight junction can be reflected by the transepithelial electrical resistance (TEER). The higher the TEER, the tighter the junctions that give a higher resistance for transport of molecules. Generally, epithelia with resistances in the range of 10–100 Ω cm^2 are considered leaky, whereas those with resistance ranging from 300 to 10,000 Ω cm^2 are "tight." The cornea is generally classified as a moderately tight or moderately leaky tissue (400–1000 Ω cm^2). A comparison of the electrophysiology and permeability of the cornea with other tissues is shown in Table 2 and 3, respectively (10).

The cornea also shows permselectivity (11). It has an isoelectric point (pI) of 3.2. At pHs above the pI, it carries a negative charge and is selective to positively charged molecules. On the other hand, at pHs below the pI, it

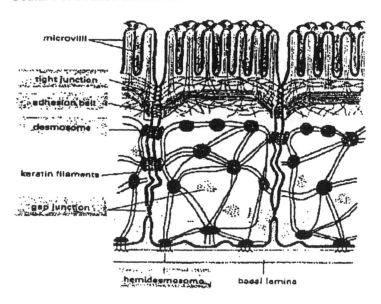

microvilli

tight junction

adhesion belt

desmosome

keratin filaments

gap junction

hemidesmosome   basal lamina

Figure 3 Summary of the various cell junctions found in animal cell epithelia. (From Ref. 9.)

Table 2 Comparative Permeability Coefficients of Several Drugs Between Cornea and Other Tissues

Permanent	MW	Permeability coefficient (cm/s)		
		Rabbit/dog buccal	Rabbit cornea	Human skin
Water	18	3.7×10^{-5} (rabbit) 2.6×10^{-5} (dog)	1.5×10^{-4}	1.4×10^{-7}
Glycerol	92	6.0×10^{-7}	4.5×10^{-6}	
Benzylamine	107	1.4×10^{-5}	1.76×10^{-5}	
Octanol	130	2.2×10^{-5}		1.4×10^{-5}
Amphetamine	135	1.5×10^{-5}		3.9×10^{-9}
salicylic acid	138	9.3×10^{-7}	7.4×10^{-6}	
Estradiol	272	6.6×10^{-6}		
Progesterone	314	8.9×10^{-6}	1.8×10^{-5}	4.2×10^{-7}
Ouabain	584	6.5×10^{-6}		1.1×10^{-9}

Source: Adapted from Ref. 10.

Table 3 Electrical Resistances and Permselective of Various Epithelia

Tissue	Species	Resistances (Ω cm^2)	P_K	P_{NA}	P_{Cl}
Proximal renal tube	Dog	6–7	1.10	1.00	0.72
Gall bladder	Rabbit	20	2.30	1.00	0.23
Small intestine					
Duodenum	Rat	98			
Jejunum	Rat	51	1.60	1.00	0.20
Ileum	Rabbit	100	1.14	1.00	0.20
Colon	Rabbit	385	1.00	1.00	
Gastric mucosa					
Antrum	Necturus	1,730	1.00		0.86
Fundus	Necturus	2,230			
Urinary bladder	Toad	3,755	1.40	1.00	0.72
Amphibian skin	Toad	763			
	Frog	8,700	1.33	1.00	4.46
Cornea	Rabbit	989	0.12	1.00	0.1
Free solution			1.47	1.00	1.52

Source: Ref. 10.

carries a net positive charge. As a result, a positively charged molecule can pass across the cornea more effectively at physiological pH (7.4).

The transcellular pathway is a path that a solute uses to diffuse through the apical lipid matrix of the epithelial membrane continuing through the cytoplasm and across the basolateral membrane. The ability of a solute to pass across the cell using this pathway depends on the interaction of the solute with plasma membrane components, e.g., lipids, cell surface receptors. For a molecule that adopts a passive transport mechanism, partitioning is a crucial step since this is a prerequisite for a molecule to enter the cell. As a result, the partition coefficient becomes a key factor in determining its transport across the epithelium. The optimum partition coefficients for corneal absorption has been reported to be in the range of 10–100 (12), indicating lipophilic molecules are preferred. However, other factors such as size, charge, etc. may also play a role. Theoretically, a small and lipophilic molecule can pass across the cornea effectively. However, this may not always be the case, as can be easily understood when the histology of the cornea is taken into account. The cornea is composed of three layers (Fig. 4) (8). The outermost layer is the epithelium, which is lipophilic in nature and has tight junctions. The middle layer is an acellular matrix, which contains about 85% water and is therefore hydrophilic in nature.

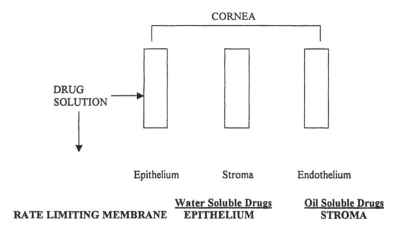

Figure 4 A simplified diagram of histology of the cornea. (Modified from Ref. 8.)

The innermost layer is the endothelium. Although the endothelium is lipophilic, it is leaky and does not give any significant resistance to the transport of molecules. It is believed that the epithelium provides the major resistance for hydrophilic/charged molecules and gives minimal resistance to small lipophilic molecules. However, after passing across the epithelium, further movement of these lipophilic molecules is limited by the matrix, which is hydrophilic in nature. As a result, in order to pass across the whole cornea, the molecule has to have a balance between its lipophilic and hydrophilic character.

Other transport mechanisms such as carrier-mediated transport, endocytosis, etc. may also be involved in transcellular transport but they are poorly understood.

IV. MECHANISMS OF OCULAR PENETRATION ENHANCERS

A detailed mechanistic description of penetration enhancement is beyond the scope of this chapter and can be found elsewhere (13). Our main focus is on ocular penetration enhancement (14). Ideally, penetration enhancers should have the following characteristics (15):

1. The absorbing-enhancing action should be immediate and uni-directional, and the duration should be specific and predictable.
2. There is immediate recovery of the tissue after removing the absorption enhancers.
3. There is no systemic and local effect associated with the enhancers.

4. The enhancers should be physically and chemically compatible with a wide range of drugs and excipients.

However, currently available penetration enhancers are far from satisfying the above requirements. None have yet been approved by the FDA presumably because of safety concerns. In order to design an efficient and safe penetration enhancer, it is necessary to have a thorough understanding of the mechanisms of penetration enhancement. Basically, penetration enhancers work by one or more of the following mechanisms (13):

1. Altering membrane structure and enhancing transcellular transport by extracting membrane components and/or increasing fluidity.
2. Enhancing paracellular transport:
   Chelating calcium ions leads to opening of tight junctions;
   Inducing high osmotic pressure that transiently opens tight junctions;
   Introducing agents to disrupt the structure of tight junctions.
3. Altering mucus structure and rheology so that this diffusion barrier is weakened
4. Modifying the physical properties of the drug-enhancer entity
5. Inhibiting enzyme activity

A summary of ocular penetration enhancers is shown in Table 4 (14). Typically, ocular penetration enhancement falls into two categories: paracellular and transcellular.

A. Enhanced Paracellular Transport

As mentioned earlier, tight junctions are the major determinant of paracellular transport. In other words, tight junctions are the primary targets for a penetration enhancer to act on in order to improve paracellular transport. The most well-known penetration enhancer to improve paracellular transport is EDTA, which is a calcium chelator commonly used as a preservative. It is well known that proper functioning of tight junctions depends on calcium ions. In the absence of calcium ions, there is a widening of tight junctions, resulting in an increase in paracellular permeability (8). EDTA can remove divalent ions by its chelating action. Therefore, there is no surprise that it has a permeabilizing effect on biological membranes (16). However, its action on the cornea is believed to be much more complicated. Rojanasakul et al. (17) showed that severe membrane damage is evident in corneas treated with EDTA, bile salts, and surfactants. This disruption of plasma membrane structures by EDTA is somewhat unexpected since it is believed that EDTA only interferes with the ability of calcium to maintain

Table 4 A Summary of Ophthalmic Penetration Enhancers

Enhancers	Concentration	Drugs	Animal	Effect
Surfactants				
Spans 20, 40 and 85, Tweens 20, 40 and 81, Aptet 100, G 1045, Brji 35 and 58, Myrj 52 and 53	1%	Fluorescein	Human	Enhanced aqueous humor concentration; Tween 20 and Brji 35 at HLB 16–17 are most effective and dose dependent
BL-9	0.1%	Atenolol, Timolol, Levobunolol, Betaxolol	Rabbit	Enhanced Papp 3.4 times for atenolol and 7.3 times for timolol
Brji 35, 48	0.05%	Atenolol, Timolol, Levobunolol, Betaxolol	Rabbit	Enhanced Papp 3.9–10.5 times for atenolol and 1.5–3.9 times for timolol
Brji 98	0.05%	Atenolol, Timolol, Levobunlool, Betaxolol	Rabbit	Enhanced Papp 2 times for betaxolol
Bile Acids				
Deoxycholic acid	0.05%	Atenolol, Timolol, Levobunolol, Betaxolol	Rabbit	Enhanced Papp, 1.9 times for atenolol, 5.3 times for timolol, 1.4 times for levobunlool, and 2.2 times for betaxolol
	0.025–0.1%	Timolol	Rabbit	Enhanced Papp 2.5–8.3 times
Taurocholic acid	1%	Atenol, Carteolol, Tilisolol, Timolol, Befunolol	Rabbit	Enhanced 2.4 times for atenolol, 1.5 times for carteolol, 1.4 times for tilisolol, and 2.1 times for timolol
	1%	FD-4, FD-10	Rabbit	Enhanced Papp 4.5 times for FD-4 and 7.1 times for FD-10

Table 4 Continued

Enhancers	Concentration	Drugs	Animal	Effect
	10 mM	6-Carboxyfluorescein	Rabbit	Enhanced penetrated amount 7.2 times
	2–10 mM	FD-4	Rabbit	Enhanced penetrated amount slightly
Taurodeoxycholic acid	0.05%	Atenolol, Timolol, Levobunolol, Betaxolol	Rabbit	Enhanced Papp 5.8 times for atenolol and 1.6 times for timolol
	0.075–0.1%	Timolol	Rabbit	Enhanced Papp 5.2–5.5 times
	10 mM	6-Carboxyfluorescein	Rabbit	Enhanced penetrated amount 593 times
	2–10 mM	FD-4	Rabbit	Enhanced penetrated amount 30.9–61.5 times
Urodeoxycholic acid	0.05%	Atenolol, Timolol, Levobunolol, Betaxolol	Rabbit	Enhanced Papp 2.1 times for timolol and 1.6 times for betaxolol
	0.075–0.1%	Timolol	Rabbit	Enhanced Papp 8.3–11.0 times
Tauroursodeoxycholic acid	0.05%	Atenolol, Timolol, Levobunolol, Betaxolol	Rabbit	Enhanced Papp 3.0 times for atenolol and 1.5 times for betaxolol
	0.075–0.1%	Timolol	Rabbit	Enhanced Papp 3.3 times at 0.1%
Fatty acids Capric acid	0.5%	Atenolol, Carteolol, Tilisolol, Timolol, Befunolol	Rabbit	Enhanced Papp 20.3 times for atenolol, 8.9 times for carteolol, 5.1 times for tilisolol, and 3.0 times for timolol

Preservatives

Benzalkonium chloride	0.01%	Prostaglandin $F_{2\alpha}$, Pilocarpine, Dexamethasone	Pig	Enhanced Papp 7.2 times for prostaglandin $F_{2\alpha}$, 1.7 times for pilocarpine, and 3.3 times for dexamethasone
	0.01%	Tilisolol, FD-4, FD-10	Rabbit	Enhanced Papp 3.5 times for tilisolol, 28.8 times for FD-4, and 37.1 times for FD-10
	0.02%	Atenolol, Timolol, Levobunolol, Betaxolol	Rabbit	Enhanced Papp 5.2 times for atenolol, 2.7 times for timolol, and 1.3 times for betaxolol
	0.05%	FD-4, FD-10	Rabbit	Enhanced Papp 43.6 times for FDA and 60.6 times for FD-10
	0.005–0.02%	Fluorescein	Rabbit	Increased permeability 4–2.5 times 0.02%
	0.01–0.03%	Carbachol	Rabbit	Enhanced miotic response about 20 times
	0.025%	Titmolol	Rabbit	Enhanced the ocular absorption about 80% and the systemic absorption about 40%
Chlorhexidine digluconate	0.01%	Pilocarpine, Dexamethasone	Pig	Enhanced Papp 1.5 times for dexamethasone
	0.0025–0.05%	Fluorescein	Rabbit, Human	Enhanced permeability significantly over at 0.005%
Benzyl alcohol	0.5%	Tilisolol, FD-4, FD-10	Rabbit	Enhanced Papp 2.6 times for FDA and 8.1 times for FD-10
Chlorbutanol	0.5%	Pilocarpine, Dexamethasone	Pig	Enhanced Papp 1.8 times for pilocarpine and 4.7 times for dexamethasone

Table 4 Continued

Enhancers	Concentration	Drugs	Animal	Effect
2-Phenylethanol	0.5%	Tilisolol, FD-4, FD-10	Rabbit	Enhanced Papp 2.7 times for tilisolol, 5.6 times for FD-4, and 4.8 times for FD-10
Paraben	0.04%	Tilisolol, FD-4, FD-10	Rabbit	Enhanced Papp 1.9 times for FD-10
Propyl paraben	0.02%	Dexamethasone	Pig	Enhanced Papp 1.5 times
Chelating Agents EDTA	0.5%	Atenolol, Timolol, Levobunolol, Betaxolol	Rabbit	Enhanced Papp 1.4 times for atenolol
	0.5%	Atenolol, Carteolol, Tilisolol, Timolol, Befunolol	Rabbit	Enhanced Papp 1.7 times for atenolol, 2.9 times for carteolol, 2.3 times for timolol, and 1.6 times for befunolol
	0.5%	FD-4, FD-10	Rabbit	Enhanced Papp 15.5 times for FDA and 39.0 times for FD-10
	0.1–0.5%	Atenolol, Timolol, Levobunolol, Betaxolol	Rabbit	Enhanced Papp 31 times for atenolol and 1.9 times for timolol at 0.5%
	0.05%	Timolol	Rabbit	Enhanced ocular and systemic absorption significantly
Others Azone	0.025–1.0%	Cimetidine	Rabbit	Enhanced Papp 14.1–87.0 times

Enhancer	Concentration	Drug	Species	Effect
	0.1–0.5%	Acetazolamide, Sulfacetamide, Guanethidine, Cimetidine, Bunolol, Predisolone, Flurbiprofen Amide	Rabit	Enhanced Papp 29.1 times for acetazolamide, 16.3 times for guanethidine, >87.3 times for guanethidine, 31.3 times for cimetidine, 2.2 times for bunolol, and 2.2 times for prednisolone
	0.025–0.1%	Cimetidine	Rabbit	Enhanced ocular bioavailability 3.9–22.0 times after instillation in rabbits
	5%	Cyclosporine	Rabbit	Enhanced penetration into the cornea and rapidly achieved state-steady state drug level
Hexamethylene Lauramide	0.025–1.0%	Cimetidine	Rabbit	Enhanced Papp 17.4–64.3 times
Hexamethylene Octanamide	0.025–1.0%	Cimetidine	Rabbit	Enhanced Papp 5.7–100.3 times
Decylmethylsulfoxide	0.025–1.0%	Cimetidine	Rabbit	Enhanced Papp 25–77 times
Saponin	0.05%	Atenolol, Timolol, Levobunolol, Betaxolol	Rabbit	Enhanced Papp 16.5 times for atenolol, 11.0 times for timolol, 1.3 times for levobunolol, 2.0 times for betaxolol
	0.01–0.025%	Timolol	Rabbit	Enhanced Papp 2.1 times at 0.01%, 3.3 times at 0.015%, and 8.3 times at 0.025%

Table 4 Continued

Enhancers	Concentration	Drugs	Animal	Effect
	0.5%	Atenolol, Carteolol, Tilisolol, Befunolol	Rabbit	Enhanced Papp 31.9 times for atenolol, 13.2 times for carteolol, 7.6 times for tilisolol, 3.3 times for timolol, 2.7 times for befunolol
	0.5%	FD-4, FD-10	Rabbit	Enhanced Papp 100 times for FD-4 and 114 times for FD-10.

FD-4: FITC-dextran (average molecular weight 4400); FD-10: FITC-dextran (average molecular weight 9400); Papp: apparent permeability coefficient.
Source: Modified from Ref. 14.

intercellular integrity, but the effect may be due to concentration and contact time. Nishihata et al. (18) showed that EDTA caused leakage of cell proteins from rectal epithelia. Therefore, there is a possibility that EDTA can exert multiple effects on biological membranes. However, it is believed that its primary action is still on the integrity of tight junctions since it fails to improve delivery of progesterone, which appears to penetrate the cornea primarily by the transcellular route (16).

Cytochalasins are a group of small molecules that bind specifically to actin microfilaments, the major component of the cytoskeleton. It has been shown that the cytoskeleton participates in regulation of epithelial permeability in a variety of conditions (19). Therefore, it is a reasonable strategy to design a penetration enhancer to act specifically on the cytoskeleton in order to improve paracellular transport. Rojanaskul et al. (17) showed that cytochalasin B decreases TEER of the cornea in a dose-dependent manner. They also studied the safety profile of cytochalasin B in vitro. Confocal microscopy showed that cytochalasin B produced negligible damage effect on the cell membrane. Moreover, replacement of cytochalasin B after 30-minute treatment with drug-free GBR results in a complete restoration of TEER, a process that is completed within 30 minutes after solution replacement. However, prolonged exposure time (e.g., > 1 hour) results in permanent damage with incomplete recovery within the time frame of the experiment. It is obvious that cytochalasin B is a relatively specific and safe ocular penetration enhancer compared with other classical penetration enhancers such as bile salts, surfactants, etc.

Another strategy to improve paracellular transport is to make use of active transport systems. Active transport of glucose or amino acids, which is coupled to sodium transport, across the intestinal mucosa into the intercellular lateral spaces creates an osmotic force for fluid flow, and this in turns triggers contraction of the perijunctional actomyosin, resulting in increased paracellular permeability (decreased TEER) (20). Martinez-Palomo (21) showed that a hypertonic lysine solution induced a reversible opening of the tight junction of the toad urinary bladder without gross deformation of tight junctions. The decreased TEER was reversed when an isotonic solution was replaced on the apical side of the epithelium. Due to complete reversibility, it appears that increased paracellular transport by applying a hypertonic solution works in isolated tissues. However, a hypertonic solution may irritate the eye and induce tear production, which flushes away the applied drug. Therefore, the practicality of this approach is questionable and has yet to be confirmed.

B. Enhanced Transcellular Transport

Enhancers that increase transcellular permeability to drugs probably do so by affecting membrane lipids and protein components. It is shown that fatty acids and their derivatives have been found to act primarily on the phospholipid component of membranes thereby creating disorder, resulting in increased permeability (22).

Membrane cholesterol is another target for enhanced transcellular delivery. It was postulated that extraction of cholesterol out of the epithelial membrane by medium chain monoglycerides, glyceryl-monooctanoate, glyceryl-1-monodecanoate, and glyceryl-monododecanoate promoted rectal cefoxitin absorption. However, some fatty acids act on the protein component in membranes. This is certainly the case for caprylate (22).

Nonprotein thios are another membrane component where certain enhancers can act. The good correlation between reduced nonprotein thiols and enhanced transport of hydrophilic compounds suggests an important role for nonprotein thiols in preventing the transport of hydrophilic compounds (22). Murakami et al. (23) showed that depletion of these nonprotein thiols by treating with SH-modifying agents like diethyl maleate, diethyl ethoxymethylenemalonate, ethanol, or alicylates enhanced the mucosal to serosal transport of many hydrophilic compounds including cefoxitin and phenol red in rat intestinal tissue.

V. NEW PENETRATION ENHANCERS

Typically, classical penetration enhancers have a nonspecific action on biological membranes. They work by reversibly or permanently damaging the membranes so that their safety is questionable. Newer penetration enhancers have been introduced in ocular drug delivery recently with an aim to solving this problem.

A. Cyclodextrin

Cyclodextrins are a group of homologous cyclic oligosaccharides consisting of six, seven, and eight glucose units, namely, α-, β-, and γ-cyclodextrin (Fig. 5) (24), respectively. Typically, cyclodextrins act as true carriers by keeping hydrophobic molecules in solution by their hydrophobic cores, i.e., complexation between hydrophobic molecules and the inner hydrophobic core of cyclodextrins. In other words, they are not capable of modifying the permeability of a biological barrier. On the other hand, drug absorption may be limited by the release of the drug from the drug-cyclodextrin com-

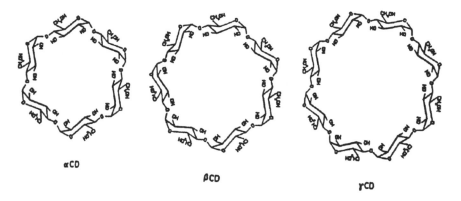

Figure 5 Structures of α-, β-, and γ-cyclodextrins. (From Ref. 24.)

plex. As a result, addition of a cyclodextrin in an ophthalmic formulation does not necessarily increase the ocular bioavailability. It may adversely affect drug absorption (25,26).

However, a recent study showed that α-cyclodextrin has a significant penetration-enhancing effect (10-fold) on the corneal permeability of pilocarpine (27). It was speculated that such an effect was achieved by direct interaction of the α-cyclodextrin with the corneal epithelium, which led to subsequent destabilization of the cell membrane since the same effect was also observed when the cornea was pretreated with the α-cyclodextrin before the transport study. Although α-cyclodextrin only produced minimal damaging effect on the cornea at low concentration (8%), the toxic effect at higher concentration (13% in this study) is still not known.

B. 1-Dodecylazacycloheptan-2-one (Azone®)

Although Azone® was extensively studied as a percutaneous penetration enhancer (28–30), its use in the ocular route is still in its infancy. The exact mechanism of the penetration enhancer effect is not known. However, it can be speculated in terms of its lipophilicity (31). Azone® is highly lipophilic (log $P > 7$), which can incorporate into lipoidal cell membrane and exert a penetration enhancing effect. It is interesting to note that 0.1% can enhance corneal penetration of hydrophilic compounds by at least 20-fold but inhibit corneal penetration of lipophilic compounds such as flurbiprofen. This was further supported by an earlier study that demonstrated that Azone® did not improve the ocular bioavailability of levobunolol (32). It was speculated that insertion of Azone® into the corneal epithelium changed the structure and fluidity of the cell membrane.

Loosening of tight junctions and subsequent water (corneal swelling was observed in the study) and drug influx might also be one of the possible mechanisms. It was believed that retardation of absorption of lipophilic molecules was due to creation of a more hydrated barrier, which retards entry of lipophilic molecules. However, this is a pure speculation, and further experiments need to be done to clarify the exact mechanism.

Safety is still the major concern in using Azone® as an ocular penetration enhancer. It is necessary to keep the Azone® concentration to a minimum (< 0.1%) since higher concentrations might cause ocular discomfort, conjunctival hyperemia, and epithelial thinning as a result of erosion and/or atrophy (33). Fortunately, in vitro experiments showed that 0.1% was enough to enhance penetration for most of the compounds under investigation to a significant extent (33).

C. Saponin

Saponin is a type of polysaccharide isolated from the bark of the Quillaja saponaria tree. Saponin is an amphiphilic compound that has surface activity. As a result, although the exact mechanism of the penetration enhancing effect is not well understood, it is believed that the penetration enhancing effect relies solely on its detergent action. 0.5% Saponin increased corneal permeability of atenolol by two- to threefold but only slightly improved the delivery of relatively lipophilic timolol and befunolol. Saponin was also extensively studied as a penetration promoter for systemic delivery of macromolecules via the eye. Saponin demonstrated improvement in the systemic delivery of insulin and glucagon via the ocular route in various species (34–39). It was shown that the penetration-enhancing effect of saponin was simply a direct detergent action since there did not exist a linear correlation between efficacy and surfactant strength. Therefore, the exact mechanism is still a mystery. The major concern in using saponin in an ophthalmic product is still safety. Concentrations higher than 0.5% are irritating to the eye (35).

VI. NOVEL PENETRATION ENHANCERS

A. α-Amino Acid

Most of classical penetration enhancers improve the paracellular transport across a biological membrane by damaging the tight junctions to varying degrees by their nonspecific actions. As a result, few of them are approved by the FDA because of safety concern. Emisphere Technologies synthesized a series of small molecular weight α-amino acids, which are used to promote oral delivery (Fig. 6) (40,41). These delivery agents successfully increased absorption of several macromolecules in vivo in rats and primates, including humans, such as salmon calcitonin (42), interferon-α (43), heparin (44), and human growth hormone (hgH) (45). Wu (41) showed that these carriers can increase the permeability coefficient of human growth hormone across Caco-2 monolayers by 10-fold. Although it did have some effects on paracellular transport, the major pathway was observed to be transcellular. Failure of these carriers to improve the transport of hydrocortisone, a transcellular marker, in Caco-2 monolayers showed that these carriers have a specific interaction with hGH, which makes the hGH more transportable, and such an interaction does not exist in the case of hydrocortisone. It was clearly established that these carriers do not damage cell membranes and thus are not classical penetration enhancers. Moreover, the carrier-drug complex is not absorbed by an active transport process.

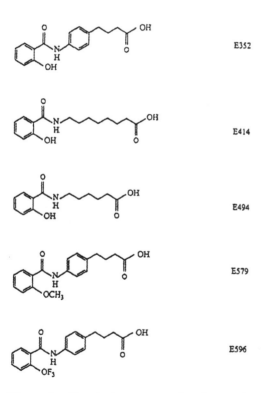

Figure 6 Chemical structures of various amino acid derivative carriers. (From Ref. 41.)

The working mechanistic assumption is that the carrier shields those hydrophilic groups on the molecule that restrain absorption.

Previous work in our laboratory showed that these carriers increase the permeability coefficient of hGH across the cornea of a rabbit by 10-fold (46). Further study is ongoing in our laboratory to confirm the efficacy and toxicity of these carriers as delivery agents/carriers for ocular drug delivery.

B. Pz-Peptide

Pz-peptide (4-phenylazobenzoxycarbonyl-Pro-Leu-Gly-Pro-D-Arg) is a hydrophilic collagenase-labile pentapeptide with a molecular weight of 777 daltons, which is capable of triggering opening of tight junctions in a transient, reversible manner. As a result, it can facilitate paracellular transport in rabbit intestinal segments and Caco-2 monolayers (47,48). Interestingly, it also facilitates its own transport.

The enhancement effect of Pz-peptide on permeability of drug across the cornea and conjunctiva was studied by Chung et al. (49). Pz-peptide increases penetration across the cornea and conjunctiva for a wide range of compounds such as atenolol, propranolol, mannitol, fluorescein, FITC-Dextran 4000, etc. Compared with other traditional penetration enhancers such as a cytochalasin B and EDTA, Pz-peptide is less potent in facilitating paracellular transport since it fails to improve the penetration of FITC-Dextran 10000 across the cornea.

The mechanism of enhancement is believed to involve stimulation of transepithelial Na^+ flux at the level of the amiloride-sensitive Na^+ channel and then triggering biochemical changes, which result in opening of tight junctions. This was demonstrated in colonic segments of rabbits and Caco-2 cell monolayers (50). However, this may not be the case in ocular tissues. Amiloride (a Na^+ channel blocker), hexamethylene amiloride (Na^+/H^+ exchange blocker), ouabain (a Na^+/K^+ ATPase inhibitor), and replacement of Na^+ with choline chloride fails to inhibit Pz-peptide penetration (49). In addition, Pz-peptide can unexpectedly enhance the penetration of propranolol, which transports across a biological membrane solely via a transcellular pathway. This may be due to inhibition of $P_{gp}170$ drug efflux pump, which was found in the conjunctiva (51), since propranolol is a substrate for this efflux system. Further investigation has to be carried out to clarify its exact mechanism of enhancement.

Although the enhancement effect of Pz-peptide is promising in vitro ($2.4-5.1\times$ for cornea, $1.8-2.0\times$ for the conjunctiva in the case of atenolol and propranolol), its effect is much less pronounced in vivo. Pz-peptide fails to enhance ocular absorption of propranolol and only improves the absorption of atenolol by 1.4–2.0 times. This may be due to the dilution effect of resident tears on Pz-peptide and the applied dose or binding of Pz-peptide to mucin in other tears proteins.

C. Multifunctional Approach (Polymeric Penetration Enhancers)

1. Colloidal Systems

Colloidal systems have been extensively studied as carriers for ocular drug delivery (52). The mechanism of enhancement is generally believed to be related to prolonged residence time in the cul-de-sac. However, enhanced penetration may also be one of the explanations for improved ocular delivery. Poly-ε-caprolactone nanoparticles, nanocapsules, and submicron emulsions improved ocular bioavailability of indomethacin when compared with aqueous solutions and with a suspension of microparticles (53). It is believed that the colloidal nature, rather than the inner structure or the specific composition of the colloidal carriers, plays a key role in the enhancement since all three colloidal carriers improve the ocular bioavailability of indomethacin to a similar extent. Confocal microscopy showed that the colloidal carriers penetrate into the epithelial cells of the cornea without causing damage to the cell membrane. This suggests that these carriers enter the epithelium via endocytosis. Therefore, these carriers act as a penetration enhancer or an endocytotic stimulator.

2. Bioadhesives

A mentioned earlier, in order to improve ocular bioavailability, either k_{eli} or k_{abs} have to be increased two- to threefold. Various means have been attempted to prolong residence time (1–4). Obviously, it is desirable to have a delivery system that can stay in the precorneal area for an extended period of time but at the same time enhance corneal penetration. A number of bioadhesive polymers have such properties. Typically, these are macromolecules that have already been approved by FDA for other purposes. Therefore, safety should not be a big problem.

3. Polyacrylates

Poly(acrylic acid) derivatives such as Carbomer and Polycarbol are used extensively as bioadhesives (54). They do have a membrane-penetrating enhancing effect, although the exact mechanism is not well understood. It was demonstrated that polyacrylic acid gel significantly increased the influx of water in the rat rectum (55). It was speculated that this solvent drag was responsible for the enhanced absorption of low molecular weight compounds. Reduction of mucus on the microvillus and dilatation of the intercellular space was also observed 5–10 minutes after administration of polyacrylic acid gel into the rat rectum. However, these changes were reversible and returned to normal relatively soon. It was not likely that polyacrylic acid gel enhanced penetration solely by its detergent action since it inhibited rather than induced hemolysis, which is commonly observed with surfactants. Another possible mechanism is related to its chelating activity. Polycarbopol and other polyacrylic acid–based polymers are able to chelate calcium (56), which is an essential component for proper functioning of tight junctions. In addition, chelation of cations that are essential for normal activity of enzymes further improves bioavailability. However, this inhibitory effect may be too weak to account for the improved bioavailability (57). In the case of ocular drug delivery, there is reported to be only a minimum amount of metabolizing enzymes in the precorneal area. As a result, there is not likely to be a drastic improvement in ocular bioavailability because of this enzyme inhibitory effect.

4. Chitosan and Derivatives

Chitosan (poly[β-(1-4)-2-amino-2-deoxy-D-glucopyranose]) (58) is a hydrophilic, biocompatible, biodegradable polymer of low toxicity. It is widely used as a pharmaceutical excipient for direct compression of tablets, controlled release rate of drugs from a dosage form, enhanced dissolution, etc. (58). It also shows strong mucoadhesive properties (59). Chitosan was evaluated as a delivery system to increase precorneal drug residence times (60). The positively charged chitosan can reduce the elimination rate from the precorneal area by increasing viscosity and by its interaction with negatively charged mucus (mucoadhesive). The presence of chitosan with tobramycin can bring an improvement in AUC and $t_{1/2}$ in the precorneal area. Moreover, this preparation is well tolerated with minimal toxicity.

Besides increasing residence time of a drug in the precorneal area, chitosan can be used as a potential penetration enhancer to improve delivery across the cornea. Dodane et al. (61) showed that chitosan caused a reversible, time and dose-dependent decrease in TEER in Caco-2 cell monolayers. The increase in permeability was further confirmed by increased mannitol permeability. They suggested that the above effects might be due to partial alteration of the cytoskeleton, but the exact mechanism is not known. The slight perturbation of the plasma membrane was evident by the rise in extracellular LDH release. However, complete recovery was observed 24 hours after exposure to a low concentration of chitosan (0.005%) for a short period of time (< 60 min). Moreover, the chitosan did not affect cell viability as shown by the trypan blue exclusion test.

Conjugation of an enzyme inhibitor to chitosan is another strategy to improve drug delivery (62,63). However, due to the limited amounts of enzymes in the precorneal area, this strategy may not be beneficial in ocular drug delivery.

It was shown that mucus may inhibit the binding of chitosan to an epithelia surface and hence decreases its absorption-enhancing effect in intestinal epithelia. The absorption-enhancing effect of chitosan has not been evaluated in the eye. The extent of inhibition of chitosan binding to mucus in the precorneal area has yet to be determined.

VII. CONCLUSIONS

The use of penetration enhancers in ocular drug delivery has been studied for more than a decade, but none has been approved by the FDA mainly due to their nonspecific actions, which often give an unfavorable safety profile. In order to design a more specific penetration enhancer, it is necessary to have a better understanding of membrane transport, physiology of tight junctions, etc. Another alternative is to reversibly modify physicochemical properties of a drug so that it becomes more transportable (e.g., prodrugs or carriers).

Obviously, penetration enhancement has its limit. It is not possible to increase drug bioavailability indefinitely by use of penetration enhancement alone. Other approaches such as increased residence time and inhibition of metabolizing enzymes should be used in conjunction with penetration enhancement. We hope that the coming biomaterial era will bring us such a drug delivery system.

REFERENCES

1. Sieg, J. W., and Robinson, J. R. Vehicle effects on ocular drug bioavailability. 1. Evaluation of fluorometholone. J. Pharm. Sci. 64:931–936, 1975.
2. Patton, T. F., and Robinson, J. R., Ocular evaluation of polyvinyl alcohol vehicle in rabbits. J. Pharm. Sci. 64:1312–1316, 1975.
3. Robinson, J. R., and Mlynek, G. M. Bioadhesive and phase-change polymers for ocular drug delivery. Adv. Drug. Delivery Rev. 16:45–50, 1995.
4. Salminen, L., and Urtti, H. Prolonged pulse-entry of pilocarpine with a soluble drug insert. Graefes Arch. Clin. Exp. Ophthalmol. 221:96, 1983.
5. Worakul, N., and Robinson, J. R. Ocular pharmacokinetics/pharmacodynamics. Eur. J. Pharm. Biopharm. 44:71–83, 1997.

6. Keister, J. C., Cooper, E. R., Missel, P. J., Lang, J. C., and Hager, D. F. Limits on optimizing ocular drug delivery. J. Pharm. Sci. 80:50–53, 1990.

7. Harris, D., and Robinson, J. R. Bioadhesive polymers in peptide drug delivery. Biomaterials 11:652–658, 1990.

8. Grass, G. M. Mechanisms of Corneal Drug Penetration. Ph.D. thesis, School of Pharmacy, University of Wisconsin–Madison, 1985.

9. Alberts, B., Bray, D., Lewis, J., Raff, M., Roberts, K., and Watson, J. D. Molecular Biology of the Cell, 3rd ed., Garland Publishing, Inc., New York, 1994.

10. Liaw, J., and Robinson, J. R. Ocular penetration enhancers. In: Ophthalmic Drug Delivery Systems (Mitra A., ed.), Marcel Dekker, New York, 1993, pp. 369–381.

11. Rojanasakul, Y., and Robinson, J. R. Transport mechanisms of the cornea: Characterization of barrier permselectivity. Int. J. Pharm. 55:237–246, 1989.

12. Lee, V. H. L., and Robinson, J. R. Review: Topical ocular drug delivery: Recent developments and future challenges. J. Ocular Pharmacol. 2:67–108, 1986.

13. Robinson, J. R., and Yang, X. Absorption enhancers. In: Encyclopedia of Pharmaceutical Technology, Vol. 18 (Swarbrick J. and Boylan J. C. (eds.), Marcel Dekker, New York, 1999, pp. 1–27.

14. Sasaki, H., Yamamura, K., Mukai, Nishida, K., Nakamura, J., Nakashima, M., and Ichikawa, M. Enhancement of ocular drug penetration, Crit. Rev. Drug Carrier Syst. 16:85–146, 1999.

15. Junginger, H. E., and Verhoef, J. C. Macromolecules as safe penetration enhancers for hydrophilic drugs—a fiction? Pharmaceut. Sci. Technol. Today 1:370–376, 1998.

16. Grass, G. M., Wood, R. W., and Robinson, J. R. Effects of calcium chelating agents on corneal permeability. Invest. Ophthalmol. Vis. Sci. 26:110–113, 1985.

17. Rojanasakul, Y., Liaw, J. and Robinson, J. R. Mechanisms of action of some penetration enhancers in the cornea: laser scanning confocal microscopic and electrophysiological studies. Int. J. Pharm. 66:131–142, 1990.

18. Nishihata, T., Tomida, H., Frederick, G., Rytting, J. H., and Higuchi, T. Comparison of the effects of sodium salicylate, disodium ethylenediamine tetraacetic acid and polyoxylene-23-lauryl ether as adjuvants for the rectal absorption of sodium cefoxitin. J. Pharm. Sci. 37:159, 1985.

19. Frederiksen, O., and Leyssac, P. P. Effects of cytochalasin B. and dimethylsulsulfoxide on isoosmotic transport by rabbit gall-bladder in vitro. J. Facial (Lund.) 265:103–118, 1977.

20. Madara, J. L., et al. Effects of cytochalasin D on occluding junctions of intestinal absorptive cells: Further evidence that the cytoskeleton may influence paracellular permeability and junctional charge selectivity. J. Cell Biol. 102:2125, 1986.

21. Martinez-Palomo, A. Structure of tight junctions in epithelia with different permeability. Proc. Natl. Acad. Sci. USA 72:4487–4491, 1975.

22. Lee, V. H. L., ed. Peptides and Proteins Drug Delivery. Marcel Dekker, New York, 1990.

23. Murakami, M., et al. Intestinal absorption enhanced by unsaturated fatty acids: Inhibitory effect of sulfhydryl modifiers. Biochim. Biophys. Acta 293:238, 1988.

24. Cyclodextrins in Pharmacy (Fromming, K.-H., and Szejtli, J., eds.), Kluwer Academic Publishers, Boston, 1994.

25. Davies, N. M., Wang, G., and Tucker, I. G. Evaluation of a hydrocortisone/hydroxypropyl-beta-cyclodextrin solution for ocular drug delivery. Int. J. Pharm. 156:201–209, 1997.

26. Jarho, P., Jarvinen, K., Urtti, A., Stella, V. J., and Jarvinen, T. Use of cyclodextrins in ophthalmic formulations of dipivefrin. Int. J. Pharm. 153:225–233, 1997.

27. Siefert, B., and Keipert, S. Influence of alpha-cyclodextrin and hydroxyalkylated β-cyclodextrin derivatives on the in vitro corneal uptake and permeation of aqueous pilocarpine-HCl solutions. J. Pharm. Sci. 86:716–720, 1997.

28. Michniak, B. B., Player, M. R., Godwin, D. A., Lockhart, C. C., and Sowell, J. W. In vitro evaluation of azone analogs as dermal penetration enhancers. Part 5. Miscellaneous compounds. Int. J. Pharm. 161:169–178, 1998.

29. Valenta, C., and Wedenig, S. Effects of penetration enhancer on the in vitro percutaneous absorption of progesterone. J. Pharm. Pharmacol. 49:955–959, 1997.

30. Chatterjee, D. J., Li, W. Y., and Koda, R. T. Effect of vehicles and penetration enhancers on the in vitro and in vivo percutaneous absorption of methotrexate and edatrexate through hairless mouse skin. Pharm. Res. 14:1058–1065, 1997.

31. Tang-Liu, D. D-S., Richman, J. B., Weinkam, R. J., and Takruri, H. Effects of four penetration enhancers on corneal permeability of drugs in vitro. J. Pharm. Sci. 83:85–90, 1994.

32. Tang-Liu, D. D.-S., and Burke, J. The effect of Azone® on ocular levobunolol absorption: Calculating the area under the curve and its standard error using tissue sampling compartments. Pharm. Res. 5:238–241, 1988.

33. Ismail, I. M., Chen, C.-C., Richman, J. B., Andersen, J. S., and Tang-Liu, D. D.-S. Comparison of azone and hexamethylene lauramide in toxicological effects and penetration enhancement of cimetidine in rabbit eyes. Pharm. Res. 9:817–821, 1992.

34. Chiou, G. C. Y., Chang, C. Y., and Chang, M. S. Systemic delivery of insulin through eyes to lower the glucose concentration. J. Ocular Pharmacol. 5:81–91, 1989.

35. Pillion, D. J., Atchison, J. A., Stott, J., McCracken, D. L., Gargiulo, C., and Meezan, E. Efficacy of insulin eyedrops. J. Ocular Pharmacol. 10:461–470, 1994.

36. Pillion, D. J., McCracken, D. L., Yang, M., and Atchison, J. A. Glucagon administration to the rat via eye drops. J. Ocular Pharmacol. 4:349–358, 1992.

37. Pillion, D. J., Amsden, J. A., Kensil, C. R., and Recchia, J. Structure-function relationship among Quillaja saponins serving as excipients for nasal and ocular delivery of insulin. J. Pharm. Sci. 85:518–524, 1996.

38. Morgan, R. V. Delivery of systemic regular insulin via the ocular route in cats. J. Ocular Pharmacol. 11:565–573, 1995.

39. Morgan, R. V., and Huntzicker, M. A. Delivery of systemic regular insulin via the ocular route in dogs. J. Ocular Pharmacol. 12:515–526, 1996.

40. Steiner, S., and Rosen, R. Delivery System for Pharmacological Agents Encapsulated Proteinoids. U.S. Patent, 1990.

41. Wu, S.-Y. Mechanistic studies on the enhanced mucosal transport of human growth hormone by certain amino acid derivatives. Ph.D. thesis, School of Pharmacy, University of Wisconsin–Madison, 1999.

42. Leone-Bay, A., McInnes, C., Wang, N., DeMorin, F., Achan, D., Lercara, C., Sarubbi, D., Haas, S., Press, J., Barantsevich, E., O'Broin, B., Milstein, S., and Patron, D. Microsphere formation in a series of derivatized α-amino acids: Properties, molecular modeling, and oral delivery of salmon calcitonin. J. Med. Chem. 38:4257–4262, 1995.

43. Leone-Bay, A., Santiago, N., Achan, D., Chaudhary, K., DeMorin, F., Falzarano, L., Haas, S., Kalbag, D., Leipold, H., Lercara, C., O'Toole, D., Rivera, T., Rosado, C., Sarubbi, D., Vuocolo, E., Wang, N., Milstein, S., and Baughman, R. A. N-acylated α-amino acids as novel oral delivery agents for proteins. J. Med. Chem. 38:4263–4269, 1995.

44. Brayden D., Creed E., O'Connell A., Leipold, H., Lercara C., Agarwal R., and Leone-Bay A. Heparin absorption across the intestine: Effects of sodium N-[8(2-hydroxybenzoyl)amino]caprylate in Caco-2 monolayers and in rat in situ intestinal instillations. Pharm. Res. 14:1772–1779, 1997.

45. Leone-Bay, A., Ho, K., Agarwal, R., Baughman, R. A., Chaudhary, K., DeMorin, F., Genoble, L., McInnes, C., Lercara, C., Milstein, S., O'Toole, D., Sarubbi, D., Variano, B., and Paton, D. R. 4-[4-[(2-Hydroxybenzoyl)amino]phenyl]butyric acid as a novel oral delivery agent for recombinant human growth hormone. J. Med. Chem. 39:2571–2578, 1996.

46. Robinson, J. R., unpublished data, 1998.

47. Yen, W.-C., and Lee, V. H. L. Paracellular transport of a proteolytically labile pentapeptide across the colonic and other intestinal segments of the albino rabbit: Implications for peptide drug design. J. Contr. Rel. 28:97–109, 1994.

48. Yen, W.-C., and Lee, V. H. L. Penetration enhancement effect of Pz-peptide, a paracellularly transported peptide, in rabbit intestinal segments and Caco-2 cell monolayers. J Contr. Rel. 36:25–37, 1995.

49. Chung, Y. B., Han, K., Nishiura, A., and Lee, V. H. L. Ocular absorption of Pz-peptide and its effect on the ocular and systemic pharmacokinetics of topically applied drugs in the rabbit. Pharm. Res. 15:1882–1887, 1998.

50. Yen, W.-C., and Lee, V. H. L. Role of Na$^+$ in the asymmetric paracellular transport of 4-phenylazobenzyloxycarbonyl-L-Pro-L-Leu-Gly-L-Pro-D-Arg across rabbit colonic segments and Caco-2 cell monolayers. J. Pharmacol. Exp. Ther. J. Contr. Rel. 36:25–37, 275:114–119, 1995.

51. Saha, P., Yang, J., and Lee, V. H. L. Existence of a P-glycoprotein drug efflux pump in cultured rabbit conjunctival epithelial cells. Invest. Ophthalmol. Vis. Sci. 39:1221–1226, 1998.

52. Zimmer, A., and Kreuter, J. Microcapsules and nanoparticles used in ocular delivery systems. Adv. Drug Delivery Rev. 16:61–73, 1995.

53. Calvo, P., Alonson, M. J., Vila-Jato, J. L., and Robinson, J. R. Improved ocular bioavailability of indomethacin by novel ocular drug carriers. J. Pharm. Pharmacol. 48:1147–1152, 1996.

54. Yang, X., and Robinson, J. R. Bioadhesion in mucosal drug delivery. In: Biomaterials for Drug Delivery (Okano, T., ed.), Elsevier, Amsterdam, 1998.

55. Morimoto, K., Iwamoto, T., and Morisaka, K. Possible mechanisms for the enhancement of rectal absorption of hydrophilic drugs and polypeptides by aqueous polyacrylic acid gel. J. Pharmacobio-Dyn. 10:85–91, 1987.

56. Kriwet, B., and Kissel, T. Interactions between bioadhesive poly(acrylic acid) and calcium ions. Int. J. Pharm. 127:135–145, 1996.

57. Lußen, H. L., Bohner, V., Pe'rard, D., Langguth, P., Verhoef, J. C., de Boer, A. G., Merkle, H. P., and Junginger, H. E. Mucoadhesive polymers in peroral peptide drug delivery: V. Effect of poly(acrylates) on the enzymatic degradation of peptide drugs by intestinal brush border membrane vesicles. Int. J. Pharm. 141:39, 1996.

58. Illum, L. Chitosan and its use as a pharmaceutical excipient. Pharm. Res. 15:1326–1331, 1998.

59. Yoshiaki, K., Yamamoto, H., Takeuchi, H., and Kuno, Y. Mucoadhesive dl-lactide/glycolide copolymer nanospheres coated with chitosan to improve oral delivery elcatonin. Pharm. Dev. Tech. 5:77–85, 2000.

60. Felt, O., Furrer, P., Mayer, J. M., Plazonnet, B., Buri, P., and Gurny, R. Topical use of chitosan in ophthalmology: tolerance assessment and evaluation of precorneal retention. Int. J. Pharm. 180:185–193, 1999.

61. Dodane, V., Khan, A. M., and Merwin, J. R. Effect of chitosan on epithelial permeability and structure. Int. J. Pharm. 182:21–32, 1999.

62. Bernkop-Schnurch, A., Paikl, C., and Pasta, M. Novel bioadhesive chitosan-EDTA conjugate protects leucine enkephalin from degradation by aminopeptidase N. Pharm. Res. 14:917–922, 1997.

63. Bernkop-Schnurch, A., and Pasta, M. Intestinal peptide and protein delivery: Novel bioadhesive drug-carrier matrix shielding from enzymatic attack. J. Pharm. Sci. 87:430–434, 1998.

10

Corneal Collagen Shields for Ocular Drug Delivery

Shiro Higaki, Marvin E. Myles, Jeannette M. Loutsch, and James M. Hill
LSU Eye and Vision Center of Excellence, Louisiana State University Health Science Center, New Orleans, Louisiana, U.S.A.

I. HISTORICAL ASPECTS

A. Soft Contact Lens for Ocular Drug Delivery

Bandage soft contact lenses made of hydrophilic polymers are widely used to protect eyes with various problems, including recurrent corneal erosions and epithelial defects after corneal transplantation or refractive surgery. Although these bandage soft contact lenses may enhance healing while allowing the eye to remain open, they can be inserted and removed only in the ophthalmologist's office. Additionally, soft contact lenses may harbor pathogens, which can cause ocular infection.

The idea of using bandage soft contact lenses to deliver drugs to the cornea was proposed as far back as 1971 by Kaufman (1). In this procedure, the hydrophilic lens was placed on the cornea and the drug was administered topically onto the surface of the lens. The contact lens was thought to act as a carrier vehicle, binding the drug and releasing it slowly, thereby increasing retention of the therapeutic agent in the tear film and at the corneal surface. However, Busin and Spitznas (2) and Matoba and McCulley (3) showed that hydrogen contact lenses hydrated with drug are nearly devoid of drug after only 1 or 2 hours on the cornea. These soft contact lenses, therefore, are not the ideal approach for sustained, continuous ocular drug delivery.

B. Collagen Used to Enhance Drug Delivery

Bloomfield et al. (4) were the first to suggest that collagen might provide a suitable carrier for sustained ocular drug delivery. They showed that wafer-shaped collagen inserts impregnated with gentamicin produced higher levels of drug in the tear film and tissue in the rabbit eye compared to drops, ointment, or subconjunctival injection.

Fyodorov et al. (5) suggested substituting collagen for hydrophilic polymer in a contact lens shape. His purpose, however, was not drug delivery but the creation of a temporary protective device to enhance healing of the cornea. In the mid-1980s, Fyodorov and colleagues (5,6) introduced the collagen shield for use as a bandage lens and showed that the shields enhance corneal epithelial healing after radial keratotomy and other anterior segment surgical procedures.

Numerous vision researchers saw the collagen shield as an extension of and improvement on Bloomfield's collagen inserts (4)—a potential new vehicle for the sustained administration of drugs to the cornea. Over the next several years, various drugs were incorporated into the collagen shield matrix during manufacture, absorbed into the shields during rehydration, and/or applied in topical drops directly onto shields in situ. Studies in animal models (described below) showed that as the drug dissolved in the shield, it was released gradually into the tear film, resulting in increased contact time with the cornea and increased penetration into both the cornea and the aqueous humor. Clinical studies demonstrated that the collagen shield is easy to use in the ophthalmologist's office, prevents delay in beginning therapy, and maintains therapeutic concentrations of drug in the eye without the need for frequent topical instillation of drops.

II. CORNEAL COLLAGEN SHIELD: PHYSICAL PROPERTIES

A. Properties of Collagen

The safety of collagen for human use is evidenced by its diverse uses and biomedical applications. Collagen is a common constituent in soaps, shampoos, facial creams, body lotions, and food-grade gelatin. In medicine, collagen has been used in cardiovascular surgery, plastic surgery, orthopedics, urology, neurosurgery, and ophthalmology. The major medical application of collagen is catgut suture, which is derived from intestinal collagen (7). Twenty-five percent of the total body protein in mammals is collagen; it is the major protein of connective tissue, cartilage, and bone. The secondary and tertiary structures of human, porcine, and bovine collagen are very similar, making it possible to use collagen derived from animal sources in humans. Biologically, collagen is suggested to promote wound healing (7). Nearly all studies on collagen have shown very low or no immunogenicity (7). Of the 10 collagen types that have been characterized, types 1, 3, and 5 are the most desirable for biomedical applications because of their high biocompatibility and low immunogenicity.

A collagen molecule consists of three polypeptide chains, called α-chains, which form a helix connected by interchain hydrogen bonds. This domain of collagen, called tropocollagen, forms a rodlike unit, 2600–26,000 Å in length and 15 Å in diameter. The molecular weight of the tropocollagen is 300,000 daltons. Collagen has a characteristic amino acid sequence: glycine appears in approximately every third position. Proline and hydroxyproline make up approximately 25% of the total amino acid content. The hydroxyproline residues are from interchain, noncovalent cross-linkages. Newly synthesized collagen contains only a few cross-linked tropocollagen fibers. However, with increased age, there is an increase in the percentage of cross-linking (7).

In the manufacture of corneal collagen shields, the ability to control the amount of cross-linking in the collagen subunits by exposure to ultraviolet (UV) light is an important physicochemical property, because the amount of cross-linking is related to the dissolution time of the shield on the cornea. Kuwano et al. (8) investigated the effect of collagen cross-linking on ofloxacin bioavailability. In this study, the collagen shields were not impregnated with drug, but drops were instilled after application of the collagen shield. They found the dissolution times for the cross-linked collagen shield were longer than those of the non–cross-linked type, thereby prolonging drug delivery times. They concluded that cross-linked collagen shields might be useful ocular drug delivery devices because they can allow drug concentrations to achieve high levels in the cornea and aqueous humor.

B. Properties of Commercial Corneal Collagen Shields

The collagen shield was designed to be a disposable, short-term therapeutic bandage lens for the cornea. It conforms to the shape of the eye, protects the corneal surface, and provides lubrication as it dissolves. Unlike the hydrophilic plastic bandage lenses, the collagen shield offers no refractive benefit; in fact, because it is not optically clear, it reduces visual acuity to the 20/80–20/200 range. Also, the collagen shield causes some discomfort.

Bio-Cor (Bausch & Lomb Surgical, Inc., Claremont, CA) was the first commercially available shield that was introduced in 1986. The diameter, base curve, oxygen permeability, thickness, water content, and other physicochemical characteristics of Bio-Cor collagen shield have been described

Table 1 Comparison of Characteristics of Two Collagen Shields

Brand name	ProShield[a]	SurgiLens[b]
Origin of collagen	Porcine sclera	Bovine corium
Dissolution time (h)	Rapid dissolution, 12, 24, 72	12
Diameter (mm)	14.0	14.5, 16.0
Base curve (mm)	9.0	ND (8.7–9.5)
Dry weight (mg)	5.1–7.9	9.0–11.0
Wet weight (mg)	14.0–52.0	ND
Water content (% H_2O)	75	80
Surface pH	ND	5.5–7.5

ND = not determined.
[a] Data obtained from Alcon Surgical (Fort Worth, TX). Allergan, Inc. (Irvine, California) and Oasis have a similar product called KeraShield and SoftShield, respectively.
[b] Data obtained from Bausch & Lomb Surgical, Inc. (Claremont, CA).

elsewhere (9–11). Bausch & Lomb Surgical, Inc. is selling only SurgiLens now. The shields are derived from bovine collagen and are 14.5 mm in diameter. Dissolution time, determined by UV irradiation during manufacture, is about 12 hours (Table 1). The shields are sterilized by gamma-irradiation, then dehydrated and individually packaged for storage and shipping (12). Alcon Laboratories, Inc. (Fort Worth, TX) is selling ProShield. The rapid dissolution as well as 12-, 24-, and 72-hour shields are available. The shields have a diameter of 14 mm and a compound base curve that is approximately 9 mm when hydrated. The water content is approximately 75% (Table 1).

III. DRUG DELIVERY BY COLLAGEN SHIELDS: EXPERIMENTAL STUDIES

A variety of studies have described the pharmacokinetics of ocular delivery of dyes and drugs by collagen shields as well as the use of the shields in the chemotherapy of various disorders. These studies are reviewed below and summarized in Tables 2 and 3 (13,14).

A. Fluorescein, a Water-Soluble Dye

To determine the ocular penetration of water-soluble compounds delivered by collagen shields, Reidy et al. (15) applied shields hydrated in a solution of sodium fluorescein to normal eyes of volunteers and measured the fluorescence in the anterior chamber by fluorophotometry. The shields delivered significantly larger amounts of dye to the aqueous humor at 2 and 4 hours compared with drops of the same concentration instilled every 30 minutes over 4 hours, as well as in comparison with daily wear soft contact lenses presoaked in 0.01% fluorescein. The collagen shields did not induce any damage to the corneal epithelium over a 2-hour period. These results demonstrate that the collagen shield is superior to topical drops and some soft contact lenses in delivering fluorescein to the cornea and aqueous humor. The collagen shields might also successfully deliver other water-soluble compounds, such as antibiotics, to the eye in amounts comparable to or greater than the amounts delivered by drops over the same period of time.

B. Antibacterial Agents

Ideally, chemotherapy for bacterial keratitis would delivery antibiotics rapidly to both the cornea and aqueous humor, produce concentrations of antibiotic significantly above the minimum inhibitory concentration (MIC) or minimum bactericidal concentration (MBC) of ocular pathogens, and sustain this high concentration for many hours. However, there are numerous problems associated with achieving this ideal, and numerous approaches have been taken to solve these problems (13,16,17).

Various investigators have examined the utility of the collagen shield for the delivery of antibiotics to the cornea and aqueous humor. In one of the earliest pharmacokinetic studies, Unterman et al. (18) assessed the pharmacokinetics of tobramycin delivered to rabbit eyes by means of collagen shields hydrated in solutions of either 40 or 200 mg/mL of tobramycin. Tobramycin concentrations in the cornea and aqueous humor were determined at 2, 4, and 8 hours after application. No toxicity was observed with shields hydrated in the 40 mg/mL solution at any time. Eight hours after application, the corneas with shields hydrated in the 200 mg/mL solution of tobramycin had some epithelial defects. At all times and with either hydration solution, the concentration of tobramycin in the cornea and aqueous humor exceeded the MIC for most aminoglycoside-sensitive strains of *Pseudomonas*.

O'Brien et al. (19) compared collagen shields with soft contact lenses in pharmacokinetic studies of the ocular penetration of tobramycin. Three groups were compared: (a) eyes with collagen shields rehydrated in 3 mg/mL of tobramycin, (b) eyes with therapeutic soft contact lenses, and (c) eyes with neither lenses nor shields. Topical tobramycin (3 mg/mL) was applied to all eyes every 5 minutes for a total of six doses. Aqueous humor samples

Table 2 Studies of Collagen Shield Drug Delivery

Ref.	Drug	Compared with Collagen shield (CS)	Assay site	Overall result with collagen shield (CS)
Phinney et al., 1988 (30)	Gentamicin	Loading dose + frequent drops	Tears Cornea Aqueous	CS comparable at all sites
Phinney et al., 1988 (30)	Vancomycin	Loading dose + frequent drops	Tears Cornea Aqueous	CS comparable at all sites
O'Brien et al., 1988 (18) Unterman et al., 1988 (17)	Tobramycin Tobramycin	Soft contact lens Subconjunctival injection	Aqueous Cornea Aqueous	CS superior CS comparable at both sites
Hwang et al., 1989 (32)	Dexamethasone	Single drop	Cornea Aqueous Iris Vitreous	CS superior at all sites
Hwang et al., 1989 (32)	Dexamethasone	Frequent drops	Cornea Aqueous Iris Vitreous	CS superior at all sites
Hwang et al., 1989 (32)	Dexamethasone	CS + frequent drops versus frequent drops	Cornea Aqueous Iris Vitreous	CS superior at all sites
Sawusch et al., 1989 (33)	Prednisolone	Single drop	Cornea Aqueous	CS superior at both sites

Reference	Drug	Delivery	Site	Result
Reidy et al., 1990 (13)	Fluorescein	Frequent drops Soft contact lens	Anterior chamber	CS superior to both
Schwartz et al., 1990 (40)	Amphotericin B	Frequent drops	Cornea Aqueous	CS comparable at both sites
Reidy et al., 1990 (44)	Cyclosporin A	Frequent drops	Cornea Aqueous	CS superior CS comparable
Murray et al., 1990 (42)	Heparin	Subconjunctival injection	Aqueous	CS Superior
Gussler et al., 1990 (47)	Trifluorothymidine	Drops CS + drops	Aqueous	Cornea with epithelial defect: CS + drops superior CS superior from 0–2 h Drops superior from 4–8 h
Chen et al., 1990 (46)	Tobramycin	Drops	Cornea Aqueous Conjunctiva	CS superior at all sites
Taravella et al., 1998 (65)	Tobramycin	Three drops	Aqueous	No difference
Kuster et al., 1998 (42)	Trifluorothymidine	Drops	Cornea Aqueous	CS higher
Taravella et al., 1999 (64)	Ofloxacin	Three drops	Aqueous	CS superior

Table 3 Studies of Collagen Shield Drug Delivery in Rabbit Models of Disease

Ref.	Experimental model	Drug	Compared with collagen shield (CS)	Result
Sawusch et al., 1988 (21)	*Pseudomonas* keratitis	Tobramycin	CS + frequent drops versus frequent drops	Enhanced antimicrobial effect with CS
Hobden et al., 1988 (20)	*Pseudomonas* keratitis	Tobramycin	Frequent drops	CS comparable antimicrobial effect
			CS + delayed drops versus second CS	CS comparable antimicrobial effect
Hobden et al., 1990 (29)	Aminoglycoside-resistant *Pseudomonas* keratitis	Ciprofloxacin Norfloxacin Tobramycin	CS with vehicle CS with water	Ciprofloxacin > norfloxacin for antimicrobial effect Tobramycin, vehicle, water—no effect
Chen et al., 1990 (19)	High-risk keratoplasty	Cyclosporine A	Drops Drops	CS superior preventive effect on graft rejection CS superior therapeutic effect on graft rejection
Hagenah et al., 1990 (52)	Epithelial wound healing	EGF, aFGF	CS alone Untreated corneas	aFGF and CS alone superior to untreated EGF and CS comparable to untreated
Clinch et al., 1992 (22)	*Pseudomonas* keratitis	Tobramycin	CS + frequent drops versus frequent drops	Enhanced antimicrobial effect with CS

Reference	Condition/Model	Drug	Comparison	Findings
Silbiger et al., 1992 (24)	*Pseudomonas* keratitis	Gentamicin	CS + frequent drops versus frequent drops	CS with topical drops every 3 hours was effective, but less effective than the topical drops every half hour
Baziuk et al., 1992 (28)	Lensectomy and vitrectomy	Gentamicin	Frequent eye drops (every 30 minutes)	CS: gentamicin concentrations were lower than frequent eye drops in aqueous humor
Murray et al., 1992 (43)	Anterior chamber fibrin clot	Tissue plasminogen activator	tPA-hydrated CS versus control CS	CS + tPA significantly shortened the time to fibrin clot lysis
Assil et al., 1992 (23)	*Pseudomonas* keratitis	Tobramycin	Eye drops	No significant difference in efficacy
Pleyer et al., 1992 (41)	*Candida albicans* keratitis	Amphotericin B	Eye drops (hourly)	CS group had significantly lower fungal counts
Callegan et al., 1994 (31)	*Staphylococcus aureus* keratitis	Tobramycin	CS + frequent drops versus frequent drops	Enhanced antimicrobial effect with CS

were taken 15 and 60 minutes following the last dose. At both times, the eyes with the collagen shields had a significantly greater concentration of tobramycin than the eyes with soft contact lenses or the eyes that received topical drops only.

Chen et al. (20) compared the ocular bioavailability in rabbits of 0.3% tobramycin applied with a collagen shield with topical drop application of tobramycin. Groups of rabbits received either a collagen shield presoaked in tobramycin with a tobramycin drop before and after shield application or three drops of tobramycin. The collagen shield group had higher tobramycin levels in the cornea, aqueous humor, and conjunctiva than the second group. They concluded that the use of collagen shields together with standard ophthalmic concentrations of tobramycin is useful in achieving higher concentrations of topically delivered drugs into the anterior segment of the eye.

Hobden et al. (21), Sawusch et al. (22), and Clinch et al. (23) reported the efficacy of collagen shields rehydrated with tobramycin in the therapy of experimental *Pseudomonas* keratitis in rabbit eyes. Hobden et al. (21) demonstrated that collagen shields hydrated in 4% tobramycin were as efficacious as 4% topical drops given every 30 minutes over a 4-hour period; the number of colony-forming units in both the shield-treated and drop-treated corneas were reduced 4–5 log. Also, eyes with antibiotic-hydrated collagen shields plus one topical application of tobramycin drops over the shield halfway through the 9-hour experimental period were compared to eyes with shields in which the shield was replaced half way through the experimental period. No difference in the number of bacteria was seen. Additionally, these studies showed that the shield alone does not enhance bacterial growth; the number of bacteria was no greater in infected corneas treated with collagen shields hydrated in distilled water (or balanced saline solution) than in untreated control corneas. The overall results provided support for the efficacy and convenience of collagen shields rehydrated in a water-soluble antibiotic such as tobramycin for the treatment of *Pseudomonas* keratitis.

Assil et al. (24) compared the efficacy of a fortified (14 mg/mL) tobramycin-soaked collagen shield to the efficacy of a single loading dose (four 50 µL drops) of fortified tobramycin eyedrops in the treatment of rabbits with *Pseudomonas aeruginosa*–induced keratitis. Six hours after a single treatment, significantly fewer colony-forming units of *Pseudomonas* were present in the corneas of all three drug-treated groups as compared to the number of colonies in the corneas of balanced salt solution–treated control rabbits. However, no significant difference was found between a collagen shield presoaked in tobramycin and a single loading dose of tobramycin eyedrops in terms of the ability to reduce *Pseudomonas*.

Silbiger and Stern (25) studied the effectiveness of topical gentamicin treatment, with and without the use of corneal collagen shields, in a rabbit model of *Pseudomonas* keratitis. A 13.6 mg/mL solution of gentamicin was topically administered, and collagen shields were soaked in 13.6 mg/mL gentamicin for 5 minutes before being placed on the cornea. One hour after the end of the treatment, the corneas were obtained and cultured. The use of an antibiotic-impregnated collagen shield supplemented with topical therapy was more effective than the use of topical treatment alone. However, the collagen shield augmented with topical treatment every 3 hours was significantly less effective than the topical treatment every half hour. They concluded that the use of antibiotic-impregnated collagen shields should not replace the use of topical treatment every half hour with fortified antibiotics as a mainstay of initial drug treatment. However, Liang et al. (26) reported that shield therapy provided significantly higher gentamicin levels in the cornea and aqueous humor than the hourly drop treatment at 0.5 and 2 hours after the end of the treatment in uninfected rabbit eyes.

Callegan et al. (27) compared the efficacy of topical fortified tobramycin (1.36%) administered by collagen shields or in topical drop form to rabbit corneas infected with *Staphylococcus aureus*. Eyes were treated with shields hydrated in and supplemented with fortified tobramycin drops applied every 1, 2, 5 or 10 hours after infection. For topical treatment alone, tobramycin was applied following the identical regimen. Shields supplemented with tobramycin drops applied every 1, 2, or 5 hours and topical delivery of tobramycin ever hour sterilized all corneas. Collagen shield delivery of tobramycin with supplemental topical drops can eradicate staphylococci in rabbits with less frequent dosing intervals than required with topical therapy alone.

Dorigo et al. (28) studied collagen shield delivery of netilmicin, an aminoglycoside antibiotic, in rabbits. Collagen shields were immersed for 10 minutes in a commercially available solution of netilmicin, at the standard concentration of 3 mg/mL. The drug levels remained above the MIC for the usual pathogens for 18 hours in the cornea and for 6 hours in the aqueous humor. The study showed that a very concentrated drug solution is not required to obtain high and persistent levels of netilmicin in the cornea.

Baziuk et al. (29) investigated the intraocular drug delivery of collagen shield and fortified eye drops in rabbits that had undergone bilateral lensectomy and vitrectomy. The left eyes were fitted with collagen shields that had been soaked for 5 minutes in 2.0 mL of gentamicin solution (40 mg/mL) and compared with the right eyes treated with fortified gentamicin drops (13.6 mg/mL) every 30 minutes for 12 hours. The gentamicin concentration was higher in the aqueous humor of all eyes treated with fortified gentamicin drops.

Hobden et al. (30) reported the use of collagen shields hydrated with various fluoroquinolones for chemotherapy of aminoglycoside-resistant *Pseudomonas*. The fluoroquinolones used were norfloxacin (40 mg/mL) and ciprofloxacin (25 mg/mL), and the aminoglycoside control was tobramycin (40 mg/mL). In these experiments, *Pseudomonas* was made aminoglycoside-resistant by conjugal transfer of a plasmid. The MICs were 31.25 μg/mL for tobramycin, 0.25 μg/mL for ciprofloxacin, and 0.48 μg/mL for norfloxacin. The colony-forming units from rabbit corneas treated with ciprofloxacin were reduced by 4 log compared to corneas treated with collagen shields containing tobramycin or untreated corneas. Norfloxacin, which decreased the colony-forming units approximately 2 log, was not as effective as ciprofloxacin.

Phinney et al. (31) were the first to report the delivery of two antibiotics in combination (gentamicin and vancomycin) to uninfected rabbit eyes using the collagen shield. Tear, corneal, and aqueous humor concentrations of each of the two antibiotics were generally higher than, or at least similar to, those achieved by frequent topical application. Combinations of antibiotics have the potential to cover a broad spectrum of infectious agents, but care must be taken to test for pharmacological compatibility to avoid potential therapeutic interference and/or toxicity.

In conclusion, these results suggested that collagen shields containing an antibiotic could serve as a vehicle for drug delivery and could be used for preoperative and postoperative antibiotic prophylaxis and initial treatment of bacterial keratitis (32).

C. Anti-Inflammatory Agents

Hwang et al. (33) and Sawusch et al. (34) used collagen shields to enhance the penetration of anti-inflammatory agents. Hwang et al. (33) compared the deliver of dexamethasone to the cornea and aqueous humor in normal rabbit eyes by four methods: single 0.1% dexamethasone drop, hourly drops, collagen shields hydrated in 0.1% dexamethasone, and collagen shields hydrated in 0.1% dexamethasone followed by hourly topical 0.1% drops. Treatment with the drug-hydrated collagen shields plus hourly drops resulted in both peak and cumulative drug concentrations in the cornea and aqueous humor that were two- to fourfold greater than the concentration achieved by hourly drops alone. Collagen shields without accompanying drops yielded drug concentrations either equal to or greater than the peak and cumulative drug concentrations produced by hourly drops. The authors concluded that collagen shields significantly enhance dexamethasone penetration and would be useful for maximizing the delivery of this anti-inflammatory agent. They also suggested that the use of collagen shields would decrease the requirement for frequent topical drops.

Sawusch et al. (34) compared (a) collagen shields hydrated in 1% prednisolone, (b) collagen shields receiving topical drops in situ, and (c) topical application of 1% prednisolone drops alone. Cornea and aqueous humor were assessed for prednisolone acetate at 30 and 120 minutes after drug application. Both collagen shield delivery systems produced significantly greater drug levels than topical drops alone at both times. Thus, both these reports support the potential for collagen shield delivery of corticosteroid anti-inflammatory agents (33,34).

D. Combination Therapy

In clinical cases, combinations of drugs are often used. Milani et al. (35) investigated the ability of collagen shields impregnated with gentamicin sulfate and dexamethasone to deliver medication to rabbit eyes. They compared collagen shields with subconjunctival injection therapy. The collagen shields produced aqueous humor levels of gentamicin and dexamethasone that were lower than those produced by subconjunctival injection therapy at 30 and 60 minutes, respectively, but that were comparable to subconjunctival injection at 3, 6, and 10 hours. They concluded that collagen shield deliver of gentamicin-dexamethasone might be comparable to subconjunctival injections and provide an alternative therapy after intraocular surgery. Renard et al. (36) used collagen shields soaked in gentamicin and dexamethasone for patients after cataract surgery. No adverse effect was reported.

Mahlberg et al. (37) studied the aggregate formation of tobramycin sulfate in combination with methylprednisolone acetate or dexamethasone sodium phosphate on collagen shields. Aggregates were formed on the surface of the shields when they were immersed in methylprednisolone acetate and tobramycin. Dexamethasone sodium phosphate and tobramycin resulted in a completely transparent shield. To avoid undesired side effects, such as epithelial sloughing and corneal edema after collagen shield application, antibiotics and steroids must be carefully selected. Combinations of gentamicin and methylprednisolone sodium succinate or gentamicin and cefazolin on collagen shield also result in precipitates (38). Additionally, care must be taken when mixing drugs to prevent adverse reactions. An aminoglycoside such as gentamicin and a penicillin such as mezlocillin should not be combined because of inactivation of the aminoglycoside by the penicillin (39).

E. Antifungal Agents

Schwartz et al. (40) compared the delivery of amphotericin B in collagen shields hydrated in a 0.5% drug solution with frequent topical drops (0.15%) in uninfected rabbit eyes. Drops were applied every 5 minutes for the first half hour and at hourly intervals thereafter. The corneas and aqeous humor were assessed at 1, 2, 3, and 6 hours following the initiation of drug delivery. Drug levels in the shield-treated corneas were significantly higher than levels in the drop-treated corneas at 1 and 2 hours after therapy began. At 3 hours, the concentrations of the antifungal drug in the corneal tissues were similar for both delivery methods. At 6 hours, both groups had significant concentrations of the antifungal agent, but the amount of the drug was greater in the drop-treated corneas than in the shield-treated corneas. Drug levels in the aqueous humor did not differ between the two groups at any time. The results suggest that amphotericin B can be delivered to the cornea via collagen shields at a rate that is comparable with frequent drop deliver.

Pleyer et al. (41) evaluated the effect of collagen shields presoaked with amphotericin B on the treatment of experimental *Candida albicans*–induced keratitis. Treatment results were compared to those of amphotericin B eyedrops instilled hourly in rabbits. Treatment groups were (a) hourly instillation of 0.15% amphotericin B drops, (b) application of a collagen shield presoaked in 0.5% amphotericin B for one hour, and (c) hourly instillation of saline drops. Rabbit eyes treated with amphotericin B–soaked collagen shields had significantly lower fungal counts compared with eyes receiving hourly amphotericin B drops at days 1 and 3 after the beginning of treatment. They concluded that collagen shields soaked in amphotericin B could be a useful and convenient treatment device in keratomycosis such as that caused by *Candida albicans*.

F. Anticoagulant Therapy

Heparin, a large molecule with a molecular weight between 6000 and 20,000 daltons, has been studied experimentally as a possible agent for the reduction of postoperative fibrin formation after vitrectomy. The intravenous route of administration, however, can be associated with increased postoperative hemorrhage. In an attempt to discover a vehicle that would permit more localized drug delivery, Murray et al. (42) examined the pharmacokinetics and anticoagulation efficacy of heparin delivered by collagen shields. Collagen shields hydrated with radiolabeled heparin were applied to rabbit eyes, and the amount of heparin in aqueous humor, cornea, and iris was measured at intervals from 15 minutes to 6 hours. The peak of radioactivity was detected in the cornea and aqueous humor 1 hour after application. Also in this study, 12-hour collagen shields hydrated with heparin were compared to subconjunctival heparin injection. The highest biological activity was seen 30 minutes after application of the collagen shield, and there was a significant amount of anticoagulant activity in the aqueous humor 6 hours after application. At no time was any anticoagulant activity seen in the aqueous humor following subconjunctival injection. The results of this study demonstrate that a high molecular weight compound such as heparin can be delivered by 12- or 24-hour collagen shields, producing significant levels in the aqueous humor. This suggests that collagen shields hydrated with heparin might be effective in the prevention of treatment of fibrin formation in the aqueous humor.

Murray et al. (43) also studied collagen shield delivery of tissue plasminogen activator (tPA) to the anterior segment and vitreous of rabbit eyes. Time to complete lysis of anterior chamber fibrin clots in the eyes treated with balanced salt solution-hydrated collagen shields was 149 ± 18 hours. Treatment with tPA-hydrated collagen shields shortened the mean time to clot clearance by approximately 50% (clearance time $= 49 \pm 23$ hours). Elevated aqueous tPA levels were first measured 18 hours after application of tPA-hydrated collagen shields. Aqueous tPA levels peaked at 36 hours and remained elevated throughout the 48-hour study period. Vitreous tPA levels were elevated by 2 hours, peaked at 24 hours, and also remained elevated throughout the study period. These results document the efficacy and safety of tPA delivery to the aqueous and vitreous humor via a hydrated collagen shield in the rabbit.

G. Immunosuppressive Agents

Cyclosporine has been used successfully to prevent graft rejection in many types of transplantation. The side effects of systemic administration, however, are considerable, and the systemic dose needed to provide sufficient drug in the cornea makes this route less than useful to prevent rejection of corneal transplants. Also, the drug penetrates the cornea poorly, frustrating the efforts at topical administration. Reidy et al. (44) demonstrated that collagen shields with 4 mg of cyclosporin A incorporated during manufacture delivered significantly higher concentrations of drug to the cornea and aqueous humor than an equivalent amount of cyclosporin A prepared in olive oil and given as drops at 15-minute intervals. Four hours after application of the collagen shield, the corneas contained almost 2500 ng of the drug and the aqueous humor contained about 250 ng. At all times, the concentration of the drug in the aqueous humor was higher in rabbits receiving cyclosporin A via collagen shields compared to drops.

Kanpolat et al. (45) also investigated the penetration of cyclosporin A into the rabbit cornea and aqueous humor after topical drop and collagen shield administration. The rabbits were divided into three groups. The first group received 6 mg of cyclosporin A in castor oil and the second group received 6 mg of cyclosporin A in olive oil applied as topical drops to rabbit eyes within 12 hours. In the third group 12-hour collagen shields soaked in 6 mg of cyclosporin A in olive oil were applied. The cyclosporin A of castor oil drops were higher than those obtained with olive oil drops. In eyes with collagen shields, cyclosporin A levels were higher than olive oil drops but nearly equal to the castor oil drops. In an extension of the studies, Chen et al. (46) showed that cyclosporin A–containing collagen shields suppress corneal allograft rejection. Rabbit eyes with penetrating keratoplasty grafts were placed in vascularized beds to enhance the possibility of graft rejection. The grafts were treated with equivalent amounts of cyclosporin A in the collagen shields or in olive oil drops. The mean survival time of shield-treated grafts was significantly longer than that of drop-treated grafts. Grafts showing early signs of graft reaction treated with cyclosporin–containing shields showed reversal of the rejection process. The results of these two studies indicate that the collagen shield is an effective delivery system for cyclosporin A and that the drug delivered in this manner can both suppress the initiation of graft rejection and reverse a graft reaction in progress.

H. Antiviral Agent

Gussler et al. (47) investigated the delivery of trifluorothymidine (TFT) in collagen shields and topical drops in normal rabbit corneas and corneas with experimental epithelial defects. Collagen shields hydrated in 1% TFT and 1% topical drops were used. The eyes were treated with either collagen shields hydrated with TFT, TFT drops, or a combination of collagen shields and drops. Rabbits with normal corneas showed no difference among the treatment groups in terms of TFT levels in the cornea or aqueous humor 30 minutes and 2, 4, and 8 hours after application of the antiviral. Among the rabbits with experimental epithelial defects, the highest drug concentrations were found in the eyes treated with the combination of shields and drops, and the second highest tissue concentrations were seen in the eyes treated with collagen shields hydrated in TFT. Treatment with drops alone produced lower concentrations of TFT than either treatment involving the collagen shields. The authors suggested that this method of drug delivery may be useful to enhance the eradication of herpes simplex virus in eyes with epithelial defects. The authors noted, however, the need for studies of corneal toxicity and efficacy in herpes-infected eyes before a definitive therapeutic regimen can be established.

I. Wound Healing

After Fyodorov et al. (5) first described the clinical use of collagen shields for the protection and enhancement of epithelial healing, a number of experimental studies were published confirming their findings. Frantz et al. (48) showed that rabbit eyes with 6 mm superficial keratectomies treated with collagen shields healed significantly faster than untreated eyes. Simsek et al. (49) studied the effects of collagen shields and therapeutic contact lenses on corneal wound healing in rabbits. A corneal wound was created by mechanical removal of the central 6 mm zone of the corneal epithelium and basement membrane. The healing rate was found to be 0.52 ± 0.08 mm^2/hour with the collagen shield, 0.54 ± 0.05 mm^2/hour with the therapeutic lens, and 0.43 ± 0.06 mm^2/hour in the control group. Comparison of the study groups revealed no statistically significant difference between the collagen shield and the therapeutic lens group at any time, whereas a significantly larger wound size was observed in the control group compared with the treatment groups. In conclusion, these results indicated that both collagen shields and therapeutic lenses enhance wound healing in rabbit eyes.

On the other hand, the results of some studies suggested that more evidence would be needed to establish effectiveness of collagen shields in promoting wound healing (50,51). Shaker et al. (50) reported that cat eyes treated with non–cross-linked porcine collagen shields had a significantly greater healing response than untreated eyes. However, there was no difference in the slope of the healing curve, suggesting that the shield did not increase the speed of epithelial cell migration. Callizo et al. (51) suggested that collagen shields might be ineffective or have adverse effects in deeply injured rabbit corneas. They performed bilateral keratectomies, then treated only the left eye with a collagen shield. No differences were seen in the time course of the healing process between control (untreated) and treated eyes. More polymorphonuclear infiltration, mainly composed of eosinophils, was shown in treated eyes. They concluded that the usefulness of collagen shields should be reappraised, especially in injured corneas.

Additional studies combined the healing properties of collagen shields with delivery of growth factors to influence the rate of reepithelialization. Hagenah et al. (52) used rabbit eyes with superficial keratectomies to examine the effect of collagen shields alone or in combination with epidermal growth factor (EGF) or acidic fibroblastic growth factor on epithelial wound healing. Eyes treated with collagen shields alone or collagen shields hydrated with a fibroblastic growth factor healed significantly faster than untreated controls. Shields containing EGF had no enhanced effect. Although it is apparent from this and other studies that the shields alone promote healing, the utility of growth factors in and of themselves, including optimal dosage, timing, and duration of application, is still uncertain. Therefore, even if the shields enhance the delivery of growth factors, it is not clear at this time how such enhanced delivery can be used to improve epithelial healing.

J. Other Uses

Wentworth et al. (53) determined the impact of collagen shields on ulceration of rabbit corneas after alkali burn. After a 60-second sodium hydroxide burn to rabbit corneas, 24-hour collagen shields were replaced once daily for 21 days. They showed daily use of 24-hour collagen shields after a severe alkali burn to the rabbit cornea exacerbates the progression of corneal ulceration and perforation. They thought that the harmful effects of collagen shields might have resulted from the repeated removal and insertion of the shields. The trapping of activated polymorphonuclear leukocytes in the collagen shields that were in contact with the corneal surface caused a locally high concentration of metalloproteinases.

IV. CLINICAL STUDIES

The effect of collagen shields on healing and antibacterial or other chemotherapeutic effects in human eyes has been reported.

A. Therapy to Assist Wound Healing

Aquavella et al. (54) reported the use of porcine collagen shields hydrated with ophthalmic drugs to treat patients following penetrating keratoplasty and cataract extraction. The drugs included tobramycin, gentamicin, pilocarpine, dexamethasone, and flurbiprofen. No adverse effects were noted. In another study by this group (55), collagen shields used as bandage lenses appeared to accelerate corneal reepithelialization after keratoplasty or other types of anterior segment surgery.

Poland and Kaufman (56) reported the use of collagen shields hydrated with tobramycin in patients who had cataract extraction, penetrating keratoplasty, epikeratophakia, or nonsurgical epithelial healing problems. All surgical patients showed more rapid healing of epithelial defects. Acute nonsurgical epithelial problems with impaired healing also benefited from the use of collagen shields. In contrast, chronic epithelial defects responded poorly. No infections occurred in any of the patients.

Similarly, Groden and White (57) found that 24-hour porcine collagen shields did not contribute to healing of persistent (chronic) epithelial defects following penetrating keratoplasty. They defined a persistent defect as an epithelial erosion (noninfectious) that did not heal in 2 weeks with patching, frequent lubrication, and/or temporary tape tarsorrhaphy. Patients with such defects were assigned to either collagen shield treatment or treatment with a hydrophilic bandage soft contact lens. When none of the collagen shield–treated defects healed, this approach was abandoned and bandage contact lens treatment instituted for all patients. The authors suggested that a longer-lasting corneal shield (72 hours dissolution time) might be more effective.

Marmer (58) described postsurgical healing in human eyes with porcine collagen shields after radial keratotomy. The patients who were treated with the collagen shields reported less glare and discomfort than patients who did not receive shields. Also, the eyes with shields showed less inflammatory reaction and edema.

Palmer and McDonald (59) used a disposable soft contact lens piggybacked onto a medicated, 12-hour corneal collagen shield after corneal surgery in three patients known to have poor corneal epithelial wound healing characteristics. This piggyback lens/shield system delivered sustained high levels of medication and promoted epithelial healing in the acute postoperative period without unnecessary postoperative orbital manipulation.

In a different kind of healing study, Fourman and Wiley (60) reported the results of treating a glaucoma filter bleb with a 24-hour collagen shield hydrated in 4 mg/mL of gentamicin. The shield was placed over the leaking site; the bleb leak was sealed within 2 days and remained sealed 2 months later. The collagen shield was helpful in the management of filter bleb leak.

B.　Antibacterial or Antiviral Efficacy

Lois and Molino (61) treated a case of *Mycobacterium chelonae* keratitis with topical fortified amikacin, with no response. They then debrided the epithelial and stromal lesions, and applied an amikacin-soaked corneal collagen shield, supplemented every 4 hours with topical fortified amikacin drops. After this treatment, clinical and laboratory examinations showed that no infectious organisms could be detected.

Kuster et al. (62) investigated the ability of collagen shields to deliver TFT to human cornea and aqueous humor. Collagen shields were soaked in commercially prepared TFT. Patients undergoing penetrating kerato-plasty wore a presoaked collagen shield for at least 30 minutes preopera-tively. Control patients received drops of TFT only. Cornea and aqueous samples were obtained during surgery. Collagen shields did not enhance delivery of TFT to the cornea with an intact epithelium. In corneas with poor epithelium, drug penetration was higher but variable. They concluded that the role of collagen shields as a drug delivery system for the treatment of herpes simplex keratitis remains to be determined.

C. Postoperative Application

Renard et al. (36) compared the effectiveness of subconjunctival injections and collagen shields in delivering anti-inflammatory agents and antibiotics after cataract surgery. The occurrence of folds in Descemet's membrane was less frequent and aqueous flare less severe in the collagen shield–treated group than in those treated with subconjunctival injections.

Haaskjold et al. (63) compared the efficacy of collagen shields with that of peribulbar/retrobulbar injection after cataract surgery. Collagen shields were saturated with an antibiotic and a steroid and placed over the cornea postoperatively. The second group received the same drugs through a peribulbar/retrobulbar injection. One day after surgery, the shield group had significantly less corneal edema, conjunctival hemor-rhage, postoperative pain, and fewer corneal opacities. They suggested that using collagen shields for drug delivery after cataract surgery decreases tissue damage and increases patient comfort without adverse side effects.

Taravella et al. (64) investigated whether collagen shields are more effective than topical eye drops for infection prophylaxis after cataract surgery. In their studies, the patients were divided into two groups: the first received three postoperative drops of commercially available topical ofloxacin (0.3%) given 10 minutes apart; the second had a collagen shield soaked in the same medication applied to the eye before surgery. Aqueous humor was extracted immediately before surgery for analysis. Aqueous concentration of ofloxacin in the shield group was significantly higher than that in the drop group. The MICs of ofloxacin for many common ocular pathogens were reached or exceeded in the shield group. However, in a similar study using tobramycin, the ocular penetration of the anti-biotic into the anterior chamber of the human eye in the shield group was not different from that in the drop group (65). The aqueous concentration did not approach the MIC of tobramycin for many common ocular patho-gens.

D. Dry Eye

Though collagen shields have a lubricating effect, they are not useful as a treatment for keratoconjunctivitis sicca because they must be applied in the physician's office and they are not transparent. Kaufman et al. (66) tested a similar system, with the addition of therapeutic agents during manufacturing (Collasomes), for drug delivery to the ocular surface. The size of Collasomes was 1 mm × 0.1 mm × 2 mm. Ease of application and minimal interference with vision were the advantages of this system.

E. Clinical Uses for Corneal Collagen Shields

At the LSU Eye Center, our ocular ophthalmologists performing cataract surgeries, corneal transplants, and other invasive corneal procedures use the corneal collagen shields as a bandage. Most often they will use antibiotics and anti-inflammatories and hydrate the shields in the solution for 3 minutes. This is the most common use of the corneal collagen shields following many surgical procedures. Since the eye is bandaged, there is no problem involving visual acuity and often only one shield is used until the bandage is removed (24–48 hours) and the patient's eye is evaluated.

Another use for the collagen shield is when an ophthalmologist has decided to hospitalize a patient with suspected ocular infection and there is concern about compliance for administering antibiotic drops. In the office, the ophthalmologist can hydrate the shield in a solution of fortified tobramycin or commercially available fluoroquinolone and then apply the corneal collagen shield. Patients are instructed to apply drops every 5 or 10 minutes until they are admitted and are being administered antibiotics as a single entity or in combinations in a hospital setting. The placing of the collagen shield hydrated with fortified antibiotics assures that a reliable amount of antibiotic will be in contact with the corneal surface over the next 2–4 hours. The shield should be removed after 3–5 hours if antibiotics are not administered. It is important not to have any oxygen deprivation of a cornea suspected to have an infection.

V. CONCLUSIONS

Collagen is a protein that can be safely applied to the body for a variety of medical and cosmetic purposes. The creation of the corneal collagen shield has provided a means to promote wound healing and, perhaps more importantly, to deliver a variety of medications to the cornea and other ocular tissues. There are many indications that the shields deliver drugs as well as, if not better than, topical drops. The simplicity of use and convenience afforded by shields make them an attractive delivery device. Although collagen shields produce some discomfort and interfere with vision, corneal collagen shields could become a commonly employed technological improvement in ophthalmic drug delivery.

ACKNOWLEDGMENTS

The authors wish to acknowledge the editorial assistance and research collaboration of A. K. Mitra, Ph.D. Specific research from the laboratory of Dr. Hill was supported in part by U.S. Public Health Service grant EY06311 and EY08871 (JMH); EY02377 (Eye Center Core Grant); an unrestricted grant from Research to Prevent Blindness (RPB); Dr. Hill is an RPB Scientific Investigator Award recipient. The authors wish to acknowledge the secretarial assistance of Mrs. Carole Hoth. The authors also wish to acknowledge special thanks to Ms. Kristina Braud and Ms. Kathy Vu. None of the authors have any financial or proprietary interest in any agents or devices mentioned in this review.

REFERENCES

1. Kaufman, H. E. (1988). Guest editorial: Collagen shield symposium, *J. Cataract Refract. Surg.*, *14*:487–488.
2. Busin, M., and Spitznas, M. (1988). Sustained gentamicin release by presoaked medicated bandage contact lense, *Ophthalmology*, *95*:796–798.
3. Matoba, A. Y., and McCulley, J. P. (1985). The effect of therapeutic soft contact lenses on antibiotic delivery to the cornea, *Ophthalmology*, *92*:97–99.
4. Bloomfield, S. E., Miyata, T., Dunn, M. W., Bueser, N., Stenzel, K. H., and Rubin, A. L. (1978). Soluble gentacin ophthalmic inserts as a drug delivery system, *Arch. Ophthalmol.*, *96*:885–887.
5. Fyodorov, S. N., Moroz, Z. I., Kramskaya, Z. I., Bagrov, S. N., Amstislavskaya, T. S., and Zolotarevsky, A. V. (1985). Comprehensive conservative treatment of dystrophia endothelialis et epithelialis cornea, using a therapeutic collagen coating, *Vestn. Oftalmol.*, *101*:33–36.
6. Ivashina, A. I. (1987). Radial keratotomy as a method of surgical correction of myopia. In: *Microsurgery of the Eye: Main Aspects* (S. N. Fyodorov, ed.), Mir Publishers, Moscow, p. 45.
7. Chvapil, M., Kronenthal, R. L., and van Winkle, Jr., W. (1973). Medical and surgical applications of collagen, *Int. Rev. connect. Tissue Res.*, *6*:1.

8. Kuwano, M., Horibe, Y., and Kawashima, Y. (1997). Effect of collagen cross-linking in collagen corneal shields on ocular drug delivery, *J. Ocul. Pharmacol. Ther.*, *13*:31–40.

9. Weissman, B. A., and Lee, D. A. (1988). Oxygen transmissibility, thickness, and water content of three types of collagen shields, *Arch. Ophthalmol.*, *106*:1706–1708.

10. Weissman, B. A., Brennan, N. A., Lee, D. A., and Fatt, I. (1990). Oxygen permeability of collagen shields, *Invest. Ophthalmol. Vis. Sci.*, *31*:334–338.

11. Hill, J. M., O'Callaghan, R. J., Hobden, J. A., Kaufman, H. E. (1993). Corneal collagen shields for ocular deliver. In: *Ophthalmic Drug Delivery Systems* (A. K. Mitra, ed.), Marcel Dekker, Inc., New York, pp. 261–273.

12. Artandi, C. (1964). Production experiences with radiation sterilization, *Bull. Parenteral Drug Assoc.*, *18*:2.

13. Hill, J. M., O'Callaghan, R. J., and Hobden, J. A. (1993). Ocular iontophoresis. In: *Ophthalmic Drug Delivery Systems* (A. K. Mitra, ed.), Marcel Dekker, Inc., New York, pp. 331–354.

14. Friedberg, M. L., Pleyer, U., and Mondiono, B. J. (1991). Device drug delivery to the eye. Collagen shields, iontophoresis, and pumps, *Ophthalmology*, *98*:725–732.

15. Reidy, J. J., Limberg, M., and Kaufman, H. E. (1990). Delivery of fluorescein to the anterior chamber using the corneal collagen shield, *Ophthalmology*, *97*:1201–1203.

16. Myles, M. M., Loutsch, J. M., Higaki, S., and Hill, J. M. Ocular iontophoresis. In: *Ophthalmic Drug Delivery Systems.* (A. K. Mitra, ed.), Marcel Dekker, Inc., New York, Chapter 12.

17. Zheng, X., Marquart, M. E., Mitra, A. K., and Hill, J. M. (2002). Unique ocular drug delivery systems. In: *Textbook of Ophthalmology* (S. Agarwal, et al., eds.), Vaybee Brothers Medical Publishers, Ltd., New Delhi, India, pp. 2076–2086.

18. Unterman, S. R., Rootman, D. S., Hill, J. M., Parelman, J. J., Thompson, H. W., and Kaufman, H. E. (1988). Collagen shield drug delivery: Therapeutic concentrations of tobramycin in the rabbit cornea and aqueous humor, *J. Cataract Refract. Surg.*, *14*:500–504.

19. O'Brien, T. P., Sawusch, M. R., Dick, J. D., Hamburg, T. R., and Gottsch, J. D. (1988). Use of collagen corneal shields versus soft contact lenses to enhance penetration of topical tobramycin, *J. Cataract Refract. Surg.*, *14*:505–507.

20. Chen, C. C., Taarui, H., and Duzman, E. (1993). Enhancement of the ocular bipability of topical tobramycin with use of a collagen shield, *J. Cataract Refract. Surg.*, 19:242–245.

21. Hobden, J. A. Reidy, J. J., O'Callaghan, R. J., Hill, J. M., Insler, M. S., and Rootman, D. S. (1988). Treatment of experimental *Pseudomonas* keratitis using collagen shields containing tobramycin, *Arch. Ophthalmol.*, *106*:1605–1607.

22. Sawusch, M. R., O'Brien, T. P., Dick, J. D., and Gottsch, J. D. (1988). Quinolones in collagen shields to treat aminoglycoside-resistant *Pseudomonas* keratitis, *Invest. Ophthalmol. Vis. Sci.*, *31*:2241.

23. Clinch, T. E., Hobden, J. A., Hill, J. M., O'Callaghan, R. J., Engel, L. S., and Kaufmann H. E. (1992). Collagen shields containing tobramycin for sustained therapy (24 hours) of experimental *Pseudomonas* keratitis, *CLAO J.*, *18*:245–247.

24. Assil, K. K., Zarnegar, S. R., Fouraker, B. D., and Schanzlin, D. J. (1992). Efficacy of tobramycin-soaked collagen shields vs tobramycin eyedrop loading dose for sustained treatment of experimental *Pseudomonas aeruginosa*-induced keratitis in rabbits, *Am. J. Ophthalmol.*, *113*:418–423.

25. Silbiger, J., and Stern, G. A. (1992). Evaluation of corneal collagen shields as a drug delivery device for the treatment of experimental *pseudomonas* keratitis, *Ophthalmology*, *99*:889–892.

26. Liang, F. Q., Viola, R. S., del Cerro, M., and Aquavella, J. V. (1992). Noncross-linked collagen discs and cross-linked collagen shields in the delivery of gentamicin to rabbits eyes, *Invest. Ophthalmol. Vis. Sci.*, *33*:2194–2198.

27. Callegan, M. C., Engel, L. S., Clinch, T. E., Hill, J. M., Kaufman, H. E., and O'Callaghan, R. J. (1994). Efficacy of tobramycin drops applied to collagen shields for experimental staphylococcal keratitis, *Curr. Eye Res.*, *13*:875–878.

28. Dorigo, M. T., De Natale, R., and Miglioli, P. A. (1995). Collagen shields delivery of netilmicin: a study of ocular pharmacokinetics, *Chemotherapy*, *41*:1.

29. Baziuk, N., Gremillion, C. M., Peyman, G. A., and Cho, H. K. (1992). Collagen shields and intraocular drug delivery: concentration of gentamicin in the aqueous and vitreous of a rabbit eye after lensectomy and vitrectomy, *Int. Ophthalmol.*, *16*:101–107.

30. Hobden, J. A., Reidy, J. J., O'Callaghan, R. J., Insler, M. S., and Hill, J. M. (1990). Quinolones in collagen shields to treat aminoglycoside-resistant pseudomonal keratitis, *Invest. Ophthalmol. Vis. Sci.*, *31*:2241–2243.

31. Phinney, R. B., Schwartz, S. D., Lee, D. A., and Mondino, B. J. (1988). Collagen-shield delivery of gentamicin and vancomycin, *Arch. Ophthalmol.*, *106*:1559–1604.

32. Callegan, M. C., O'Callaghan, R. J., and Hill, J. M. (1994). Pharmacokinetic considerations in the treatment of bacterial keratitis, *Clin. Pharmacokin.*, *27*:129.

33. Hwang, D. G., Stern, W. H., Hwang, P. H., and MacGowan-smith, L. A. (1989). Collagen shield enhancement of topical dexamethasone penetration, *Arch. Ophthalmol.*, *107*:1375–1380.

34. Sawusch, M. R., O'Brien, T. P., and Updegraff, S. A. (1989). Collagen corneal shields enhance penetration of topical prednisolone acetate, *J. Cataract Refract. Surg.*, *15*:625–628.

35. Milani, J. K., Verbukh, I., Pleyer, U., Sumner, H., Adamu, S. A., Halabi, H. P., Chou, H. J., Lee, D. A., and Mondino, B. J. (1993). Collagen shields impregnated with gentamicin-dexamethasone as a potential drug delivery device, *Am. J. Ophthalmol.*, *116*:622–627.

36. Renard, G., Bennani, N., Lutaj, P., Richard, C., and Trinquand, C. (1993). Comparative study of a collagen corneal shield and a subconjunctival injection at the end of cataract surgery, *J. Cataract Refract. Surg.*, *19*:48–51.

37. Mahlberg, K., Krootila, K., and Uusitalo, R. (1997). Compatibility of corticosteroids and antibiotics in combination, *J. Cataract Refract. Surg.*, *23*:878–882.

38. Phinney, R. B., Schwartz, S. D., Lee, D. A., and Mondino, B. J. (1988). Collagen-shield delivery of gentamicin and vancomycin, *Arch. Ophthalmol.*, *106*:1599–1604.

39. Mondino, B. J. (1991). Collagen shields, *Am. J. Ophthalmol.*, *112*:587–590.

40. Schwartz, S. D., Harrison, S. A., Engstrom, R. E., Bawdon, R. E., Lee, D. A., and Mondino, B. J. (1990). Collagen shield delivery of amphotericin B, *Am. J. Ophthalmol.*, *109*:701–704.

41. Pleyer, U., Legmann, A., Mondino, B. J., and Lee, D. A. (1992). Use of collagen shields containing amphotericin B in the treatment of experimental *Candida albicans*-induced keratomycosis in rabbits, *Am. J. Ophthalmol.*, *113*:303–307.

42. Murray, T. G., Stern, W. H., Chin, D. H., and MacGowan-Smith, E. A. (1990). Collagen shield heparin delivery for prevention of postoperative fibrin, *Arch. Ophthalmol.*, *108:104–106*.

43. Murray, T. G., Jaffe, G. J., McKay, B. S., Han, D. P., Burke, J. M., and Abrams, G. W. (1992). Collagen shield delivery of tissue plasminogen activator: functional and pharmacokinetic studies of anterior segment delivery, *Refract. Corneal Surg.*, *8*:44–48.

44. Reidy, J. J., Gebhardt, B. M., and Kaufman, H. E. (1990). The collagen shield: A new vehicle for delivery of cyclosporin A to the eye, *Cornea*, *9*:196–199.

45. Kanpolat, A., Batioglu, F., Yilmaz, M., and Akbas, F. (1994). Penetration of cyclosporin A into the rabbit cornea and aqueous humor after topical drop and collagen shield administration, *CLAO J.*, *20*:119–122.

46. Chen, Y. F., Gebhardt, B. M., Reidy, J. J., and Kaufman, H. E. (1990) > Cyclosporin-containing collagen shields suppress corneal allograft rejection, *Am. J. Ophthalmol.*, *109*:132–137.

47. Gussler, J. R., Ashton, P., VanMeter, W. S., and Smith, T. J. (1990). Collagen shield delivery of trifluorothymidine, *J. Cataract Refract. Surg.*, *16*:719–722.

48. Frantz, J. M., Dupuy, B. M., Kaufman, H. E., and Beuerman, R. W. (1989). The effect of collagen shields on epithelial wound healing in rabbits, *Am. J. Ophthalmol.*, *108*:524–528.

49. Simsek, N. A., Ay, G. M., Tugal-Tutkun, I., Basar, D., and Bilgin, L. K. (1996). An experimental study on the effect of collagen shields and therapeutic contact lenses on corneal wound healing, *Cornea*, *15*:612–616.

50. Shaker, G. J., Ueda, S., LoCascio, J., and Aquavella, J. V. (1989). Effect of a collagen shield on cat corneal epithelial wound healing, *Invest. Ophthalmol. Vis. Sci.*, *30*:1565–1568.

51. Callizo, J., Cervello, I., Mayano, E., and Mallol, J. (1996). Inefficacy of collagen shields in the rabbit corneal wound-healing process, *Cornea*, *15*:258–262.

52. Hagenah, M., Lopez, J. G., and Insler, M. S. (1990). Effect of EGF, FGF, and collagen shields on corneal epithelial wound healing following lamellar keratectomy, *Invest. Ophthalmol. Vis. Sci. Suppl.*, *31*:225.

53. Wentworth, J. S., Paterson, C. A., Wells, J. T., Tilki, N., Gray, R. S., and McCartney, M. D. (1993) Collagen shields exacerbate ulceration of alkali-burned rabbit corneas, *Arch. Ophthalmol.*, *111*:389–392.

54. Aquavella, J. V., Ruffini, J. J., and LoCascio, J. A. (1988). Use of collagen shields as a surgical adjunct, *J. Cataract Refract. Surg.*, *14*:492–495.

55. Aquavella, J. V., Musco, P. S., Ueda, S., and LoCascio, J. A. (1988). Therapeutic applications of collagen bandage lens: A preliminary report, *CLAO J.*, *14*:47–50.

56. Poland, D. E., and Kaufman, H. E. (1990). Clinical uses of collagen shields, *J. Cataract Refract. Surg.*, *14*:489–491.

57. Groden, L. R., and White, W. (1990). Porcine collagen corneal shield treatment of persistent epithelial defects following penetrating keratoplasty, *CLAO J.*, *16*:95–97.

58. Marmer, R. H. (1988). Therapeutic and protective properties of the corneal collagen shield, *J. Cataract Refract. Surg.*, *14*:496–499.

59. Palmer, R. M., and McDonald, M. B. (1995). A corneal lens/shield system to promote postoperative corneal epithelial healing, *J. Cataracat Refract. Surg.*, *21*:125.

60. Fourman, S., and Wiley, L. (1989). Use of a collagen shield to treat a glaucoma filter bleb leak, *Am. J. Ophthalmol.*, *107*:673–674.

61. Lois, N., and Molino, M. L. P. (1994). *Mycobacterium chelonae* keratitis: resolution after debridement and presoaked collagen shields, *Cornea*, *14*:536–539.

62. Kuster, P., Taravella, M., Gelinas, M., and Stepp, P. (1998). Delivery of trifluridine to human cornea and aqueous using collagen shields, *CLAO J.*, *24*:122–124.

63. Haaskjold, E., Ohrstrom, A., Uusitalo, R. J., Krootila, K., Sandvig, K. U., Sonne, H., and Mahlberg, K. (1994). Use of collagen shields in cataract surgery, *J. Cataract Refract. Surg.*, *20*:150–153.

64. Taravella, M. J., Balentine, J., Young, D. A., and Stepp, P. (1999). Collagen shield delivery of ofloxacin to the human eye, *J. Cataract Refract. Surg.*, *25*:562–565.

65. Taravella, M. J., Stepp, P., and Young, D. A. (1998). Collagen shield delivery of tobramycin to the human eye, *CLAO J.*, *24*:166–168.

66. Kaufman, H. E., Steinemann, T. L., Lehman, E., Thompson, H. W., Varnell, E. D., Jacob-Labarre J. T., and Gebhardt, B. M. (1994). Collagen-based drug delivery and artificial tears, *J. Ocul. Pharmacol.*, *10*:17–27.

11

The Noncorneal Route in Ocular Drug Delivery

Imran Ahmed
Pfizer Global R&D—Groton Laboratories, Groton, Connecticut, U.S.A.

I. INTRODUCTION

It is now generally accepted that topically applied drugs can enter the eye by both a corneal and a noncorneal pathway. Although the corneal pathway is the primary route of intraocular entry for most drugs, penetration through the conjunctiva and sclera can also be important (1–3) and, under some circumstances, could be more important than the corneal route (4–22). Ahmed and Patton (5,6), using blocking techniques, showed that the noncorneal pathway was the dominant route for intraocular entry of inulin, a molecule that is poorly absorbed across the cornea. This group was also the first to suggest that it might be possible to exploit the conjunctival/scleral absorption route to promote site-specific delivery of drugs to intraocular tissues in the back of the eye (23). The increasing interest in intraocular delivery of peptide and protein drugs, drug therapy targeting posterior segment eye disease, and the advent of new chemical entities and novel ophthalmic drug delivery systems necessitates a thorough understanding of the noncorneal pathway and approaches of exploiting this route in ocular therapy.

Recently there has been considerable progress in efforts to characterize the permeability properties and permselectivity of the conjunctiva and the sclera. A greater mechanistic understanding of drug transport in the ocular epithelia has further enhanced this research. It has been established that compared with the cornea, the conjunctiva is generally more permeable to drugs (24). This is primarily due to a leakier epithelium in the conjunctiva

(25–32). Furthermore, the conjunctiva plays an active role in drug transport facilitated by the existence of a variety of drug transporters and ion transport processes (33–37). There has been extensive work on elucidating the diffusional barrier properties of the sclera (38–47) and conjunctiva (48–54). Systemic loss of drug via absorption into the ocular blood vessels is believed to significantly diminish the contribution of the scleral/conjunctival route in ocular drug delivery. Factors affecting the systemic absorption of ocularly applied drugs (55–65) have been studied, as well as approaches to minimize non-productive loss (66–74) and the possibility of using the eye as a portal for systemic drug delivery (75–85). Several excellent reviews discussing the pharmacokinetic and pharmacodynamic considerations in ocular drug delivery have been published over the years (86–94).

This chapter reviews the recent progress in the understanding of the noncorneal penetration route towards creating a framework for rational design of drug delivery systems for therapeutic agents that are poorly absorbed across the cornea or require delivery to posterior segment of the eye. Drug delivery across the conjunctiva and sclera is examined with reference to (a) physicochemical drug properties that may make the noncorneal route significant, (b) approaches of optimizing this route by understanding the mechanism by which this occurs, and (c) opportunities for taking advantage of this route in the design and evaluation of ocular drug delivery systems.

II. OCULAR ANATOMY AND PHYSIOLOGY RELEVANT TO THE NONCORNEAL ROUTE

The ocular anatomy and physiology relevant to ocular drug delivery was reviewed by Robinson (95). Some of the main points relevant to noncorneal drug delivery are summarized below.

A. Noncorneal Drug Penetration and Tissue Distribution

The shape of the eye in humans and rabbits, the primary animal model used in ocular research, approximates that of a globe, as shown in Figure 1. From the perspective of ocular drug delivery, the eye can be regarded as consisting of two parts: an anterior and a posterior segment. The tear fluid, the cornea, anterior chamber filled with aqueous humor, iris-ciliary body, and the lens comprise the anterior segment. The posterior segment of the eye consists of

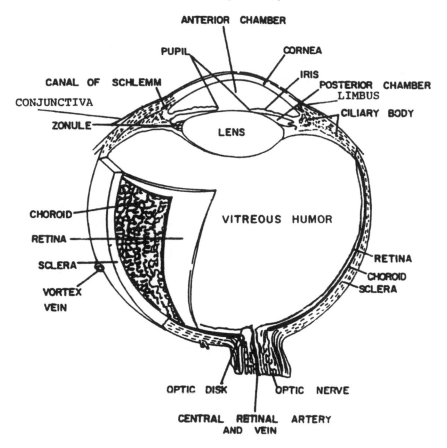

Figure 1 Anatomy of the eye. (Adapted from Ref. 154.)

four structures—the conjunctiva, sclera, choroid, and retina—surrounding the vitreous cavity that contains the vitreous humor. Taking into consideration the geometry of the eyeball and the diffusional pathways, drug penetrating via the corneal route has direct access to the anterior segment tissues, providing high levels in the cornea, aqueous humor, and the iris-ciliary body. In contrast, drug entering via the noncorneal route traverses the conjunctiva and sclera entering the choroid, retina, and eventually the vitreous humor. This selective tissue distribution of drugs entering the eye via the noncorneal route may be promising for drug delivery targeting the posterior eye (23,96).

B. Barriers to Noncorneal Drug Penetration

Intraocular entry via the noncorneal route requires drug penetration across the conjunctiva and the sclera. There are are three factors that can be barriers to the noncorneal penetration of ocularly applied drugs: (a) drug removal from the precorneal areas due to lacrimation and tear drainage, (b) the barriers to drug diffusion offered by the structures making up the outer coat of the eye, and (c) drug loss to the systemic circulation via the ocular vasculature.

1. Precorneal Fluid Dynamics

Topically applied drugs are commonly administered as an eye drop formulated as a solution, suspension, gel, ointment, and occasionally as a solid insert (86–94). The first barrier to intraocular penetration of topically applied drugs is tear turnover in the precorneal area. Under normal, unanesthetized conditions, the human tear volume averages 7 µL, with the estimated maximum volume that the cul-de-sac can momentarily contain with eye drop administration at about 30 µL (97). The human tear film is a lightly buffered aqueous fluid with a pH of approximately 7.2–7.5 and with an estimated thickness of 4–9 µm (98,99). The average tear turnover rate in humans is about 16% per minute under basal conditions but may be increased to 30% per minute due to stimulation resulting from drop instillation. The restoration of normal tear volume in the human requires an estimated 2–3 minutes, with 80% or more of the administered eye drops lost to drainage in the first 15–30 seconds after instillation (98). The resulting short contact times of drugs with absorbing membranes of the eye is the primary reason that typically less than 5% of a topically applied drug reaches the intraocular tissues (87–89).

2. Diffusion Across Ocular Membranes

a. Conjunctiva   The conjunctiva is a thin, transparent mucous membrane that starts at the corneoscleral junction (limbus) and extends to the eyelid margin. The portion of the conjunctiva loosely attached to the anterior surface of the globe is referred to as the bulbar conjunctiva. The more firmly adhering segment lining the inside of the eyelids is called the tarsal or palpebral conjunctiva. The conjunctiva can be divided into three layers: (a) an outer epithelium, forming a permeability barrier, (b) the substantia propria, containing structural and cellular elements, nerves, lymphatics and blood vessels, and (c) the submucosa, providing a loose attachment to the underlying sclera. The conjunctival epithelium is a stratified epithelium, squamous at the lids and columnar towards the cornea.

It is nonkeratized and has tight junctions that can present a permeability barrier to the diffusion of drugs. The thickness of the conjunctiva varies from region to region, being 10–15 layers thick towards the cornea and 5–6 layers thick at the eyelids. The conjunctival epithelium possesses dense microvilli covered with glycoclayx and a mucus layer (100–102). The area of the conjunctival sac in humans has been estimated at 16 cm^2, of which the cornea constitutes about 10%, whereas that in rabbits is approximately 12–13 cm^2, of which the cornea accounts for about 20% (103,104). Therefore, the conjunctival surface area exceeds that of the cornea by over fourfold. Unlike the cornea the conjunctiva is highly vascularized. Systemic loss can significantly reduce the fraction of drug available for penetration via the scleral/conjunctival route.

b. The Sclera The sclera, which is the white, tough outer coat of the eye, is composed largely of connective tissue (105). It has a protective function and maintains the shape of the eyeball by resisting intraocular pressure (106). The sclera is continuous with the cornea and extends posteriorly from the limbus, representing nearly 80% of the total surface area of the globe. The relatively softer, outer layer of the sclera is called the episclera. In rabbits, the sclera adjacent to the limbus is about 0.5 mm thick, thinning to as little as 0.2 mm in some areas (107). Structurally, the sclera is very similar to the corneal stroma and is made up of primarily collagen and mucopolysaccharides (108). Numerous channels through which fluid drainage occurs perforate the sclera. Blood vessels enter the uvea and the retina, but the sclera is itself poorly vascularized (109).

3. Systemic Loss via the Ocular Vasculature

Although the blood-ocular barrier prevents most systemically administered drugs from penetrating into the eye (65), ocularly applied drugs can enter the systemic circulation with relative ease. In excess of 70% of the instilled dose of an eye drop can enter the systemic circulation via absorption into the vasculature of the conjunctival and nasal mucosae (62–65). The nasal route is believed to be the primary contributor to the systemic loss of eye drops. For example,the nasal mucosa was 2.5 times more efficient than the conjunctival mucosa in contributing the systemic level of timolol (62). Whereas tight junctions between the endothelial cells of the microvessels result in a very low permeability to most solutes in the retina, the capillaries in the choroid and the ciliary processes there are fenestrated and the permeability to low molecular weight compounds is high. By injecting labeled proteins intravenously in rabbits and maintaining a steady-state concentration, Bill et al. (59) showed that the permeability of proteins in the choroid and the ciliary body were high compared to other ocular tissues.

Table 1   Blood Flow in Ocular Tissues of Primates

Tissue	Blood flow in whole tissue (mean ± S.E.) (mg/min)	Blood flow (mean ± S.E.) (g/min/tissue)
Retina	34 ± 2^a ($N = 15$)	
Iris	8 ± 1 ($N = 15$)	56 ± 8 ($N = 15$)
Ciliary body	81 ± 6 ($N = 15$)	150 ± 12 ($N = 13$)
Ciliary processes	677 ± 67 ($N = 15$)	227 ± 17 ($N = 8$)
Ciliary muscle		163 ± 26 ($N = 8$)

N = Number of determinations.
[a] Standard Error of Mean.
Source: Ref. 59.

Radiolabeled microspheres and indicator-dilution techniques have been used to measure ocular hemodynamics (55–57). The blood flow rate through various parts of the eye in primates is reported in Table 1. The kinetic constant of drug transfer from the eye to the circulation usually has a value of 20–50 h^{-1} from conventional dosage forms (64). Systemic loss via the ocular vasculature is a major deterrent to noncorneal drug delivery and must be factored into calculating the fraction of drug available for intraocular absorption. Minimizing the systemic loss there can also help to reduce adverse systemic effect following ocular application of potent compounds (66–75).

III.   NONCORNEAL ROUTES IN OCULAR DRUG DELIVERY

Ahmed and Patton (5) proposed a schematic for the pathways for the intraocular penetration of topically applied drugs, as shown in Figure 2. Modeling of the intraocular penetration routes and implication on ocular pharmacokinetics and pharmacodynamics was recently reviewed by Worakul and Robinson (14).

Although several investigators had reported a minor route of intraocular drug entry via the sclera and the conjunctiva (1–3), Bito and Baroody were the first to present evidence that this noncorneal route may, at least under some circumstances, be more important than the corneal route (4). They showed that after topical ^{3}H-PGF$_{2\alpha}$ application, the choroid, anterior sclera, and the ciliary body contained higher drug concentrations than the aqueous, indicating that the drug was entering the eye by some route other than through the cornea.

(a)

(b)

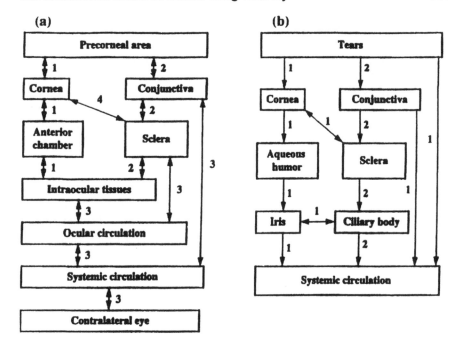

Figure 2 Intraocular penetration routes.

Over the past two decades there have been several investigations to further examine the conjunctival/scleral pathway for intraocular entry of drugs. The preferred method has been to mechanically block the cornea from the conjunctiva and sclera in situ with the use of a cylindrical well and introducing a drug solution either inside or outside the well. Hence, the disappearance of drug from the reservoir as well as the appearance of drug in intraocular tissues can be determined to compare the rate and extent of drug penetration via the corneal versus the conjunctival/scleral pathway. This method was employed by Schoenwald et al. (15) to study the ocular penetration pathway for methazolamide analogs, 6-carboxyfluorescein and rhodamine. The conjunctival/scleral route of entry produced higher iris/ciliary body concentrations for all compounds except for the lipophilic rhodamine. Confocal microscopy results suggested that drug gained entry into the ciliary body through uptake into the blood vessels of the sclera. The clinical implication of the scleral/conjunctival pathway may be important for antiglaucoma drugs where a quicker route to the iris-ciliary body via the blood vessels may result in a faster onset of action. Sasaki et al. (11) used the in situ technique to show that while the β-blocker tilisolol entered the aqueous humor primarily via the corneal route, the access to the vitreous body was four times more effective through the sclera than through the cornea. The application of tilisolol in the conjunctiva or the sclera also showed a high concentration in plasma whereas corneal application produced no systemic levels.

The physicochemical drug properties important to noncorneal penetration of topically applied drugs appear to be lipophilicity and molecular size. Using a series of β-blockers Sasaki et al. (16) showed that the permeability of penetrants is strongly dependent on lipophilicity for the cornea but less so for the conjunctiva and the sclera (Fig. 3). Chien et al. (10) studied α_2-adrenergic agents of varying lipophilicity and observed that the conjunctival/scleral pathway was the predominant route for delivery of least lipophilic molecule, p-aminoclonidine. The investigators also reported evidence of lateral diffusion of drug from the conjunctiva to the cornea. Pech et al. (18) evaluated a series of amphiphilic timolol prodrugs and observed that the transcleral absorption was the highest with the longest aliphatic chain prodrugs, which also had the most amphiphilic/lipophilic character. Hence, the in vitro studies suggest that solute lipophilicity is less important for noncorneal drug penetration than it is for transcorneal drug penetration. However, the effect of lipophilicity on the extent of noncorneal penetration

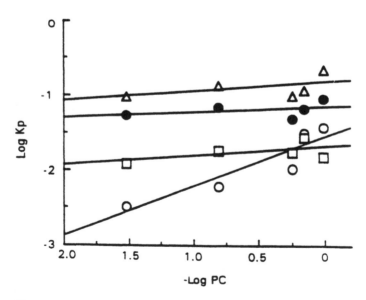

Figure 3 Relationship between logarithmic values of the octanol/water partition coefficient (PC) and permeability coefficient (K_p). (0) Cornea; (Δ) conjunctiva; (□) sclera; (●) scraped cornea.

of topically applied drugs in vivo may be difficult to predict from in vitro studies alone. This requires information on the permeability of the drug across the conjunctiva, sclera, and ocular blood vessels, as well as drug binding to ocular tissues. A suitable predictive model that accounts for all these factors is not yet available.

There is also strong evidence that the noncorneal route may be the preferred pathway for intraocular entry of large, polar molecules that have poor corneal permeability. Ahmed and Patton (5,6) used corneal blocking techniques to demonstrate that the noncorneal pathway was the primary route of intraocular entry for inulin, a molecule that was poorly absorbed across the cornea (Table 2). The permeability of large molecules in conjunctiva and sclera is typically higher than in the cornea, suggesting that the noncorneal route may contribute more to the intraocular absorption of large molecules than the corneal route. The permeability of the sclera and conjunctiva will be discussed later in the chapter.

Table 2 Concentration of Inulin in Various Ocular Tissues 20 Minutes Following the Topical Instillation of 25 μL of a 0.65% Inulin Solution, in the Presence and Absence of Corneal Access

	Concentration (μg/g)		
	With corneal access	Without corneal access	Percent (with/without) × 100
Aqueous humor	2.10[a] (0.420,9)	0.03 (0.020,6)	1.4
Cornea	22.8 (4.00,9)	1.87 (0.210,9)	8
Lens	ND	ND	
Vitreous humor	0.03 (0.008,9)	0.02 (0.003,9)	67
Iris-ciliary body	0.79 (0.162,9)	0.63 (0.087,9)	80
Sclera	7.82 (2.354,6)	8.45 (2.280,6)	108
Bulbar conjunctiva	177 (34.9,6)	273 (24.9,6)	154

[a]The mean; standard error of the mean and the number of eyes in parentheses.
ND = Not detectable.
Source: Ref. 5.

Systemic loss via drug absorption into the ocular blood vessels of the conjunctiva is a nonproductive pathway that diminishes the fraction of drug available for intraocular penetration via the noncorneal route. Accordingly, delivery methods that maximize the drug concentration at the conjunctival surface and minimize nonproductive systemic loss are also expected to improve noncorneal drug penetration. This hypothesis has been supported by some recent studies. Urtti and coworkers (7) presented evidence of application site–dependent noncorneal entry of timolol in rabbit from a topical device that released timolol at 7.2 µg/h. When the device was placed in the inferior conjunctival sac, the resulting timolol concentration in the aqueous humor was nearly 100-fold lower than in the iris-ciliary body. Romanelli et al. (20) showed that bendazac was absorbed into the retina-choroid via the scleral/conjunctival route when delivered topically in polysaccharide vehicles. It was noted that transcorneal penetration of bendazac was hindered not only by the epithelial barrier but also by the strong binding of the drug to the stroma. In another study, Lehr et al. (21) reported formulating gentamicin in the mucoadhesive polymer, polycarbophil, facilitated the noncorneal penetration of gentamicin probably by intensified contact between the polymer and the underlying bulbar conjunctiva. Dosage design considerations for noncorneal delivery will be discussed in a subsequent section.

IV. PERMEABILITY OF THE CONJUNCTIVA AND THE SCLERA

The recognition that noncorneal penetration may be a productive route of intraocular entry for some drugs has triggered extensive research to understand the barrier properties of the conjunctiva and the sclera and the physicochemical determinants of drug permeability across these membranes. In vitro and in situ permeability studies have proven to be a useful approach in estimating drug transport for in vivo conditions. In general, permeability characteristics of ocular membranes correlate well with the intraocular absorption of drugs.

A. Methodology

Four methods have been commonly used for measuring permeability across ocular membranes. The first method is based on the measurement of steady-state permeability of drugs across the isolated ocular membrane using a side-by-side diffusion cell or a modified two-chamber Ussing apparatus.

Accordingly, the membrane permeability coefficients may be calculated using the following equation:

$$P = V_R \Delta C / \Delta t . A . C_D$$

where $\Delta C / \Delta t$ is the change in the concentration with time represented by the slope of the linear part of the amount of drug accumulated versus time curve, V_R is the volume of the receiver chamber, A is the surface area of the mounted membrane, and C_D is the initial concentration of the drug in the donor chamber. This method assumes sink conditions. As pointed out by Maurice (32) in his critique of such techniques, it is important to ensure that the in vivo characteristics of the membranes are maintained as closely as possible. This requires care during the dissection to avoid folding or damage to the surfaces of the membranes and preservation of the tissue during the course of the experiment using physiologically relevant buffer systems (e.g., oxygenated glutathione bicarbonate Ringers solution) to maintain tissue viability. It is also important to measure, confirm, and report the integrity of the barrier based on electrical properties, hydration level, and diffusion of marker substances. Another alert is interspecies differences and caution in overinterpreting data obtained from animals to humans.

The second method is in situ perfusion technique that enables quantitation of drug uptake in live animals. This method was originally utilized for measuring corneal permeation and uptake of drugs (110,111) and subsequently applied to study the conjunctival and scleral uptake of various compounds (10,11,16). The technique involves affixing a cylindrical well on the surface of the eye near the corneoscleral junction using surgical adhesives (Fig. 4). A drug solution is then placed either inside the well bathing the cornea or outside the well bathing the remainder of the conjunctival sac. The rate of mass flux in the system can be described by:

$$dC_s V_s / dt = Cl_s . C_s$$

where C_s is the concentration of drug in the systeml, V_s is the volume of fluid in the reservoir and Cl_s is a clearance parameter describing the loss of drug from the system. This method can be utilized to study the effect of physical-chemical drug properties while avoiding some of the problems associated with in vitro studies on isolated membranes as previously described. The primary disadvantage is the difficulty in extracting a true permeability coefficient or mechanistic information from such experiments.

A third is a flow-through permeation chamber where the excised tissue is mounted horizontally method (43,46,112). A small volume of the drug solution is applied on the external surface of the membrane and the internal surface is perfused with a physiological receptor solution. In this method the flux across the membrane can be calculated using the following equation:

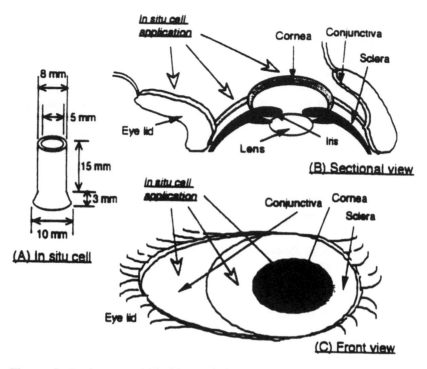

Figure 4   In situ corneal blocking technique.

$$V\partial C/\partial t = JS - QC$$

where V is the volume of the receiver compartment, C is the concentration in the receiver compartment, S is the exposed surface area, J is the flux at the membrane surface on the receptor side, Q is the flow rate out of the receptor compartment, and t is the time. This method is appropriate for the measurement and prediction of transient transport across the ocular membrane simulating more realistic ocular drug delivery scenarios. For example, it has been shown that the predictions of transscleral transport based on steady-state measurements may significantly overpredict the amount of drug delivered into the eye because the lag time for transport across the sclera is similar or longer than the drug-sclera contact time from an eye drop (43). Drug binding to the sclera may also prolong the lag time. A disadvantage of non–steady-state experiments is that the data treatment and mathematics is complicated.

The fourth method is the use of cell culture and physical models. During the past decade advances in cell culture techniques have resulted in the development of a primary culture model of rabbit conjunctival epithelial cells exhibiting tight barrier properties (112–115). There has been an attempt to develop physical models to describe the transport of molecules through the cornea and the sclera by taking into account the ultrastructure of these tissues (44). The use of intestinal tissues to predict ocular permeability and ex vivo models based on isolated perfused tissue has also been reported (118). These techniques may offer an alternative to the use of animals in research and an opportunity for gaining a greater mechanistic understanding of transport processes. However, the practical application and scope of these methods remain to be determined.

B. Permeability of the Sclera and Conjunctiva

1. Sclera

The permeability of the sclera to small molecules is comparable to that of the corneal stroma. There was no significant difference between the corneal stroma and the sclera of the beef eye in their permeability to a variety of small solute (24). Even large molecules can move across the sclera by the way of perivascular spaces but also by diffusion through interfibrillary spaces (38). Maurice and Polgar measured the movement of a number of anionic and cationic dyes, as well as small ions, proteins, and biologically active molecules across the isolated beef sclera using a two-chamber diffusion cell (39). Only anionic dyes of small molecular weights were able to cross the sclera, but the sclera offered little obstacle to the penetration of drugs into the eye.

Prausnitz and Noonan (24) recently published a comprehensive database of ocular tissue permeability measurements found in a review of the literature. There was no apparent dependence on distribution coefficient but a strong dependence of penetrant size on scleral permeability. The scleral permeability to tracers of various molecular sizes in rabbit and humans is shown in Table 3. Ambati et al. (47) showed that molecular radius was a better predictor of scleral permeability than molecular weight, and large molecules, such as IgG, diffuse across the sclera in a manner consistent with porous diffusion through a fiber matrix. Edwards and Prausnitz supported this assertion with a fiber matrix model to predict the permeability of the sclera to water and solute (44). Unlu and Robinson (45) observed that the scleral permeability of radiolabeled hydrocortisone and mannitol across the isolated rabbit sclera was five times greater than the corneal permeability. The low activation energy of scleral transport of hydrocortisone suggested an aqueous pore pathway. Hamalainen (30) used a modified two-chamber Ussing apparatus to characterize quantitatively the paracellular permeation routes in the rabbit cornea, conjunctiva, and sclera using poly-

Table 3 Permeability of Sclera to Tracers of Various Molecular Sizes in Rabbits and Humans

Tracer	Molecular weight (D)	Molecular radius (nm)	Permeability coefficient $\times 10^{-6}$ cm/s (SD)	
			Rabbit	Human
Water	18		54.4 919)[a]	44.6 (13)[a]
Mannitol	182		28.3 (3.7)[d]	
Sucrose	342		42.2 (13.7)[e]	21.6 (6.0)[b]
Hydrocortisone	362		21.8 (4.3)[d]	
Dexamethasone	396		12.7 (2.3)[a]	18.2 (5.8)[a]
				23.5 (7.7)[b]
Sodium fluorescein	376	0.5	84.5 (16.1)[c]	
Carboxyfluorescein			13.0 (3.4)[a]	11.8 (1.37)[a]
Dextran, 4 kDa	4,400	1.3	25.2 (5.1)[c]	
Inulin	5000–5,250		2.54 (0.35)[e]	9.0 (2.2)[b]
Dextran, 10 kDa	10,000			6.4 (1.7)[b]
Dextran, 20 kDa	19,600	3.2	6.79 (4.18)[c]	
Dextran, 40 kDa	38,900	4.5	2.79 (1.58)[c]	4.9 (2.4)[b]
Dextran, 70 kDa	71,200	6.4	1.39 (0.88)[c]	1.9 (0.4)[b]
Dextran, 150 kDa	150,000	8.25	1.34 (0.88)[c]	

SD = Standard deviation.
[a] From Ref. 46.
[b] From Ref. 42.
[c] From Ref. 47.
[d] From Ref. 45.
[e] From Ref. 40.

ethylene glycol (PEG) oligomers. The scleral permeability was 15–25 times more than that of the cornea but about half that of the conjunctiva. The permeability of PEGs decreased linearly with increasing molecular weight, for example, decreasing threefold from a value of 8.80×10^{-6} cm/s for PEG 238 to 3.08×10^{-6} cm/s for PEG 942.

There have been several reports comparing the permeability of the sclera, conjunctiva, and cornea to penetrant lipophilicity. The comparative permeability of a series of β-blockers across isolated rabbit ocular membranes is shown in Table 4. Ahmed et al. (40) showed that the conjunctival and corneal permeabilities for timolol were comparable but fourfold lower than the scleral permeability. Sasaki and coworkers (54) reported that the in vitro permeability of a series of β-blockers across the isolated rabbit sclera and conjunctiva was not affected by penetrant lipophilicity. Edelhauser and Maren (41) compared the scleral versus corneal permeability of the carbonic

Table 4 Differential Permeability of β-Blockers Across Isolated Ocular Membranes in Rabbit

| Compound | MW | Log PC | Permeability (cm/s $\times$ 10^6) | | |
			Cornea	Conjunctiva	Sclera
Atenolol	266	−0.11	1.1, 0.68	52	
Sotalol	272	0.23			68
Nadolol	309	0.23	14, 7, 1.6	53	39
Metroprolol	267	1.20	28, 24	62	
Timolol	316	1.61	12, 18, 8, 12	52	41
Acetobutolol	336	1.63	1.1, 0.85	50	
Pindolol	248	1.67	10	15	
Oxyprenolol	265	1.69	28	9	
Betaxolol	307	2.17	27, 54	42	
Levobunolol	291	2.26	29, 23, 17	51	
Labetalol	328	2.50	14	60	
Alprenolol	249	2.65	29	24	
Propranolol	259	2.75	31, 34, 46, 58	20	58
Penbutolol	291	4.04	22, 60		71

Source: Adapted from Ref. 24.

anhydrase inhibitors ethoxzolamide and methazolamide and concluded that the permeability was six times greater in the sclera than in the cornea for the less lipophilic methazolamide but similar for the more lipophilic ethoxzolamide.

2. Conjunctiva

Unlike the sclera, the conjunctiva shares an important attribute with the cornea in that both contain an outer lining of stratified squamous epithelium continuous with each other at the corneoscleral limbus. However, the cornea is avascular while the conjunctival epithelium overlies a loose, highly vascular connective tissue, the substantia propria.

Characteristic of any epithelial tissue, both paracellular and transcellular transport is possible across the conjunctiva. In both the cornea and the conjunctiva, lipophilic drugs prefer the transcellular route, while the paracellular route is preferred by hydrophilic drugs (36). The ratio of the permeability coefficients of a series of β-adrenergic blockers in the cornea and those in the conjunctiva exhibited a sigmoidal correlation with log partition coefficient, as shown in Figure 5 (51). This indicates that while the conjunctiva is leakier than the cornea, the differential permeability of the conjunctiva to the cornea is higher for hydrophilic compounds than for lipophilic compounds. The data presented in Table 5, which shows that the permeability of peptides in conjunctiva is higher than in the cornea, support this conclusion (52,53).

Several authors have studied the effect of molecular size on conjunctival permeability. Horibe et al. (31) characterized the conjunctival permeability to polar solutes ranging from 182 to 167,000 daltons in molecular weight and concluded that solutes up to 40 kDa traverse the conjunctival epithelial barrier primarily by restricted diffusion through equivalent pores of 5.5 nm. Polar solutes of greater than 70 kDa may cross the barrier primarily via nondiffusional pathways, such as nonspecific endocytosis. Huang et al. (27) and Kahn et al. (28) also studied the solute size effect on conjunctival penetration. They estimated the limiting size of solutes that can pass the conjunctival barrier by paracellular transport at between 20 and 40 kDa. Hamalainen et al. (29) reported that the conjunctival epithelia in the rabbit have 2 times larger pores and 16 times higher pore density than the cornea. They estimated that intercellular space in the cornea is 0.3×10^{-3} mm^2, whereas it is 7×10^{-3} mm^2 in rabbit conjunctiva. Finally, there is some evidence that human conjunctiva may be more permeable to hydrophilic solutes than rabbit conjunctiva (32)

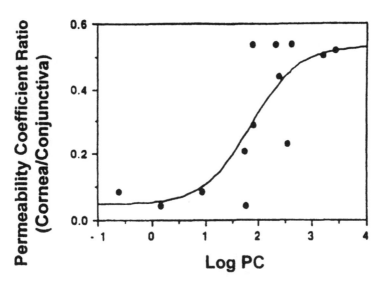

Figure 5 Permeability coefficient ratio (cornea/conjunctiva) as a function of the log partition coefficient

Table 5 Permeability Ratio of Peptides Across Ocular Membranes in Rabbit

Compound	MS	Log PC	Permeability ratio Conjunctiva/Cornea
Diglycine	132	1.89	10
Triglycine	189	1.74	93
Tetraglycine	246	1.70	5
Pentaglycine	303	0.77	9
TRH	362	1.59	22
PNP	950		17
LHRH	1182		47

Source: Adapted from Refs. 36, 53.

V. DESIGN OF DRUG DELIVERY SYSTEMS TARGETING THE NONCORNEAL ROUTE

There are limited reports of practical examples of noncorneal drug delivery dosage forms and drug delivery systems. As noted previously, the noncorneal pathway may be best suited to deliver large, polar molecules, which have poor permeability across the cornea and which are less likely to be extensively cleared by systemic loss via absorption into the ocular blood vessels. However, effective noncorneal drug delivery is likely to require special considerations in dosage form design and methods of administration that can minimize precorneal and retain high concentrations of drug at the absorptive surfaces or the conjunctiva or sclera. Delivery system options may include bioadhesive polymeric vehicles, controlled release inserts, prodrugs, microparticulates, and scleral implants. The method of administration that is most likely to maximize the opportunity to deliver drugs via the noncorneal route is suprachoroidal delivery via subconjunctival or sub-Tenon's injection or implantation, as these methods are best suited to administer the drug in close proximity of the absorbing surface as a depot form. Iontophoretic delivery is an option that has not yet been explored for noncorneal deliver, as is the approach of minimizing systemic drug loss via absorption into the conjunctival blood vessels by using vasoconstrictors.

A. Custom Vehicles

Romanelli et al. (20) studied the absorption, distribution, and elimination of bendazac in ocular tissues after topical administration as eye drops formulated with different polysaccharide vehicles. Based on spatial and temporal distribution of drug in ocular tissues, they concluded that bendazac entered the retina-choroid and the iris-ciliary body by a sclero-conjunctival route. Lehr et al. (21) investigated the use of polycarbophil, a mucoadhesive polymer, to improve the ocular delivery of gentamicin formulated in eye drops. A twofold increase in bulbar conjunctival levels was noted. Based on the rank-order of peak concentrations and peak times in ocular tissues, the authors proposed that gentamicin formulated in polycarbophil-containing eyedrops reach the anterior chamber primarily via the noncorneal route.

B. Conjunctival Inserts

Urtti et al. (7) showed that application site–dependent absorption of timolol formulated in a silicone cylindrical device that released drug at 7.2 μ/h. Very low timolol concentrations in the aqueous humor following placement of the device in the inferior conjunctival sac and high drug concentrations in parts of each tissue that was closer to the site of application was presented as evidence of noncorneal entry.

C. Microparticulates

Ahmed et al. (23) showed evidence of site-specific, noncorneal delivery of inulin to the posterior eye from topical application of multilamellar liposomes. It is reasonable to expect that noncorneal delivery of some drugs using nanoparticulates may be feasible.

D. Prodrugs and Enhancers

In a preliminary evaluation of a series of amphiphilic timolol prodrugs, Pech et al. (18) presented possible evidence of transscleral absorption. The potential of a drug latentiation as a means to promote selective noncorneal entry was also presented in the in vitro evaluation of polyethylene glycol esters of hydrocortisone 21-succinate as ocular prodrugs (120). Chien et al. reported improved permeability across the conjunctiva for prostaglandin $F_{2\alpha}$ prodrugs (19). Noncorneal enhancers may be agents that reduce systemic loss or increase conjunctival permeability. Epinephrine pretreatment did not significantly affect the concentrations of topically applied timolol in the cornea, aqueous humor, iris-ciliary body, and conjunctiva of rabbits but resulted in significantly higher concentrations in the sclera (67). Although not explicitly stated, this approach of minimizing systemic loss with vasoconstrictors may render noncorneal entry of selective drugs more favorable. There have been some exciting leads in approaches and entities to transiently enhance the epithelial permeability of ocular membranes (122–124). The technology of enhancing the conjunctival permeability may become available in the near future.

E.   Devices and Novel Administration Methods

Arguably the most promising approach to noncorneal delivery is deposition of drug, preferably as a depot or as a biodegradable implant at, or in the near proximity of the episclera. Kunou et al. (119) formulated betamethasone phosphate in a biodegradable, polylactic glycolic acid scleral implant and showed that the drug concentrations in the retina-choroid stayed in the therapeutic range for one month. Further, the concentrations in the retina-choroid were consistently greater than in the vitreous, which is evidence of noncorneal entry. Transcleral penetration of drugs following subconjunctival and sub-Tenon's injection is precedented and is considered to be a viable approach for delivering drugs to the posterior tissues of the eye (125–127). Advances in iontophoretic techniques present the possibility that transscleral iontophoresis may replace or supplement intravitreal injection of antibiotics for the treatment of endophthalmitis (128–130).

VI.   CONCLUSIONS/FUTURE DIRECTION

Based on the current understanding it is possible to put the conjunctival/scleral pathway for intraocular entry of drugs in perspective vis-a-vis ocular drug delivery. First, the noncorneal penetration pathway involves the permeation of drug across the conjunctiva and sclera and may contribute significantly to drug penetration into intraocular tissues for some drugs. Second, drug entering the eye via the cornea enters the aqueous humor and provides high drug levels to the anterior segment tissues, as described earlier. In contrast, the fraction of drug entering the eye via the noncorneal route may bypass the anterior chamber and access tissues of the posterior segment of the eye, such as the uveal tract, choroid, and retina and, to a lesser extent, the vitreous humor. The differential spatial distribution of drug entering the eye via the corneal versus conjunctival/scleral pathway has exciting implications in terms of ocular drug delivery. For example, whereas the corneal route may be preferred for treating anterior segment eye disease (e.g., glaucoma), the noncorneal route may be considered for drug therapy targeting the posterior segment of the eye (e.g., uveitis, choroidal neovascular membrane formation, viral retinitis, age-related macular degeneration). Third, the nonproductive loss of ocularly applied drugs to the systemic circulation diminishes the fraction of drug that can enter the eye via the noncorneal route. Since the cornea is nonvascularized, the conjunctival/scleral entry is a minor pathway for most small, semipolar heterocycles that represent the majority of commonly used ophthalmic drugs. However, the noncorneal pathway may become significant for large, polar molecules, administration methods that can minimize precorneal and systemic loss, drugs susceptible to degradation during diffusion across the cornea, and for delivery systems that can retain high concentrations of drug at the absorptive surfaces or the conjunctiva or sclera.

Recent advances in drug delivery systems that minimize precorneal loss and can retain high concentrations of drug at the absorptive surfaces of the conjunctiva or sclera may be particularly suited for noncorneal delivery. These include bioadhesive vehicles, microparticulates, and controlled release conjunctival inserts. Suprachoroidal delivery of drugs via subconjunctival and sub-Tenon's injection, scleral and suprachoroidal implants, may be the most promising approach to noncorneal delivery. Prodrugs and permeation enhancers and vasoconstrictors are plausible concepts, but they require further investigation.

Much progress has been made over the past two decades towards understanding the fundamental basis of drug penetration via the noncorneal pathway. The challenge for the future is to creatively apply the available knowledge to the practical design of drugs and drug delivery systems for ocular therapy. Noncorneal delivery is not a panacea and will probably have niche utility in ocular drug delivery. The greatest potential for the concept appears to be in the area of intraocular delivery of polar molecules, peptides and protein drugs, and directed drug delivery to treat posterior segment eye disease.

REFERENCES

1. McCartney, H. J., Drysdale, I. O., Gornall, A. G., and Basau, P. K. (1965). An auto-radiographic study of the penetration of subconjunctivally injected hydrocortisone into the normal and inflamed rabbit eyes, *Invest. Ophthalmol.*, 4:297.
2. Bienfang, D. C. (1973). Sector pupillary dilation with an epinephrine strip, *Am. J. Ophthalmol.*, 75:883.
3. Doane, M. G., Jensen, A. D., and Dohlman, C. H. (1978). Penetration routes of topically applied eye medications, *Am. J. Ophthalmol.*, 85:383–386.
4. Bito, L. Z., and Baroody, R. A. (1981). The penetration of exogenous prostaglandin and arachidonic acid into, and their distribution within, the mammalian eye, *Curr. Eye Res.*, 1:659–669.
5. Ahmed, I., and Patton, T. F. (1985). Importance of the noncorneal absorption route in topical ophthalmic drug delivery, *Invest. Ophthal. Vis. Sci.*, 26:584–587.
6. Ahmed, I., and Patton, T. F. (1987). Disposition of timolol and inulin in the rabbit eye following corneal versus non-corneal absorption, *Int. J. Pharm.*, 38:9–21.

7. Urtti, A., Sondo, T., Pipkin, J. D., Rork, G., and Repta, A. J. (1988). Application site dependent ocular absorption of timolol, *J. Ocul. Pharmacol.*, *4*:335–343.
8. Ashton, P., and Lee, V. H. L. (1989). Role of drug lipophilicity in determining the contribution of noncorneal penetration in ocular drug absorption, *Pharm. Res.*, *6*:S114.
9. Lee, V. H. L., Ashton, P., Bundgaard, H., and Heuer, D. K. (1990). Noncorneal route of drug penetration role of drug lipophilicity in determining its contribution to the ocular absorption of beta blockers and timolol prodrugs, *Invest. Ophthal. Vis. Sci.*, *31*:403.
10. Chien, D.-S., Homsy, J. J., Gluchowski, C., and Tang-Liu, D. (1990). Corneal and conjunctival/scleral penetration of p-aminoclonidine, AGN 190342, and clonidine in rabbit eyes, *Curr. Eye Res.*, *9*:1051–1059.
11. Sasaki, H., Ichikawa, M., Kawakami, S., Yamamura, K., Nishida, K., and Nakamura, J. (1996). In situ ocular absorption of tilisolol through ocular membranes in albino rabbits, *J. Pharm. Sci.*, *85*:940–943.
12. Rabiah, P. K., Fiscella, R. G., and Tessler, H. H. (1996). Intraocular penetration of periocular ketorolac and efficacy in experimental uveitis, *Invest. Ophthal. Vis. Sci.*, *37*:613–618.
13. Kurmala, P., Wilson, G. C., Foulds, W. S., Dhillon, B., Kamal, A., and Rao, L. S. (1997). Suprachoroidal route of drug delivery to the posterior segment of the eye, *J. Pharm. Pharmacol.*, *49*:83.
14. Worakul, N., and Robinson, J. R. (1997). Review: Ocular pharmacokinetics/pharmacodynamics, *Eur. J. Pharm. Biopharm.*, *44*:71–83.
15. Schoenwald, R. D., Deshpande, G. S., Rethwisch, D. G., and Barfknecht, C. F. (1997). Penetration into the anterior chamber via the conjunctival/scleral pathway, *J. Ocul. Pharmacol. Therap.*, *13*:41–59.
16. Sasaki, H., Icikawa, M., Kawakami, S., Yamamura, K., and Mukai, T. (1997). In situ ocular absorption of ophthalmic β-blockers through ocular membranes in albino rabbits, *J. Pharm. Pharmacol.*, *49*:140–144.
17. Conroy, C. W., and Maren, T. H. (1998). The ocular distribution of methazolamide after corneal and sclera administration: Effect of ionization state, *J. Ocul. Pharmacol. Therap.*, *14*:565–573.
18. Pech, B., Chetoni, P., Saettone, M. F., Duval, O., and Benoit, J.-P. (1993). Preliminary evaluation of a series of amphiphilic timolol prodrugs: Possible evidence for transscleral absorption, *J. Ocular Pharmacol.*, *9*:141–150.
19. Chien, D. S., TangLiu, D. D. S., and Woodward, D. F. (1997). Ocular penetration and bioconversion of prostaglandin F2 alpha prodrugs in rabbit cornea and conjunctiva, *J. Pharm. Sci.*, *86*:1180–1186.
20. Romanelli, L., Valeri, P., Morrone, L. A., Pimpinella, G., Graziani, G., and Tita, B. (1994). Ocular absorption and distribution of bendazac after topical administration to rabbits with different vehicles, *Life Sci.*, *54*:877–885.
21. Lehr, C. M., Lee, Y.-H., and Lee, V. H. L. (1992). Effect of mucoadhesive polymer polycarbophil on ocular penetration of gentamicin, *Pharm. Weekbl. Sci. Ed.*, *14*: F31.

22. Shiue, M. H. I., Kim, K. J., and Lee, V. H. L. (1998). Modulation of chloride secretion across the pigmented rabbit conjunctiva, *Curr. Eye. Res.*, *14*:927–935.

23. Ahmed, I., and Patton, T. F. (1986). Selective intraocular delivery of liposome-encapsulated inulin via the non-corneal absorption route, *Int. J. Pharm.*, *34*:163–167.

24. Prausnitz, M. R., and Noonan, J. S. (1998). Permeability of the cornea, sclera, and conjunctiva: A literature analysis for drug delivery to the eye, *J. Pharm. Sci.*, *87*:1479–1488.

25. Lee, V. H. L., Carson, L. W., and Takemoto, K. A. (1986). Macromolecular drug absorption in the albino rabbit eye, *Int. J. Pharm.*, *29*:43–51.

26. Ashton, P., Lee, V. H. L. (1989). Para- and transcellular pathways of drug penetration across the cornea and conjunctiva of the pigmented rabbit, *Pharm. Res.*, *6*: S590.

27. Huang, A. J. W., Tseng, S. C. G., and Kenyon, K. R. (1990). Paracellular permeability of corneal and conjunctival epithelia, *Invest. Ophthalmol. Vis. Sci.*, *30*:684–689.

28. Kahn, M., Barney, N. P., Briggs, R. M., Bloch, K. J., and Allansmith, M. R. (1990). Penetrating the conjunctival barrier: The role of molecular weight, *Invest. Ophthalmol. Vis. Sci.*, *31*:258–261.

29. Hamalainen, K. M., Kananen, K., Auriola, S., Kontturi, K., and Urtti, A. (1997). Characterization of paracellular and aqueous penetration routes in cornea, conjunctival and sclera, *Invest. Ophthal. Vis. Sci.*, *38*:627–634.

30. Hamalainen, K. M. (1997). Characterization of the paracellular penetration route—reply, *Invest. Ophthal. Vis. Sci.*, *38*:2179–2180.

31. Horibe, Y., Hosoya, K., Kim, K. J., Ogiso, T., and Lee, V. H. L. (1997). Polar solute transport across the pigmented rabbit conjunctiva: size dependence and the influence of 8-bromo cyclic ademosine monophosphate, *Pharm. Res.*, *14*:1246–1251.

32. Maurice, D. M. (1997). Letter: Characterization of paracellular penetration routes, *Invest. Ophthalmol. Vis. Sci.*, *38*:2177–2179.

33. Kompella, U., Kim, K. J., and Lee, V. H. L. (1992). Active ion and nutrient transport mechanisms of the pigmented rabbit conjunctiva, *Pharm. Res.*, *9* (Suppl. 3).

34. Kompella, U., Kim, K. J., and Lee, V. H. L. (1993). Active chloride transport in the pigmented rabbit conjunctiva, *Curr. Eye Res.*, *12*:1041–1048.

35. Kompella, U., Kim, K. J., and Lee, V. H. L. (1995). Possible existence of Na$^+$ coupled amino acid transport in the pigmented rabbit conjunctiva, *Life Sci.*, *57*:1427–1431.

36. Lee, V. H. L. (1996). Ocular epithelial models, *Pharm Biotech.*, *8*:425–436.

37. Kompella, U. B., and Lee, V. H. L. (1998). Barriers to drug transport in the ocular epithelia, in *Transport Processes in Pharmaceutical Systems* (G. L. Amidon, P. I. Lee, and E. M. Topp, eds.), Marcel Dekker, New York, pp. 317–375.

38. Bill, A. (1965). Movement of albumin and dextran through the sclera, *Arch. Ophthalmol.*, *74*:248–252.

39. Maurice, D. M., and Polgar, J. (1977). Diffusion across the sclera, *Exp. Eye. Res.*, *25*:577–582.

40. Ahmed, I., Gokhale, R. D., Shah, M. V., and Pattom, T. F. (1987). Physicochemical determinants of drug diffusion across the conjunctiva, sclera and cornea, *J. Pharm. Sci.*, *76*:583–586.

41. Edelhauser, H. F., and Maren, T. H. (1988). Permeability of the human cornea and sclera to sulfonamide carbonic anhydrase inhibitors, *Arch. Ophthalmol.*, *106*:1110–1115.

42. Olsen, T. W., Edelhauser, H. F., Lim, J. I., and Geroski, D. H. (1995). Human scleral permeability: effects of age, cryotherapy, transscleral diode laser and surgical thinning, *Invest. Ophthalmol. Vis. Sci.*, *36*:1893–1903.

43. Prausnitz, M. R., Edwards, A., Noonan, J. S., Rudnick, D. E., Edelhauser, H. F., and Geroski, D. H. (1998). Measurement and prediction of transient transport across the sclera for drug delivery to the eye, *Ind. Eng. Chem. Res.*, *37*:2903–2907.

44. Edwards, A., and Prausnitz, M. R. (1998). Fiber matrix model of sclera and corneal stroma for drug delivery to the eye, *AIChE J.*, *44*:214–225.

45. Unlu, N., and Robinson, J. R. (1998). Scleral permeability to hydrocortisone and mannitol in the albino rabbit eye, *J. Ocul. Pharm. Ther.*, *14*:273–281.

46. Rudnick, D. E., Noonan, J. S., Geroski, D. H., Praunitz, M. R., and Edelhuser, H. F. (1999). The effect of intraocular pressure on human and scleral permeability, *Invest. Ophthal. Vis. Sci.*, *40*:3054–3058.

47. Ambati, J., Canakis, C. S., Miller, J. W., Gragoudas, E. S., Edward, A., Weissgold, D. J., Kim, I., Delor, F. C., and Adamis, A. P. (2000). Diffusion of high molecular weight compounds through the sclera, *Invest. Ophthal. Vis. Sci.*, *41*:1181–1185.

48. Maurice, D. M. (1973). Electrical potential and ion transport, *Exp. Eye Res.*, *15*:527–532.

49. Sorensen, T., and Jensen, F. T. (1979). Conjunctival transport of technetium-99m pertechnetate, *Acta Opthalmol.*, *57*:691–699.

50. Sasaki, H., Chien, D. S., and Lee, V. H. L. (1988). Differential conjunctival and corneal permeability to beta-blockers and its influence on the ratio of systemic to ocular drug absorption, *Pharm. Res.*, *5*:S98.

51. Wang, W., Sasaki, H., Chien, D.-S., and Lee, V. H. L. (1991). Lipophilicity influence on conjunctival drug penetration in the pigmented rabbit: A comparison with corneal penetration, *Curr. Eye. Res.*, *10*:571–579.

52. Sasaki, H., Igarashi, Y., Nagano, T., Yamamura, K., Nishida, K., and Nakamura, J. (1995). Penetration of beta-blockers through ocular membranes in albino rabbits, *J. Pharm. Pharmacol.*, *47*:17–21.

53. Sasaki, H., Icikawa, M., Yamamura, K., Nishida, K., and Nakamura, J. (1997). Ocular membrane permeability of hydrophilic drugs for ocular peptide delivery, *J. Pharm. Pharmacol.*, *49*:135–139.

54. Sasaki, H., Masataka, I., Shigeru, K., Keno, Y., Takahiro, M., Koyo, N., and Junzo, N. (1997). Ocular absorption of ophthalmic beta-blockers through ocular membranes in albino rabbits, *J. Pharm. Pharmacol.*, *49*:140–144.

55. Alm, A., and Bill, A. (1973). The effect of pilocarpine and neostigmine on blood flow through the anterior uvea in monkeys. A study with radiolabelled microspheres, *Exp. Eye. Res*, *15*:31–36.

56. Green, K., Wynn, H., and Padgett, D. (1978). Effects of 9-Tetrahydrocannabinol on ocular blood flow and aqueous humor formation, *Exp. Eye Res.*, *26*:65–69.

57. Riva, C. E., and Ben-Sira, I. (1974). Injection method for ocular hemodynamic studies in man, *Invest. Ophthalmol.*, *13*:77–79.

58. Lee, V. H. L., and Robinson, J. R. (1979). Mechanistic and quantitative evaluation of precorneal pilocarpine disposition in albino rabbits, *J. Pharm. Sci.*, *68*:673.

59. Bill, A., Tornquist, P., and Alm, A. (1980). Permeability of the intraocular blood vessels, *Trans. Ophthalmol. Soc. U.K.*, *100*:332–336.

60. Lee, V. H. L., Takemoto, K. A., and Iimoto, D. S. (1984). Precorneal factors influencing the ocular distribution of topically applied inulin, *Curr. Eye Res.*, *3*:585–592.

61. Ziada, G., El-Haddad, S., Fatouh, M., Mustafa, H., and Mahfouz, M. (1985). Radionuclide study of the blood ocular barrier, *Eur. J. Drug Met. Pharmacokin.*, *10*:325–328.

62. Chang, S.-C., and Lee, V. H. L. (1987). Nasal and conjunctival contribution to the systemic absorption of topical timolol in the pigmented rabbit implications in the design of strategies to maximize the ratio of ocular to systemic absorption, *J. Ocul. Pharmacol.*, *3*:159–170.

63. Maitani, Y., Yamamoto, T., Takayama, K., Peppas, N. A., and Nagai, T. (1995). A modelling analysis of drug absorption and administration from ocular, nasolacrimal duct, and nasal routes, *Int. J. Pharm.*, *126*:89–94.

64. Yoshi, M., Nagai, T., Kollias, K., and Peppas, N. (1997). Design of ocular/lacrimal and nasal systems through analysis of drug administration and absorption, *J. Contr. Rel.*, *49*:185–192.

65. Cunha-Vaz, J. G. (1997). The blood-ocular barriers: Past, present, and future, Doc. Ophthalmol. *93*:149–157.

66. Kyyronen, K., and Urtti, A. (1990). Improved ocular-systemic absorption ratio of timolol by viscous vehicle and phenylephrine, *Invest. Ophthal. Vis. Sci.*, *31*:1827–1833.

67. Kyyronen, K., and Urtti, A., (1990). Effects of epinephrine pretreatment and solution pH on ocular and systemic absorption of ocularly applied timolol in rabbits, *J. Pharm. Sci.*, *79*:688–691.

68. Finne, U., Vaisanen, V., and Urtti, A. (1990). Modification of ocular and systemic absorption of timolol from ocular inserts by a buffering agent and a vasoconstrictor, *Int. J. Pharm.*, *65*:19–27.

69. Ohdo, S., Grass, G. M., and Lee, V. H. L. (1991). Improving the ocular to systemic ratio of topical timolol by varying the dosing time, *Invest. Ophthal. Vis. Sci.*, *32*:2790–2798.

70. Jarvinen, K., Vartianen, E., and Urtti, A. (1992). Optimizing the systemic and ocular absorption of timolol from eye drops, *STP Pharma Sci.*, *2*:105–110.

71. Urtti, A., and Salminen, L. (1993). Review: Minimizing systemic absorption of topically administered ophthalmic drugs, *Surv. Ophthalmol.*, *37*:435–456.

72. Lee, Y.-H., and Lee, V. H. L. (1993). Formulation influence on ocular and systemic absorption of topically applied atenolol in the pigmented rabbit, *J. Ocular Pharmacol.*, *9*:47–58.

73. Urtti, A. (1994). Delivery of antiglaucoma drugs: ocular versus systemic absorption, *J. Ocul. Pharmacol.*, *10*:349–357.

74. Jones, A. L., Keighley, J. E., Gold, W., and Good, A. M. (1996). Review: eye drops—the hidden poison, *Scott. Med. J.*, *41*:110–112.

75. Jay, W. M., Aziz, M. J., and Green, K. (1985). The effect of retrobulbar epinephrine injection on ocular and optic nerve blood flow, *Curr. Eye. Res.*, *4*:55–58.

76. Chast, F., Bardin, C., Sauvageon-Martre, H., Callaert, S., and Chaumeil, J. C. (1991). Systemic morphine pharmacokinetics after ocular administration, *J. Pharm. Sci.*, *80*:911–917.

77. Losa, C., Alonson, M. J., Vila, J. L., Orallo, F., Martinez, J., Saavedra, J. A., and Pastor, J. C. (1992). Reduction of cardiovascular side-effects associated with ocular administration of metipranolol by inclusion in polymeric nano-capsules, *J. Ocul. Pharmacol.*, *8*:191–198.

78. Li, B. H. P., and Chiou, G. C. Y. (1992). Systemic administration of calcitonin through the ocular route, *Life Sci.*, *50*:349–354.

79. Chiou, G. C. Y., Shen, Z. F., Zheng, Y. Q., and Chen, Y. J. (1992). Enhancement of systemic delivery of peptide drugs via the ocular route with surfactants, *Drug Dev. Res.*, *27*:177–183.

80. Harris, D., Liaw, J. H., and Robinson, J. R. (1992). Routes of delivery: case studies. (7). Ocular delivery of peptide and protein drugs, *Adv. Drug Delivery Rev.*, *8*:331–339.

81. Chiou, G. C. Y. (1994). Systemic delivery of polypeptide drugs through ocular route, *J. Ocul. Pharmacol.*, *10*:93–99.

82. Morgan, R. V. (1995). Delivery of systemic regular insulin via the ocular route in cats, *J. Ocul. Pharmacol. Ther.*, *11*:565–573.

83. Morgan, R. V., and Huntzicker, M. A. (1996). Delivery of systemic regular insulin via the ocular route in dogs, *J. Ocul. Pharmacol. Ther.*, *12*:515–526.

84. Friedrich, S. W., Saville, B. A., Cheng, Y.-L., and Rootman, D. S. (1996). Pharmacokinetic differences between ocular inserts and eye drops, *J. Ocul. Pharmacol.*, *12*:5–18.

85. Lee, Y. C., and Yalkowski, S. H. (1999). Effect of formulation on the systemic absorption of insulin from enhancer-free ocular device, *Int. J. Pharm.*, *185*:199–204.

86. Mishima, S. (1981). Clinical pharmacokinetics of the eye, *Invest. Ophthalmol. Vis. Sci.*, *21*:504–541.
87. Shell, J. W. (1982). Pharmacokinetics of topically applied ophthalmic drugs, *Surv. Ophthalmol.*, *26*:207–218.
88. Mikkelson, T. J. (1984). Review: Ophthalmic drug delivery, *Pharm. Tech.*, *8*:90–98.
89. Lee, V. H. L. (1985). Review: Topical ocular drug delivery—recent advances and future perspectives, *Pharm. Int.*, *6*:135–138.
90. Lee, V. H. L., and Robinson, J. R. (1986). Review: Topical ocular drug delivery: Recent developments and future challenges, *J. Ocul. Pharmacol.*, *2*:67–108.
91. Schoenwald, R. D. (1990). Review: Ocular drug delivery-Pharmacokinetic considerations, *Clin. Pharmacokin.*, *18*:255–269.
92. Lee, V. H. L. (1990). Review: New directions in the optimization of ocular drug delivery, *J. Ocul. Pharmacol.*, *6*:157–164.
93. Ding, S. (1998). Review: Recent advances in ophthalmic drug delivery, *Pharm. Sci. Technol. Today.*, *1*:328–335.
94. Boutlais, C. L., Acar, L., Zia, H., Sado, P. A., Needham, T., and Leverge, R. (1998). Ophthalmic drug delivery systems—recent advances, *Prog. Retinal Eye Res.*, *17*:33–58.
95. Robinson, J. C. (1993). Ocular anatomy and physiology relevant to ocular drug delivery. *Drugs Pharm. Sci.*, *58*:29–57.
96. Hosoya, K., and Lee, V. H. L. (1997). Cidofovir transport in the pigmented rabbit conjunctiva, *Curr. Eye Res.*, *16*:693–697.
97. Mishima, S., Gasset, A., Klyce, S. D., and Baum, J. L. (1966). Determination of the tear volume and tear flow, *Invest. Ophthalmol.*, *5*:264–276.
98. Maurice, D. M. (1967). The use of fluorescein in ophthalmic research, *Invest. Ophthalmol.*, *6*:464.
99. Holly, F. J. (1973). Formation and stability of the tear film, *Int. Ophthalmol. Clin.*, *13*:73.
100. Pfister, R. R. (1975). The normal surface of the conjunctival epithelium: A scanning electron microscopic study, *Invest. Ophthalmol.*, *14*:267.
101. Kessing, S. V. (1968). Mucus gland system of the conjunctiva, *Acta Ophthalmol. (Suppl.)*, *95*:133.
102. Nichols, B., Davson, C. R., and Togni, B. (1983). Surface features of the conjunctiva and cornea, *Invest. Ophthalmol. Vis. Sci.*, *24*:570–576.
103. Watsky, M. A., Jablonski, M. M., and Edelhauser, H. F. (1988). Comparison of conjunctival and corneal surface areas in rabbit and human, *Curr. Eye Res.*, *7*:483–486.
104. Ehlers, N. (1965). On the size of the conjunctival sac, *Acta Ophthalmol.*, *43*:205–210.
105. Maurice, D. M. (1984). The cornea and sclera in *The Eye* (H. Davson, ed.), Academic Press, New York, pp. 1–158.
106. Battagliolo, J. L., and Kamm, R. D. (1984). Measurements of the compressive properties of scleral tissue, *Invest. Ophthalmol. Vis. Sci.*, *25*:59–65.

107. Olsen, T. W., Aaberg, S. Y., Geroski, D. H., Edelhauser, H. F. (1998). Human sclera: thickness and surface area, *Am. J. Ophthalmol.*, *125*:237–241.
108. Keeley, F. W., Morin, J. D., and Vesely, S. (1984). Characterization of collagen from normal human sclera, *Exp. Eye Res.*, *39*:533–542.
109. Kleinstein, R. N., and Fatt, I. (1977). Pressure dependency of transscleral flow, *Exp. Eye Res.*, *24*:335–340.
110. Francoeur, M., and Patton, T. F. (1979). Kinetics of corneal drug up-take studied by corneal perfusion in situ I. Evaluation of system and up-take of ethyl p-aminobenzoate in rabbits, *Int. J. Pharmaceut.*, *2*:337–342.
111. Olejnik, O., Davis, S. S., and Wilson, C. G. (1981). A non-invasive perfusion technique for measuring the corneal permeation of drugs, *J. Pharm. Pharmacol.*
112. Krohn, D. L., and Breitfeller, J. M. (1974). Transport of pilocarpine by isolated cornea, *Invest. Ophthalmol.*, *13*:312–316.
113. Gegge, H. S., and Gipson, I. K. (1985). Removal of viable sheets of conjunctival epithelium with dipase II, *Invest. Ophthalmol. Vis. Sci.*, *26*:15–22.
114. Saha, P., Kim, K. J., and Lee, V. H. L. (1996). A primary culture model of rabbit conjunctival epithelial cells exhibiting tight barrier properties, *Curr. Eye. Res.*, *15*:1163–1169.
115. Goskonde, V. R., Khan, M. A., Hutak, C. M., and Reddy, I. K. (1999). Permeability characteristics of novel mydriatic agents using an in vitro cell culture model that utilizes sirc rabbit corneal cells, *J. Pharm. Sci.*, *88*:180–184.
116. Yang, J. J. Ueda, H., Kim, K. J., and Lee, V. H. L. (2000). Meeting future challenges in topical ocular drug delivery: Development of an air interfaced primary culture of rabbit conjunctival epithelial cells on a permeable support for drug transport studies, *J. Contr. Rel.*, *65*:1–11.
117. Sasaki, H., Igarashi, Y., Nishida, K., and Nakamura, J. (1994). Intestinal permeability of ophthalmic beta-blockers for predicting ocular permeability, *J. Pharm. Sci.*, *83*:1335–1338.
118. Zhu, Y. P., Wilson, W. S. (1996). An ex vivo model for the assessment of drug delivery to the eye: isolated bovine perfusion system, *Eur. J. Pharm. Biopharm.*, *42*:405–410.
119. Kunou, N., Ogura, Y., Honda, Y., Hyon, S. H., and Ikada, Y. (2000). Biodegradable scleral implant for controlled intraocular delivery of beta-methasone phosphate, *J. Biomed. Mat. Res.*, *51*:634–641.
120. Foroutan, S. M., and Watson, D. G. (1999). In vitro evaluation of polyethylene glycol esters of hydrocortisone esters of hydrocortisone 21-succinate as ocular prodrugs, *Int. J. Pharm.*, *182*:79–92.
121. Sasaki, H., Igarashi, Y., Nishida, K., and Nakamura, J. (1993). Ocular delivery of the beta-blocker, tilisolol, through the prodrug approach, *Int. J. Pharm.*, *93*:49–60.
122. Hamalainen, K. M., Ranta, V. P., Auriola, S., and Urtti, A. (2000). Enzymatic and permeation barrier of [D-ala (2)]-met-enkephalinamide in the anterior membranes of the albino rabbit eye, *Eur. J. Pharm. Sci.*, *9*:265–270.

123. Madhu, C., Rix, P., Nguyen, T., Chien, D. S., Woodward, D. F., and TangLiu, D. D. S. (1998). Penetration of natural prostaglandins and their ester prodrugs and analogs across human ocular tissues in vitro, *J. Ocul. Pharm. Ther.*, *14*:389–399.
124. Sasaki, H., Nagano, T., Yamamura, K., Nishida, K., and Nakamura, J. (1995). Ophthalmic preservatives as absorption promoters for ocular drug delivery, *J. Pharm. Pharmacol.*, *47*:703–707.
125. Sasaki, H., Yamamura, K., Tei, C., Nishida, K., and Nakamura, J. (1995). Ocular permeability of FITC-dextran with absorption promoter for ocular delivery of peptide drugs, *J. Drug Targeting*, *3*:129–135.
126. Chung, Y. B., Nishiura, A., and Lee, V. H. L. (1993). Pz-peptide as a novel enhancer of ocular epithelial paracellular permeability in the rabbit, *Pharm. Res.*, *10*:204.
127. Bok, C. Y., Kun, H., Akio, N., and Lee, V. H. L. (1998). Ocular absorption of pz-peptide and its effect on the ocular systemic pharmacokinetics of topically applied drugs in the rabbit, *Pharm. Res.*, *15*:1882–1887.
128. Peyman, G. A., and Ganiban, G. J. (1995). Delivery systems for intraocular routes, *Adv. Drug Delivery Rev.*, *16*:107–123.
129. Geroski, D. H., and Edelhauser, H. F. (2000). Review: Drug delivery for posterior segment eye disease, *Invest. Ophthal. Vis. Sci.*: 961–964.
130. Coltrust, M. J., Williams, R. L., Hiscott, P. S., and Grierson, I. (2000). Review: Biomaterials used in posterior segment of the eye, *Biomaterials.*, *21*:649–665.
131. Peyman, G. A., and Ganiban, G. J. (1995). Review: Delivery systems for intraocular routes, *Adv. Drug Delivery Rev.*, *16*:107–123.
132. Velez, G., and Whitcup, S. M. (1999). New developments in sustained release drug delivery for the treatment of intraocular disease, *Br. J. Ophthalmol.*, *83*:1225–1229.
133. Conroy, C. W. (1997). Sulfonamides do not reach the retina in therapeutic amounts after topical application to the cornea, *J. Ocul. Pharmacol.*, 13:465–472.
134. Lim, J. I., Maguire, A. M., John, G., Mohler, M. A., and Fiscella, R. G. (1993). Intraocular tissue plasminogen-activator concentrations after subconjunctival delivery, *Ophthalmology*, 100:373–376.
135. Pakes, S. P. (1998). V. A., Grant: Implantation of a sub-tenon drug delivery device loaded with a test article in rabbits and distribution of the test article in ocular tissues. Dept. of Veterans Administration Grant, 1998.
136. Adamis, A. P., Gragoudas, E. S., and Miller, J. W. (1999). Patent: Targeted trans-scleral controlled release drug delivery to the retina and choroid, WO 2000US207.
137. Sasaki, H., Kashiwagi, S., Mukai, T., Nishida, K., Nakamura, J., Nakashima, M., and Ichikawa, M. (1999). Drug absorption behavior after periocular injections, *Biol. Pharm. Bull.*, *22*:956–960.

138. Blair, J. M., Gionfriddo, J. R., Polazzi, L. M., Sojka, J. E., Pfaff, A. M., and Bingaman, D. P. (1999). Subconjunctivally implanted micro-osmotic pumps for continuous ocular treatment in forses, *Am. J. Vet. Res.*, *60*:1102–1105.

139. LaFranco, D. M., Tao, T. V., Yan, G. C., and Herbert, C. P. (1999). Posterior sub-Tenon's steroid injection for the treatment of posterior ocular inflammation: Indications, efficacy and side-effects, *Graefe's Arch. Clin. Exp. Ophthal.*, *237*:289–295.

140. Kunow, N., Ogura, Y., Honda, Y., Hyon, S. H., and Ikada, Y. (2000). Biodegradable sclera implant for controlled intraocular delivery of betamethasone phosphate, *J. Biomed. Res.*, *51*:635–641.

141. Schulman, J. A., Peyman, G. A., and Liu, J. (1987). The intraocular penetration of acyclovir after subconjunctival administration, *Ophthal. Surg.*, *18*:111–114.

142. Kurmala, P., Wilson, C. G., Dhillon, B., Kamal, A., and Rao, L. S. (1997). A comparison of intraocular delivery routes for an acyclovir implant using an arterially perfused sheep eye, *Pharm. Res.*, 14:S46.

143. Callegan, M. C., Mobden, J. A., O'Callaghan, R. J., and Hill, J. M. (1995). Ocular drug delivery: A comparison of transcorneal iontophoresis to corneal collagen shields, *Int. J. Pharm.*, *123*:173–179.

144. Sarraf, D., and Lee, D. A. (1994). Review: The role of iontophoresis in ocular drug delivery, *J. Ocul. Pharmacol.*, *10*:69–81.

145. Frucht, P. J., Solomon, A., Doron, R., Ever-Hadani, P., Manor, O., and Shapiro, M. (1996). Efficacy of iontophoresis in the rat cornea, *Graefe's Arch. Clin. Exp. Ophthal.*, *234*:765–769.

146. Friedberg, M. L., Pleyer, U., and Mondino, B. J. (1991). Device drug delivery to the eye. Collagen shields, iontophoresis, and pumps, *Ophthalmology.*, *98*:725–732.

147. Hill, J. M. (1991). Symposium on drug delivery. V. Ocular drug delivery; corneal collagen shields and ocular iontophoresis, *Proc. Soc. Exp. biol. Med.*, *196*:365.

148. Burstein, N., and Anderson, J. A. (1985). Review: Corneal penetration and ocular bioavailability of drugs, *J. Ocular Pharmacol.*, *1*:309–326.

149. Munjusha, M., and Majumdar, D. K. (1997). In vitro transcorneal penetration of ketorolac tromethamine from buffered and unbuffered aqueous ocular drops, *Indian J. Exp. Biol.*, *35*:941–947.

150. DeSantis, L. M., and Schoenwald, R. D. (1978). Lack of influence of rabbit nectitating membrane on miosis effect of pilocarpine, *J. Pharm. Sci.*, *67*:1189–1190.

151. Burstein, N. L., and Anderson, J. A. (1985). Review: Corneal penetration and ocular bioavailability of drugs, *J. Ocular Pharmacol.*, *3*:309–326.

152. Klyce, S. D., and Beuerman, R. W. (1988). Structure and function of the cornea, in *The Cornea* (H. E. Kaufman, B. A. Barron, M. B. McDonald, S. R. Waltman, eds.), Churchill Livingstone, New York, pp. 3–54.

153. Pepose, J. S., and Ubels, J. L. (1992). The cornea, in *Alder's Physiology of the Eye* (W. Hart, ed.), Mosby Year book, New York, pp. 29–70.

154. A. K. Mitra. Ophthalmic drug delivery. In: P. Tyle, ed. Drug Delivery Devices. New York: Marcel Dekker, 1988.

12

Ocular Iontophoresis

Marvin E. Myles, Jeannette M. Loutsch, Shiro Higaki, and James M. Hill
LSU Eye and Vision Center of Excellence, Louisiana State University Health Science Center, New Orleans, Louisiana, U.S.A.

I. IONTOPHORESIS

A. Introduction, Literature Reviews, and Citations

Iontophoresis is the use of a direct electrical current to drive topically applied ionized substances into or through a tissue (1). Iontophoresis is based on the physical principle that ions with the same charge repel (electrorepulsion) and ions with opposite charge attract (electroosmosis) (2). Iontophoresis usually employs low voltage (10 V or less) to supply a continuous direct current of 0.5 mA/cm^2 or less (1). These basic operational guidelines have enabled iontophoresis to be used to enhance drug delivery in a wide variety of conditions. The symmetry of the procedure also permits its application to the noninvasive sampling of biologically important subcutaneous fluids or for blood monitoring (3). Table 1 lists reviews on the topic and selected citations that highlight some of the innovative ways in which this modality is being used in the treatment and diagnosis of various conditions.

B. Basic Concepts and Electrical Laws

Iontophoresis causes increased transport of ionized substances into or through a tissue by application of an external electric current (14,15). Iontophoretic transport results from the passage of a current from electrodes into an electrolyte solution and thus into the skin or body. The

Table 1   Iontophoresis Reviews

Topic	Author(s)	Year	Ref.
Historical	Duke-Elder	1962	4
	Harris	1967	5
General aspects	Hughes and Maurice	1984	72
	Banga and Chien	1988	6
Principles	Singh and Maibach	1994	1
	Nair et al.	1999	7
	Guy et al.	2000	2
Dermatology	Kassan et al.	1996	33
Anesthesia	Zempsky and Ashburn	1998	61
Devices/technology	Tyle	1986	8
	Garrison	1998	9
Peptides and proteins	Hirvonen et al.	1996	10
Ocular therapy	Shofner et al.	1989	11
	Sarraf and Lee	1994	12
	Sasaki et al.	1999	13

basic electrical principle that oppositely charged ions attract and same charged ions repel is the central tenet of iontophoresis. Thus, positive ions (cations) are attracted to the negative electrode (or cathode) and repelled by the positive electrode (or anode). Conversely, negative ions (anions) are attracted to the positive electrode and repelled by the negative electrode. When iontophoresis is used therapeutically, the ions of importance are charged molecules of the drug or other bioactive substances. The ionized substances are driven into the tissues by electrorepulsion at either the anode (if they carry a positive charge) or the cathode (if they carry a negative charge) (2).

A few laws of physics and chemistry will help to delineate the important parameters in iontophoretic transport. Those parameters are the amount of drug transported, the current rate, and the amount of time that current is applied. The first law is Ohm's law:

$$V = IR$$

where V is the electromotive force in volts, I is the current in milliamperes (mA), and R is the resistance in ohms. At constant voltage, any change in resistance results in a change in the current. With iontophoresis, resistance decreases during the procedure. The result is that the current (mA) increases and must be reduced to maintain a constant current over time.

A second law important for iontophoresis is Coulomb's law:

$$Q = IT$$

where Q is the quantity of electricity, I is the current in mA, and T is the time in minutes. Thus, Q, which is the total current dosage, can be expressed as mA-minutes. Precise conditions for specific iontophoretic applications can be expressed as a minimum, maximum, or a range of mA-minutes.

Finally, a third important physical principle is Faraday's law:

$$D = \frac{IT}{IZIF}$$

where D is the drug delivered in gram-equivalents, I is the current in mA, T is the time in minutes, IZI is the valence of the drug, and F is Faraday's constant. Faraday's constant is the electrical charge carried by 1 gram-equivalent of a substance. The importance of this proportional relationship is that if more current is applied (either by increasing the current rate or increasing the time of application of a constant low current), more of the drug enters the tissue.

C. Design of Iontophoresis Devices

Iontophoretic devices vary in complexity, but the basic design is a unit with a power source (either a battery or an on-line unit with a voltage regulator), a milliampere meter to measure the current, a rheostat to control the amount of current flowing through the system, and two electrodes. Platinum is the material of choice for the electrodes, since it releases almost no ions, undergoes degradation at a slow rate, and is nontoxic.

A variety of iontophoretic apparatuses exist for use in ocular iontophoresis. They mainly consist of either an eyecup or an applicator probe. Figure 1 shows a diagram of ocular iontophoresis of a positively charged drug in a rabbit. The eyecup, with an internal diameter of ~ 1 cm, is placed over the cornea and filled with the drug solution. A metal electrode that is connected to a direct current power supply is submerged in the solution in the eyecup without making contact with the surface of the eye. The ground electrode, connected to the other terminal of the power supply, is attached to the ear of the rabbit via wet (0.9% NaCl) gauze to ensure a good connection. With the hand-held applicator probe, the metal (platinum) electrode extends into the eyecup that is filled with the drug solution. The eyecup is placed against the eye and is held in place throughout the entire iontophoresis procedure. Iontophoresis requires a complete electrical circuit with direct current passing from the anode to the cathode and from the cathode back to the anode. The two electrodes are placed as anatomically close to each other as possible on the body, which is an excellent conductor of electricity, to complete the circuit.

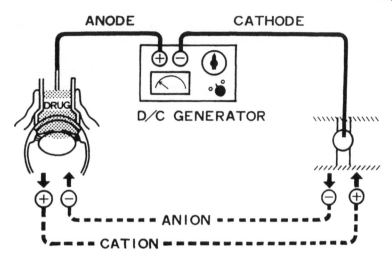

Figure 1 Ocular iontophoresis in the rabbit. The drug is placed in a cylindrical eye cup with a central diameter of 9–12 mm; the inner circumference of the eye cup fits within the corneoscleral limbus. The current is controlled by a rheostat on the direct current transformer. In general, the current should not exceed 2.0 mA and the time be no longer than 10 min. In the case illustrated here, the drug molecules (cations) have a positive charge. Therefore, the platinum electrode connected to the anode (the positively charged pole) is placed in contact with the solution. The other electrode (cathode) is connected to the ear or front leg of the rabbit to complete the circuit. The positively charged anode drives the positively charged drug molecules from the solution into the eye at a greater rate than would be observed with simple diffusion.

The drug solution or preparation to be iontophoresed should be devoid or have a minimum of extraneous ions. Drugs with one or more pKa values either below pH 6 or above pH 8 are generally excellent candidates for iontophoresis into the eye because these drugs will be in the ionized form at the physiological pH of the eye (12). The salt form of a drug is also preferred for iontophoresis since the dissociated salt is highly soluble. The drug is driven into the ocular tissue with an electrode carrying the same charge as the drug while the ground electrode, which is of the opposite charge, is placed elsewhere on the body (usually the ear) to complete the circuit. The drug or bioactive substance serves as a conductor of the current through the ocular tissue. The transported drugs or bioactive substance either remain in the tissue until they are altered/metabolized or are carried away by the blood vascular network.

II. MEDICAL APPLICATIONS OF IONTOPHORESIS

A. Archival Studies

The use of the shock of the torpedo, an electric fish, for the treatment of gout was described by Aetius, a Greek physician, more than 1000 years ago (14). In 1747, Veratti enunciated the concept of applying an electric current to increase the penetration of drugs into surface tissues (15). In 1898, Morton demonstrated that finely powdered graphite could be driven into his arm under the positive electrode and produced small black spots that persisted for weeks (16). In 1900, Leduc reported the first controlled studies of iontophoresis as a therapeutic modality (17,18). Leduc showed that transcutaneous iontophoretic delivery of strychnine and cyanide ions into rabbits produced fatal tetanic seizures and cyanide poisoning.

The earliest description of ocular iontophoresis was published in 1908 by the German investigator Wirtz (19), who performed iontophoresis of zinc salts for the treatment of corneal ulcers. In 1927, Morisot (20) enumerated many successful ophthalmological applications of iontophoresis including iontophoresis of magnesium for treatment of glaucoma, iontophoresis of ammonium chloride for treatment of cataract, and iontophoresis of phosphoric acid for treatment of optic atrophy. Erlanger was one of the first ophthalmologists to introduce iontophoresis to England and the United States. In 1936, he delivered barium chloride iontophoretically into the eyes of guinea pigs and observed cataract formation 48 hours later (21). He went on to describe the usefulness of iontophoresis in the clinical treatment of corneal ulcers, conjunctivitis, scleritis, glaucoma, and cataract (22,23).

During the 1940s in the United States, Ludwig von Sallmann, a prominent ophthalmologist, was one of the pioneers in the clinical use of ocular iontophoresis. Von Sallmann showed that transcorneal iontophoresis of penicillin was more effective than subconjunctival injection for the delivery of penicillin into the aqueous humor (24,25) and demonstrated modest success in the treatment of intraocular staphylococcal infection (26). In 1956, Witzel and his colleagues (27) published a report on the use of ocular iontophoresis as a drug delivery system for a variety of antibiotics. They found that iontophoresis was effective in the delivery of streptomycin, neomycin, and penicillin.

Despite its widespread use and study during the first 60 years of the twentieth century, iontophoresis was never fully adopted as a standard procedure. The lack of carefully controlled trials and the paucity of toxicity data were among the reasons that precluded its acceptance as a viable alternative for drug delivery. However, over the past 30–40 years, iontophoresis has been adapted for use in a variety of medical specialties, including anesthesiology, dermatology, dentistry, and ophthalmology. Table 1 provides a list of selected reviews and reports describing the recent evolution of this procedure and highlighting some of its medical applications.

B. Iontophoresis in General Medicine and Dentistry

1. Diagnosis of Cystic Fibrosis: Pilocarpine Iontophoresis

Iontophoresis of pilocarpine (28) to induce sweating to measure sweat sodium and chloride concentration is the basis of the "sweat test" that is used to diagnose cystic fibrosis (29–31). High concentrations of both sodium and chloride ions in the sweat are considered as unequivocal evidence of the disease. Although essential criteria have been established for a positive test result in both children (30) and adults (31), pilocarpine iontophoresis should be used in conjunction with other clinical features to make a definitive diagnosis. This procedure is particularly useful in children younger than 1 year old because it is essentially painless and takes only 3–5 minutes to complete.

2. Treatment of Hyperhidrosis: Tap-Water Iontophoresis

The first dermatological application of iontophoresis was to treat hyperhidrosis (32). Hyperhidrosis is a condition characterized by pathologically excessive sweating due to abnormal secretion of the eccrine sweat glands in various parts of the body [primarily the palms, soles and axillae (33–35)]. Iontophoresis of tap water has been very effective (≥90% of patients) in inhibiting palmar and plantar hyperhidrosis, but the results are less rewarding for axillary hyperhidrosis (33,35).

3. Treatment of Hypersensitive Teeth: NaF Iontophoresis

Iontophoresis of sodium fluoride to treat teeth that have become thermosensitive is a very useful and successful therapy in dentistry (36,37). Teeth previously shown to be hypersensitive to cold lose their sensitivity to heat and cold immediately after iontophoresis of sodium fluoride, and the effects are long lasting. The mechanisms by which teeth become hypersensitive and by which iontophoresis alleviates this condition are not fully understood. One theory is that exposed dentin allows fluid movement through microtubules that stretch from the pulp. Occlusion of the patent dentinal tubules would appear to be one mechanism by which sodium fluoride iontophoresis could have a beneficial effect.

4. Pediatric Anesthesia: Lidocaine Iontophoresis

Iontophoresis of anesthetics for induction of local anesthesia in pediatric office patients has been very successful (38–40). Randomized studies have found lidocaine iontophoresis to be more effective than EMLA (eutetic mixture of local anesthetics) cream or topical lidocaine (38,41), and its effectiveness has been documented for placement of pediatric intravenous catheters (39). Iontophoresis is advantageous in pediatric patients because it alleviates the pain and anxiety due to needle injections and works more rapidly than topically applied anesthetics, which take a long time to become effective (up to 1 h) and often provide incomplete anesthesia. Squire et al. (41) demonstrated that the time to accomplish topical anesthesia was shorter with iontophoresis of 2% lidocaine with epinephrine 1:100,000 (13 min) compared to a surface-applied EMLA cream [60 min (41)]. Iontophoresis of lidocaine with epinephrine is a safe, rapid, and effective method of local anesthesia delivery for pediatric procedures.

C. Iontophoretic Therapies in Ophthalmology

Table 2 provides a list of the drugs, dyes, and other charged molecules summarized below. The cations (positive ions) are used in anodal (positive electrode) iontophoresis, whereas the anions (negative ions) are used in cathodal (negative electrode) iontophoresis. Iontophoresis of the various classes of drugs (antibiotics, antivirals, antifungal, antimetabolite, adrenergic, steroid, anesthetic, and dyes) can be delivered by two approaches. *Transcorneal iontophoresis* (described earlier and in diagrammatic form in Fig. 1) delivers a high concentration of drug to the anterior segment of the eye (cornea, aqueous humor, ciliary body, and lens). In phakic animals, the lens-iris diaphragm limits penetration of a drug to the posterior tissues of the eye such as posterior vitreous and retina. This barrier can be overcome by applying the current through the pars plana (*transscleral iontophoresis*), which can produce significantly high and sustained drug concentration in the vitreous and retina. For transscleral iontophoresis, the drug solution is contained in a narrow tube within an eyecup held to the conjunctiva by suction. The tube is placed over the pars plana to avoid current damage to the retina. This technique circumvents the lens-iris barrier and delivers drugs into the vitreous or retina. Figure 2 shows a diagram of a transscleral iontophoresis device and setup.

Within the past 10 years, a number of excellent articles/chapters have reviewed the application of iontophoresis in therapeutic approaches in ophthalmology (11,12,42–44). Current research in ocular iontophoresis is aimed at resolving the delivery problems associated with newly developed

Table 2 Drugs Used in Ocular Iontophoresis

Class	Drug	Site	Ion	Application	Ref.
Antibiotic	Gentamicin	Transcorneal	Cation	Tx Pseudomonal keratitis	70–78
	Tobramycin	Transcorneal	Cation	Tx Pseudomonal keratitis	79–82
	Ciprofloxacin	Transscleral	Cation	Tx Pseudomonal keratitis	83–85
	Vancomycin	Transcorneal	Cation	Tx Pseudomonal keratitis	86
	Ticarcillin	Transscleral	Anion	Tx Endophthalmitis	75
	Cefazolin	Transscleral	Anion	Tx Endophthalmitis	75
Antiviral	Foscarnet	Transscleral	Anion	Tx CMV retinitis	91–101
	Ara-AMP	Transcorneal	Anion	Tx Herpes keratitis; stromal disease	104–106
	Iododeoxyuridine	Transcorneal	Anion	Tx Herpes keratitis	107
	Acyclovir	Transcorneal	Anion	Tx Herpes stromal disease	107
Antifungal	Ketoconazole	Transcorneal	Cation	Tx Fungal infection	87
Antimetabolite	5-Fluorouracil	Transscleral	Anion	Glaucoma surgery, Tx ocular tumors	59,60
Adrenergic	Epinephrine	Transcorneal	Cation	HSV-1 shedding	110,115–126
	Timolol maleate	Transcorneal	Cation	HSV-1 shedding	127–129
	β-Propranolol	Transcorneal	Cation	HSV-1 shedding	130–133
	6-Hydroxydopamine	Transcorneal	Cation	Tx glaucoma	54–57
	α-Methylparatyrosine	Transcorneal	Cation	Tx glaucoma	58
Steroid	Dexamethasone	Transscleral	Anion	Tx Inflammation	64–69
	Hydrocortisone	Transcorneal		Tx Inflammation	64
Generic	Lidocaine	Transcorneal	Cation	Anesthesia	61–63
Dyes	Lysophosphatidic acid	Transcorneal	Anion	HSV-1 reactivation	163
	Fluorescein	Transcorneal	Anion	Study aqueous humor dynamics	45–48
	Methylene blue	Transscleral	Cation	Laser sclerostomy; Tx glaucoma	49–52
	reactive black 5	Transscleral	Anion	Laser sclerostomy; Tx glaucoma	53

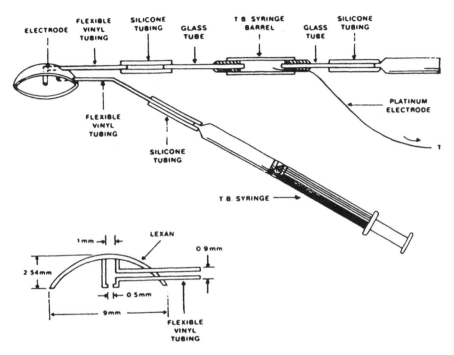

Figure 2 Diagram of apparatus used for transscleral iontophoresis. (Adapted from Ref. 75.)

drugs, techniques, and therapies. This section discusses the literature concerning the use of iontophoresis for delivery of anesthetics to the eye and in the treatment/study of glaucoma, ocular infections, ocular inflammation, and ocular herpes infection.

1. Glaucoma

a. Fluorescein for Studies of Aqueous Humor Dynamics Fluorescein is an orange-colored dye that is soluble in water and has a negative charge in solution. In 1966, Jones and Maurice (45) published a new procedure for measuring the rate of flow of the aqueous humor in patients using iontophoresis of fluorescein (10% solution) and a slit-lamp fluorophotometer. The solution was iontophoresed for 10–15 seconds with a current of 0.2 mA. Other early investigators included Starr (46), who reported results similar to those of Jones and Maurice (45) using iontophoresis of fluorescein at 0.2 mA for 30–60 seconds (s), and Holm (47), who observed pupillary flow of fluorescein after saturating the anterior chamber by iontophoresis (0.5 mA for 4 min) through a cotton-wick electrode.

A review of the procedures and techniques used to study the flow of aqueous humor in the eye was published by Brubaker in 1982 (48). He noted that these methods were essentially equivalent to those described by Jones and Maurice (45). After application of topical anesthesia, a gel 5 mm in diameter containing 2% agar and 10% fluorescein was placed on the central cornea. The power source was a 45 V battery. The agar gel constituted the negative electrode, and to complete the circuit, the patient held the positive electrode in his hand. The current (0.2 mA) was applied for 5–7 seconds. In more than 10,000 iontophoretic applications of fluorescein, no obvious side effects of the iontophoretic procedure were observed.

b. Dyes for Laser Sclerostomy   Pulsed dye laser sclerostomy is an adjunctive procedure used in the treatment of glaucoma (49). The pulsed dye laser procedure uses a gonioscopic approach for the ab interno delivery of visible laser light. The procedure requires a full thickness penetration of a dye throughout a 1–2 mm^2 area of scleral tissue for adequate absorption of the visible light energy. The light beam is transmitted through the cornea, crosses the anterior chamber, and ablates stained limbal scleral tissue with the formation of a fistula [a filtration channel for intraocular pressure (IOP) release (49)].

Methylene blue dye is water soluble and has a positive electrical charge in solution. It has an absorption peak of 668 nm and is used to enhance the optical absorption of scleral tissue (49). Latina et al. (50) iontophoresed 1% methylene blue at the limbal region of 35 glaucoma patients. The current applied was 5.0 μA for a duration of 4–8 minutes. To create the sclerostomy, the laser energy (200–250 mJ), delivered by a slit-lamp, was focused onto the dyed sclera, using a goniolens, so that only a light beam penetrated the eye. The red wavelength of 660 nm generated by the laser was maximally absorbed by the stained sclera and created a complete sclerostomy. Successful sclerostomies were achieved in 21 of 35 patients (~60%) with a reduction in IOP from a mean preoperative value of 35 mmHg to a mean postoperative value (at 9 months) of 22 mmHg. Melamed (51) obtained similar results with a 58% success rate for complete sclerostomies and a reduction in IOP from a mean preoperative IOP of 36.6 mmHg to a mean postoperative IOP of 23.7 mmHg. Grossman et al. (52) examined the stability of iontophoresed methylene blue in rabbit eyes. Decreased dye concentration of over 50% within 2 hours and a complete disappearance of dye within 24 hours were demonstrated. They also noted that the stain tended to bleach from the laser dye exposure. This prevented further absorption of the laser energy, resulting in incomplete scleral ablation and fistula formation. Melamed (51) reported blanching of the stained sclera after the first laser shots, which adversely affected the efficacy of subsequent shots.

Reactive black-5 (RB5) is a water-soluble black dye that is negatively charged at the physiological pH of the eye. RB5 has been proposed as an alternative dye to stain the scleral tissue (53). RB5 stain was subjected to a number of different conditions simulating laser treatment of the sclera. The stain was stable over time (72 h) and stable when exposed to high temperature (120°C), to scleral breakdown products (collagen), to strong oxidants (1.5% H_2O_2), and to laser light energy (53). Optimal parameters for iontophoretic delivery of RB5 into limbal scleral tissue were also determined. Ideal parameters for iontophoresis included a probe tip surface area between 0.1 and 0.7 mm^2, a current of 0.5 mA, and a duration of 5 minutes. Using these parameters for iontophoresis, the maximum concentration of RB5 achieved in sclera was 0.15% (53). This value is considerably greater than the threshold for ablation of 0.001% RB5 using a laser energy of 250 mJ. Thus, iontophoresis can deliver an amount of RB5 stain to the sclera that is more than sufficient for laser ablation. This approach obviates conjunctival dissection and decreases the stimulus for episcleral scarring that eventually could cause reelevation of intraocular pressure (49,52,53).

c. Adrenergic Agents for Treatment of Glaucoma 6-Hydroxydopamine and α-methylparatyrosine are two pharmacological agents that block the synthesis of norepinephrine. 6-Hydroxydopamine, a congener of norepinephrine, causes the reversible destruction of nerve terminals in the anterior segment. In the early to mid-1970s, a number of investigators (54–58) used iontophoresis to deliver these substances to the eyes of rabbits, normal volunteers, and glaucoma patients with primary open-angle glaucoma. The theory behind the treatment involved the depletion of ocular norepinephrine, which would result in an increased sensitivity to glaucoma drugs such as epinephrine.

Kitazawa et al. (54,55) were the first to report the results of iontophoresis of 6-hydroxydopamine in rabbits and human eyes. A 1% solution of 6-hydroxydopamine was iontophoresed at 0.75 mA for 3 minutes. High concentrations of 6-hydroxydopamine were achieved in ocular tissues in rabbits, and intraocular pressure was reduced in normal human eyes. Subsequently, Kitazawa et al. (56) treated patients with primary open-angle glaucoma with a combination therapy of iontophoresed 6-hydroxydopamine and topical epinephrine. The results led them to conclude that this combination therapy had clinical value in the management of open-angle glaucoma.

Iontophoresis of 6-hydroxydopamine to treat primary open-angle glaucoma was also examined by Watanabe et al. (57). For the patients for whom they had sufficient data for analysis (49/100), this procedure was therapeutically effective in 41%, questionable in 31%, and ineffective in 28%.

Colasanti and Trotter (58) performed ocular iontophoresis of α-methylparatyrosine in rabbits. A 4.0% α-methylparatyrosine solution was iontophoresed at a current of 3 mA for 5 minutes. This drug is similar to 6-hydroxydopamine, and it also produced a significant decrease in the norepinephrine concentration in rabbit ocular tissues. No clinical studies with α-methylparatyrosine were done in normal human eyes or in patients with primary open-angle glaucoma.

These results demonstrated that iontophoresis of 6-hydroxydopamine was a viable method of sensitizing the eyes to glaucoma drugs and that this procedure had some clinical value in the management of this disease. However, with the advent of long-acting antiglaucoma drugs such as timolol, levobunolol, and betaxolol, iontophoresis of 6-hydroxydopamine for the therapy of glaucoma was discontinued.

d. 5-Fluorouracil for Control of Cellular Proliferation After Glaucoma Surgery 5-Fluorouracil (5-FU) acts as an antiproliferative agent to prevent cellular replication. The concentration of 5-FU required for 50% inhibition of rabbit conjunctival fibroblasts in culture is 0.2–0.5 μg/mL (59). 5-FU is a small, negatively charged molecule with a pKa of ∼ 8. Kondo and Araie (60) were the first to report iontophoresis of 5-FU to the rabbit eye. A 5% solution of 5-FU containing 8.47% tris(hydroxymethyl)aminomethane was delivered transsclerally at 0.5 mA for 30 seconds. An electrode 7 mm in diameter was placed on the bulbar conjunctiva 4 mm posterior to the limbus in the superior temporal quadrant. Iontophoresis of 30-second duration delivered enough 5-FU into ocular tissue such that 30 minutes later the drug concentration was 50 μg/g and 21 μg/g in conjunctival and scleral tissue, respectively. Over the next 10 hours, the amount of 5-FU decreased to 0.6 μg/g in the conjunctiva and 1.2 μg/g in the sclera. These concentrations are still high enough to have a therapeutic effect.

Transscleral iontophoresis of 5-FU would eliminate the need for subconjunctival injection and its unwanted complications (risk of bleeding, infections, scarring, and drug penetration into other ocular tissues). Iontophoretically delivered 5-FU may improve the efficacy of antiglaucoma surgery (e.g., sclerostomy) by interfering with healing and thereby maintaining patency of the fistulas. To date, however, no studies have been done in experimental models of disease or in human eyes.

2. Ocular Anesthesia

The deliver of local anesthetics by iontophoresis has been very successful (61–63). Iontophoretically delivered anesthetics can provide topical anesthesia within 5–15 minutes with limited systemic absorption (61). The anesthetic solutions used most often are a combination of lidocaine and epinephrine.

Sisler (62) iontophoresed anesthetic solutions containing either 4% lidocaine with 1:1000 epinephrine or 2% lidocaine with 1:2000 epinephrine to patients with lesions of the tarsus and tarsal conjunctiva prior to surgical excision of conjunctival plaques. A current 0.5 mA was applied for 10 minutes. Twenty-seven patients were treated. None of the patients reported any discomfort in the eyelids or the arm to which the negative electrode was attached; only a mild sensation was described. Three patients with lesions in the deeper portion of the tarsus reported pain and were given an injection to achieve local anesthesia. This is the only report describing iontophoretic delivery of an anesthetic agent to adnexal areas for pain prevention.

Meyer et al. (63) iontophoresed a 4% lidocaine solution to eyelids of patients for local anesthesia prior to blepharoplasty or ptosis repair. A current of 2 mA was applied for 12 minutes. Ten normal volunteers were used so as to compare pain sensations after anesthesia by iontophoresis or topical application of the anesthetic. Both surgical patients and volunteers reported significantly less pain after iontophoresis of the anesthetic. No side effects of this iontophoresis procedure were observed.

3. Ocular Inflammation

Corticosteroids are the most common drugs used in treating ocular inflammatory disorders (64–67). Topical drop application is preferred to avoid the serious systemic side effects of steroids (68). However, this mode of administration does not allow for sufficient drug delivery to the posterior segment of the eye. Iontophoretic delivery of anti-inflammatory drugs into the eye has been examined in human and various animal models and offers a viable alternative to topical or systemic administration.

Lachaud (65) iontophoresed hydrocortisone acetate (0.1% solution) into rabbit eyes with a current of 3 mA for 10 minutes. He demonstrated that iontophoresis could deliver higher concentrations of steroid to rabbit ocular tissue than either topical drops (0.5%) or subconjunctival injection (0.1 mL, 2.5%). In human studies, Lachaud iontophoresed dexamethasone acetate (7 mg%, 1–2 mA, 20 min) to treat a variety of clinical conditions, including idiopathic uveitis. He reported that a significant proportion of the patients with uveitis benefited in terms of more rapid recovery and/or increased comfort. Lachaud (65) concluded that iontophoresis resulted in therapeutic concentrations of the steroid(s) in ocular tissue. However, it must be noted that this open clinical study did not involve comparisons with eyes receiving other therapies or with untreated control eyes.

Lam et al. (66) iontophoresed a 30% dexamethasone solution transsclerally into rabbit eyes using 1.6 mA for 25 minutes. The diameter of the cylinder holding the drug solution in contact with the sclera was 0.7 mm. They compared peak steroid concentrations in the choroid-retinal tissue following iontophoresis, subconjunctival injection (1 mg) or retrobulbar injection (1 mg). The peak steroid concentration (µg/g tissue) for iontophoresis was 122, for subconjunctival injection 18.1, and for retrobulbar injection 6.6. In the vitreous humor the values were 140, 0.2, and 0.3 µg/mL, respectively. Even at 24 hours after iontophoresis, significant therapeutic levels of dexamethasone remained 3.3 µg/mL in the vitreous and 3.9 µg/g in the choroid-retina.

Behar-Cohen et al. (67) investigated the efficacy of iontophoretic delivery of dexamethasone for the treatment of endotoxin-induced uveitis in the rat. Dexamethasone was delivered by concurrent transcorneal-transscleral iontophoresis (1% at 0.4 mA for 4 min) using a 1 mL reservoir electrode that covered the cornea, the limbus, and the first millimeter of the sclera. They showed that administration of dexamethasone by iontophoresis inhibited anterior and posterior signs of intraocular inflammation (protein exudation, cellular infiltration) as effectively as systemic administration. Cytokine (TNF-α) (69) expression was inhibited in the anterior as well as the posterior segment of the eye. No clinical or histological damage was caused by iontophoresis. Thus, iontophoresis can deliver therapeutic doses of this anti-inflammatory drug to the posterior as well as the anterior segment of the eye and may be a viable alternative to systemic administration of corticoids in severe ocular inflammation.

4. Ocular Infection

Transcorneal iontophoresis of antibiotics is an effective means of treatment for bacterial keratitis and other anterior segment infections. Transcorneal iontophoresis delivers therapeutic concentrations of antibiotics to the cornea and aqueous humor. In phakic animals, the lens-iris diaphragm limits penetration of the drug into the posterior tissues of the eye such as posterior vitreous and retina. Transscleral iontophoresis circumvents the lens-iris barrier and delivers drugs into the vitreous or retina in amounts high enough to be therapeutic in the treatment of posterior segment infections, such as endophthalmitis. Numerous studies have documented successful iontophoretic delivery of various antibiotics into ocular tissues of animal models. Examples are summarized below.

a. Gentamicin: Transcorneal and/or Transscleral The aminoglycoside gentamicin has a molecular weight of approximately 430 daltons, is lipid insoluble, and bears two positive charges at physiologic pH (70). It possesses bactericidal properties against a wide variety of gram-negative and gram-positive bacteria (71). Gentamicin concentrations of 5 mg/mL inhibit over 90% of *Pseudomonas* (71), *Proteus rettgeri, P. vulgaris,* and *P. morganii* strains, as well as 99% of *Staphylococcus* strains (70). These molecular features, combined with the extreme sensitivity of the target organisms, make gentamicin an ideal drug for iontophoresis.

Hughes and Maurice (72) found that transcorneal iontophoresis of gentamicin in the rabbit eye increased permeability to the antibiotic more than 100-fold, compared with control eyes in which topical application was performed under the same iontophoretic conditions but with no current applied. Grossman et al. (70) iontophoresed 10% gentamicin in a 2% agar solution into rabbit corneas. They demonstrated that significantly higher and longer-lasting gentamicin concentrations were achieved in the cornea with iontophoresis as compared to subconjunctival injection of a 20 mg dose. Frucht-Pery et al. (73) showed that higher current density did not significantly enhance antibiotic penetration into rabbit cornea, but bactericidal concentrations of gentamicin could be obtained. Frucht-Pery et al. (74) also described the distribution of transcorneally iontophoresed gentamicin in the rabbit cornea. They found that the highest concentrations of the drug were in the central cornea, while the midperipheral cornea(s) had higher levels than peripheral cornea(s).

Fishman et al. (71) described iontophoresis of gentamicin to uninfected aphakic rabbit eyes. Gentamicin iontophoresis (50 mg/mL at 0.75 mA for 10 min) yielded peak corneal (71 μg/g of tissue) and aqueous humor (78 μg/mL) concentrations 30 minutes after treatment. The peak vitreous concentration (10.4 mg/mL) was observed 16 hours after treatment. Therapeutic concentrations of gentamicin were still present in the vitreous 24 hours after iontophoresis. This study suggests that even transcorneal iontophoresis has the potential to deliver high concentrations of gentamicin to the posterior segment in aphakic eyes. Since many patients with endophthalmitis are aphakic, transcorneal iontophoresis could be a suitable route of administration of antibiotics for therapeutic management of this disease.

Barza et al. (75) modified the standard transcorneal procedures to achieve direct delivery of high concentrations of gentamicin into the vitreous by transscleral iontophoresis. First, a reservoir holding the drug was placed over the pars plana, thereby bypassing the lens-iris barrier. Second, the contact area of the fluid that delivered both the antibiotic and the current was kept small (approximately 1 mm in diameter). They reported that transscleral iontophoresis delivered therapeutic concentrations (94–207 μg/mL) of gentamicin to the vitreous humor of uninfected rabbit eyes, thus obviating the need for intraocular injections.

Another study from the same laboratory (76) demonstrated that transscleral iontophoresis of gentamicin is a useful adjunct to intravitreal injections for the treatment of endophthalmitis caused by *pseudomonas aeruginosa*. They showed that rabbits receiving both intravitreal injection and transscleral iontophoresis of gentamicin had lower bacteria counts at each treatment interval compared to rabbits that received gentamicin by a single intravitreal injection of a 100 µg dose. These results support the use of iontophoresis of gentamicin as a useful supplement to intravitreal injection for the treatment of bacterial endophthalmitis.

Grossman et al. (70) reported that transscleral iontophoresis of gentamicin produced results similar to their findings with transcorneal iontophoresis described above. Iontophoresis of 10% gentamicin in 2% agar solution at 2 mA for 10 minutes with a contact area of 2 mm in diameter delivered very high concentrations of gentamicin to the vitreous humor of rabbit eyes. Vitreous concentrations peaked (53.4 µg/mL) 16 hours after iontophoresis and remained at inhibitory levels even at 24 hours. As with transcorneal iontophoresis (70), no ocular tissue toxicity or damage was observed with transscleral iontophoresis.

Burstein et al. (77) reported that transscleral iontophoresis of gentamicin into uninfected rabbit eyes resulted in antibiotic concentrations of 10–20 µg/mL in the vitreous humor. These concentrations are significantly lower than the concentration range (94–207 µg/mL) reported by Barza et al. (75) in rabbit eyes. The authors found that the total surface area of the electrode is inversely proportional to the amount of antibiotic delivered, e.g., a 4.5 mm^2 applicator delivers approximately 20 times more drug to the vitreous than a 28 mm^2 applicator. This result reinforced the conclusion of Barza et al. (75,76) that a small area of contact in iontophoresis results in a higher concentration of drug in the eye.

Barza's research group (78) also reported the first use of a nonhuman primate (the cynomolgus monkey) to study the pharmacokinetics of transsclerally delivered gentamicin and/or potential histological damage of transscleral iontophoresis. High and sustained concentrations of antibiotics were achieved in the vitreous. Although small burns were observed in the area of the pars plana where the electrode was applied, all electroretinograms were normal. The results suggest that transscleral iontophoresis is well tolerated in the primate eye and that investigations with human eyes may yield alternative treatment options. The absence of side effects with the agar-based delivery system of Grossman et al. (70) is noteworthy. This formulation may facilitate the use of transscleral iontophoresis as a treatment of choice for patients with bacterial endophthalmitis or other clinical conditions that require high concentrations of antibiotics in the posterior segment.

b. Tobramycin: Transcorneal Transcorneal iontophoresis of the aminoglycoside tobramycin has been examined by our group in studies with the normal rabbit eye. Rootman et al. (79) were the first to demonstrate the efficacy of iontophoresed tobramycin for the treatment of experimental *Pseudomonas* keratitis. Rabbit corneas were infected with 10^3 colony-forming units of *P. aeruginosa*. Transcorneal iontophoresis of a 2.5% tobramycin solution at 0.8 mA for 10 minutes was performed at 22, 27, and 32 hours after inoculation. On average, the treated corneas had a 6 log reduction in colony-forming units relative to untreated corneas. At 32 hours postinoculation, 67% of the corneas had no viable bacteria (i.e., were sterile). Topically applied or subconjunctival injection of tobramycin did not yield corneas free of viable (infectious) *Pseudomonas*.

In other studies, Hill and associates examined the pharmacokinetics of iontophoresed tobramycin and/or potential toxicity to the corneal epithelium of transcorneal iontophoresis (80,81). In uninfected, mock-infected, and *P. aeruginosa*–infected rabbit corneas, transcorneal iontophoresis produced high and sustained concentration of the antibiotic in the corneal epithelium, corneal stroma, and aqueous humor (80,81). Iontophoresis delivered five times more drug than bathing the cornea with a 2.5% tobramycin solution and 20 times more the applying 1.36% tobramycin as fortified drops (80). No permanent abnormalities were observed by slit-lamp biomicroscopy, scanning electron microscopy, or light microscopy (81). After 10 minutes of iontophoresis, the epithelium showed focal edema and disruption of all cell layers. Histological specimens obtained 8 and 16 hours after iontophoresis showed no defects in the corneal epithelium.

The efficacy of iontophoretically delivered tobramycin was examined using a tobramycin-resistant strain of *Pseudomonas* (82). A strain of *P. aeruginosa* with a minimum inhibitory concentration (MIC) for tobramycin of 31 μg/mL was injected into the corneal stroma in rabbit eyes. Transcorneal iontophoresis of 2.5% tobramycin resulted in a 3 log reduction in the number of bacteria. These results show that transcorneal iontophoresis can deliver concentrations of tobramycin high enough to combat a clinically tobramycin-resistant strain of *Pseudomonas*.

c. Ciprofloxacin: Transcorneal/Transscleral Ciprofloxacin, a very potent fluoroquinolone antibiotic, is active against a broad spectrum of gram-positive and gram-negative bacteria (83). Hobden et al. (84) used transcorneal iontophoresis to deliver ciprofloxacin to rabbit corneas infected with an aminoglycoside-resistant strain of *Pseudomonas*. Iontophoresis of 1% or 2.5% ciprofloxacin reduced the number of colony-forming units by more than 5 log relative to untreated controls. This level of inhibition was significantly greater than either topically applied drops (0.75%

ciprofloxacin) or corneal bathing with an eyecup containing 2.5% cipro-floxacin for 10 minutes. The concentration of ciprofloxacin in the aqueous humor following iontophoresis (84 µg/mL) was significantly higher than that with drops (30 µg/mL) or corneal bathing (25 µg/mL). This was the first report of iontophoresis of a fluoroquinolone for therapy of experi-mental *Pseudomonas* keratitis (84).

Yoshizumi et al. (85) used transscleral iontophoresis to deliver cipro-floxacin to the aqueous humor and vitreous body of the rabbit eye. Ciprofloxacin molecules carrying either a positive or negative charge were tested. Therapeutic concentrations of antibiotic were achieved in the ante-rior chamber only when the negatively charged drug molecule was used. Transscleral iontophoresis did not deliver therapeutic concentrations of either charged form (+ or =) of the molecule to the posterior segment. Peak concentrations were obtained in the aqueous (0.62 µg/mL) and vit-reous bodies (0.19 µg/mL) one hour after transscleral iontophoresis of nega-tively charged ciprofloxacin at 5 mA for 15 minutes. These concentrations reached the MIC_{90} for several organisms that commonly cause endophthal-mitis: *Staphyloccus aureus* (0.5 µg/mL), *Staphylcoccus epidermidis* (0.5 µg/mL), and *Pseudomonas aeruginosa* (0.5 µg/mL) (85).

d. Vancomycin: Transcorneal/Transscleral Vancomycin, a complex glycopolypeptide antibiotic with a high molecular weight (1448 daltons), is very active against gram-positive bacteria. Choi and Lee (86) were the first to report that vancomycin could be applied to the eye by transcorneal iontophoresis. A 5% solution of the antibiotic was iontophoresed at 0.5 mA for 5 minutes with an area of contact between the drug solution and the cornea of 30 mm^2. Peak antibiotic levels in the cornea (12.4 µg/mL) were obtained 30 minutes after transcorneal iontophoresis. By compari-son, a 25 mg subconjunctival injection resulted in a peak concentration of 14.7 µg/mL. This study demonstrated that iontophoresis could be used to deliver therapeutic concentrations of a high molecular weight antibiotic to the cornea and is a viable alternative to subconjunctival injection.

These investigators also studied transscleral iontophoresis for delivery of vancomycin to the vitreous humor (86). The contact area was approxi-mately 25–30 mm^2 of the temporal sclera overlying the pars plana. A 5% vancomycin solution was iontophoresed at 3.5 mA for 10 minutes. Peak antibiotic concentration (13.4 µg/mL) in the vitreous was reached 2 hours after iontophoresis. Even at 16 hours postiontophoresis, the concentration of vancomycin in the vitreous was still relatively high (3 µg/mL). This study reported that bactericidal concentrations for gram-positive organisms iso-lated from patients with endophthalmitis were less than or equal to 4 µg/mL (86). Thus, iontophoresis clearly delivered enough antibiotic to be therapeutically useful. This is the first report of transscleral iontophoresis of a high molecular weight glycopolypeptide antibiotic.

e. Cefazolin and Ticarcillin: Transscleral Barza et al. (75), using the modifications previously described, also reported that therapeutic concentrations of cefazolin and ticarcillin could be delivered to the vitreous humor of uninfected rabbit eyes by transscleral iontophoresis instead of intraocular injection. Cefazolin, a first-generation cephalosporin, has excellent gram-positive and gram-negative antibacterial activity. Ticarcillin, the disodium salt of penicillin, is particularly useful in treating *P. aeruginosa* infections. Cefazolin and ticarcillin bear negative charges (one and two, respectively) and were applied with the negative electrode in the antibiotic solution. Application of 2 mA for 10 minutes yielded mean vitreal concentrations of 94–207 mg/mL in the normal rabbit eye. Drug penetration correlated with strength of current (0.1–2 mA) and duration of iontophoresis (1–10 min). A two- to fourfold variation in the concentration of the drug solution did not alter the total amount of drug delivered under constant current and time. The authors concluded that the concentrations produced in the rabbit eye are in the range expected from intravitreal injection in humans. However, the volume of vitreous humor in an adult human eye is about three times that of the rabbit eye. Therefore, the expected peak concentrations in humans would be about one third of those obtained in the rabbit.

f. Ketoconazole: Transcorneal/Transscleral Ketoconazole is a relatively nontoxic, broad-spectrum, imidazole antifungal agent that is used in the treatment of various forms of ocular fungal keratitis, including *Candida albicans*, histoplasmosis, and *Cryptococcus neoformans*. Grossman et al. (87) performed both transcorneal and transscleral iontophoresis of ketoconazole and measured the resulting drug concentrations in the aqueous and vitreous humor as well as the cornea of the rabbit eye. Transcorneal iontophoresis (1.5 mA for 15 min) resulted in peak corneal ketoconazole concentrations of 27.6 µg/mL and peak aqueous concentrations of 1.4 µg/mL 1 hour posttreatment. These drug levels are inhibitory for many fungal pathogens and transcorneal iontophoresis of ketoconazole may be an effective means of treating anterior segment fungal infections.

Transscleral iontophoresis (4–6 mA for 15 min) resulted in peak aqueous ketoconazole concentrations of 10.2 µg/mL 1 hour after iontophoresis and fungicidal levels were present even after 8 hours. Both the aqueous and corneal concentrations of ketoconazole were significantly higher after iontophoresis than after subconjunctival injection. Transscleral iontophoresis resulted in peak vitreal ketoconazole concentrations of 0.1 µg/mL 1–2 hours posttreatment. By comparison, a subconjunctival injection of ketoconazole produced a peak concentration of 0.7 µg/mL 1 hour after injection. Since neither of these values is sufficient for therapeutic fungicidal activity, the treatment of endophthalmitis by transscleral iontophoresis or subconjunctival injection of ketoconazole is questionable at best.

5. Antiviral Agent for Treatment of Cytomegalovirus Retinitis

Human cytomegalovirus is a member of the herpesvirus family, which also includes the herpes simplex (discussed below), varicella zoster, and Epstein-Barr viruses (88,89). Cytomegalovirus (CMV) and herpes simplex are the most studied of the microorganisms responsible for the opportunistic infections associated with acquired immunodeficiency syndrome (AIDS) (90). Cytomegalovirus infection in AIDS patients is most commonly manifested as retinitis (CMV retinopathy) and is the most common cause of blindness in AIDS patients (90).

Foscarnet (trisodium phosphonoformate) inhibits all human herpes viruses in vitro, including CMV (91), and intravenously administered foscarnet is currently available for treatment of CMV infections and/or retinitis (92,93). The treatment regimen for CMV retinitis consists of an initial induction dose (180 mg/kg of body mass per day for 2 weeks) followed by a maintenance dose (120 mg/kg/day indefinitely) (92,93). Since foscarnet prevents replication of the viral DNA but does not eliminate the virus from the tissues, CMV eventually reactivates and the lesions enlarge so that higher doses of the drug have to be administered. This mode of administering foscarnet may result in serious systemic toxicity (92,93). Intravitreal injection of foscarnet has been reported but also suffers from many of the same complications (endophthalmitis, increased intraocular pressure, retinal detachment, etc.) associated with other modes of ocular injection (94–96). Foscarnet is an ideal candidate for iontophoresis, since it is ionized at the physiological pH of the eye, is soluble in water, and has a molecular weight of 300.1 (91,97).

Sarraf et al. (97) studied the vitreous pharmacokinetics of foscarnet (24 mg/mL solution) after transscleral iontophoresis into normal rabbit eyes. The iontophoretic probe was applied perpendicular over the conjunctiva 1–3 mm posterior to the corneoscleral limbus. The surface area of the probe was $\sim$0.2 mm^2. The current applied was 1.0 mA for a 10-minute duration. Intravitreal samples were obtained at 12 time points (15 and 30 min and 1, 2, 4, 8, 16, 24, 32, 40, 48, and 60 h) after iontophoresis or subconjunctival injection and analyzed by HPLC. Mean vitreous concentrations of foscarnet were within the therapeutic range (25–800 µM) (91) for inhibition of CMV as early as 15 minutes posttreatment. A peak vitreal foscarnet concentration of 200 ± 311 µM was observed 4 hours after iontophoresis. This concentration is well below the concentration reported to cause retinal toxicity (>2000 μM) (94). Therapeutic levels of foscarnet for CMV retinitis were maintained for up to 60 hours posttreatment. These levels were well above the range (10–25 μM) at which foscarnet is active against HIV (93). No toxic effects to the sclera, cornea, anterior chamber, or lens were observed by biomicroscopy.

Yoshizumi et al. (98) characterized the utility of foscarnet iontophoresis for the treatment of CMV retinitis. The possible retinotoxic effects of transscleral iontophoresis of foscarnet were examined by slit-lamp biomicroscopy, indirect ophthalmicroscopy, light and electron microscopy, and electroretinography (ERG) (98). Slit-lamp examination (SLE) revealed no toxic effects for any of the treated eyes. Indirect ophthalmicroscopy showed retinal and choroidal burns 1–3 mm in diameter at the site of iontophoresis. Light and electron microscopy showed focal retinal, retinal pigment epithelial, and choroidal necrosis at the site of iontophoresis but no abnormalities elsewhere. ERG studies showed no changes in the response between foscarnet-treated eyes and saline-treated control eyes. The lesions reported were minimal and judged to be equivalent to or less than those that would have been created by an intravitreal injection or surgical implantation of an intraocular drug delivery device (99).

Another study from Yoshizumi's group (100) demonstrated that ocular iontophoresis of foscarnet could supplement intravenous injection of foscarnet in the management of CMV retinopathy. Foscarnet (120 or 180 mg/kg) was injected intravenously into one group of rabbits and peak concentrations in the serum and vitreous were determined at 1, 4, 8, 24, 60, and 120 hours after injection. A second group of rabbits, injected with the same dose of foscarnet, received ocular foscarnet iontophoresis 1 hour after the injection. Vitreous humor samples were obtained at the same time points as for group one. Maximum serum and vitreous humor concentrations were obtained 1 hour after each intravenous dose. Peak vitreous humor concentrations were obtained 4 hours after the 120 mg/kg intravenous dose plus iontophoresis and 8 hours after the 180 mg/kg intravenous dose plus iontophoresis. Vitreous humor levels of foscarnet were significantly higher in eyes receiving intravenous foscarnet plus ocular foscarnet iontophoresis than in those receiving intravenous foscarnet alone (126.77 μM vs. 7.63 μM for the group receiving 120 mg/kg; $p < 0.00001$ and 86.92 μM vs. 7.43 μM for the group receiving 180 μg/kg; $p < 0.00001$). The difference in vitreous humor levels observed in eyes receiving the intravenous dose plus iontophoresis (either 120 or 180 mg/kg) was not significant ($p < 0.1$). Although the intravenous dose was administered 1 hour prior to ocular iontophoresis, it did not significantly affect the levels obtained after ocular iontophoresis ($p < 0.1$). The authors concluded that the increased foscarnet concentrations obtained with ocular iontophoresis could be a valuable adjunct to intravenous injection in the treatment of CMV retinitis.

A subsequent study from Yoshizumi and associates examined the ocular toxicity of multiple applications of foscarnet iontophoresis (101). They performed multiple ocular iontophoretic applications of foscarnet at the same paralimbal site for a total of seven treatments over a period of 21 days (one treatment every 3 days). This was done to mimic the repeated treatments that may be necessary for long-term iontophoretic therapy for treatment of CMV retinitis and/or AIDS (92,93). The mean concentration of foscarnet in the vitreous humor 4 hours after the seventh ocular iontophoresis was 189 ± 50.6 μM. These levels are clearly within the therapeutic range (25–800 μM) needed for treatment of CMV retinitis (91). Moreover, the values are comparable to those obtained in eyes treated with only a single foscarnet iontophoresis. Electroretinography and slit-lamp examination revealed no evidence of ocular toxicity. Examination of the retinas and choroid revealed a single small burn in the retina and choroid corresponding to the iontophoresis probe contact site, which was similar to the lesion resulting from a single iontophoretic application (98). These results suggest that repeated ocular iontophoresis of foscarnet could be an effective means of achieving enhanced, localized treatment of CMV retinitis in humans.

6. Herpes Simplex Virus Infection

Herpes viruses are among the most well-studied microorganisms that cause chronic infection and are a well-described cause of ocular diseases (89,102). Ocular degeneration due to infection with herpes simplex type 1 (HSV-1) and herpes simplex type 2 (HSV-2) is a leading cause of blinding keratitis in industrialized countries (102,103). Analysis of ocular viral isolates demonstrated that HSV-1 is responsible for about 85% of ocular HSV infections (102,103). Ocular HSV-1 infection consists of an acute keratoconjunctivitis followed by a lifelong cycle of latency, reactivation, and recurrent infection (102,103). This section reviews research on herpetic eye infection and the use of iontophoresis to deliver therapeutic doses of antiviral agents and/or agents that cause experimental reactivation of latent HSV-1.

a. Antivirals for Treatment of Epithelial Keratitis   Hill et al. (104) were the first to report the transdermal delivery of antiviral agents by iontophoresis. They demonstrated that the antiviral agents iododeoxyuridine (IDU), phosphonoacetic acid (PPA), and vidarabine monophosphate (Ara-AMP) could be iontophoresed across mouse epidermis with enough efficiency to achieve long-lasting and potentially therapeutic concentrations of drug.

A subsequent study (105) examined the pharmacokinetics of ionto-phoresed Ara-AMP. Ara-AMP was chosen because the parent compound, vidarabine, was shown to be effective in the treatment of HSV-1 infection after topical or systemic administration. Ara-AMP is phosphorylated and highly charged and thus an excellent candidate for iontophoresis. Tritium-labeled Ara-AMP was applied either topically or iontophoresed into unin-fected rabbit eyes. Transcorneal iontophoresis was performed at 0.5 mA for 4 minutes with the cathode in contact with the drug solution. Iontophoresis resulted in drug concentrations in the cornea, aqueous humor, and iris which were 3–12 times higher than those obtained with topical application. No obvious corneal damage was observed. The results showed that ionto-phoresis increased corneal penetration of an antiviral agent in comparison to topical application.

Kwon et al. (106) were the first to demonstrate that iontophoresed Ara-AMP retained its antiviral properties. They studied the virucidal effects of iontophoretically applied Ara-AMP on experimental HSV keratitis in rabbits infected with HSV-1 McKrae strain. Transcorneal iontophoresis of Ara-AMP (0.3 M, 3.4%) was done in both eyes at 24, 48, and 72 hours postinoculation. A second group of infected rabbits served as a con-trol for the procedure and were iontophoresed with a 0.9% sodium chloride solution. Additional groups of rabbits received either topical 10% Ara-AMP, 0.5% IDU, or 0.9% sodium chloride five times daily for 4 days. Slit-lamp examination was performed daily for 10 consecutive days after initiation of treatment and the severity of the disease was scored. Mean lesion scores for the eyes treated by iontophoresis of Ara-AMP were sig-nificantly lower (i.e., less severe disease of shorter duration) compared to the scores of eyes treated with iontophoresis of sodium chloride or topically with Ara-AMP, IDU, or sodium chloride.

b. Antivirals for Treatment of Stromal Disease   Hill et al. (107) ex-tended these studies by comparing the efficacy of transcorneal iontophor-esis versus intravenous injection of either acyclovir or Ara-AMP (alone or in combination) for the treatment of HSV-1 stromal infection in rabbits. Herpetic infection was achieved by an intrasomal injection of purified HSV-1 McKrae strain. Treatments (iontophoresis of either Ara-AMP, acyclovir, or sodium chloride; or intravenous infusion of acyclovir or so-dium chloride) were initiated 24 hours later. Two ophthalmologists per-formed slit-lamp examination daily for up to 22 days postinoculation and recorded the severity of the disease.

Iontophoresis itself did not have any effect on the severity of the disease. Iontophoresis of acyclovir or Ara-AMP significantly shortened the duration of the disease compared to iontophoresis of sodium chloride, and iontophoresed Ara-AMP was as effective as iontophoresed acyclovir. Acyclovir significantly reduced the severity of the disease whether it was delivered iontophoretically or by intravenous injection. Intravenous administration of acyclovir resulted in significantly higher levels of drug in ocular tissues than that obtained with iontophoresis, but iontophoresis delivered a dose that achieved the same therapeutic effect. These results suggested that iontophoresis of acyclovir or Ara-AMP (with or without intravenous supplementation) could be a valuable treatment option for patients with HSV-1 stromal keratitis.

c. Adrenergic Agents for Experimental Reactivation of HSV-1 in the Study of Ocular Herpetic Disease Primary HSV infection is an acute inflammatory response. While the acute infection is occurring, HSV travels along neuronal axons to regional sensory ganglia where it enters a state of dormancy (i.e., latency) (108–110). The exact stimulus that triggers HSV reactivation is unknown, but certain environmental factors (stress, irradiation, hypo- or hyperthermia) result in the appearance of infectious virus at the site of primary infection and a recurrence of the disease (110–113). The rabbit eye model has allowed investigators to study the pathogenesis of HSV latency and reactivation (102,114). In this model, viral latency can be established by inoculation of the cornea with 17Syn$^+$, McKrae, or other strains of HSV-1 (102,115,116). Viral reactivation can be induced by iontophoresis of adrenergic agents and monitored by viral shedding on the ocular surface (102,116,117).

Clinicians had noted for some time the relationship between physical stress and the appearance of fever blisters (cold sores) or genital herpetic lesions. This suggested a role for epinephrine in the process, and various investigators showed that topical or intravenous applications of epinephrine could cause reactivation of HSV-1 in rabbits. Researchers from Hill's group (118,119) were the first to report that transcorneal iontophoresis of this agent could induce viral shedding in rabbits harboring latent HSV-1. They inoculated rabbits with HSV-1 and 60 days later performed epinephrine iontophoresis on one eye from each rabbit. A 0.01% epinephrine solution was iontophoresed (0.8 mA for 8 min) once daily for 3 consecutive days. Viral shedding was verified by ocular swabbing and culturing the tear film in cell culture. Antigenic and/or nucleic acid analysis was used to confirm the identity of the viral isolate. Epinephrine iontophoresis resulted in HSV-1 viral shedding in all treated eyes (118). A follow-up report from this group (119) validated these results and demonstrated that the HSV-1 titers rose, peaked, and fell with time after iontophoresis. This reliable and efficient means of inducing viral shedding served as the basis for the development of other animal models for the study of herpetic disease (120–123).

These models have been used to study the kinetics, pathogenesis, and molecular biology of HSV-1 latency, reactivation, and recurrence of clinical disease.

A subsequent study from this group (124) characterized the appearance of HSV-1 in the nerves and ganglia after reactivation by epinephrine iontophoresis. Hill et al. (124) showed that the presence of infectious virus could be detected more rapidly from cultured neuronal tissue from rabbits that had undergone epinephrine iontophoresis than from their untreated counterparts.

Shimomura et al. (125) modified the epinephrine iontophoresis protocol so as to eliminate the need to anesthetize animals once daily for 3 consecutive days. They developed a method that was based on a single iontophoresis of 6-hydroxydopamine followed by topical application of epinephrine over several days. The rationale for this came from studies using iontophoresed 6-hydroxydopamine to treat glaucoma. As described above, 6-hydroxydopamine causes a selective and reversible degeneration of sympathetic nerve terminals in the anterior segment, after which the innervated structures of the eye are exquisitely sensitive to extremely dilute solutions of epinephrine. With this method, viral shedding was induced by a single iontophoresis of a 1% solution of 6-hydroxydopamine under various conditions (0.5–0.75 mA for 3–8 min). Two drops of 2% epinephrine were applied 6 hours after iontophoresis and twice daily for the next 4 days. All treated eyes (17/17; 100%) shed HSV-1, regardless of the iontophoretic conditions.

Hill et al. (115,126) used this modified procedure to further characterize ocular HSV-1 shedding induced by 6-hydroxydopamine iontophoresis plus topical epinephrine. They were the first to quantify the number of plaque-forming units of HSV-1 shed into the tear film following 6-hydroxydopamine iontophoresis plus topical epinephrine-induced reactivation (126). Titers ranged up to 10^5 plaque-forming units/eye. A subsequent study (115) showed that dipivefrin hydrochloride could be used in place of epinephrine in this reactivation model. Dipivefrin hydrochloride is a prodrug of epinephrine, which has increased corneal penetration compared to epinephrine. In clinical studies, 0.1% dipivefrin hydrochloride was as effective as topical 1 or 2% epinephrine. Hill et al. (115) demonstrated that iontophoresed 6-hydroxydopamine followed by topical application of 0.1% dipivefrin hydrochloride resulted in HSV-1 ocular shedding and recurrent HSV-1 corneal lesions. This was the first report showing that an adrenergic drug could induce both HSV-1 ocular shedding (reactivation) and HSV-1 corneal epithelial lesions (recurrence) in rabbits harboring latent virus.

Rivera et al. (110) used epinephrine iontophoresis to study the temporal relationship between viral reactivation and the presence of viral particles or virions in corneal nerves or the cornea, respectively. Transmission electron microscopy revealed viral particles (in low abundance) in unmyelinated axons, but no enveloped virions were found. This study suggests that ocular iontophoresis of epinephrine reactivates HSV-1 in the ganglia and that the virus is translocated from the sensory ganglia (trigeminal and/or superior cervical) to the cornea by anterograde axonal transport mechanisms.

Hill et al. (117) demonstrated that levo(-)epinephrine was significantly more potent than dextro(+)epinephrine for inducing HSV-1 ocular shedding. The data suggested that the mechanism of induction of HSV-1 ocular shedding by epinephrine is correlated with the receptor potency of levo(-)epinephrine. Epinephrine activates both α- and β-adrenergic receptors in the eye. If the signal for viral reactivation was transmitted exclusively through a β-adrenergic receptor, a β-adrenergic receptor antagonist should inhibit epinephrine-induced reactivation.

Studies from Hill's group (127–129) assessed the effect of topically applied timolol maleate, a nonspecific β_1,β_2-adenergic receptor blocking agent, on ocular HSV-1 reactivation in rabbit eyes. Timolol maleate was applied following iontophoresis of 6-hydroxydopamine or by direct transcorneal iontophoresis. It was discovered that timolol iontophoresis for 3 consecutive days could cause corneal epithelial lesions (127). However, a single direct transcorneal iontophoresis of timolol induced ocular HSV-1 shedding (128). The data suggest that both timolol (a β-adrenergic receptor antagonist) and epinephrine (an α,β-adrenergic receptor agonist) could induce ocular HSV-1 shedding. The results of these studies demonstrated that specific receptor occupancy of epinephrine alone is not an exclusive signal for viral reactivation. We are unable to explain why iontophoresis of this agonist/antagonist pair of adrenergic agents induces viral reactivation in animals that harbor latent HSV-1 strain McKrae.

Studies with propranolol, also a β-adrenergic antagonist, have yielded paradoxical results. Kaufman et al. (130) showed that propranolol suppressed both ocular HSV-1 recurrence and severity following spontaneous reactivation in the rabbit. Gebhardt and Kaufman (131) demonstrated that propranolol blocked the HSV-1 reactivation following hyperthermic induction in latently infected mice. Garza and Hill (132) examined the effect of propranolol on HSV-1 reactivation in latently infected rabbits following induction either by epinephrine iontophoresis (stress pathway) or by systemic immunosuppression (nonstress pathway). Immunosuppression was produced by injection of cyclophosphamide and dexamethasone (133). Propranolol was given intramuscularly by injection in doses of 5, 20, or 200 mg/kg twice daily. Propranolol had no effect at any concentration on blocking HSV-1 induction, either by transcorneal iontophoresis of epinephrine or by systemic immunosuppression due to cyclcophosphamide plus dexamethasone treatment. These results suggest that (a) propranolol can specifically block the induction pathway in the mouse model but not the rabbit model, or (b) propranolol is not a broad/potent enough inhibitor to prevent HSV-1 induction in the rabbit.

    d. Epinephrine Iontophoresis and the Study of LATs   Initial studies in murine models of HSV infection demonstrated the presence of novel HSV RNA transcripts in sensory neurons of mice harboring a latent HSV infection (134–136). These mRNA species resulted from transcription of the only region of the HSV genome that is transcriptionally active during the latent phase of HSV infection (134,137–139). Latency-associated transcripts (LATs RNA) have also been demonstrated in rabbits (140,141) and humans (135,142,143). Three "major" LATs (2, 1.55, and 1.45 kb) as well as a "minor" transcript (8.3 kb) have been detected in ganglia latently infected with HSV-1 (134,136,144–146). The "major" LATs are highly expressed and poly(A)$^-$, whereas the "minor" LAT has low level expression and is poly(A)$^+$. LATs are expressed at similar levels in sensory neurons of mice, rabbits, and humans (136,140,142). Although LAT is not essential for latency, it remains the only known molecular marker for latent HSV infection (134,139,147,148).

    Epinephrine iontophoresis and/or the rabbit eye model have been used in conjunction with various mutant strains of HSV to examine the role of LATs in the process of establishment, maintenance, and reactivation of latent HSV infection. HSV constructs that contain genetic alterations in the LAT locus were compared to unmodified (wild-type) or marker rescued (LAT-positive) viruses for their ability to establish latency and/or reactivate from latency (134,136). Hill et al. (149,150) used mutant HSV-1 strains (X10-13 or 17ΔSty) that could not produce a latently associated transcript (LAT-negative) and genetically engineered LAT-positive mutants (XC-20 or 17ΔSty-Res) to demonstrate that the LAT-positive strains, which are similar to the parent HSV-1 strains 17Syn$^+$, could be reactivated by iontophoresis with high efficiency. The LAT-negative strains showed very limited or significantly reduced reactivation. The results suggested a role for the latently associated transcript in viral reactivation. All the mutants (LAT-negative or LAT-positive) were able to establish and maintain latency in sensory ganglia (149,150).

    Bloom et al. (151) demonstrated that HSV-1 mutants with deletions encompassing the LAT promoter area have significantly reduced ocular reactivation following transcorneally iontophoresed epinephrine induction. 17ΔPst (LAT-negative) has a 202 bp deletion in the LAT promoter in an area encompassing the TATA box, cAMP response element (CRE), upstream stimulatory factor, and transcription start sites, which significantly reduces LAT transcription (147,151). They demonstrated that although this virus established latency with the same kinetics as its parent, 17Syn[+], spontaneous and adrenergically induced reactivation is significantly reduced. This evidence suggested that expression of LATs was important in regulating HSV-1 reactivation. Bloom et al. (152) also examined the LAT promoter region at a more precise level. HSV-1 mutants containing a mutated CRE-1 element were shown to be significantly impaired in their ability to reactivate either spontaneously or by induction following epinephrine iontophoresis in the rabbit eye model (152). This evidence suggested a role for CRE-1 (CRE-1 binding factors) (134,136,153) in the reactivation process.

Similar studies have provided evidence that viral strains exhibit varying sensitivities to genetic alterations within the LAT domain. Loutsch et al. (154) used mutant strains of McKrae and 17Syn[+] that had identical 371-base-pair deletion mutations in the LAT genes to examine spontaneous in vivo reactivation kinetics. They were able to demonstrate that an identical deletion resulted in different in vivo reactivation phenotypes. The results suggest a difference in genetic background of McKrae and 17Syn[+] resulting in different in vivo reactivation phenotypes.

Zheng et al. (155) recently investigated the ability of LAT-positive and LAT-negative strains of HSV-1 to establish latent infection in rabbit corneas following penetrating keratoplasty. 17ΔPst (LAT-negative, low reactivation) and 17Pr (LAT-positive, high reactivation recusant of 17ΔPst) were inoculated into rabbit corneas. Latently infected rabbits received corneal allografts from naive rabbits, and naive rabbits received grafts from latently infected rabbits. Penetrating keratoplasty of latently infected and naive rabbits made it possible to study the migration of HSV from a site of latency to other tissues. They demonstrated that corneas from latently infected rabbits contain HSV-1 DNA that can replicate after viral reactivation by transcorneal epinephrine iontophoresis. The LAT negative strain also had a significantly reduced ability to replicate. The data showed that HSV-1 in latently infected rabbit sensory ganglia could be induced by epinephrine iontophoresis and migrate into other uninfected tissues (i.e., the transplanted cornea of a naive rabbit). The LAT-negative strain had a reduced ability to migrate. The results suggest that HSV-1 can migrate in both anterograde and retrograde directions between the site of viral latency (the trigeminal ganglion in the rabbit) and corneal tissues following epinephrine-induced reactivation. This is the first report to provide evidence to support the concept of corneal HSV-1 latency and reactivation (156,157).

Numerous other studies have used iontophoresis to study viral reactivation, as well as the treatment and prevention of recurrent herpetic disease (158–164). In summary, these studies validate the accuracy, reliability, and reproducibility of iontophoresis as a noninvasive mode of drug delivery and suggest that the iontophoretic model may be beneficial in the development of new, designer drugs to replace or supplement current herpetic disease regimens. Experimentally, ocular iontophoresis and the rabbit eye model are mainstays in the study of HSV-1 latency and reactivation.

III. COMMERCIALLY AVAILABLE IONTOPHORETIC DEVICES

A variety of iontophoretic devices are available with different types of power sources that vary in complexity from the simple battery-rheostat type to modern electronic circuitry (8,9). Table 3 provides a list of companies that produce iontophoresis equipment, their addresses and phone numbers, as well as a brief description of one specific model manufactured by each company. The commercial devices are safe, portable, and work well for the intended purpose.

IV. CONCLUSIONS

The last 10–20 years have seen the development and optimization of the technology of iontophoresis as a noninvasive method of drug delivery. Peptide and protein drugs (e.g., insulin and vasopressin) have been delivered iontophoretically without the pain and side effects associated with traditional subcutaneous injection (10,165,166). Iontophoresis also has the potential to revolutionize clinical diagnosis and monitoring procedures in that it offers an avenue for extracting information from the body without the need for invasive procedures (3,167,168). Iontophoresis is already used clinically in physical therapy clinics, and an allergy patch test is close to commercial reality (33,169).

Ocular iontophoresis is fast, painless, safe, and, in most cases, results in the delivery of a high concentration of the drug to a specific ocular site. Experimentally, iontophoresis has proven extremely useful as a reliable system for inducing reactivation of herpes simplex virus in various animal models of this ocular disease. Clinically, ocular iontophoresis is potentially a valuable adjunctive treatment for cytomegalovirus retinitis. In glaucoma studies, iontophoresis of fluorescein, adrenergic agents, and 5-fluorouracil has facilitated the study of aqueous humor dynamics, treatment of glaucoma, and the control of cellular proliferation of glaucoma surgery. Anesthetics and antibiotic/antifungal agents can be delivered transcorneally or transsclerally according to the site of infection. Ocular iontophoresis has

Table 3 Iontophoresis Equipment and Suppliers

Company	Model number/description
IOMED, Inc. 2441 South 3850 West, Suite A Salt Lake city, UT 84120 (801) 975-1191 (800) 621-3347 Fax (801) 975-7366	Phoresor II Auto model number PM900. This model provides an effective, safe, and easy to use system with a preset dose (40 mAmp-Mins) for iontophoretic drug application to the skin. This model is compact, easy to operate, fast to set-up, and portable. E-mail: es@iomed,com Website: www.iomed.com
Life-Tech, Inc. 4235 Greenbrier Drive Stafford, TX 77477 (713) 495-9411 (800) 231-9841 Fax (281) 492-6646	Iontophor-II model number 6111 PM/DX. This model provides a painless, safe, and effective method of delivering high concentrations of drug into a localized skin area. This unit is battery operated, compact, and portable. It is an excellent unit for maintaining constant current. This model has dual site treatment function that enables you to treat two sites simultaneously. E-mail: admin@life-tech.com Website: www.life-tech.com
General Medical Company 1935 Armacost Avenue Los Angeles, CA 90025 (310) 820-5881 (800) 432-5362 Fax (310) 826-5778	The Drionic unit. This compact iontophoresis unit has FDA approval for home treatment of hyperhidrosis. Battery-generated direct current. E-mail: drionic@generalmedical.com Website: www.drionic.com
Wescor, Inc. 459 South Main Street Logan, UT 84321 (435) 752-6011 (800) 453-2725 Fax (435) 752-4127	Macroduct model 3700. This model is used for sweat stimulation (pilocarpine iontophoresis), collection and analysis (via a sweat analyzer). It is easy to operate and provides accurate and reliable sweat testing. E-mail: billie@wescor.com Website: www.dataloggersinc.com
Fischer Co., Inc 517 Commercial Street Glendale, CA 91203 (818) 241-1178 (800) 525-3467 Fax (323) 245-2748	Fischer Galvanic Unit, Model MD-1a is a high-output iontophoretic device ideally suited for treatment of large areas (hyperhidrosis patients). It produces DC current in two ranges (0–10mAmp and 0–50mAmp). Available to physicians or by prescription only. E-mail: info@rafischer. com Website: www.rafischer. com

Table 3 Continued

Company	Model number/description
Dagan Corporation 2855 Park Avenue Minneapolis, MN 55407 (612) 827-5959 Fax (612) 827-6535	Dagan 6400 Advanced model. Micro-Iontophoresis current generator. Delivers precise drug delivery without batteries. Power is 100 to 115 volts AC. Current range is 0–1000 n/Amp. E-mail: sales@dagan. com Website: www.dagan.com
MedTherm Corporation 2604 Newby Road Huntsville, AL 35805 (205) 837-2000	Electro-Medicator Model A1 (Distributed by Pamir Electronics corp.: 603 N. Gordon Drive, Exton PA 19341; (610) 594-8537). This model is used for dental research and clinical practice. It is easy to operate and has AC charging or direct use of AC. E-mail: pamir@pamir.com Website: www.pamir.com
Parkell 155 Schmitt Boulevard Farmingdale, NY 11735 (631) 249-1134 (800) 243-7446 Fax (631) 249-1242	Desensitron II model number ID643DGC. This model is used for treating hypersensitive teeth by iontophoresis of fluoride ions. Current range is 0–0.5mAmp. E-mail: info@parkell.com Website: www.parkell.com
McdTronic, Inc. 7000 Central Ave., NE Minneapolis, MN 55432 (612) 574-4000 (800) 525-5552 Fax (612) 785-6541	Model 9820. This iontophoretic device is part of complete system (Model 9800) for sweat analysis after pilocarpine iontophoresis. E-mail Website: www.medtronic.com

also been used to introduce genes into the anterior and posterior segments of the rabbit eye (170).

There are several ongoing ocular iontophoresis studies that are particularly pertinent to this discussion and should be noted. Chapon et al. (171), using rabbits, have shown that transscleral iontophoresis delivered 15 times more of the anti-CMV agent ganciclovir to the retina and 6.5 times more to the choroid (6 h posttreatment 370 and 828 ng/mg, respectively) than topical administration. At 3 days posttreatment, retinal levels of ganciclovir remained significantly higher than those achieved by oral administration, intravenous injection, topical application, or intravitreal injection. Chauvaud et al. (172) presented initial findings of a Phase II clinical trial for transscleral iontophoresis of the anti-inflammatory corticosteroid SoluMedrol (hemisuccinate methylprednisolone). Transscleral iontophoresis of SoluMedrol was safe, well tolerated, and easily applicable to the treatment of severe ocular inflammation thereby reducing the systemic side effects of corticotherapy. Hayden et al. (173) studied transscleral iontophoresis of the anticancer drug carboplatin in transgenic mice with hereditary retinoblastoma. A dose-dependent inhibition of intraocular tumor formation was observed following repetitive iontophoretic treatment. These results suggest that transscleral iontophoresis of carboplatin may be useful, as well as advantageous, in the treatment of intraocular pediatric retinoblastoma. Ocular iontophoresis is not a panacea for all eye disorders, but it is a viable alternative delivery system for those substances that are not amenable to topical application and/or require repeated administration over an extended period of time.

ACKNOWLEDGMENTS

Louis P. Gangarosa, D.D.S., Ph.D., is acknowledged as the person who introduced iontophoresis to one of the authors (JMH). The authors wish to acknowledge the editorial assistance and research collaboration of A. K. Mitra, Ph.D. Specific research from the laboratory of JMH was supported in part by U.S. Public Health Service grant EY06311 and EY08871; EY02377 (Eye Center Core Grant); an unrestricted grant from Research to Prevent Blindness (RPB); Dr. Hill is an RPB Scientific Investigator Award recipient. The authors wish to acknowledge the secretarial assistance of Mrs. Carole Hoth. The authors also wish to acknowledge the student workers with special thanks to Ms. Kristina Braud and Ms. Kathy Vu. None of the authors have any financial or proprietary interest in any agents or devices mentioned in this review.

REFERENCES

1. Sing, P., and Maibach, H. I. (1994). Iontophoresis in drug delivery: Basic principles and applications. *Crit. Rev. Therp. Drug Carrier Systems, 11*:161–213.
2. Guy, R. H., Kalia, Y. N., Delgado-Charro, M. B., Merino, V., Lopez, A., and Marro, D. (2000). Iontophoresis: electrorepulsion and electroosmosis. *J. Control Release, 64*:129–132.
3. Merino, V., Kalia, Y. N., and Guy, R. H. (1997). Transdermal therapy and diagnosis by iontophoresis. *Trends Biotechnol, 15*:288–290.

4. Duke-Elder, S. (1962). Iontophoresis. In *The Foundations of Ophthalmology*, Vol. VII. C. V. Mosby, St. Louis, pp. 507–514.
5. Harris, R. (1967). Iontophoresis, in *Therapeutic Electricity and Ultraviolet Radiation* (S. Licht, ed.), Waverly Press, Baltimore, pp. 156–178.
6. Banga, A. K., and Chien, Y. W. (1988). Iontophoretic delivery of drugs: fundamentals, development and biomedical applications. *J. Control Release*, 7:1–24.
7. Nair, V, Pillai, O, Poduri, R., and Panchagnula, R. (1999). Transdermal iontophoresis. Part I: Basic principles and considerations. *Meth. Find. Exp. Clin. Pharmacol.*, *21*:139–151.
8. Tyle, P. (1986). Iontophoretic devices for drug delivery. *Review. Pharm. Res.*, *3*:318–326.
9. Garrison, J. (1998). Iontophoresis: an alternative drug-delivery system. *Med. Device Technol.*, *9*:32–36.
10. Hirvonen, J., Kalia, Y. N., and Guy, R. H. (1996). Transdermal delivery of peptides by iontophoresis. *Nature Biotechnol.*, *14*:1710–1713.
11. Shofner, R. S., Kaufman, H. E., and Hill, J. M. (1989). New horizons in ocular drug delivery. *Ophthalmol. Clin. North Am.*, *2*:15–24.
12. Sarraf, D., and Lee, D. A. (1994). The role of iontophoresis in ocular drug delivery. *J. Ocular Pharm.*, *10*:69–81.
13. Sasaki, H., Yamamura, K., Mukai, T., Nishida, K., Nakamura, J., Nakashima, M., and Ichikawa, M. (1999). Enhancement of ocular drug penetration. *Crit. Rev. Ther. Drug Carrier Syst.*, *16*:85–146.
14. Shriber, W. J. (1975). The direct current and ion transfer. In: *A Manual of Electrotherapy* (W. J. Shriber, ed.). Lea & Febiger, Philadelphia, p. 124.
15. Turrell, W. J. (1921). Therapeutic action of the constant current. *Proc. R. Soc. Med.*, *14*:41–52.
16. Morton, W. J. (1898). *Cataphoresis of Electric Medicament Surgery*. American Technical Book, New York.
17. Leduc, S. (1900). Introduction of medicinal substances into the depth of tissues by electric current. *Ann. Electrobiol.*, *3*:545–550.
18. Leduc, S. (1908). *Electric Ions and Their Use in Medicine*. Rebman Ltd., London.
19. Wirtz, R. (1908). Die Ionentherapie in der Augenheilkunde. *Klin. Monatsbl. Augenheilkd.*, *46*:543–579.
20. Morisot, L. (1927). L'iontherapie ou ionisation appliquee au traitement des affections ocu-laires. *Clin. Ophthalmol.*, *31*:5–16.
21. Erlanger, G. (1936). On the scientific and practical value of ionization in ophthalmology. Recent advances and researchers. *Br. J. Ophthalmol.*, *20*:213–229.
22. Erlanger, G. (1939). Iontophoretic medication in ophthalmology. Theoretic and practical aspects. *Arch. Phys. Ther.*, *20*:16–24.
23. Erlanger, G. (1954). Iontophoresis: a scientific and practical tool in ophthalmology. *Ophthalmologica*, *128*:232–246.

24. Von Sallmann, L., and Meyer, K. (1944). Penetration of penicillin into the eye. *Arch. Ophthalmol., 31*:1–7.

25. Von Sallmann, L. (1944). Penicillin and sulfadiazine in the treatment of experimental intraocular infections with *Staphylococcus aureus* and *Clostridium welchii. Arch. Ophthalmol., 31*:54–61.

26. Von Sallmann, L. (1945). Penetration of penicillin into the eye. *Arch. Ophthalmol., 34*:195–201.

27. Witzel, S. H., Fielding, I. Z., and Ormsby, H. L. (1956). Ocular penetration of antibiotics by iontophoresis. *Am. J. Ophthalmol., 42*:89–95.

28. Ichihashi, T. (1936). Effect of drugs on the sweat glands by cataphoresis and an effective method for suppression of local sweating: Observation on the effect of diaphoretics and adiaphoretics. *J. Oriental Med., 25*:101–102.

29. Gibson, L. E., and Cooke, R. E. (1959). A test for concentration of electrolytes in sweat in cystic fibrosis of the pancreas utilizing pilocarpine by iontophoresis. *Pediatrics., 23*:545–549.

30. Carter, E. P., Barrett, A. D., Heeley, A. F., and Kuzemko, J. A. (1984). Improved sweat test method for the diagnosis of cystic fibrosis. *Arch. Dis. Child., 59*:919–922.

31. Hall, S. K., Stableforth, D. E., and Green, A. (1990). Sweat sodium and chloride concentrations—essential criteria for the diagnosis of cystic fibrosis in adults. *Ann. Clin. Biochem., 27*:318–320.

32. Sloan, J. B., and Soltani, K. (1986). Iontophoresis in dermatology: A review. *J. Am. Acad. Dermatol., 15*:671–684.

33. Kassan, D. G., Lynch, A. M., and Stiller, M. J. (1996). Physical enhancement of dermatologic drug delivery: Iontophoresis and phonophoresis. *J. Am. Acad. Dermatol., 34*:657–666.

34. Stolman, L. P. (1998). Treatment of hyperhidrosis. *Dermatol. Clin., 16*:863–869.

35. Murphy, R., and Harrington, C.I. (2000). Treating hyperhidrosis: Iontophoresis should be tried before other treatments (letter). *BMJ, 321*:702–703.

36. Gangarosa, L. P., and Park, N. H. (1978). Practical considerations in iontophoresis of fluoride for desensitizing dentin. *J. Prosthet. Dent., 39*:173–178.

37. Krauser, J. T. (1986). Hypersensitive teeth. Part II: Treatment. *J. Prosthet. Dent., 56*(3):307–311.

38. Greenbaum, S. S., and Bernstein, E. F. (1994). Comparison of iontophoresis of lidocaine with a eutetic mixture of lidocaine and prilocaine (EMLA) for topically administered local anesthesia. *J. Dermatol. Surg. Oncol., 20*:579–583.

39. Zempsky, W. T., Anand, K. J. S., Sullivan, K. M., Fraser, D., and Cucina, K. (1998). Lidocaine iontophoresis for topical anesthesia before intravenous line placement in children. *J. Pediatr., 132*:1061–1063.

40. DeCou, J. M., Abrams, R. S., Hammond, J. H., Lowder, L. R., and Gauderer, W. L. (1999). Iontophoresis: a needle-free, electrical system of local anesthesia delivery for pediatric surgical office procedures. *J. Pediatr. Surg., 34*:946–949.

41. Squire, S. J., Kirchhoff, K. T., and Hissong, K. (2000). Comparing two methods of topical anesthesia used before intravenous cannulation in pediatric patients. *J. Pediatr. Health Care.*, *14*:68–72.

42. Hill, J. M., O'Callaghan, R. J., and Hobden, J. A. (1993). Ocular iontophoresis. In: *Ophthalmic Drug Delivery Systems* (A. K. Mitra, ed.). Marcel Dekker, New York, pp. 331–354.

43. Callegan, M. C., O'Callaghan, R. J., and Hill, J. M. (1994). Pharmacokinetic considerations in the treatment of bacterial keratitis. *Clin. Pharmacokinet.*, *27*:129–149.

44. Pillai, O., Nair, V., Poduri, R., and Panchagnula, R. (1999). Transdermal iontophoresis. Part II: Peptide and protein delivery. *Methods Find. Exp. Clin. Pharmacol.*, *21*:229–240.

45. Jones, R. F., and Maurice, D. M. (1966). New methods of measuring the rate of aqueous flow in man with fluorescein. *Exp. Eye Res.*, *5*:208–220.

46. Starr, P. A. J. (1966). Changes in aqueous flow determined by fluorophotometry. *Trans. Ophthalmol. Soc. U.K.*, *86*:639–646.

47. Holm, O. (1968). A photogrammetric method for estimation of the pupillary aqueous flow in the living human eye. I. *Acta Ophthalmol.*, *46*:254–277.

48. Brubaker, R. F. (1982). The flow of aqueous humor in the human eye. *Trans. Am. Ophthalmol. Soc.*, *80*:391–474.

49. Latina, M. A., Dobrogowski, M., March, W. F., and Birngruber, R. (1990). Laser sclerostomy by pulsed-dye laser and goniolens. *Arch. Ophthalmol.*, *108*:1745–1750.

50. Latina, M. A., Melamed, S., March, W. F., Kass, M. A., and Kolker, A. E. (1992). Gonioscopic Ab Interno Laser Sclerostomy. A pilot study in glaucoma patients. *Ophthalmology*, *99*:1736–1744.

51. Melamed, S., Solomon, A., Neumann, D., Hirsch, A., Blumenthal, M., and Belkin, M. (1993). Internal sclerostomy using laser ablation of dyed sclera in glaucoma patients: a pilot study. *Br. J. Ophthalmol.*, *77*;139–144.

52. Grossman, R. E., Sarraf, D., and Lee, D. A. (1993). Iontophoresis of methylene blue for gonioscopic pulsed dye laser sclerostomy. *J. Ocul. Pharmacol.*, *9*:277–285.

53. Sarraf, D., and Lee, D. A. (1993). Iontophoresis of reactive black 5 for pulsed dye laser sclerostomy. *J. Ocul Pharmacol. Ther.*, *9*:25–33.

54. Kitazawa, Y., Nose, H., and Horie, T. (1973). The effects of chemical sympathectomy on intraocular pressure of the normal human subjects. *Acta Soc. Ophthalmol. Jpn.*, *77*:1901–1903.

55. Kitazawa, Y., and Horie, T. (1974). Denervation supersensitivity induced by chemical sympathectomy with 6-hydroxydopamine. *Jpn. J. Ophthalmol.*, *18*:109–118.

56. Kitazawa, Y., Nose, H., and Horie, T. (1975). Chemical sympathectomy with 6-hydroxydopamine in the treatment of primary open-angle glaucoma. *Am. J. Ophthalmol.*, *79*:98–103.

57. Watanabe, H., Levene, R. Z., and Bernstein, M. R. (1977). 6-Hydroxydopamine therapy in glaucoma. *Trans. Am. Acad. Ophthalmol. Otolaryngol.*, *83*:69–77.

58. Colasanti, B. K., and Trotter, R. R. (1977). Enhanced ocular penetration of the methyl ester of alpha-methyl-para-tyrosine after iontophoresis. *Arch. Int. Pharmacodyn. Ther.*, *228*:171–176.

59. Blumenkranz, M. S., Clafin, A., and Hajek, A. S. (1984). Selection of therapeutic agents for intraocular proliferative disease. *Arch. Ophthalmol.*, *102*:598–604.

60. Kondo, M., and Araie, M. (1989). Iontophoresis of 5-fluorouracil into the conjunctiva and sclera. *Invest. Ophthalmol. Vis. Sci.*, *30*:583–585.

61. Zempsky, W. T., and Ashburn, M. A. (1998). Iontophoresis: noninvasive drug delivery. *Am. J. Anesthesiol.*, *25*:158–162.

62. Sisler, H. A. (1978). Iontophoretic local anesthesia for conjunctival surgery. *Ann. Ophthalmol.*, *10*:597–598.

63. Meyer, D. R., Lindberg, J. V., and Vasquez, R. J. (1990). Iontophoresis for eyelid anesthesia. *Ophthalmic Surg.*, *21*:845–848.

64. Havener, W. H. (1978). Corticosteroid therapy. In: *Ocular Pharmacology*, 4th ed. CV Mosby, St. Louis, pp. 143–174.

65. Lachaud, J. P. (1965). Considerations on the use of corticosteroids by ionization in certain ocular diseases. *Bull. Soc. Ophthalmol. France*, *65*:84–89.

66. Lam, T. T., Edward, D. P., Zhu, X., and Tso, M. O. M. (1989). Transscleral iontophoresis of dexamethasone. *Arch. Ophthalmol.*, *107*:1368–1371.

67. Behar-Cohen, F. F., Parel, J.-M., Pouliquen, Y., Thillaye-Goldenberg, B., Goureau, O., Heydolph, S., Courtois, Y., and DeKozak, Y. (1997). Iontophoresis of dexamethasone in the treatment of endotoxin-induced-uveitis in rats. *Exp. Eye Res.*, *65*:533–545.

68. Pagano, G., Bruno, A., Cavallo-Perin, P., Cesco, L., and Imbimbo, B. (1989). Glucose intolerance after short-term administration of corticosteroids in healthy subjects. *Arch. Int. Med.*, *149*:1098–1091.

69. Yoshida, M., Yoshimura, N., Hangai, M., Tanihara, H., and Honda, Y. (1994). Interleukin-1 α, interleukin-1 β, and tumor necrosis factor gene expression in endotoxin-induced uveitis. *Invest. Ophthalmol. Vis. Sci.*, *35*:1107–1113.

70. Grossman, R. E., Chu, D. F., and Lee, D. A. (1990). Regional ocular gentamicin levels after transcorneal and transscleral iontophoresis. *Invest. Ophthalmol. Vis. Sci.*, *31*:909–916.

71. Fishman, P. H., Jay, W. M., Hill, J. M., Rissing, J. P., and Shockley, R. K. (1984). Iontophoresis of gentamicin into aphakic rabbit eyes: sustained vitreal levels. *Invest. Ophthalmol. Vis. Sci.*, *25*:343–345.

72. Hughes, L., and Maurice, D. (1984). A fresh look at iontophoresis. *Arch. Ophthalmol.*, *102*;1825–1829.

73. Frucht-Pery, J., Solomon, A., Doron, R., Ever-Hadani, P., Manor, O., and Shapiro, M. (1996). Efficacy of iontophoresis in the rat cornea. *Graefes Arch. Clin. Exp. Ophthalmol.*, *234*:765–769.

74. Frucht-Pery, J., Goren, D., Solomon, A., Siganos, C. S., Mechoulam, H., Ever-Hadani, P., and Shapiro, M. (1999). The distribution of gentamicin in the rabbit cornea following iontophoresis to the central cornea. *J. Ocular Pharm. Therapeut.*, *15*:251–256.

75. Barza, M., Peckman, C., and Baum, J. (1986). Transscleral iontophoresis of cefazolin, ticarcillin, and gentamicin in the rabbit. *Ophthalmology*, *93*:133–139.

76. Barza, M., Peckman, C., and Baum, J. (1987). Transscleral iontophoresis as an adjunctive treatment for experimental endophthalmitis. *Arch. Ophthalmol.*, *105*:1418–1420.

77. Burstein, N. L., Leopold, I. H., and Bernaacchii, D. B. (1985). Transscleral iontophoresis of gentamicin. *J. Ocul. Pharmacol.*, *1*:363–368.

78. Barza, M. M., Peckman, C., and Baum, J. (1987). Transscleral iontophoresis of gentamicin in monkeys. *Invest. Ophthalmol. Vis. Sci.*, *28*:1033–1036.

79. Rootman, D. S., Hobden, J. A., Jantzen, J. A., Gonzales, V. R., O'Callaghan, R. J., and Hill, J. M. (1988). Iontophoresis of tobramycin for the treatment of experimental *Pseudomonas* keratitis in the rabbit. *Arch. Ophthalmol.*, *106*:262–265.

80. Hobden, J. A., Rootman, D. S., O'Callaghan, R. J., and Hill, J. M. (1988). Iontophoretic application of tobramycin to uninfected and *Pseudomonas aeruginosa*-infected rabbit corneas. *Antimicrob. Agents Chemother.*, *32*:978–981.

81. Rootman, D. S., Jantzen, J. A., Gonzalez, J. R. Fischer, M., Beuerman, R., and Hill, J. M. (1988). Pharmacokinetics and safety of transcorneal iontophoresis of tobramycin in the rabbit. *Invest. Ophthalmol. Vis. Sci.*, *29*:1397–1401.

82. Hobden, J. A., O'Callaghan, R. J., Hill, J. M., Reidy, J. J., Rootman, D. S., and Thompson, H. W. (1989). Tobramycin iontophoresis into corneas infected with drug-resistant *Pseudomonas aeruginosa*. *Curr. Eye Res.*, *8*:1163–1169.

83. *Physician's Desk Reference*. (1977). Medical Economics Company, Montvale, N.J.

84. Hobden, J. A., Reidy, J. J., O'Callaghan, R. J., and Hill, J. M. (1990). Ciprofloxacin iontophoresis for aminoglycoside-resistant *Pseudomonas* keratitis. *Invest. Ophthalmol. Vis. Sci.*, *31*:1940–1944.

85. Yoshizumi, M. O., Cohen, D., Verbukh, I., Leinwand, M., Kim, J., and Lee, D. A. (1991). Experimental transscleral iontophoresis of ciprofloxacin. *J. Ocular Pharm.*, *7*:163–167.

86. Choi, T. B., and Lee, D. A. (1988). Transscleral and transcorneal iontophoresis of vancomycin in rabbit eyes. *J. Ocular Pharmacol.*, *4*:153–164.

87. Grossman, R., and Lee, D. A. (1989). Transscleral and transcorneal iontophoresis of ketoconazole in the rabbit eye. *Ophthalmology*, *96*:724–729.

88. Boniuk, I. (1972). The cytomegaloviruses and the eye. *Int. Ophthalmol. Clin.*, *12*:169–190.

89. Miller, R. F., Howard, M. R., Frith, P., Perrons, C. J., Pecorella, I., and Lucas, S. B. (2000). Herpes-virus infection of eye and brain in HIV. *Sex. Transm. Inf.*, *76*:282–286.

90. Friedman, A. H., Orellana, J., Freeman, W. R., Luntz, M. H., Starr, M. B., Tapper, M. L., et al. (1983). Cytomegalovirus retinitis: a manifestation of the acquired immune deficiency syndrome (AIDS). *Br. J. Ophthalmol.*, *67*:372–380.

91. Oberg, B. (1983). Antiviral effects of phosphonoformate (PFA foscarnet sodium). *Pharmacol. Ther.*, *19*:387–415.

92. Fannibg, M. M., Read, S.. E., Benson, M., Vas, S., Rachlis, A., Kozousek, V., et al. (1990). Foscarnet therapy of cytomegalovirus retinitis in AIDS. *J. Acquir. Immune Defic. Syndr.*, *3*:472–479.

93. Jacobson, M. A., and O'Donnell, J. J. (1991). Approaches to the treatment of cytomegalovirus retinitis: Ganciclovir and Foscarnet. *J. Acquir. Immune Defic.*, *Syndr.*, *4* (Suppl. 1):S11–S15.

94. She, S.-C., Peyman, G. A., and Schulman, J. A. (1988). Toxicity of intravitreal injection of foscarnet in the rabbit eye. *Int. Ophthalmol.*, *12*:151–154.

95. Diaz-Llopis, M., Chipont, E., Sanchez, S., Espana, E., Navea, A., and Menezo, J. L. (1992). Intravitreal foscarnet for cytomegalovirus retinitis in a patient with acquired immunodeficiency syndrome. *Am. J. Ophthalmol.*, *114*:742–747.

96. Kreiger, A. E., Foos, R. Y., and Yoshizumi, M. O. (1992). Intravitreous granulation tissue and retinal detachment following pars plana injection for cytomegalovirus retinopathy. *Graefe's Arch. Clin. Exp. Ophthalmol.*, *230*:197–198.

97. Sarraf, D., Equi, R. A., Holland, G. N., Yoshizumi, M. O., and Lee, D. A. (1993). Transscleral iontophoresis of foscarnet. *Am. J. Ophthalmol.*, *115*:748–754.

98. Yoshizumi, M. O., Lee, D. A., Sarraf, D. A., Equi, R. A., and Verdon, W. (1995). Ocular toxicity of iontophoretic foscarnet in rabbits. *J. Ocul. Pharmacol. Ther.*, *11*:183–189.

99. Anand, R., Nightingale, S. D., Fish, R. H., Smith, T. J., and Ashton, P. (1993). Control of cytomegalovirus retinitis using sustained release of intra-ocular ganciclovir. *Arch., Ophthalmol.*, *111*:223–227.

100. Yoshizumi, M. O., Roca, J. A., Lee, D. A., Lee, G., and Gomez, I. (1996). Ocular iontophoretic supplementation of intravenous foscarnet therapy. *Am. J. Ophthalmol.*, *122*:86–90.

101. Yoshizumi, M. O., Dessouki, A., Lee, D. A., and Lee, G. (1997). Determination of Ocular toxicity in multiple applications of foscarnet ionto-phoresis. *J. ocular Pharmacol. Therapeut.*, *13*:529–536.

102. Hill, J. M., Wen, R., and Halford, W. P. (1998). Pathogenesis and molecular biology of ocular HSV in the rabbit. In: *Herpes Simplex Virus Protocols* (MS Brown, AR Maclean, eds.). Humana Press, Inc., Totowa, NJ, pp. 291–315.

103. Kaufman, H. E., and Rayfield, M. A. (1988). In: *The Cornea: Viral Conjunctivitis and Keratitis* (H. E. Kaufman, B. A. Barron, M. B.

McDonald, and S. R. Waltman, eds.). Churchill Livingstone, New York, pp. 299–331.

104. Hill, J. M., Gangarosa, L. P., and Park, N. H. (1977). Iontophoretic application of antiviral chemotherapeutic agents. *Ann. NY Acad. Sci., 284*:604–612.

105. Hill, J. M., Park, N. H., Gangarosa, L. P., Hull, D. S., Tuggle, C. L., Bowman, K., and Green, K. (1978). Iontophoretic application of vidarabine monophosphate into rabbit eyes. *Invest. Ophthalmol. Vis. Sci., 17*:473–476.

106. Kwon, B. S., Gangarosa, L. P., Park, N. H., Hull, D. S., Fineberg, E., Wiggins, C., and Hill, J. M. (1979). Effects of iontophoretic and topical application of antiviral agents in treatment of experimental HSV-1 keratitis in rabbits. *Invest. Ophthalmol. Vis. Sci., 18*:984–988.

107. Hill, J. M., Kwon, B. S., Burch, K. D., deBack, J., Whang, I., Jones, G. T., Luke, B., Andrews, P., Harp, R., Shimomura, Y., Hull, D. S., and Gangarosa, L. P. (1982). Acyclovir and vidarabine monophosphate: a comparison of iontophoretic and intravenous administration for the treatment of HSV-1 stromal keratitis. *Am. J. Med., 73*:300–304.

108. Stevens, J. G., Newburn, A. B., and Cook, M. L. (1972). Latent herpes simplex virus from trigeminal ganglia of rabbits with recurrent eye infection. *Nature (New Biology), 235*:216–217.

109. Stevens, J. G. (1994). Overview of herpesvirus latency. *Semi. Virol., 5*:191–196.

110. Rivera, L., Beuerman, R. W., and Hill, J. M. (1988). Corneal nerves contain intra-axonal HSV-1 after virus reactivation by epinephrine iontophoresis. *Curr. Eye Res., 7*:1001–1008.

111. Schmidt, D. D., Zyzanski, S., Ellner, J., Kumar, M. L., and Arno, J. (1985). Stress as a precipitating factor in subjects with recurrent herpes labialis. *J. Family Pract., 20*:359–366.

112. Varnell, E. D., Kaufman, H. E., Hill, J. M., and Thompson, H. W. (1995). Cold stress-induced recurrences of herpetic keratitis in the squirrel monkey. *Invest. Ophthalmol. Vis. Sci., 36*:1181–1183.

113. Hill, J. M., Garza, H. H., Helmy, M. F., Cook, S. D., Osborne, P. A., Johnson, E. M., Thompson, H. W., Green, L. C., O'Callaghan, R. J., and Gebhardt, B. M. (1997). Nerve growth factor antibody stimulates reactivation of ocular herpes simplex virus type 1 in latently infected rabbits. *J. Neurovirol., 3*:206–211.

114. Stanberry, L. R. (1994). Animal models and HSV latency. *Sem. Virol., 5*:213–219.

115. Hill, J. M., Haruta, Y., and Rootman, D. S. (1987). Adrenergically induced recurrent HSV-1 corneal epithelial lesions. *Curr. Eye Res., 6*:1065–1071.

116. Hill, J. M., Rayfield, M. A., and Haruta, Y. (1987). Strain specificity of spontaneous and adrenergically induced HSV-1 ocular reactivation in latently infected rabbits. *Curr. Eye Res., 6*:91–97.

117. Hill, J. M., Shimomura, Y., Kwon, B. S., and Gangarosa, L. P. (1986). Iontophoresis of epinephrine isomers to rabbit eyes induced HSV-1 ocular shedding. *Invest. Ophthalmol. Vis. Sci., 26*:1299–1303.

118. Kwon, B. S., Gangarosa, L. P., Burch, K. D., deBack, J., and Hill, J. M. (1981). Induction of ocular herpes simplex virus shedding by iontophoresis of epinephrine into rabbit cornea. *Invest. Ophthalmol. Vis. Sci., 21*:442–449.

119. Kwon, B. S., Gangarosa, L. P., Green, K., and Hill, J. M. (1982). Kinetics of ocular herpes simplex virus shedding induced by epinephrine iontophoresis. *Invest. Ophthalmol. Vis. Sci., 22*:818–821.

120. Willey, D. E., Trousdale, M. D., and Nesburn, A. B. (1984). Reactivation of murine latent HSV infection by epinephrine iontophoresis. *Invest. Ophthalmol. Vis. Sci., 25*: 945–950.

121. Gordon, Y. J., Araullo-Cruz, T. P., Romanowski, E., Ruziczka, L., Balouris, C., Oren, J., Cheng, K. P., and Kim, S. (1986). The development of an improved murine iontophoresis reactivation model for the study of HSV-1 latency. *Invest. Ophthalmol. Vis. Sci., 27*:1230–1234.

122. Varnell E. D., Kaufman, H. E., Hill, J. M., and Wolf, R. H. (1987). A primate model for acute and recurrent herpetic keratitis. *Curr. Eye Res., 6*:277–279.

123. Rootman, D. S., Haruta, Y., and Hill, J. M. (1990). Reactivation of HSV-1 in primates by transcorneal iontophoresis of adrenergic agents. *Invest. Ophthalmol. Vis. Sci., 31*:597–600.

124. Hill, J. M., Kwon, B. S., Shimomura, Y., Colborn, G. L., Yaghmai, F., and Gangarosa, L. P. (1983). Herpes simplex virus recovery in neural tissues after ocular HSV shedding induced by epinephrine iontophoresis to the rabbit cornea. *Invest. Ophthalmol. Vis. Sci., 24*:243–247.

125. Shimomura, Y., Gangarosa, L. P., Sr., Kataoka, M., and Hill, J. M. (1983). HSV-1 shedding by iontophoresis of 6-hydroxydopamine followed by topical epinephrine. *Invest Ophthalmol Vis. Sci., 24*:1588–1594.

126. Hill, J. M., Dudley, J. B., Shimomura, Y., and Kaufman, H. E. (1986). Quantitation and kinetics of induced HSV-1 ocular shedding. *Curr. Eye. Res., 5*:241–246.

127. Haruta, Y., Rootman, D. S., and Hill, J. M. (1988). Recurrent HSV-1 corneal epithelial lesions by timolol iontophoresis in latently infected rabbits. *Invest. Ophthalmol. Vis. Sci., 29*:387–392.

128. Hill, J. M., Shimomura, Y., Dudley, J. B., Berman, E., Haruta, Y., Kwon, B. S., and Maguire, L. J. (1987). Timolol induces HSV-1 ocular shedding in the latently infected rabbit. *Invest. Ophthalmol. Vis. Sci., 28*:585–590.

129. Rootman, D. S., Haruta, Y., Hill, J. M., and Kaufman, H. E. (1989). Trifluridine decreases ocular HSV-1 recovery, not recurrent HSV-1 lesions following timolol iontophoresis in the rabbit. *Invest. Ophthalmol. Vis. Sci., 30*:678–683.

130. Kaufman, H. E., Varnell, E. D., Gebhardt, B. M., Thompson, H. W., and Hill, J. M. (1996). Propranolol suppression of ocular HSV-1 recurrence and associated corneal lesions following spontaneous reactivation in the rabbit. *Curr. Eye Res., 9*:1015–1021.

131. Gebhardt, B. M., and Kaufman, H. E. (1995). Propranolol suppresses reactivation of herpesvirus. *Antiviral Res., 27*:255–261.

132. Garza, H. H., Jr., and Hill, J. M. (1997). Effect of a beta-adrenergic antagonist, propranolol, on induced HSV-1 ocular recurrence in latently infected rabbits. *Curr. Eye Res.*, *16*:453–458.

133. Haruta, Y., Rootman, D. S., Xie, L., Kiritoshi, A., and Hill, J. M. (1989). Recurrent HSV-1 corneal lesions in rabbits induced by cyclophosphamide and dexamethasone. *Invest. Ophthalmol. Vis. Sci.*, *30*:371–376.

134. Wagner, E. K., and Bloom, D. C. (1997). Experimental investigation of herpes simplex virus latency. *Clin. Microbiol. Rev.*, *10*:419–443.

135. Miller, C. S., Danaher, R. J., and Jacob, R. J. (1998). Molecular aspects of herpes simplex virus I latency, reactivation, and recurrence. *Crit. Rev. Oral Biol. Med.*, *9*:541–562.

136. Millhouse, S., and Wigdhal, B. (2000). Molecular circuitry regulating herpes simplex virus type 1 latency in neurons. *J. Neurovirol.*, *6*:6–24.

137. Stevens, J. G., Wagner, E. K., Devi-Rao, G. B., Cook, M. L., and Feldman, L. T. (1987). RNA complementary to a herpesvirus α gene mRNA is prominent in latently infected neurons. *Science*, *235*:1056–1059.

138. Spivak, J. G., and Fraser, N. W. (1987). Detection of herpes simplex virus type 1 transcripts during latent infection in mice. *J. Virol.*, *61*:3841–3847.

139. Javier, R. T., Stevens, J. G., Dissette, V. B., and Wagner, E. K. (1988). A herpes simplex virus transcript abundant in latently infected neurons is dispensable for establishment of the latent state. *Virology*, *166*:254–257.

140. Stevens, J. G. (1989). Human herpesviruses: a consideration of the latent state. *Microbiol. Rev.*, *53*:318–332.

141. Rock, D. L., Nesburn, A. B., Ghiasi, H., Ong, I., Lewis, T. L., Lokensgard, J. R., and Wechsler, S. L. (1987). Detection of latency-related viral RNAs in trigeminal ganglia of rabbits latently infected with herpcs simplex virus type 1. *J. Virol.*, *61*:3820–3826.

142. Cook, S. D., Hill, J. M., Lynas, C., and Maitland, N. J. (1991). Latency-associated transcripts in corneas and ganglia of HSV-1 infected rabbits. *Br. J. Ophthalmol.*, *75*:644–648.

143. Croen, K. D., Ostrove, J. M., Dragovic, L. J., Smialek, J. E., and Straus, S. E. (1987). Latent herpes simplex virus in human trigeminal ganglia. Detection of an immediate early gene "anti-sense" transcript by in situ hybridization. *N. Engl. J. Med.*, *317*:1427–1432.

144. Kaye, S. B., Lynas, C., Patterson, A., Risk, J. M., McCarthy, K., and Hart, C. A. (1991). Evidence of herpes simplex viral latency in the human cornea. *Br. J. Ophthalmol.*, *75*:195–200.

145. Fraser, N. W., Block, T. M., and Spivak, J. G. (1992). The latency-associated transcripts of herpes simplex virus: RNA in search of a function. *Virology* *191*:1–8.

146. Wagner, E. K., Flanagan, W. M., Devi-Rao, G., Zhang, Y. F., Hill, J. M., Anderson, K. P., and Stevens, J. G. (1988). The herpes simplex virus latency-associated transcript is spliced during the latent phase of infection. *J. Virol.*, *62*:4577–4585.

147. Block, T. M., and Hill, J. M. (1997). The latency associated transcripts (LAT) of herpes simplex virus: still no end in sight. *J. Neurovirol.*, *3*:313–321.

148. Farrell, M. J., Dobson, A. T., and Feldman, L. T. (1991). Herpes simplex virus-latency-associated transcript is a stable intron. *Proc. Natl. Acad. Sci. USA*, *88*:790–794.

149. Hill, J. M., Sedarati, F., Javier, R. T., Wagner, E. K., and Stevens, J. G. (1990). Herpes simplex virus latent phase transcription facilitates in vivo reactivation. *Virology*, *174*:117–125.

150. Hill, J. M., Maggioncalda, J. B., Garza, H. H., Jr., Su, Y.-H., Fraser, N. W., and Block, T. M. (1996). In vivo epinephrine reactivation of ocular herpes simplex virus type 1 in the rabbit is correlated to a 370-base-pair region located between the promoter and the 5' end of the 2.0-kilobase latency-associated transcript. *J. Virol.*, *70*:7270–7274.

151. Bloom, D. C., Devi-Rao, G. B., Hill, J. M., Stevens, J. G., and Wagner, E. K. (1994). Molecular analysis of herpes simplex virus type 1 during epinephrine-induced reactivation of latently infected rabbits in vivo. *J. Virol.*, *68*:1283–1292.

152. Bloom, D. C., Stevens, J. G., Hill, J. M., and Tran, R. K. (1997). Mutagenesis of a cAMP response element within the latency-associated transcript promoter of HSV-1 reduces adrenergic reactivation. *Virology*, *236*:202–207.

153. Colgin, M. A., Smith, R. L., and Wilcox, C. L. (2001). Inducible cyclic AMP early repressor produces reactivation of latent herpes simplex virus type 1 in neurons in vitro. *J. Virol.*, *75*:2912–2920.

154. Loutsch, J. M., Perng, G.-C., Hill, J. M., Zheng, X., Marquart, M. E., Block, T. M., Ghiasi, H., Nesburn, A. B., and Wechsler, S. L. (1999). Identical 371-base-pair deletion mutations in the LAT genes of herpes simplex virus type 1 McKrae and 17syn+ result in different in vivo reactivation phenotypes. *J. Virol.*, *73*:767–771.

155. Zheng, X., Marquart, M. E., Loutsch, J. M., Shah, P., Sainz, B., Ray, A., O'Callaghan, R. J., Kaufman, H. E., and Hill, J. M. (1999). HSV-1 migration in latently infected and naive rabbits after penetrating keratoplasty. *Invest. Ophthalmol. Vis. Sci.*, *40*:2490–2497.

156. McGill, J. (1991). Herpes simplex latency and the eye. *Br. J. Ophthalmol.*, *75*:641–642.

157. Cook, S. D., Ophth, F. C., and Hill, J. M. (1991). Herpes simplex virus: molecular biology and the possibility of corneal latency. *Surv. Ophthalmol.*, *36*:140–148.

158. Bloom, D. C., Hill, J. M., Devi-Rao, G., Wagner, E. K., Feldman, L. T., and Stevens, J. G. (1996). A 348-base pair region in the latency-associated transcript facilitates herpes simplex virus type 1 reactivation. *J. Virol.*, *70*:2449–2459.

159. Perng, G.-C., Slanina, S. M., Ghiasi, H., Nesburn, A. B., and Wechsler, S. L. (1996). A 371-nucleotide region between the herpes simplex virus type 1 (HSV-1) LAT promoter and the 2-kilobase LAT is not essential for efficient spontaneous reactivation of latent HSV-1. *J. Virol.*, *70*:2014–2018.

160. Hill, J. M., Garza, H. H., Su, Y. H., Meegalla, R., Hanna, L. A., Loutsch, J. M., Thompson, H. W., Varnell, E. D., Bloom, D. C., and Block, T. M. (1997). A 437-base pair deletion at the beginning of the latency-associated transcript promoter significantly reduced adrenergically induced herpes simplex virus type 1 ocular reactivation in latently infected rabbits. *J. Virol., 71*:6555–6559.

161. Devi-Rao, G. B., Aquilar, J. S., Rice, M. K., Garza, H. H., Jr., Bloom, D. C., Hill, J. M., and Wagner, E. K. (1997). Herpes simplex virus genome replication and transcription during induced reactivation in the rabbit eye. *J. Virol., 71*:7039–7047.

162. Behar-Cohen, F. F., Savoldelli, M., Parel, J. M., Goureau, O., Thillaye-Goldenberg, B., Courtois, Y., Pouliquen, Y., and de Kozak, Y. (1998). Reduction of corneal edema in endotoxin-induced uveitis after application of L-NAME as nitric oxide synthase inhibitor in rats by iontophoresis. *Invest. Ophthalmol. Vis. Sci., 39*:897–904.

163. Martin, R. E., Loutsch, J. M., Garza, H. H., Jr., Boedeker, D. J., and Hill, J. M. (1999). Iontophoresis of lysophosphatidic acid into rabbit cornea induces HSV-1 reactivation: evidence that neuronal signaling changes after infection. *Mol. Vis., 5*:36, *www.molvis.org/molvis/v5/p36/*.

164. Dowd, N. P., Day, F., Timon, D., Cunningham, A. J., and Brown, L. (1999). Iontophoretic vincristine in the treatment of postherpetic neuralgia: A double-blind, randomized, controlled trial. *J. Pain Symptom Manage., 17*:175–180.

165. Santi, P., Volpato, N. M., Bettini, R., Catellani, P. L., Massimo, G., and Colombo, P. (1997). Transdermal iontophoresis of salmon calcitonin can reproduce the hypocalcemic effect of intravenous administration. *Farmaco, 52*:445–448.

166. Chang, S. L., Hofmann, G. A., Zhang, L., Deftos, L. J., and Banga, A. K. (2000). Transdermal iontophoretic delivery of salmon calcitonin. *Int. J. Pharm., 200*:107–113.

167. Mize, N. K., Buttery, M., Daddona, P., Morales, C., and Cormier, M. (1997). Reverse iontophoresis: monitoring prostaglandin E2 associated with cutaneous inflammation in vivo. *Exp. Dermatol., 6*:298–302.

168. Merino, V., Lopez, A., Hochstrasser, D., and Guy, R. H. (1999). Noninvasive sampling of phenylalanine by reverse iontophoresis. *J. Control Release, 61*:65–69.

169. Brasch, J., Huttemann, M., and Proksch, E. (2000). Iontophoresis of nickel elicits a delayed cutaneous response in sensitized individuals that is similar to an allergic patch test reaction. *Contact Dermatitis, 42*:36–41.

170. Asahara, T., Shinomiya, K., Naito, T., and Shiota, H. (1999). Induction of genes into the rabbit eye by iontophoresis. *Acta Soc. Ophthalmol. Jpn., 103*:178–186.

171. Chapon, P., Voigt, M., Gautier, S., Behar-Cohen, F., O'Grady, G., and Parel, J.-M. (1999). Intraocular tissues pharmacokinetics of ganciclovir transscleral Coulomb Controlled iontophoresis in rabbits (abstr). *IOVS/ARVO, 40*(4):S189.

172. Chauvaud, D., Behar-Cohen, F., Parel, J. M., and Renard, G. (2000). Transscleral iontophoresis of corticosteroids: Phase II clinical trial (abstr). *IOVS/ARVO 41*(4):S79.
173. Hayden, B. C., Voigt, M., Murray, T. G., Hernandez, E., Parel, J.-M., Cicciarelli, N., Feuer, W., Fulton, L., and O'Brien, J. M. (2000). Iontophoretic delivery of carboplatin in the treatment of murine transgenic retinoblastoma (abstr). *IOVS/ARVO 41*(4):S788.

13

Mucoadhesive Polymers in Ophthalmic Drug Delivery

Thomas P. Johnston, Clapton S. Dias, and Ashim K. Mitra
University of Missouri–Kansas City, Kansas City, Missouri, U.S.A.

Hemant Alur
Murty Pharmaceuticals, Inc., Lexington, Kentucky, U.S.A.

I. MUCOADHESIVE DOSAGE FORMS

A. Rationale for the Use of Mucoadhesives

Mucoadhesive dosage forms can provide a localized delivery of medicinal agents to a specific site in the body. The ability of mucoadhesive dosage forms to provide an intimate contact of the delivery system with the absorbing corneal layer would undoubtedly improve ocular bioavailability. The intimate contact may result in high drug concentration in the local area and hence high drug flux through the absorbing tissue. The intimate contact may also increase the local permeability of high molecular weight drugs such as peptides and proteins (1).

   Bioadhesion is a term that is widely used in the pharmaceutical literature. For drug delivery purposes, this term refers to the attachment of a drug carrier to a specific biological tissue. The majority of bioadhesives studied for drug delivery adhere to epithelial tissue and possibly to the mucosal surface of these tissues. Coating the external surface of the globe of the eye is a thin film of glycoprotein referred to as mucin. Therefore, such bioadhesion is also referred to as mucoadhesion. We shall take this opportunity to examine the structure and function of the mucus layer and its role in the process of mucoadhesion.

1. Physiology of the Mucus Layer

Mucus is a highly viscous secretion, which forms a thin, continuous gel blanket adherent to the mucosal epithelial surface. It is continually secreted by either the goblet cells or specialized exocrine glands in various regions of the body (2). The major constituents of mucus are water (95%) and high molecular weight glucoproteins capable of forming slimy, viscoelastic gels (3,4). The mean thickness of the mucus layer varies from 50 to 450 μm in humans and about half as much in the rat (5). The exact composition of the mucus layer varies substantially depending on the anatomical location, the species, and the pathophysiological state (6). Mucus contains some nonmucin components, which aid in its protective functions. Lipids and covalently bound fatty acids are frequently found in the mucin layer.

The mucus in the eye (Fig. 1) is mainly produced by the conjunctival goblet cells, which are most abundant in the inner canthral region and the lower fornix. The maximum number of such cells per unit area is found in the palpebral conjunctiva. On the surface of the mucosal tissue, the mucin molecules are tightly packed. As one proceeds outward from the epithelial layer, the mucus layer becomes less densely packed with a corresponding lowering of viscosity and ion content. Neutral and acidic mucins are produced by the goblet cells. Once secreted onto the conjunctiva, the mucus is spread over the surface of the cornea by the upper eyelid.

The principal functions of the mucus layer are lubrication and protection of the underlying epithelial cells from dehydration and other challenges. Continuous secretion of mucus is necessary to compensate for the loss due to digestion, bacterial degradation, and solubilization of mucin molecules. Soluble mucus may form temporary unstirred layers atop the adherent mucus gel (5).

2. Composition of Mucin

Characteristically, the mucus is composed of a number of components: glycoproteins, proteins, lipids, electrolytes, inorganic salts, water, enzymes, mucopolysaccharides, among others. The mucin molecule of a polypeptide backbone, which is attached to the pendant sugar groups at periodic intervals on the peptide chain. The molecular weights of these glycoproteins vary from 2×10^6 to 14×10^6 daltons (3). In general, a major portion of the peptide backbone is covered with carbohydrates grouped in various combinations. Galactose, fucose, N-acetylglucosamine, N-acetylgalactosamine, and N-acetylneuraminic acid (sialic acid) are typically found in the mucin molecules. These carbohydrates may constitute as much as 70–90% of the total mucin weight (7). The sugar molecules can carry sulfate residues via ester linkages. Each carbohydrate chain terminates in either a sialic acid

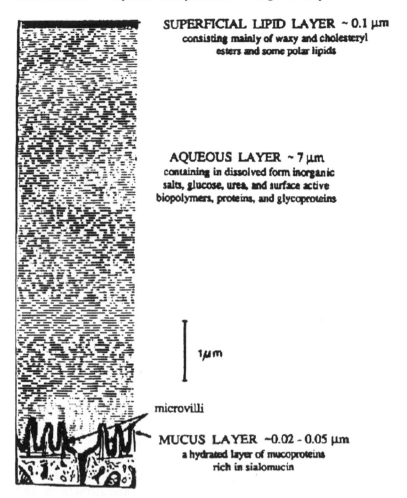

SUPERFICIAL LIPID LAYER ~ 0.1 μm
consisting mainly of waxy and cholesteryl
esters and some polar lipids

AQUEOUS LAYER ~ 7 μm
containing in dissolved form inorganic
salts, glucose, urea, and surface active
biopolymers, proteins, and glycoproteins

1μm

microvilli

MUCUS LAYER ~0.02 - 0.05 μm
a hydrated layer of mucoproteins
rich in sialomucin

Figure 1 Structure and composition of the tear film, illustrating the physicochemical properties of the mucus layer.

($pK_a = 2.6$) or with an L-fucose group. Hence, the mucin molecules behave as anionic polyelectrolytes as neutral pH (8). Because of the rather large number of sugar groups, the mucin molecule is capable of picking up almost 50–80 times its own weight in water. The oligosaccharides form a protective coat over the glycoprotein backbone by preventing the enzymatic action of proteases (9). Numerous sugar hydroxyl groups of mucin molecules have the potential to interact with other polymers by hydrogen bonds. The positions and relative amounts of amino acids in the glycoprotein backbone are important to the matrix structure of the mucus, since they confer to the overall tertiary structure and folding of the glycoprotein.

B. Mechanism of Mucoadhesion

The attachment of mucin to the epithelial surface may be considered as an interaction of a number of charged and neutral polymer groups with the mucin through noncovalent bonds. Understanding the mechanisms of mucoadhesion is fundamental to the development of mucoadhesive. One may view the entire process to be simply a physical entanglement—a currently accepted mechanism for the attachment of cross-linked polyacrylates to mucin (10). The polymer undergoes swelling in water, which permits entanglement of the polymer chains with mucin on the epithelial surface of the tissue (11). The un-ionized carboxylic acid residues on the polymer form hydrogen bonds with the mucin molecule.

The mucoadhesion phenomenon has also been explained using the mechanisms of nonbiological adhesion, such as electron transfer (12), wetting (13–16), diffusion (11,17–20), adsorption (21–23), fracture (24–25), and mechanical interlocking theories (26). Although these theories provide some insights into the mechanisms of mucoadhesion, no one theory by itself has successfully explained the phenomenon of mucoadhesion. Considering the number of factors involved in this process, this is not surprising.

Understanding molecular interactions between mucin and mucoadhesive may provide a better hypothesis for mucoadhesion. When two molecules coalesce, the interaction is composed of attractive and repulsive forces. The magnitudes of these two forces determine whether the molecules will interact or not. For mucoadhesion to occur, the attractive interaction should be larger than nonspecific repulsion. Attractive interactions result from van der Waals forces, hydrogen bonding, electrostatic attractions, and hydrophobic bonding. Repulsive interactions occur as the result of electrostatic and steric repulsions. The theories relating to these phenomena are detailed elsewhere (27).

The bioadhesive process can be conceptualized as the establishment of intimate contact, by diffusion or network expansion, of the polymer chains, with subsequent interpenetration (11). This physical model is depicted in Figure 2. In swellable hydrogels, an expanded polymer is a necessary prerequisite for adhesion, and this process may be further enhanced by viscoelastic deformation of the bioadhesive and substrate tissue by applied force or pressure.

When anionic polymers interact with anionic mucin, the maximum adhesion occurs at an acidic pH, indicating that it is the protonated form

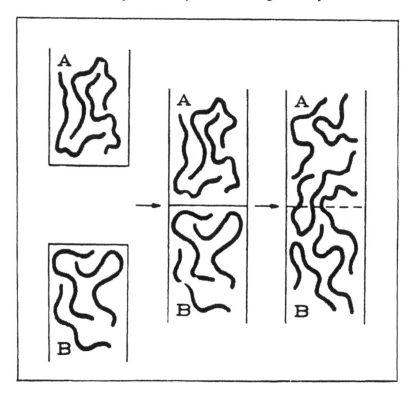

Figure 2   Schematic representation of the chain interpenetration during the bioadhesion of a polymer (A) with the mucus layer (B).

of the mucoadhesive that is responsible for the bioadhesion. Therefore, hydrogen bonding plays an important role in bioadhesion (28).

In addition, the expanded nature of both mucin and polymer networks permit mutual interpenetration. Interpenetration/interdiffusion of mucin and the adhesives results in increased contact and henceforth physical entanglement of the two different macromolecules. The physical entanglement is time dependent and may be enhanced by promoting intermolecular interactions between specific functional groups on the two polymers. Strong mucoadhesion depends on the moderate interactive forces between mucus and mucoadhesives, which will allow diffusion and subsequent entanglements among polymer chains. A number of factors may affect interpenetration; i.e., chain segment mobility, chain entanglement, cross-linking density of the networks, swelling, porosity, and compatibility of adhesives and mucin.

While a number of polymers will attach to mucin through noncovalent and covalent bonds, the former is preferred, since the strength of attachment is sufficiently strong. The removal occurs primarily through mucin turnover. The strength of adhesion between polycarbophil (partial structure shown in Fig. 3) and mucin is sufficiently stronger to resist rinsing. Forcible removal leads to rupture of mucin-mucin bonds and polymer-mucin bonds. The water-swellable yet water-insoluble systems are preferred as mucoadhesives, since predictable drug release from such systems would be easier to obtain. Moreover, toxicity concerns will also be less for an insoluble polymer. Table 1 lists some of the representative mucoadhesives.

C. Factors Relevant to Ocular Mucoadhesion

A number of variables can affect the performance of an ocular delivery system, especially when mucoadhesives are employed in the design of an ophthalmic vehicle. Satisfactory performance of a topical dosage form depends on a number of variables, which include experimental, physiological, and dosage form effects.

1. Experimental Variables

a. Mucoadhesive Polymer Characteristics.   Choice of polymer plays an important role in the release kinetics of the drug from a mucoadhesive dosage form. Ocular bioavailability from a mucoadhesive dosage form will depend on the polymer's bioadhesion properties, which, in turn, are affected by its swelling properties, hydration time, molecular weight, and degree of crosslinking. Other factors, such as pH, mucin turnover, and disease state, that affect bioadhesion will be discussed later. There are various new polymers now being introduced in the pharmaceutical market. Some of these polymers have found a place in the ophthalmic drug development industry. Recently, polyethylene oxide (PEO) has been investi-

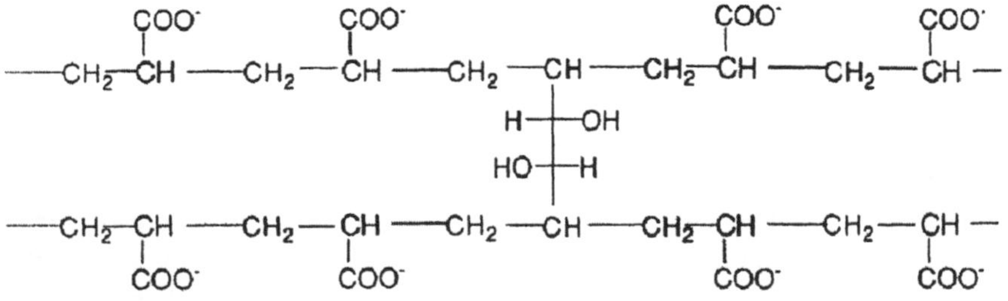

Figure 3 Partial structure of polycarbophil.

Table 1 Some Representative Mucoadhesives with Their Relative Mucoadhesive Performance

Substance	Adhesive performance
Carboxymethylcellulose	Excellent
Carbopol	Excellent
Carbopol and hydroxypropylcellulose	Good
Carbopol base with white petrolatum/hydrophilic petrolatum	Fair
Carbopol 934 and EX 55	Good
Poly(methyl methacrylate)	Excellent
Polyacrylamide	Good
Poly(acrylic acid)	Excellent
Polycarbophil	Excellent
Homopolymers and copolymers of acrylic acid and butyl acrylate	Good
Gelatin	Fair
Sodium alginate	Excellent
Dextran	Good
Pectin	Poor
Acacia	Poor
Povidone	Poor
Poly(acrylic acid) cross-linked with sucrose	Fair

gated extensively for ophthalmic purposes (29). Investigators have shown that polymer molecular weight affects the in vitro and in vivo performance of the dosage form into which it is incorporated. It is reported that for a given polymer there exists a hydration degree corresponding to an optimum polymer concentration in the gel allowing maximal interaction with the substrate (in this case, the mucous layer). Hydration time affects the bioadhesive force, and hence it is essential to determine the optimal hydration degree. At the optimum hydration, there exists an optimum polymer concentration in the gel allowing maximal interaction between the polymer and the substrate. Higher concentrations of the polymer will favor polymer-polymer interactions, whereas, at lower concentrations, the number of penetrating polymer chains per unit volume of the mucous layer is decreased, leading to a weak bioadhesive force. Studies with PEO showed that molecular weight affected the degree of hydration and, in turn, affected bioadhesion. With PEOs it was found that the mucoadhesive potential of the lower molecular weight PEOs was greater than that of the higher molecular weight PEOs, with a maximum for PEO 400. Another important factor to be considered is the affect of these polymers on the viscosity of the tear fluid. If the polymer enhances the viscosity of the tear fluid, precorneal clearance will decrease, allowing more contact time between the drug and the cornea. Viscosity of the aqueous solution increases with an increase in the polymer molecular weight. However, when formulating an ophthalmic dosage form, it is essential to strike a balance between the hydration properties and the viscosity-enhancing effects of the polymer. A polymer that enhances viscosity severalfold may not necessarily be ideal, as it may have poor hydration properties leading to weak bioadhesion and hence might fail. Higher molecular weight polymers may swell excessively in aqueous solutions leading to their limited use in the dosage form. In addition to these factors, the toxicity and degree of irritation exerted by the polymer affect the precorneal residence time of the dose. A polymer that irritates the corneal surface will cause increased tear secretion leading to dilution and elimination of the drug.

b. pH. The pH of the medium employed in the mucoadhesion studies has a profound effect on the performance of the delivery system. The effects of hydrophilicity and hydrogen bonding of polymers cannot be overemphasized in mucoadhesion, considering the fact that common functional groups found in bioadhesive polymers, i.e., carboxyl, amide, and sulfate groups, are polar and have the ability to form hydrogen bonds. This property of the polymers in turn has been shown to correlate well with the degree of hydration, which can be controlled by adjusting the pH of the medium (30). The first systematic investigation of pH effects on mucoadhesive strength was undertaken using polycarbophil and rabbit gastric tissue (Fig. 3). The experiments revealed maximum adhesive strength at or below pH 3 and a complete loss in mucoadhesive property above pH 5. The results indicated that the protonated carboxyl groups rather than the ionized carboxylate anions interact with mucin molecules through numerous hydrogen bonds. At higher pH values, the chains are fully extended owing to electrostatic repulsion of the carboxylate anions. Since the mucin molecules are negatively charged in this environment, electrostatic repulsion also occurs. Similar postulations have been forwarded by Nagai and Machida (31), where the interpolymer complex between hydroxypropylcellulose and Carbopol 934 was observed below pH 4.5 (32).

At physiological pH (pH 7.4) mucin is negatively charged owing to the presence of sialic acid groups at the terminal ends of the mucopolysaccharide chains (33). The preferential uptake of cationic liposomes by the cornea is probably evidence supporting the hypothesis of electrostatic interactions between the mucin and cationic mucoadhesives. In the case of anionic polymers, a hydrogen bonding mechanism is suggested for mucoadhesion.

At physiological pH, the hydration of the cross-linked polymers in the precorneal fluid is maximum, whereas the number of hydrogen bonds is comparatively low. Such loss in hydrogen bonding ability somewhat lowers the mucoadhesive strength in the precorneal fluid. However, the attachment is firm enough to provide some retention of the delivery system in the precorneal area.

c. Contact Time. Almost all bioadhesive polymers are solvated in aqueous medium and owe their expanding networks to hydration and subsequent swelling. Also, this swelling would increase the flexibility and mobility of the polymer chains. Swelling is an important prerequisite for the interpenetration and entanglement, i.e., strong bioadhesion.

The initial contact time between mucoadhesives and the mucus determines the extent of swelling of the mucoadhesives and the interpenetration of polymer chains. The mucoadhesive strength has been shown to increase with an increase in the initial contact time (34,35). Nevertheless, one needs to consider the optimum contact time based on the tissue viability. In the case of mucoadhesive dosage forms, which needs to be polymerized at the site of application, i.e., corneal, buccal, or nasal tissue, the initial contact time is critical for successful mucoadhesion (36).

Recent reports (37) suggest that the adhesive strength increases as the molecular weight of the bioadhesive polymer increases up to 100,000 daltons. For sodium carboxymethyl cellulose to function as an effective bioadhesive, the molecular weight should be in excess of 78,600 daltons (38). The adhesive force may be related to the critical macromolecular length required to produce entanglement and an interpenetrating layer.

d. Selection of Model Substrate. An abundance of literature exists detailing the use of tissue samples for understanding the mechanism of mucoadhesion and bioadhesion of new materials. Gastric mucosa obtained from rabbits is the most common model tissue specimen cited in the literature. However, caution needs to be exercised in terms of extrapolation of these findings to any human clinical studies.

The handling and treatment of biological substrates during the testing of mucoadhesives is an important factor. Physical and biological changes may occur in the mucus gels or tissues under the experimental conditions (38–40), which may be of major concern in optimizing the delivery systems. The viability of the biological tissue needs to be confirmed by electrophysiology or histological examinations.

2. Physiological Variables

a. Mucin Turnover. The mucin turnover is expected to limit the residence time of the mucoadhesives. This is especially significant, since the mucoadhesive will eventually be detached from the surface of the eye owing to mucin turnover. However, the turnover rate may increase in the presence of the mucoadhesive dosage form. An increase in the rate of mucus production generates a substantial amount of the soluble mucin molecules, which will interact with mucoadhesives before they have a chance to attach to the mucus layer. This phenomenon has been demonstrated to be true and unavoidable (41). The exact turnover rate of the mucus layer remains to be determined. Although the thickness of the mucus layer in contact with the epithelial cells is quite small, it is of similar magnitude to the estimated mean diffusional path on the corneal surface.

b. Choice of Animal Model. The most commonly used animal model for ocular studies has been the albino rabbit, because of its ease of handling, low cost, comparable eye size to those of humans, and a vast amount of available information on its anatomy and physiology. This animal model seems to be less sensitive to ocular availability alterations from viscosity changes in topical vehicles than humans (42). Since the blink rate of rabbits (4 times/h) (43) is significantly less than that of humans (15 times/min), humans commonly require higher viscosities than rabbits to retain the drug on the corneal surface. A very important consideration in using the rabbit model for evaluation of mucoadhesives as an ophthalmic delivery device is the size of the drainage apparatus. Rabbits have one large punctum that is capable of accommodating a large particle, whereas humans have two small punctae in each eye. Cross-linked mucoadhesives must be cleared from the eye. Thus, the drainage opening is an important consideration.

A recent report (44) documented the species differences in the effect of polymeric vehicles on the corneal membrane disrupting action of benzalkonium chloride. The report suggested that the rabbit and human corneas differed in the mucin glycocalyx domains at their surfaces. In view of this report, more work needs to be done to delineate these differences. The animal model, which may be predictive of behavior of the ocular delivery systems in humans, plays an important role in the iterative process of design and evaluation of such systems. The lack of absolute predictability of the rabbit model relative to vehicle effects on ocular drug bioavailability may be attributed in part to the differences between rabbits and human subjects with respect to the anatomy and physiology of the precorneal area and the cornea itself.

c. Disease States. The physicochemical properties of the mucus are known to change during various pathological conditions such as the common cold, bacterial and fungal infections, and inflammatory conditions of the eye (45–47). The exact structural changes taking place in mucus under these conditions are not clearly understood. The problems presented by such a complex and changing biological milieu for potential adhesion represent a unique challenge to pharmaceutical scientists. If mucoadhesives are to be used in the diseased states, the bioadhesion property needs to be evaluated under identical experimental conditions.

Many physiological factors of normal and diseased eyes affect the performance of the delivery system. The rate of tear turnover and composition of the preocular tear film changes in various pathological conditions. The vehicles used in the formulation may also contribute to direct stimulation of the epithelial layers of the cornea or conujunctiva and cause release of enzymes, glycoproteins, or immunological factors. In pathologies involving mucus-secreting epithelial cells, hypersecretion is more common than hyposecretion. Mucus hyposecretion results in disruption of the tear film and dry spot formation. An excess of mucus occurs in a number of disease states such as neuroparaly tickeratitis and keratoconjunctivitis sicca. Under these conditions, the degree of sulfation of the mucin layer is also known to increase (7). Blinking mixes the secretions and removes tear film debris. In addition, the dosage form location will contribute to the composition and rate of tear secretion in a variety of ways. Thus, in both normal and diseased eyes, the effects of the adhesive dosage form on ocular physiology may determine the ultimate therapeutic outcome.

3. Dosage Form Effects

a. Extent of Drug Incorporation.   The drug may be loaded onto the polymer matrix in a variety of ways. The most common approach is to incorporate the drug into mucoadhesive drug delivery systems, as shown in Figure 4. For water-soluble polymers, it is possible to employ the mucoadhesive as a typical polymer to coat or to laminate a device. The contact time in such cases is rate limited by the dissolution of the polymer. Such systems, however, suffer from the disadvantage of having a short shelf life, because of the undesirable release of the drug in the aqueous environment (moisture) of the storage container.

The cross-linked mucoadhesives need to become hydrated to function as an effective mucoadhesive drug delivery device. In such cases, the adhesive often detaches itself from the rate-controlling drug delivery device and causes a premature release of the drug, especially with water-soluble drugs. One solution to such a problem is through incorporation of a sparingly soluble drug inside the mucoadhesive polymer. The device can slowly provide drug release until dissolution is complete. This approach may be used for sparingly soluble salts and lipophilic prodrugs of highly water-soluble drugs.

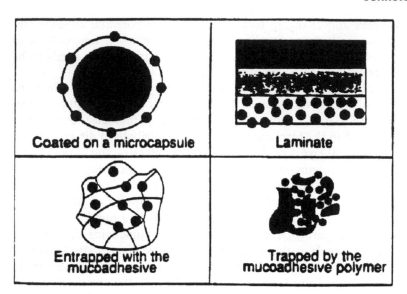

Figure 4 Approaches to incorporate drug into mucoadhesive drug delivery systems. Top panels: (●) mucoadhesive. Bottom panels: (●) drug.

Achieving high consistent loading compounds into mucoadhesive dosage forms continues to be a significant problem. A combination of a phase change and mucoadhesive concept may be used in some cases. For example, polycarbophil exhibits large changes in viscosity with pH and ionic strength. Thus, drugs either alone or with a small quantity of lipid can be suspended with the polycarbophil at the proper pH and ionic strength. When such a suspension is placed in the tear pocket of the eye, it rapidly gels, trapping the drug. The newly formed gel then releases the drug slowly over prolonged periods of time.

b. Vehicular Effects. A delivery system that would allow the drug to remain associated with a vehicle possessing enhanced precorneal retention may, therefore, provide for an attractive ocular drug delivery system. Most attention has been directed toward the influence of solution viscosity, although it has been shown that the maximum ocular availability increase obtained in rabbits by increasing the viscosity of the vehicle is approximately twice that from a simple aqueous solution (7). The viscosity effect of mucoadhesives on ocular delivery, therefore, needs to be addressed.

According to Swan (48), maintaining the lubricity and viscosity of the precorneal film is as important as maintaining the isotonicity and pH of the ophthalmic solutions. When aqueous solutions are instilled in the eye, the integrity of the precorneal film is altered. However, when 1% methylcellulose solution is instilled into the eye, it spreads evenly over the surface of the globe, imparts viscosity to the precorneal film, and causes minimal alteration in the integrity of the precorneal film. The viscosity of the methylcellulose solution prevents it from being washed rapidly from the eye and maintains the normal physiology, i.e., lacrimation. A combination of these effects increases contact time, which prolongs the absorption of drugs like homatropine (49). Oechsner and Keipert (50) have altered a polyacrylic acid (PAA) aqueous formulation for dry eyes by including a second polymer. Since PAA solutions have the disadvantage that PAA builds high viscous gels in the usual concentration of 0.2% and at physiological pH, the authors have included polyvinylpyrrolidone (PVP) in the ocular formation (50). After full hydration of the PAA polymer, a dispersion containing 2% PA was prepared and combined with an aqueous solution of PVP at a temperature of 30°C while stirring (50). A 10% aqueous solution of NaCl was then added, which resulted in a clear preparation and the formulations then made isotonic with mannitol and stabilized with 0.01% EDTA (50). The net effect of the addition of the PVP to the PAA solution was a significant reduction in the apparent viscosity of the formulation such that the preparation was nonirritating to ocular tissues (50). The mucoadhesion index (as a measure of bioadhesive strength) was determined for the experimental PAA/PVP formulations and found to possess greater mucoadhesivity compared to monopolymer formulations that employed PAA alone. It was postulated that perhaps sustained or prolonged delivery of both hydrophilic and lipophilic drugs may be possible by incorporation of either in a PAA complex with PVP (50).

Increasing contact time with methylcellulose ophthalmic vehicles has been found to be preportional to its viscosity for up to about 25 cps. This effect has been found to level off at 55 cps (51). In humans, a significant reduction in the drainage rates was observed with higher concentrations of polyvinyl alcohol (5.85%) and with 0.9% hydroxypropyl methylcellulose (42). However, it appears that in order to achieve the substantial reduction in drainage rate, abnormally high viscosities are required.

Physicochemical parameters of the viscosity-imparting agents, other than those related to viscosity effects, may also influence the corneal retention as well as ocular bioavailability from an ophthalmic product. Benedetto et al. (52) examined this effect using an in vitro model of the corneal surface and suggested that polyvinyl alcohol, but not hydroxypropyl methylcellulose, would significantly increase the thickness of the corneal tear film. However, such affects are considered to be only minimal. Davies et al., using rabbits, demonstrated not only a significant increase in the precorneal clearance, but also a significant increase in the bioavailability of pilocarpine when administered as a mucoadhesive polymeric solution (Carbopol 934P) as compared to an equivoscous, nonmucoadhesive polyvinyl alcohol (PVA) solution (53). Studies conducted to evaluate vehicle-drug (Carbopol 934P-pilocarpine) association indicated no binding of the pilocarpine to the polymer at physiological pH (53). Huupponen et al., using albino rabbits, combined the myriatic and cycloplegic agent, cyclopentolate, with either polygalacturonic or hyaluronic acid and determined whether the mydriatic response was increased compared to cyclopentolate base alone (54). Although treated eyes all demonstrated approximately the same time to reach a maximum mydriatic response when compared to cyclopentolate base alone, the cyclopentolate/polygalacturonic (CY-PGA) and cyclopentolate/hyaluronic acid (CY-HA) formulations demonstrated a significant increase in the maximal mydriatic response when compared to the base alone. However, only the CY-PGA formulation demonstrated a significant ($p < 0.05$) increase in the ocular bioavailability of cyclopentolate (54).

    Increasing the contact time in the precorneal area appears to be governed by both the mucoadhesive agent as well as the viscosity effects of the polymer. Thus, in designing the ocular drug delivery systems using mucoadhesives, one needs to find a vehicle that imparts good mucoadhesive strength as well as high viscosity at a low concentration.

II. CURRENT STATUS OF MUCOADHESIVES IN OCULAR DRUG DELIVERY

The successful development of newer mucoadhesive dosage forms for ocular delivery still poses numerable challenges. Particularly important among these are the determination of the exact nature of the interactions occurring at the tissue mucoadhesive interface and the development of an ideal, nontoxic, nonimmunogenic mucoadhesive for clinical application. Moreover, a better understanding of the exact physical structure of mucin molecules by computational chemistry may aid in the calculation of the mucoadhesive strength.

    The pioneering work of Hui and Robinson (55) illustrated the utilization of bioadhesive polymers in the enhancement of ocular bioavailability of progesterone (Fig. 5). Subsequently, several natural and synthetic polymers have been screened for their ability to adhere to mucin epithelial surfaces; however, little attention has been paid to their use in ophthalmic drug delivery.

    Saettone et al. (56) undertook a study evaluating the efficacy of a series of bioadhesive dosage forms for ocular delivery of pilocarpine and tropica-

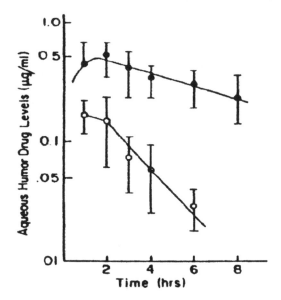

Figure 5 Progesterone levels in aqueous humour following topical administration of 0.3% suspension of progesterone-entrapped polymer (●) and 0.3% suspension of progesterone without polymer (○).

mide. From this study, hyaluronic acid emerged as the most promising mucoadhesive agent. The biological analysis data, however, revealed that the physicochemical properties of the drug itself had an impact on the efficacy of the delivery system.

To retard rapid drug loss from the precorneal area, various devices have been tested. Some of the potential candidates have been:

1. Erodible inserts of polyvinyl alcohol film or silicone rubber for the ocular delivery of pilocarpine and oxytetracycline, respectively (57,58)
2. Poly(vinyl methyl ether-maleic anhydride) matrices containing timolol (59)
3. Polycyanoacrylate nanoparticles to improve the corneal penetration of hydrophilic drugs (60)
4. An aqueous dispersion with limited water solubility (61)
5. In situ forming gel preparation (62)
6. Sustained-release liposomes coated with a mucoadhesive polymer (63)
7. Microsphere preparations (64)
8. Mucoadhesive polysaccharides (65)

Ocular inserts (cylindrical rods) fabricated from medical grade silicone rubber have also been evaluated for sustained delivery of oxytetracycline (OXT) when placed in the upper or lower conjunctival fornix (58). Cylindrical rods (diameter 0.9 mm, length 6–12 mm, weight 3–8 mg) all containing OXT were prepared from mixtures of silicone elastomer, OXT, and sodium chloride as a release modifier. A stable polyacrylic acid (PAA) or polymethacrylic acid (PMA) interpenetrating polymer network (IPN; 30% or 46% w/w) was grafted onto the insert's surface by treatment with a mixture of acrylic (or methacrylic) acid and ethylene glycol dimethacrylate in xylene at 100°C. This grafting procedure was employed since the hydrophobic silicone rubber would not be mucoadhesive to the hydrophilic palpebral and scleral mucosae. The thickness of the IPN layer was positively correlated with the strength of mucoadhesion in vitro with the PMA IPN grafting causing a lower rate of release of OXT than the IPN graft comprised of PAA (58). Release of OXT in vitro was zero-order and spanned nearly a week for some of the PMA IPN grafted silicone rods. When tested in rabbits, some of the IPN grafted inserts maintained in the lacrimal fluid an OXT concentration of 20–30 μg/mL for several days; an OXT concentration sufficient for killing microorganisms responsible for common ocular infections (58).

The use of poly(vinyl methyl ether-maleic anhydride) (PVMMA) ocular inserts containing timolol was shown to have both advantages and limitations. Timolol, a nonselective β-adrenergic antagonist widely used to treat open-angle glaucoma, can produce unwanted respiratory and cardiovascular side effects when systematically absorbed following ocular instillation. Using pigmented rabbits, Lee et al. (66) demonstrated that timolol/PVMMA inserts released the drug relatively slowly ($\cong$ 50% of the loading dose in 6 h) in vitro but increased the extent of systemic timolol absorption (AUC). The timolol/PVMMA inserts reduced the peak timolol concentration in plasma (C_{max}) and significantly delayed the time at which the timolol C_{max} was attained, raising the possibility that delayed timolol absorption occurred until the timolol/PVMMA inserts were discharged into the nasal cavity (66).

Poly(alkylcyanoacrylate) nanoparticles, specifically those formulated with poly(isobutylcyanoacrylate), have been systematically evaluated in vitro by Das et al. (67). Several formulation variables were assessed in a factorial design, including the use of dextran T40 or T70 and Pluronic™ F-68 or Tween™ 20 acting as stabilizer and surfactant, respectively, and three pH levels (2, 4, and 7). Significant effects of pH, surfactant, and stabilizer were noted on the molecular weight and size distribution of the timolol-containing nanoparticles (67). As an example, the greatest percent yield of formulated timolol nanoparticles was the Pluronic™ F-68 at pH 2. These authors concluded that formulation variables are extremely important for optimal in vivo performance of all poly(alkylcyanoacrylate)-based nanoparticles.

The aqueous dispersion upon instillation into the eye generated an apparent opaque mass, which adhered to and stayed in the lower fornix for extended periods of time. The slow dissolution of the polymer itself and diffusion of pilocarpine out of the polymeric matrix probably controls the availability of the drug for ocular absorption (68).

Similar results of pilocarpine ocular availability enhancement due to precorneal retention through mucoadhesion has been reported by Saettone et al. (69). This group investigated the use of a series of bioadhesive polymers, including hyaluronic acid, polygalacturonic acid, mesoglycan, and carboxymethylchitin.

In situ activated gel-forming systems can be described as viscous liquids, which undergo a transition to the gel phase upon exposure to certain physiological conditions like a pH change or temperature change. The systems utilize polymers that demonstrate transition from a sol to a gel phase when the dosage form is applied to the corneal surface. The phase transition occurs either due to a change in the pH (e.g., from 4.5 to 7.4) or due to a change in the temperature (from a lower temperature to the temperature of the corneal surface). Josh et al. were the first to report the use of a combination of polymers in such systems (70). They reported that a combination of polymers elicit the desired characteristics when subjected to changes in the physicochemical environment. Another factor that may affect this transition is the change in electrolyte composition. Several polymers such as carbopol, methylcellulose, pluronics, tetronics, and cellulose acetophthalate (CAP) have been used for this purpose. In order to reduce polymer content, Kumar and Himmelstein (71) developed a combination of polymers, which included polyacrylic acid (PAA) and hydroxypropylmethylcellulose (HPMC) for the release of timolol maleate. Various studies involving several different polymers have shown to increase ocular bioavailability. Rozier et al. found an improvement in the ocular absorption of timolol in the albino rabbit when administered in Gelrite, when compared with an equiviscous solution of hydroxyethylcellulose (72). Sanzigiri et al. compared various systems of methylprednisolone (MP): ester of Gelrite eyedrops, gellan-MP film, and gellan film with dispersed MP. The authors showed that the gellan eyedrops provided significant MP precorneal levels over a period of 6 hours (73).

Davies et al., using rabbits demonstrated that liposomes containing the mydriatic tropicamide and coated with either Carbopol 934P or Carbopol 1342 (a hydrophobic modified Carbopol resin) displayed a significant increase in precorneal retention at pH 5 compared to noncoated tropicamide liposomes (63). Both polymer coatings of tropicamide-containing liposomes failed to significantly increase the bioavailability of the entrapped drug relative to uncoated vesicles (63). However, in contrast to previous work (53), size and zeta potential measurements of uncoated tropicamide liposomes and liposomes coated in both polymer solutions demonstrated an association between the Carbopols and the vesicles at both pH 7.4 and pH 5, as evidenced by an increase in size and a decrease in the corresponding zeta potential. It was suggested that the prolongation in precorneal residence for Carbopol 1342–coated tropicamide liposomes was due to the formation of a three-dimensional microgel structure, which interacted with the phospholipid vesicles and subsequently increased their retention via a mechanism of adhesion to the mucin network (63).

Microsphere formulations have been evaluated for their capacity to retain ^{111}In as indium chloride in the preocular (precorneal) area of the rabbit eye (64). Clearance of the radiolabeled compound was monitored using gamma scintigraphy, and the influence of pH and prehydration of the microspheres on precorneal retention was assessed. These authors prepared microspheres of poly(acrylic acid) (Carbopol 907) cross-linked with maltose by a water-in-oil (w/o) emulsification process. Precorneal clearance of the microspheres at pH 5 and 7.4 were compared to an ^{111}In aqueous suspension (64). Clearance of the microspheres demonstrated a biphasic (α = rapid initial phase and β = slower phase) profile, and microspheres buffered at pH 5 exhibited a significantly slower β phase than microspheres buffered at pH 7.4. Presumably, the neutralized Carbopol formulation (pH 7.4) did not possess the same degree of mucoadhesive strength as the microsphere preparation formulated at pH 5. In vitro tests of mucoadhesive strength verified that the force of detachment of the microspheres formulated at pH 5 from mucus glycoprotein was significantly greater than the corresponding value for microspheres buffered at pH 7.4 (64). A significant increase in the retention of prehydrated microspheres in the preocular area was observed compared to microsphere formulations that were not hydrated prior to instillation (64).

Albasini and Ludwig (65) evaluated a series of polysaccharides for their potential inclusion in ocular dosage forms. The polysaccharides evaluated were carrageenan, locust bean gum, guar gum, xanthan gum, and scleroglucan. Measurements of the dynamic surface tension, pH, refractive index, and a visual clarity check comprised the physical measurements and determination of viscosity, viscoelasticity, effect of ionic strength on the resulting viscosity, and mucoadhesive strength (as assessed by an increase in the viscosity of a solution of the polysaccharide and mucin) comprised the rheological analysis of all the polysaccharides evaluated (65). All ocular preparations were made by adding the required amount of each polysaccharide to an aqueous iso-osmotic vehicle at 90°C and stirring the mixture mechanically until the polysaccharide was completely dissolved (65). Only scleroglucan and xanthan gum were found to demonstrate desirable viscoelastic and mucoadhesive properties suitable for instillation into the eye. The two preparations were evaluated in human volunteers and found to possess no ocular irritancy (65). Polysaccharides have also been shown to have potential for drug delivery by other routes of administration. Using a high molecular weight polysaccharide gum, *Hakea gibbosa*, isolated from a tree, Alur et al. have shown that the gum possessed both the ability to sustain the release of low molecular weight, organic-based drug substances as well as therapeutic polypeptides (salmon calcitonin) both in vitro and in vivo following application to the buccal mucosa of rabbits (74–76). This polysaccharide may hold promise for sustained delivery to the eye of both conventional drugs and newer therapeutic polypeptides requiring retention of biological activity.

The biomaterials for ocular use have been mainly synthetic polymers. Some natural biopolymers, such as collagen and hyaluronic acid, have also been examined. Of these, hyaluronic acid offers attractive possibilities (77–80). Some of the materials indicated as "ocular mucoadhesives" are mentioned below.

A. Naturally Occurring Mucoadhesives

Collagen and fibrin have been used as erodible insets for the long-term delivery of pilocarpine to the eye (81,82). The utility of these macromolecules in ophthalmic drug delivery depends largely upon their attachment capability to the drug molecules and their interaction with the glycocalyx domain of the corneal surface for maximum mucoadhesion. Among these, lectins and fibronectin are most promising.

The role of lectins as cellular-recognition mediators has been explored in great detail in the field of cellular biology. Lectins belong to a class of proteins of nonimmune origin that bind carbohydrates specifically and noncovalently (83). The most commonly studied lectin is the one derived from tomatoes. This particular lectin has been found to be nontoxic, binds specifically to the sialic acids (a major component of the mucus glycoproteins), and is transported into the cells by endocytosis (84). Such properties could be useful for the delivery of therapeutic agents into the ocular chambers.

Fibronectin is a glycoprotein and a component of the extracellular matrix. The pentapeptide backbone of this substance has been identified as having a cell-attachment property (85). Purified fibronectin has been reported to lessen the healing time of corneal ulcers (86). It has also been used in conjunction with hyaluronic acid for decreasing the healing time.

B. Synthetic Mucoadhesives

As discussed earlier, the potential of a mucoadhesive agent is determined by a number of parameters; i.e., chain length, configuration, and molecular weight. The extent of corneal adhesion of some neutral polymers has been reported to be comparable to that of natural mucins. Lemp and Szymanski (87) measured the extent of corneal adsorption of water-soluble polymers onto the epithelial surface. Among the polymers, 1.4% polyvinyl alcohol, 0.5% hydroxypropyl methyl cellulose, and 2% hydroxyethyl cellulose vehicles have shown comparable corneal adhesion to that of mucin. The study concluded that ocular therapeutic agents would be well absorbed from topical formulations containing such polymers. Since only marginal improvements (two- to threefold) in ocular bioavailability were seen with these agents, the adsorbed polymers were either unable to hold the drug or were being rapidly removed from the surface by the bathing tears. Other water-soluble polymers like polyacrylic acid also improved the ocular bioavailability of pilocarpine, albeit by a factor of two.

A polymer most effective as a mucoadhesive will be the one that can form an extended and hydrated network to allow for greater interpenetration and subsequent physical entanglement. These kinds of networks may be formed by:

1. Physical intertwining of the polymers
2. Bridging of the polymer chains
3. Cross-linking of the polymer chains

Thus, cross-linked polyacrylic acid has been shown to have an excellent mucoadhesive property, causing significant enhancement in ocular bioavailability (55). Using pigmented rabbits, Lehr et al. (88) demonstrated a twofold increase in the uptake of gentamicin by the bulbar conjunctiva when the aminoglycoside was delivered as a mucoadhesive, polycarbophil [a poly(acrylic acid)–based polymer] formulation. Two gentamicin formulations of this polymer (neutralized vs. nonneutralized) were evaluated and compared to an aqueous control formulation. While both the neutralized (pH 7.5) and nonneutralized (pH 2.5) gentamicin/polycarbophil formulations increased the uptake of the aminoglycoside antibiotic by the bulbar conjunctiva, only the nonneutralized aminoglycoside formulation provided drug penetration into the aqueous humor. Penetration of gentamicin into the aqueous humor from the nonneutralized formulation was suggested to result from drug absorption via the conjunctival-scleral pathway facilitated by intensified contact between the mucoadhesive polymer and the underlying bulbar conjunctiva (88). A partially esterified acrylic acid polymer was successful in prolonging the therapeutic effect of topically applied pilocarpine (89). Urtti et al. (90) also indicated that the use of a polyacrylamide and a copolymer of acrylamide (*N*-vinyl pyrrolidone and ethyl acrylate) as a matrix, which resulted in a threefold increase in the ocular bioavailability of pilocarpine.

Similarly, cyanoacrylates have been used in the field of opthalmology to seal corneal perforations and ulcers, to stop leakage of aqueous or vitreous humor, and to protect against external contamination (91,92). These agents have a potential as effective ocular mucoadhesive agents provided the monomer polymerization could be controlled.

III. WHAT IS IN STORE FOR THE FUTURE?

A multidisciplinary approach will be necessary to overcome the challenges associated with the development of ocular mucoadhesives. A nonbiodegradable adhesive is adequate for topical use to treat perforations and ulcerations. However, the use of a nontoxic biodegradable surgical adhesive is deemed necessary for long-term use in ocular drug delivery. Mucoadhesives can make an important contribution in this area. An ideal ocular mucoadhesive would be site specific, durable for the desired period of time, biodegradable, and above all nontoxic, nonimmunogenic, and nonirritant. It would be even better if the adhesive could serve as absorption enhancers (for therapeutic protein and peptide drugs) and/or as enzyme inhibitors.

REFERENCES

1. Harris, D., and Robinson, J. R. (1990). Bioadhesive polymers in peptide drug delivery, *Biomaterials, 11*:652.
2. Schacter, H., and Williams, D. (1982). Biosynthesis of mucus glycoproteins, *Adv. Exp. Med. Biol., 144*:3.
3. Marriot, C., and Gregory, N. P. (1990). Mucus physiology and pathology. In: *Bioadhesive Drug Delivery Systems* (V. Lenaerts and R. Gurny, eds.). CRC Press, Boca Raton, FL, p. 21.
4. Allen, A. (1981). The structure and function of gastrointestinal mucus. In: *Basic Mechanisms of Gastrointestinal Mucosal Cell Injury and Protection* (J. W. Harmon, ed.). Williams & Wilkins, Baltimore, p. 351.
5. Allen, A., and Carrol, N. J. H. (1985). Adherent and soluble mucus in the stomach and duodenum, *Dig. Dis. Sci., 30*:55s.
6. Gandhi, R. B., and Robinson, J. R. (1988). Bioadhesion in drug delivery, *Indian J. Pharm. Sci., 50*:145.

7. Marriot, C., and Hughes, D. R. L. (1989). Mucus physiology and pathology. In: *Bioadhesion: Possibilities and Future Trends* (R. Gurny and H. E. Junginger, eds.). Wissenschaftliche Verlagsgesellschaft, Stuttgart, p. 29.
8. Johnson, P. M., and Rainsford, K. D. (1978). The physical properties of mucus: Preliminary observations on the sedimentation behavior of porcine gastric mucus, *Biochim. Biophys. Acta, 286*:72.
9. Phelps, C. F. (1978). Biosynthesis of mucus glycoproteins, *Br. Med. Bull., 34*:43.
10. Robinson, J. R. (1989). Ocular drug delivery. Mechanism(s) of corneal drug transport and mucoadhesive delivery systems, *S.T.P. Pharma, 5*:839.
11. Mikos, A. G., and Peppas, N. A. (1986). Systems for controlled release of drug. V. Bioadhesive systems, *S.T.P. Pharm., 2*:705.
12. Dedaguin, B. V., Toporov, Y. P., Mueler, V. M., and Aleinikova, I. N. (1977). On the relationship between the electrostatic and the molecular component of the adhesion of elastic particles to a solid surface. *J. Colloid Interface Sci., 58*:528.
13. Baier, R.E., Shafrin, I.G., and Zisman, W.A. (1968). Adhesion: Mechanism that assist and impede it, *Science, 162*:1360.
14. Helfand, E., and Tagami, Y. (1971). Theory of the interface between immiscible polymers, *Polym. Lett., 9*:741.
15. Helfand, E., and Tagami, Y. (1972). Theory of the interface between immiscible polymers. II. *J. Chem. Phys., 56*:3592.
16. Helfand, E., and Tagami, Y. (1972). Theory of the interface between immiscible polymers, *J. Chem. Phys., 57*:1812.
17. Peppas, N. A., and Buri, P. A. (1985). Surface, interfacial and molecular aspects of polymer adhesion on soft tissues, *J. Controlled Release, 2*:257.
18. Peppas, N. A., and Lustig, B. R. (1985). The role of crosslinks, entanglements, and relaxations of the macromolecular carrier in the diffusional release of biologically active materials: Conceptual and scaling relationships, *Ann. NY Acad. Sci., 446*:26.
19. Reinhart, C. T., and Peppas, N. A. (1984). Solute diffusion in swollen membranes. II. Influence of crosslinking on diffusive properties. *J. Membr. Sci., 18*:227.
20. Peppas, N. A., and Reinhart, C. T. (1983). Solute diffusion in swollen membranes. Part I. New therapy, *J. Membr. Sci., 15*:275.
21. Tabor, D. J. (1977). Surface forces and surface interactions, *J. Colloid Interface Sci., 58*:2.
22. Kinloch, A. J. (1980). The science of adhesion: I. Surface and interfacial aspects, *J. Mater. Sci., 15*:2141.
23. Good, R. J. (1977). Surface free energy of solids and liquids: Thermodynamics, molecular forces and structure, *J. Colloid Interface Sci., 58*:398.
24. Ponchel, G., Touchard, F., Duchene, D., and Peppas, N. A. (1987). Bioadhesive analysis of controlled release systems. I. Fracture and interpene-

tration analysis in poly(acrylic acid) containing systems, *J. Controlled Release*, *5*:129.

25. Mikos, A. G., and Peppas, N. A. (1988). Polymer chain entanglements and brittle fracture, *J. Chem. Phys.*, *88*:1337.
26. Wake, W. C. (1976). Theories of adhesion and adhesive action. In: *Adhesion and Formulation of Adhesives*. Applied Science, London, p. 65.
27. Israelachvili, J. N. (1985). *Intermolecular and Surface Forces*. Academic Press, New York.
28. Pritchard, W. H. (1971). The role of hydrogen bonding in adhesion, *Aspects Adhes.*, *6*:11.
29. Colo, G. D., Bugalassi, S., Chetoni, P., Fiaschi, M. P., Zambito, Y. and Sattone, M. F. (2001). Relevance of polymer molecular weight to the in vitro/in vivo performances of ocular inserts based on poly(ethylene oxide), *Int. J. Pharmaceutics*, *220*:169.
30. Park, H., and Robinson, J. R. (1985). Physico-chemical properties of water insoluble polymers important to mucin/epithelial adhesion, *J. Controlled Release*, *2*:47.
31. Nagai, T., and Machida, Y. (1985). Advances in drug delivery. Mucosal adhesive dosage forms, *Pharma. Int. Engl. Ed., August*:196.
32. Satoh, K., Takayama, K., Machida, Y., Suzuki, Y., Nakagaki, M., and Nagai, T. (1989). Factors affecting the bioadhesive properties of tablets consisting of hydroxypropyl cellulose and carboxy vinyl polymers, *Chem. Pharm. Bull.*, *37*:1366.
33. Gottschalk, A. (1960). In: *The Chemistry and Biology of Sialic Acid and Related Substances*. Cambridge University Press, London.
34. Leonard, F., Hodge, J. W., Jr., Houston, S., and Ousterhout, D. K. (1968). Alpha cyanoacrylate adhesive bond strengths with proteinaceous and non proteinaceous substances, *J. Biomed. Mater. Res.*, *2*:173.
35. Smart, J. D., Kellaway, I. W., and Worthington, H. E. C. (1984). An in vitro investigation of mucosal adhesive materials for use in controlled drug delivery, *J. Pharm. Pharmacol.*, *36*:295.
36. Leung, S. H. S., and Robinson, J. R. (1990). Polymer structure features contributing to mucoadhesion. II., *J. Controlled Release*, *12*:187.
37. Chen, J. L., and Cyr, G. N. (1970). Compositions producing adhesion through adhesion. In: *Adhesive Biological Systems* (R. S. Manly, ed.). Academic Press, New York, p. 78.
38. Smart, J. D. (1991). An in vitro assessment of some muco-adhesive dosage forms, *Int. J. Pharm.*, *73*:69.
39. Park, K., and Park, H. (1990). Test methods of bioadhesion. In: *Bioadhesive Drug Delivery Systems* (V. Lenaerts and R. Gurny, eds.). CRC Press, Boca Raton, FL, p. 43.
40. Wang, P. Y., and Forrester, D. H. (1974). Conditions for the induced adhesion of hydrophobic polymers to soft tissue, *Trans. Am. Soc. Artif. Int. Organs*, *20*:504.

41. Teng, C. L. C., and Ho, N. F. L. (1987). Mechanistic studies in the simultaneous flow and adsorption of polymer coated latex particles on intestinal mucus. I: Methods and physical model development, *J. Controlled Release,* 6:133.

42. Zaki, I., Fitzgerald, P., Hardy, J. G., and Wilson, C. G. (1986). A comparison of the effect of viscosity in the precorneal residence of solutions in rabbit and man, *J. Pharm. Pharmacol., 38*:463.

43. Moss, R. A. (1987). The eyelids. In: *Adler's Physiology of the Eye: Clinical Applications,* 8th ed. (R. A. Moses and W. M. Hart, Jr., eds.). Mosby, St. Louis, p. 1.

44. Saettone, M. F., Giannaccinni, B., Guiducci, A., LaMarca, F., and Tota, G. (1985). Polymer effects on ocular bioavailability. II: The influence of benzalkonium chloride on the mydriatic response of tropicamide in different polymeric vehicles, *Int. J. Pharm., 25*:73.

45. Wright, P., and Mackie, I. A. (1977). Mucus in healthy and diseased eye, *Trans. Ophthalmol. Soc. UK, 91*:1.

46. Hardy, J. G., Lee, S. W., and Wilson, C. G. (1985). Intranasal drug delivery by sprays and drops, *J. Pharm. Pharmacol., 37*:294.

47. Tabachnik, N. F., Blackburn, P., and Cerami, A. (1981). Biochemical and rheological characteristics of sputum mucus from a patients with cystic fibrosis, *J. Biol. Chem., 256*:7161.

48. Swan, K. C. (1945). Use of methylcellulose in ophthalmology, *Arch. Ophthalmol., 33*:378.

49. Mueller, W. H., and Deardorff, D. L. (1956). Ophthalmic vehicles: The effect of methylcellulose on the penetration of Homatropine hydrobromide through the cornea, *J. Am. Pharm. Assoc., 45*:334.

50. Oechsner, M., and Keipert, S. (1999). Polyacrylic acid/polyvinylpyrrolidone biopolymeric systems. I. Rheological and mucoadhesive properties of formulations potentially useful for the treatment of dry-eye syndrome, *Eur. J. Pharm. Biopharm., 47*:113–118.

51. Saettone, M. F., Giannaccinni, B., Ravecca, S., La Marca, F., and Tota, G. (1984). Polymer effects of ocular bioavailability: The influence of different liquid vehicles on the mydriatic response of tropicamide in humans and in rabbits, *Int. J. Pharm., 20*:187.

52. Benedetto, D. A., Shah, D. O., and Kaufman, H. E. (1975). Instilled fluid dynamics and surface chemistry of polymers in the preocular tear film, *Invest. Ophthalmol., 14*:887.

53. Davies, N. M., Farr, S. J., Hadgraft, J., and Kellaway, I. W. (1991). Evaluation of mucoadhesive polymers in ocular drug delivery. I. Viscous solutions, *Pharm. Res., 8*:1039–1043.

54. Huupponen, R., Kaila, T., Saettone, M. F., Monti, D., Iisalo, E., Salminen, L., and Oksala, O. (1992). The effect of some macromolecular ionic complexes on the pharmacokinetics and dynamics of ocular cyclopentolate in rabbits, *J. Ocular Pharmacol., 8*:59–67.

55. Hui, H. W., and Robinson, J. R. (1985). Ocular delivery of progesterone using a bioadhesive polymer, *Int. J. Pharm., 26*:203.
56. Saettone, M. F., Chetoni, P., Torracca, M. T., Burgalassi, S., and Giannaccinni, B. (1989). Evaluation of mucoadhesive properties and in vivo activity of ophthalmic vehicles based on hyaluronic acid, *Int. J. Pharm., 51*:203.
57. Saettone, M. F., Giannaccini, B., Chetoni, P., Galli, G., and Chiellini, E. (1984). Vehicle effects on the ophthalmic bioavailability: An evaluation of polymeric inserts containing pilocarpine, *J. Pharm. Pharmacol., 36*:229.
58. Chetoni, P., Di Colo, G., Grandi, M., Morelli, M., Saettone, M. F., and Darougar, S. (1998). Silicone rubber/hydrogel composite ophthalmic inserts: Preparation and preliminary in vitro/in vivo evaluation, *Eur. J. Pharm. Biopharm., 46*:125–132.
59. Finne, U., Salivirta, J., and Urtti, A. (1991). Sodium acetate improves the ocular/systemic absorption ratio of timolol applied ocularly in monoisopropyl PVM-MA matrices, *Int. J. Pharm., 75*:R1.
60. Losa, C., Calvo, P., Castro, E., Vila-Jato, J. L., and Alono, M. J. (1991). Improvement of ocular penetration of amikacin sulphate by association to poly(butylcyanoacrylate) nanoparticles, *J. Pharm. Pharmacol., 43*:548.
61. Vanderhoff, J., El-Asser, E. R., and Urgerstad, J. (1977). U.S. Patent Application #867031.
62. Kumar, S., Haglund, B. O., and Himmelstein, K. J. (1994). In situ-forming gels for opthalmic drug delivery, *J. Ocular Pharmacol. 10*:47.
63. Davies, N. M., Farr, S. J., Hadgraft, J., and Kellaway, I. W. (1992). Evaluation of mucoadhesive polymers in ocular drug delivery. II. Polymer-coated vesicles, *Pharm. Res., 9*:1137–1144.
64. Durrani, A. M., Farr, S. J., and Kellaway, I. W. (1995). Precorneal clearance of mucoadhesive microspheres from the rabbit eye, *J. Pharm. Pharmacol., 47*:581–584.
65. Albasini, M., and Ludwig, A. (1995). Evaluation of polysaccharides intended for ophthalmic use in ocular dosage forms, *Farmaco, 50*:633–642.
66. Lee, V. H. L., Li, S. Y., Sasaki, H., Saettone, M. F., and Chetoni, P. (1994). Influence of drug release rate on systemic timolol adsorption from polymeric occular inserts in the pigmented rabbit, *J. Ocular. Pharmacol., 10*:421–429.
67. Das, S. K., Tucker, I. G., Hill, D. J. T., and Ganguly, N. (1995). Evaluation of poly(isobutylcyanoacrylate) nanoparticles for mucoadhesive ocular drug delivery. I. Effect of formulation variables on physicochemical characteristics of nanoparticles, *Pharm. Res., 12*:534–540.
68. Robinson, J. R., and Li, V. H. K. (1984). Ocular disposition and bioavailability of pilocarpine from Piloplex® and other sustained release drug delivery systems. In: *Recent Advances in Glaucoma* (U. Ticho and R. David, eds.). Excerpta Medica, Amsterdam, p. 231.
69. Saettone, M. F., Giannaccinni, B., Guidicci, A., and Savigni, P. (1986). Semisolids ophthalmic vehicles. III. An evaluation of four organic hydrogels containing pilocarpine, *Int. J. Pharm., 31*:261.

70. Joshi, A., Ding, S., and Himmelstein, K. J. Patent application U.S. 91/04104 (Publication No. WO 91/19481).

71. Kumar, S., and Himmelstein, K. J. (1995). Modification of in situ gelling behavior of carbopol solutions by hydroxypropyl methylcellulose. *J. Pharm. Sci., 84*:344.

72. Rozier, A., Mazuel, C., Grove, J., and Plazonnet, B. (1989). Gelrite: a novel, ion activated, in situ gelling polymer for ophthalmic vehicles. Effect on bioavailability of timolol, *Int. J. Pharmaceutics, 57*:163.

73. Sanzigiri, Y. D., Maschi, S., Crescenzi, V., Callegaro, L., Topp, E. M., and Stella, V. J. (1993). Gellan-based systems for ophthalmic sustained delivery of methylprednisolone. *J. Control Release, 26*:195.

74. Alur, H. H., Pather, S. I., Mitra, A. K., and Johnston, T. P. (1999). Transmucosal delivery of chlorpheniramine maleate from a buccal tablet containing a natural, mucoadhesive gum, *Int. J. Pharm., 188*:1–10.

75. Alur, H. H., Beal, J. D., Panther, S. I., Mitra, A. K., and Johnston, T. P. (1999). Evaluation of a novel, natural oligosaccharide gum as a sustained-release and mucoadhesive component of calcitonin buccal tablets, *J. Pharm. Sci., 88*:1313–1319.

76. Alur, H. H., Pather, S. I., Mitra, A. K., and Johnston, T. P. (1999). Evaluation of the gum *Hakea gibbosa* as a sustained-release and mucoadhesive component in buccal tablets, *Pharm. Develop. Technol., 4*:347–358.

77. Benditti, L. M., Kyyronen, K., Hume, L., Topp, E., and Stella, V. (1991). Steroid ester of hyaluronic acid in ophthalmic drug delivery, *Proc. Int. Symp. Controlled Release Bioact. Mater., 18*:497.

78. Saettone, M. F., Giannaccinni, B., Torracca, M. T., and Burgalassi, S. (1987). An evaluation of the bioadhesive properties of hyaluronic acid. *Proceedings of the 3rd Eur. Congress on Biopharm. Pharmacokinetics*, Vol. 1, Freiburg, April, p. 413.

79. Saettone, M. F., Chetoni, P., Torracca, M. T., Giannaccinni, B., and Ordello, G. (1986). Evaluation of hyaluronic acid as a vehicle for topical ophthalmic drugs. *Abstr. of Int. Symp. Ophthalmic Dosage Forms*, Pisa, Oct. 13–14.

80. Saettone, M. F., Chetoni, P., and Giannaccinni, B. (1985). Evaluation of hyaluronic acid as a vehicle for topical ophthalmic drugs, *Abstr. of 2nd Int. Conference on Polymers in Medicine*, Capri, June 3–7.

81. Miyazaki, S., Ishii, K., and Takada, M. (1982). Use of fibrin film as a carrier for drug delivery: A long acting delivery system for pilocarpine into the eye. *Chem. Pharm. Bull., 30*:3405.

82. Bloomfield, S. E., Miyata, T., Dunn, M. W., Bueser, N., Stenzel, K. H., and Rubin, A. L. (1978). Soluble gentamicin ophthalmic inserts as a drug delivery system, *Arch. Ophthalmol., 96*:885.

83. McCoy, J. P., Jr. (1986). Contemporary laboratory applications of lectins, *Biotechniques, 4*:252.

84. Kilpatrick, D. C., Pusztai, A., Grant, G., Graham, G., and Ewen, S. W. B. (1985). Tomato lectins resist degradation in the mammalian alimentary canal and binds to intestinal villi without deleterious effects, *FEBS Lett., 185*:299.

85. Hynes, R. O., and Yamada, K. M. (1982). Fibronectins: Multifunctional modular glycoproteins, *J. Cell Biol., 95*:369.
86. Nishida, T., Ohashi, Y., Awanta, T., and Manabe, R. (1983). Fibronectin, new therapy for corneal trophic ulcer, *Arch. Ophthalmol., 101*:1046.
87. Lemp, M. H., and Szymanski, E. S. (1975). Polymer adsorption at the ocular surface, *Arch. Ophthalmol., 99*:134.
88. Lehr, C. M., Lee, Y. H., and Lee, V. H. L. (1994). Improved ocular penetration of gentamicin by mucoadhesive polymer polycarbophil in the pigmented rabbit, *Invest. Ophthalmol. Vis. Sci., 35*:2809–2814.
89. Ticho, U., Blumenthal, M., Zonis, S., Gal, A., Blank, L., Mazor, Z. W. (1979). A clinical trial with Piloplex®—a new long-acting pilocarpine compound: Preliminary report, *Ann. Ophthalmol., April*:555.
90. Urtti, A., Salminen, L., Kujari, H., and Jantti, V. (1984). Effect of ocular pigmentation on pilocarpine pharmacology in the rabbit eye. II. Drug response, *Int. J. Pharm., 19*:53.
91. Refojo, M. F. (1982). Current status of biomaterials in ophthalmology, *Surv. Ophthalmol., 26*:257.
92. Refojo, M. F., Dohlman, C. H., and Koliopoulos, J. (1971). Adhesives in ophthalmology: A review, *Surv. Ophthalmol., 15*:217.

14

Microparticles and Nanoparticles in Ocular Drug Delivery

Murali K. Kothuri, Swathi Pinnamaneni, * **Nandita G. Das, and Sudip K. Das**
Idaho State University, Pocatello, Idaho, U.S.A.

I. INTRODUCTION

Controlled and sustained delivery of ophthalmic drugs continues to remain a major focus area in the field of pharmaceutical drug delivery with the emergence of new, more potent drugs and biological response modifiers that may also have very short biological half-lives. The major objective of clinical therapeutics is to provide and maintain adequate concentration of drugs at the site of action. In ocular drug delivery, the physiological constraints imposed by the protective mechanisms of the eye lead to poor absorption of drugs with very small fractions of the instilled dose penetrating the cornea and reaching the intraocular tissues. The reasons for inefficient drug delivery include rapid turnover, lacrimal drainage, reflex blinking, and drug dilution by tears (1,2). The limited permeability of cornea also contributes to the low absorption of ocular drugs. As shown in Figure 1, tear drainage causes a major portion of the administered dose to be transported via the nasolacrimal duct to the gastrointestinal (GI) tract, where it may be absorbed, leading to unwanted systemic side effects and occasional toxicity due to the drug (3). The rapid elimination of administered eye drops often results in a short duration of the ocular therapeutic effect, making a frequent dosing regimen necessary.

---
* *Current affiliation*: Bristol-Myers Squibb Company, New Brunswick, New Jersey, U.S.A.

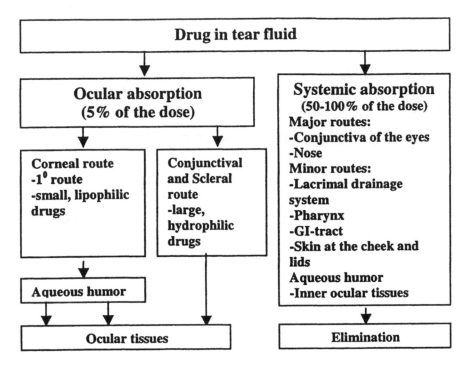

Fig. 1 Schematic diagram of ocular distribution. (From Ref. 3.)

Three main factors have to be considered when drug delivery is attempted to the intraocular tissues (4): (a) how to cross the blood-eye barrier (systemic to ocular) or cornea (external to ocular) to reach the site of action, (b) how to localize the pharmacodynamic action at the eye and minimize drug action on other tissues, and (c) how to prolong the duration of drug action such that the frequency of drug administration can be reduced. There is a clear need for effective topical formulations providing superior bioavailability of drugs along with a reasonable frequency of application, and the goals during the development of appropriate delivery systems should include increased contact time of the drug with the eye surface and promotion or facilitation of transfer of drug molecules from the tear phase into the eye tissue without causing any inconvenience to the patient. Approaches to optimize drug residence time have included prolongation of precorneal drug retention by the use of viscous gels, colloidal suspensions, and erodible or nonerodible inserts (5,6). Besides the issue of bioavailability, patient compliance and comfort considerations in drug instillation are very important factors that may impact the drug's therapeutic efficacy. Patient discomfort excludes inserts from the list of potentially popular drug delivery systems. Although adding soluble polymers to ophthalmic solutions can increase drug retention by increasing viscosity and decreasing the rate of drainage, there are problems associated with viscous solutions during their manufacture and administration that usually result in vision blurring, limiting their chances of becoming popular dosage forms. Liposomes have been extensively investigated as ocular drug delivery vehicles for over a decade as they offer potential benefits of controlled and sustained drug release and protection from metabolic processes while the therapeutic agent remains sequestered within the vesicles. But the problems associated with liposomes are possible toxicity and irritability. The primary factors that determine the relative toxicity of liposomes appear to be the lipid composition and irritability associated with the charge of liposomes (7–10). These factors may limit their chances of becoming popular ocular dosage forms of the future. Attempts to reduce systemic absorption have been made based on the design of prodrug derivatives with a higher lipophilic character (11–13). However, results obtained from these studies are inconclusive because most prodrugs are unstable in an aqueous solution.

In order to address the above-stated problems, micro- and nanotechnology involving drug-loaded polymer particles has been proposed as an ophthalmic drug delivery technique that may enhance dosage form acceptability while providing sustained release in the ocular milieu (14). Particulate drug delivery consists of systems described as microparticles, nanoparticles, microspheres, nanospheres, microcapsules, and nanocapsules. They consist of macromolecular materials and can be used therapeutically by themselves, e.g., as adjuvant in vaccines, or as drug carriers, in which the active principle (drug or biologically active material) is dissolved, entrapped, encapsulated, and/or to which active principle is absorbed, adsorbed, or attached. Particles ranging from 100 nm to the order of several hundred micrometers are included in the microparticulate category, which is divided into two broad groups (15): *microcapsules* are almost spherical entities of the order of several hundred micrometers in diameter where the drug particles or droplets are entrapped inside a polymeric membrane, and *microspheres* are polymer-drug combinations where the drug is homogeneously dispersed in the polymer matrix. Nanoparticles possess similar characteristics as microparticles, except their size is approximately three orders of magnitude smaller ($< 1\,\mu$m). Nanoparticles are also subdivided into two groups: nanospheres and nanocapsules (11). *Nanospheres* are small solid monolithic spheres constituted of a dense solid polymeric network, which develops a large specific area (16). The drug can be either incorporated or adsorbed onto the surface. *Nanocapsules* are small reservoirs consisting of a central cavity (usually an oily droplet containing dissolved drug) surrounded by a polymeric membrane. Several studies have shown nanoparticles to be more stable in biological fluids and during storage compared to other carriers that are similar in size distribution and controlled-release properties, such as liposomes. Furthermore, they can entrap and retain various drug molecules in their stable state.

Polymers used for the preparation of microparticulates may be erodible, biodegradable, nonerodible, or ion exchange resins (17). Nanoparticles made of nonbiodegradable polymers are neither digested by enzymes nor degraded in vivo through a chemical pathway (18). The risk of chronic toxicity due to the intracellular overloading of nondegradable polymers would be a limitation of their systemic administration to human beings, making these materials more suitable for removable inserts or implants. Erodible systems have an inherent advantage over other systems in that the self-eroding process of the hydrolyzable polymer obviates the need for their removal or retrieval after the drug is delivered. Upon the administration of particle suspension in the eyes, particles reside at the delivery site and the drug is released from the polymer matrix through diffusion, erosion, ion exchange, or combinations thereof (19).

Nanoparticles, when formulated properly, provide controlled drug release and prolonged therapeutic effect. To achieve these characteristics, particles must be retained in the cul-de-sac after topical administration, and the entrapped drug must be released from the particles at an appropriate rate. As mentioned before, the utility of nanoparticles as an ocular drug delivery system may depend on (19) (a) optimizing lipophilic-hydrophilic properties of the polymer-drug system, (b) optimizing rates of biodegradation in the precorneal pocket, and (c) increasing retention efficiency in the precorneal pocket. It is highly desirable to formulate the particles with bioadhesive materials in order to enhance the retention time of the particles in the ocular cul-de-sac. Without bioadhesion, nanoparticles could be eliminated as quickly as aqueous solutions from the precorneal site. Bioadhesive systems can be either polymeric solutions (20) or particulate systems (21). With several pilot studies using natural bioadhesive polymers demonstrating promising improvements in ocular bioavailability, synthetic biodegradable and bioadhesive polyalkylcyanoacrylate systems were developed, and these may prove to be the most promising particulate ocular drug delivery systems of the future. Polyalkylcyanoacrylates gained popularity because of their apparent lack of toxicity, proven by decades of safe and successful use in surgery (22), which from a toxicological point of view is a very favorable characteristic for a preferred pharmaceutical drug delivery system.

II. PARTICULATE SYSTEMS IN OCULAR DRUG DELIVERY

A. Topical Systems

The isolation of the vitreous caused by the blood-retinal and blood-aqueous barriers creates difficulties for effective drug therapy in all eye diseases (23). Systemic administration is often not feasible because only a small percentage of drugs can penetrate the ophthalmic barriers and their pharmacokinetics is complicated by fast-flowing blood supply in the posterior segment of the eye (e.g., ocular pharmacokinetics of chloramphenicol and tetracycline) (17). This necessitates large systemic doses to achieve therapeutic concentrations in ocular tissues, which brings forth the problems of unwanted side effects and potential toxicity from the drug. Therefore, regardless of the dosage form and constituents thereof, the most common route of drug delivery to the eye is topical. Drug-loaded microparticulate systems are suspended in aqueous or nonaqueous medium and instilled typically in the cul-de-sac of the eye, wherefrom drug is slowly released in the lacrimal pool by dissolution and mixing, diffusion, or mechanical disintegration and erosion of the polymer matrix (15). Microparticles for topical administration are of several types, including polymer-drug complex systems, erodible microspheres, responsive particulates, in situ gelling systems, ion-exchange systems, and nanoparticles (15).

B. Local Injectable Systems

When the vitreous cavity is targeted for drug delivery, topical, systemic, or subconjunctival drug delivery prove unsatisfactory due to their inability to target the action site and maintain sufficient, constant, and prolonged therapeutic levels of the drug (24,25). The treatment of some diseases like proliferative vitreoretinopathy, endophthalmitis, and recurrent uveitis requires repeated injection of drugs in the vitreous cavity to maintain therapeutic levels (24–28). Such multiple injections may result in clinical complications such as lens damage or retinal injury and may cause deleterious infections or bleeding in the eye, not to mention the patient discomfort and noncompliance issues that may lead to failure of therapy. Development of biodegradable particulate dosage forms for local injections may circumvent limitations of frequent intravitreal injections by providing a slow-releasing depot of drug in the vitreous cavity and reducing the frequency of injections, thereby increasing patient compliance. Microspheres made of poly(lactide/glycolide) and loaded with 5-fluorouracil (5-FU) were used for in vitro and in vivo intravitreal kinetic studies (24). 5-FU was released from the microspheres for at least 2 and up to 7 days, and microspheres were completely eroded in about 7 weeks with no adverse effects on ocular tissues. The drug was released from the polymer matrix through simultaneous polymer hydrolysis and drug diffusion.

III.   METHODS OF PREPARATION OF NANOPARTICLES

A.   Emulsion Polymerization in a Continuous Aqueous Phase

In this process monomers are dissolved in the aqueous phase and within emulsifier micelles. Additional monomers may be present as monomer droplets stabilized by emulsifier molecules. Initiation of polymerization takes place in the aqueous phase when the dissolved monomer molecules are hit by a starter molecule or by high-energy radiation (29–33). Polymerization and chain growth is maintained by further monomer molecules, which originate from the aqueous phase, the emulsifier micelles, or the monomer droplets. The monomer droplets and the emulsifier micelles therefore act mainly as reservoirs for the monomers or for the emulsifier, which later stabilize the polymer particles after phase separation and prevent coagulation. Also, to prevent excessively rapid polymerization and promote the formation of nanoparticles, emulsion polymerization is carried out at an acidic pH (1–2) (34). The drugs may be added before, during, or after polymerization and formation of particles. It has been demonstrated that pilocarpine adsorbed onto blank nanoparticles induced longer miosis compared to drug incorporated in the particles (35). On the other hand, addition before or during polymerization may lead to more drug being incorporated into the nanoparticles.

B.   Emulsion Polymerization in a Continuous Organic Phase

In this process, the conditions for the different phases are reversed compared to aqueous phase emulsion polymerization, and very water-soluble monomers are used. Because of the high amounts of organic solvents and toxic surfactants required as well as the toxic nature of the monomers, this process has limited utility (36). The drugs are dissolved in a small amount of water and solubilized by the surfactants in the organic phase. For solubilization of drugs, higher amounts of surfactants are required than for polymerization in an aqueous phase. The monomers are then added either directly to or dissolved in organic solvents (37–39).

C. Interfacial Polymerization

Interfacial polymerization of the polyalkylcyanoacrylate polymers allows the formation of nanocapsules with a shell-like wall (40). This carrier type can encapsulate drugs with lipophilic character, and the rate of encapsulation is generally related to the solubility of the drug in the oily compartment (40). The technique involves dissolving the polyalkylcyanoacrylate (PACA) monomers and lipophilic drug in an ethanolic solution or oil and slowly injecting this mixture into a well-stirred solution of 0.5% poloxamer 338 in water at pH 6 (may contain nonionic surfactant) (41). At the oil/water interface, nanoparticles with a shell-like wall are formed spontaneously by hydroxyl ion–induced polymerization, and the polymeric colloidal suspension occurs immediately.

D. Polymerization by Denaturation or Desolvation of Natural Proteins

Macromolecules such as albumin or gelatin can form nanoparticles through the desolvation and denaturation processes. Desolvation of macromolecules in aqueous solution can be induced by changes in pH, charge, or the addition of desolvating agents such as ethanol (31,41). The desolvation process induces the swollen molecules to coil tightly. At this point, the tightly coiled macromolecules can be fixed and hardened by crosslinking with glutaraldehyde to form nanoparticles rather than nanocapsules. Nanoparticles are then purified by gel filtration. The denaturation process involves preparing an emulsion from an aqueous phase containing the drug, magnetite particles, and the macromolecule and oil (cottonseed oil) (42–45). Polymerization is carried out by heat denaturation at temperatures above 120°C or by chemical crosslinking. Nanoparticles are precipitated out and washed with ether (or in the case of gelatin, acetone) and stored in the dry form.

E. Solvent Evaporation Method

Gurny et al. (46) were the first to use this process for the production of polylactic acid nanoparticles containing testosterone. In this method, the polymer of interest is dissolved in an organic solvent, suspended in a suitable water or oil medium, after which the solvent is extracted from the droplets. The particles obtained after solvent evaporation are recovered by filtration, centrifugation, or lyophilization. In general, the diameter of the particles depends on the size of the microdroplets that are formed in the emulsion before evaporation of the solvent. Chiang et al. used the solvent evaporation technique with an oil-in-oil emulsion to prepare polylactide-co-glycolide microspheres of 5-fluorouracil for ocular delivery (47). Microspheres containing cyclosporin A have been prepared with a mixture of 50 : 50 polylactic and polyglycolic acid polymers using the solvent evaporation process. The polymer and drug mixture was dissolved in a mixture of chloroform and acetone, emulsified in an aqueous solution of polyvinyl alcohol, and stirred for 24 hours to evaporate the organic solvent and yield the microparticle dispersion (48).

F. Ionic Gelation Technique

De Campos et al. developed chitosan nanoparticles using the ionic gelation technique (49). Nanoparticles were obtained upon the addition of sodium tripolyphosphate aqueous solution to an aqueous polymer solution of chitosan under magnetic stirring at room temperature. The formation of nanoparticles was a result of the interaction between the negative groups of the tripolyphosphate and the positively charged amino groups of chitosan. In this technique, drug in an acetonitrile-water mixture can be incorporated either into chitosan solution or the tripolyphosphate solution.

G. Nanoprecipitation

Fessi et al. (50) developed nanoparticles using this method. In this technique a polymer and a specified quantity of drug is dissolved in acetonitrile. The organic phase is then added dropwise to the aqueous phase and stirred magnetically at room temperature until complete evaporation of the organic phase takes place. Drug-free nanoparticles may be prepared using the same procedure by simply omitting the drug.

H. Spray-Drying

In this technique (51), microparticles are prepared by dissolving the polymer of interest in an organic solvent. The drug is added to this solution and spray-dried using a spray-dryer. The process parameters and spray nozzle size are set up as required. The spray-dried product is collected by a cyclone separator.

IV. POLYMERS USED IN THE PREPARATION OF NANOPARTICLES

A successful nanoparticulate system may be one that has a high loading capacity, thus reducing the quantity of carrier required for administration.

The drug can be either adsorbed onto the surface of performed particles or incorporated into the nanospheres during the polymerization process. Concerning the loading capacity of nanoparticles, it has been found that both the nature and quantities of the monomer used influences the absorption capacity of the carrier. Generally, the longer the chain length, the higher is the affinity of the drug to the polymer, i.e., the capacity of adsorption is related to the hydrophobicity of the polymer and to the specific area of the polymer (52).

Several types of polymeric nanoparticles are used in ophthalmic drug delivery and prepared by the methods described earlier. Polymethylmethacrylate (PMMA) nanoparticles, which are excellent adjuvants for vaccines, can be produced by the emulsion polymerization technique. In this process, monomeric methylmethacrylate is dissolved in a concentration range of 0.1–1.5% in water or phosphate–buffered saline or a solution or suspension of drugs or antigens (33). The polymerization is carried out by irradiation with γ-radiation source or by chemically initiated polymerization using potassium peroxodisulfate and heating to high temperatures. PMMA nanoparticles are generally produced without emulsifiers (12). The biologically active substance, such as drug or antigen, may be present during polymerization or can be added to previously produced nanoparticles. Polymerization in the presence of heat-sensitive materials can only be carried out by γ-radiation (53). Other polymers produced by emulsion polymerization in continuous aqueous phase include acrylic copolymer nanoparticles (54–56), polystyrene (57–59), and polyvinyl pyridine (54,60). Nanoparticles made of polyacrylamide or PMMA do not degrade either biologically or enzymatically, which makes them less attractive for ophthalmic use.

Cellulose acetate phthalate has been used for in situ gelling of latex nanoparticles (61). The preparation of these latex particles involves emulsification of polymer in organic solvent followed by solvent evaporation. This latex suspension, upon coming in contact with the lacrimal fluid at pH 7.2–7.4, gels in situ, thus averting rapid washout of the instilled solution from the eye. The disadvantage of these preparations is vision blurring.

PACA particles possess properties of biodegradation and bioadhesion, making them of considerable interest as possible drug carriers for controlled ocular drug delivery and drug targeting. Wood et al. (62) showed that PACA nanoparticles were able to adhere to the corneal and conjunctival surfaces, which represent their mucoadhesion property. This polymer has the ability to entangle in the mucin matrix and form a noncovalent or ionic bond with the mucin layer of the conjunctiva. PACA nanoparticles are prepared in the same manner as previously described for PMMA. The monomer at a concentration of 0.1–3% is added to an aqueous system or to the drug solution (33). Polymerization starts at room temperature and does not require γ-radiation or addition of special chemical initiators. This is the most significant advantage over acrylic derivatives, as these particles do not require high energy input for the polymerization process, and there is no effect on the stability of the absorbed drug. Alkyl cyanoacrylate particles polymerize according to an anionic mechanism in an aqueous medium using hydroxyl ions as the initiator. Starting with the polymeric reaction in an acidic medium and varying the pH of the medium during the polymerization process, the velocity of the polymerization and molecular weight of resultant polymer can be controlled, which in turn influences the particle size of the nanoparticles formed by this reaction (33,63). The main disadvantage of these carriers is that PACA nanoparticles penetrate into the outer layers of the corneal epithelium, causing a disruption of the cell membranes (64).

As an alternative to PACA nanoparticles, recent studies have shown that poly-ϵ-caprolactone (PECL) nanocapsules may serve as superior polymer systems for ocular drug delivery (65,66). Marchal-Heussler et al. (66) compared nanoparticles prepared by using PACA, PECL, and polylactic-co-glycolic acid with betaxolol as model drug. It was shown that the PECL nanoparticles yielded the highest pharmacological effect. This was believed to be due to the agglomeration of these nanoparticles in the conjunctival sac.

In previous studies it has been shown that regarding ocular administration, the surface charge of the nanoparticles and binding type of the drug onto the nanoparticles were much more important parameters than the drug adsorption percentage onto the nanoparticles (67). It was assumed that coating nanoparticles with positively charged bioadhesive polymers enhances the interaction between nanoparticles and the negatively charged corneal surface, but there are indications that this assumption may not always hold true (68). The bioavailability of nanoparticles coated with poly-L-lysine and chitosan (both have positive charge) were compared to that of noncoated nanoparticles. It was suggested that the specific nature of chitosan was responsible for bioavailability improvement rather than the charge. Using fluorescein-labeled chitosan, it was revealed that chitosan nanoparticles interact favorably with rabbit corneal and conjunctival epithelia and remain associated to these tissues for over 48 hours (68). By contrast, chitosan solutions were washed off the eye within a much shorter period of time.

V. BIODEGRADATION AND DRUG RELEASE FROM PARTICULATE SYSTEMS

In order to prolong the entrance of drugs into the intraocular structures, a long residence time of the particles in the cul-de-sac and a total desorption of the drug from the particles during that time have to be attained. Alkyl cyanoacrylate polymers degrade relatively rapidly in vivo when compared to other polymers used in particulate ocular drug delivery such as poly(lactic acid) and its copolymers with glycolic acid (69). The degradation time is dependent on the alkyl chain length and ranges from a few hours (when methyl cyanoacrylate is used) to approximately 3 days (when 80% of iso-butyl cyanoacrylate is used) (70). The degradation of cyanoacrylates leads to the formation of alcohol together with formaldehyde and poly(cyanoacrylic acid) compounds, which could be toxic in high concentrations (71). Too rapid a degradation can lead to a burst release of degradation products, possibly causing cytotoxic effects (70). In order to assess the relevance of the degradation products regarding possible toxic effects in humans, their rate of release during particle degradation and the maximum local concentrations must be considered (69).

The rate of degradation of cyanoacrylate particles is dependent on the alkyl chain length, and the dominating mechanism of particle degradation was found to be a surface erosion process (72,73). By this mechanism, the polymeric chain remains intact, but it gradually becomes more and more hydrophilic until it is water-soluble. Since the biodegradability of polyalk-ylcyanoacrylate particles depends on the length of the alkyl chain, it is theoretically possible to choose a monomer whose polymerized form has the desirable release characteristics (74). However, the release of a drug cannot always be attributed to polymer degradation alone. Drug desorption from the polymer surface and diffusion of the drug through the polymer matrix are other mechanisms by which a drug can be released from the nanoparticles. By using a radiolabeling technique (^{14}C-labeled nanoparticles loaded with ^{3}H-labeled actinomycin), drug release from polyisobutylcya-noacrylate nanoparticles was found to be a direct consequence of polymer bioerosion (71). The main mechanism of the interaction of PACA particles with cells in culture was found to be endocytosis, leading to intralysosomal localization of the carrier (75). As shown in Figure 2, the particles with a low drug payload and a lower negative surface charge (suspension A, suspension C) trigger a better response compared to the particles containing a greater amount of drug adsorbed onto their surface along with a more negatively charged surface (suspension B) (values are shown in Table 1).

VI. TRANSPORT PATHWAY OF NANOPARTICLES

Ocular transport of polybutylcyanoacrylate nanoparticles has been studied by Zimmer et al. (54) using fluoroscence microscopy. Nanoparticles were labeled with rhodamine 6G or propidium iodide as fluorescent dyes and

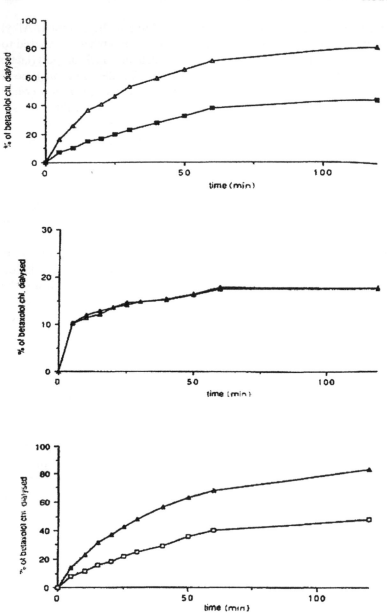

Fig. 2 Adsorption isotherms of betaxolol chlorhydrate. △, Betaxolol solution; ■, suspension A; ▲, suspension B; □, suspension C. (From Ref. 80.)

Table 1 Physicochemical Characteristics[a] of Polyalkylcyanoacrylate Nanoparticles

	Size (nm) (S.D.)	Zeta-potential (mV) (S.D.)	Adsorption percentage (S.D.)
Suspension A			
without betaxolol chl.	246 (3.6)	−15 (1)	
with betaxolol chl.	240 (4)	−11 (1.5)	30 (3)
Suspension B			
without betaxolol chl.	276 (2.8)	−45 (2.5)	
with betaxolol chl.	220 (3.1)	−30 (2.1)	65 (2)
Suspension C			
without betaxolol chl.	242 (3)	−2 (1.5)	
with betaxolol chl.	241 (3.8)	1 (1.5)	22 (3)

[a] Physicochemical characteristics of particles at 25°C and pH 7.4
S.D. = standard deviation; $n = 9$;
Suspension A = Isobutylcyanoacrylate nanoparticles in acidic aqueous solution (10^{-3} M HCl) with a stabilizer dextran 70000 (1%).
Suspension B = Isobutylcyanoacrylate nanoparticles in acidic aqueous solution (10^{-3} M HCl) with a mixture of dextran 70000 (0.8%) and dextran sulfate (0.3%)
Suspension C = Isobutylcyanoacrylate nanoparticles in acidic aqueous solution (10^{-3} M HCl) with a mixture of dextran 70000 (0.5%) and N-acetylglucosamine (0.5%).
Source: Ref. 80.

incubated with freshly excised rabbit cornea and conjunctiva for about 30 minutes in standard perfusion cells. After incubation, it was found that there is a fluorescence signal inside the cells, which indicates uptake of nanoparticles by the cornea and conjunctiva. Fluorescent particles were visually observed inside the cells in what appeared to be vesicles or granules. Thus, either endocytosis of the nanoparticles by conjunctival tissue or lysis of the cell membrane by the nanoparticle metabolic degradation products explained the results of their experiments. The authors also found that the penetration was limited to the first two cell layers of the cornea, and further penetration did not occur.

VII. OCULAR DISTRIBUTION OF NANOPARTICLES

The fate of nanoparticles in the body depends on the physicochemical properties of the nanoparticles (76). Properties such as pH, surfactant, and stabilizers influence the mucoadhesion properties to the ocular membrane and thereby modify the precorneal retention of the nanoparticles. It has been shown that the molecular weight of the polymer influences the residence time of nanoparticles in the precorneal area (Fig. 3) (77). As the molecular weight increases, the polymer becomes poorly retained, whereas low molecular weight polymers are retained for a longer time. Experimental data on the disposition of polyhexylcyanoacrylate nanoparticles in tears, the aqueous humor, cornea, and conjunctiva of albino rabbits clearly showed adhesion of nanoparticles to absorbing tissue (74). Polyalkylcyanoacrylate colloidal carriers were eliminated from the tears with a half-life of about 15–20 minutes (78). This is significantly slower than the elimination rate of aqueous drops, which show a half-life of 1–3 minutes. With pilocarpine, it was found that PACA nanoparticles were able to prolong the intraocular pressure-reducing effect of pilocarpine in rabbits for more than 9 hours (79). Similar results were obtained with betaxolol as a model drug (80). Thus, either prolonged drug release or increased contact time between the corneal tissue and drug could improve the bioavailability and the therapeutic efficiency.

Wood et al. (62) studied the disposition of ^{14}C-labeled polyhexylcyanoacrylate nanoparticles using radiotracer techniques. The concentration of nanoparticles in the cornea, conjunctiva, and aqueous humor was found to be three to five times higher in rabbit eyes in which chronic inflammation had been induced. This is an important observation that suggests that cya-

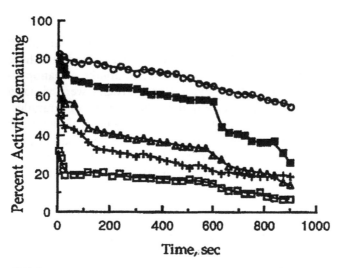

Fig. 3. Precorneal drainage profile of poly(isobutylcyanoacrylate) nanoparticles: M.W. (○) 4,275; (■) 13,178; (▲) 72,030; (+) 128,865; (□) 607,439 in g/mol. (From Ref. 77.)

noacrylates may have an enhanced bioadhesiveness to inflamed tissues. In addition, the ratio of nanoparticles between inflated and normal tissue was higher in the conjunctiva than in the cornea. This is especially favorable since various anti-inflammatory drugs are used in conjunctival inflammation, but these have some side effects after diffusion through the cornea into the aqueous humor. Marchal-Heussler et al. (80) showed that the surface charge and hydrophobicity of the drug play an important role in drug adsorption onto the particles. It has been observed that polyethylene glycol–coated (PEG) nanospheres made of polyethyl-2-cyanoacrylate (PECA) particles loaded with acyclovir showed significant improvement in bioavailability (81). The improved bioavailability is due to better interaction of the PEG-coated PECA nanospheres with the corneal epithelium, thereby increasing ocular mucoadhesion.

VIII. DRUGS USED IN PARTICULATE OCULAR DELIVERY

The first nanoparticulate system (average size, 0.3 μm) for pilocarpine was introduced by Gurny and employed cellulose acetate hydrogen phthalate (CAP) pseudolatex as the polymer (82). The formulation increased the miosis time (up to 10 h) as well as AUC of the drug by 50% compared to the drug solution by decreasing the elimination rate of the drug. This was possible by the dissolution of the polymer at pH 7.2 (pH of tears) forming a viscous polymer solution when the formulation (pH 4.5) was administered in the eye (83). It has been shown that nanodispersions made of anionic lattices with low viscosity and containing large amount of polymeric material exhibit an important increase in viscosity when neutralized with a base (84). Wesslau (85) described this effect as an inner thickening that is due to the swelling of the nanoparticles from the neutralization of the acid groups contained on the polymer chain and the absorption of water.

A polybutylcyanoacrylate nanoparticle delivery system for pilocarpine nitrate has been evaluated in comparison to the solution of the drug for pharmacokinetic and pharmacodynamic aspects (86). Emulsion polymerization technique was employed in preparing nanoparticles, and in vivo experiments were performed by application of the formulations to the eyes of New Zealand white rabbits pretreated with betamethasone to create an elevated intraocular pressure mimicking glaucoma conditions. The results indicated an increase of 23% in pilocarpine levels in aqueous humor and prolonged $t_{1/2}$ for the polybutylcyanoacrylate nanoparticle preparation compared to the aqueous control solution. It was possible to prolong the miosis with nanoparticles with lower drug content compared to the control solution. Betaxolol (80) and amikacin sulfate (87) loaded polyalkylcyanoacrylate nanoparticles have shown similar effects. The superficial charge and binding type of the drug onto the nanoparticles are important factors playing a role in the improvement of the therapeutic response. In another study, adsorption of pilocarpine onto polybutylcyanoacrylate nanoparticles enhanced the miotic response by about 22% compared to the control aqueous drug solution (35).

Diepold et al. (79) incorporated pilocarpine into polybutylcyanoacrylate nanoparticles and evaluated the aqueous humor drug levels and the intraocular pressure-lowering effects using three models (the water-loading model, the alpha-chymotrypsin model, and the betamethasone model) in rabbits. The miotic response was enhanced by about 33% while the miotic time increased from 180 to 240 minutes for nanoparticles compared to the control solution. Also, the intraocular pressure-lowering effects were prolonged to more than 9 hours in all three models mentioned. Vidmar et al. (88) showed that poly(lactic acid) microcapsules of pilocarpine hydrochloride prepared by a solvent precipitation method prolonged miosis about 4 hours in comparison to control solution (< 2 hours) in rabbits (88). A significant improvement in the bioavailability of pilocarpine was attained by co-administering the pilocarpine-loaded albumin nanoparticles with the viscous bioadhesive polymer mucin (89).

In a clinical study with Piloplex® (latex emulsion of pilocarpine hydrochloride) a lower level of the drug with less fluctuation compared to the corresponding control solution was observed on the third day of treatment. This study involving nine subjects showed a reduction by 5.25 mmHg of the average diurnal intraocular pressure value compared to the control. Only one out of 30 patients complained of a local sensitivity reaction with Piloplex in the yearlong study (90). Similar results were obtained in yet another study involving 50 patients, where 67.6% of the eyes treated with the formulation were under control, while only 45.2% were under control with the pilocarpine solution (91).

Nanocapsules for topical ocular delivery of cyclosporin A (CyA) comprising an oily core (Miglyol 840) and a poly-ϵ-caprolactone coating increased the corneal levels of the drug by 5 times compared to the oily solution of the drug when administered to the cul-de-sac of fully awake New Zealand white rabbits (92). Also, the drug levels remained higher for up to 3 days with the nanocapsule preparation. More than 90% of CyA could be encapsulated giving a maximum loading capacity of 50% (drug: polymer) (92). The enhancement in the drug levels occurred due to the increased uptake of nanocapsules by the corneal epithelial cells (93). Poly(acrylic acid) gel of nanocapsules containing 1% CyA showed a better percent absorption ($7.92 \pm 2.55\%$) compared to 1% CyA solution in olive oil ($5.81 \pm 2.04\%$) after 24-hour contact time on bovine cornea ex vivo owing to the bioadhesive behavior of poly(acrylic acid) polymer and the encapsulated form. The nanocapsules incorporated in the gel were prepared by interfacial polymer deposition method, with isobutyl-2-cyanoacrylate and Miglyol 812 forming the polymer coating and the oily core, respectively. The nanocapsule gel presents a potential ocular drug delivery system with higher absorption rate and lower risk of toxicity to the cornea (94). In a study by De Campos et al. (49), chitosan nanoparticles developed for intraocular delivery of CyA (73% association efficiency and 9% loading) by ionic gelation technique showed improved levels of the lipophilic drug in the cornea and conjunctiva on topical administration to rabbit eyes compared to an aqueous CyA suspension. The studies confirmed that CyA was preferentially accumulated on the external tissues from chitosan nanoparticles while sparing the intraocular structures (49).

Polyalkylcyanoacrylate nanoparticles could also be used for anti-inflammatory drugs to target inflamed ocular tissue as they have four times more affinity towards inflamed tissue compared to healthy tissue (95). Both indomethacin-loaded nanoparticles and nanocapsules performed better in terms of bioavailability and drug levels in the cornea compared to the commercial solution of the drug Indocollyre® when administered to rabbit eye (96). The nanocapsules were prepared by interfacial polymerization using PECL, lecithin, Miglyol 840 as oil, acetone, and poloxamer 188, while the nanoparticles were prepared omitting the oil and lecithin using a nano-precipitation method, and nanoemulsions were prepared by using spontaneous emulsification technique. The authors suggest that the colloidal particles are taken up by the corneal epithelium through an endocytic mechanism, and additionally, the colloidal nature of these formulations (nanocapsules and nanoparticles) aids in increasing the bioavailability (Fig. 4). These formulations provide a potential for treating intraocular inflammatory diseases with reduced doses of indomethacin. In another study, chitosan and poly-L-lysine (PLL)–coated PECL nanocapsules increased indomethacin levels in the cornea and aqueous humor of rabbits four times and eight times, respectively, compared to Indocollyre, the commercial eye drops (67). The positively charged PLL and chitosan coatings were employed in an attempt to increase interaction of the particles with the negatively charged corneal epithelium. However, it was found that it was the specific nature of CS and not the positive charge that was responsible for the enhanced uptake. PLL coating failed to enhance the uptake of the drug compared to the corresponding uncoated PECL nanocapsules.

Poly-ε-caprolactone nanocapsules also showed good performance in increasing the ocular availability of drugs such as metipranolol (65) and betaxolol (66) while suppressing their systemic absorption. The PECL nanocapsules of metipranolol were prepared by interfacial polymerization technique incorporating the drug in a Miglyol 840 oily core. When administered to rabbits, the nanocapsules decreased the intraocular pressure similar to the commercial ophthalmic solution of the drug, but the systemic side effects, studied by evaluation of the cardiovascular effects, were significantly suppressed with the nanocapsules. The heart rate reached normal values within an hour of administration of nanocapsules versus the commercial eye drops, which showed pronounced bradycardia for more than 2 hours (97).

Acyclovir-loaded PEG-coated polyethyl-2-cyanoacrylate (PECA) nanospheres prepared by emulsion polymerization technique showed increased drug levels in the aqueous humor compared to the free drug suspension in the rabbits (83). Polylactide and polylactide-co-glycolide biopolymers in the molecular weight range of 3000–109,000 have been employed in the preparation of microparticulate systems for intravitreal administration of acyclovir (98). Spray-drying technique was employed for the preparation and the in vivo evaluation was performed by intravitreal administration in rabbits. The poly-D, L-lactide microspheres of acyclovir were more efficient compared to the free drug in providing a sustained release of the drug in the vitreous humor in rabbits. Not only is the initial drug concentration in vitreous humor attained with microspheres higher

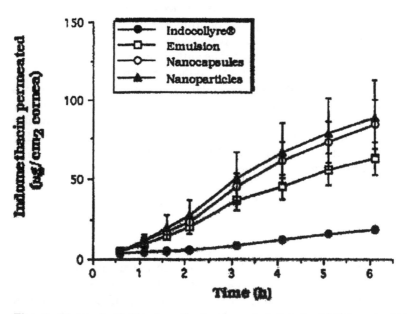

Fig. 4 Permeation of indomethacin through isolated rabbit cornea: (▲) PECL nanoparticles; (○) PECL nanocapsules; (□) submicron emulsion; and (●) commercial eye drops (Indocollyre). (From Ref. 96.)

compared to the free drug, but the drug levels with the former remained constant for 14 days, unlike the free drug. The drug concentration diminished to undetectable levels with free drug after 3 days.

PECL nanoparticles and nanocapsules (with a TiO_5 oily core) have been studied for the glaucoma drug carteolol (99). Both formulations demonstrated a pronounced decrease in the intraocular pressure compared to the commercial aqueous solution, Carteol®, in rabbits with induced intraocular hypertension. The PECL carriers increase the residence time of the drug, enhance the corneal uptake of the drug in unionized form, and decrease the systemic side effects. Moreover, the studies show that PECL nanocapsules demonstrate a better effect compared to the PECL nanoparticles for carteolol. It was concluded that the drug entrapped in the oily core is more available for corneal absorption.

[3]H-Labeled hydrocortisone-17-butyrate-21-propionate (^{3}H-HBP) loaded lipid microspheres have been shown to produce a significant increase in the drug levels in the cornea of rabbits compared to the control ^{3}H-HBP suspension after 1 and 3 hours of administration (100). Kimura et al. (101) prepared 75:25 lactide/glycolide microspheres for an antifungal agent, fluconazole, used for the treatment of endophthalmitis. Microspheres of 1–10 μm in diameter have been prepared with hyaluronate esters incorporating methylprednisolone as a model drug and by using the spray-drying technique (102,103). The carboxyl group of methylprednisolone was esterified for 50% of the drug content, while the remaining half was present as the sodium salt. From in vivo studies it was found that the drug could be delivered for long time with a lower drug peak concentration, diminished side effects, and enhanced bioavailability compared to the control suspension.

Pilocarpine-loaded albumin or gelatin microspheres (104) and acyclovir-loaded chitosan microspheres (105) have also been studied. Both microparticulate systems were found to be superior to conventional dosage forms in terms of in vivo performance. Pilocarpine-loaded albumin or gelatin microspheres with an average particle size of 30 μm were prepared by emulsification of the aqueous solution of pilocarpine nitrate together with the macromolecule in sunflower oil and subsequent crosslinking with formaldehyde (for gelatin microspheres) or heating to 150°C (for albumin microspheres). Further, the oil was removed by washing with ether. The AUC of the miosis versus time curve was increased by 2.3 and 3.3 times for the gelatin and albumin microspheres, respectively, compared to the aqueous solution of the drug (104).

Binding betaxolol to ion-resin exchange resin microparticles (Betoptic® S) increases the drug bioavailability by reducing the drug release in the tear. Betoptic S 0.25% and Betoptic solution 0.5% are considered bioequivalent. Since introduction in the market, Betoptic S has increased patient compliance by reducing the dose and frequency of dosing (106). Marchal-Heussler et al. (66) studied betaxolol-loaded nanospheres or nanocapsules using three different polymers: polyisobutylcyanoacrylate, a copolymer of lactic and glycolic acid, and PECL. The intraocular pressure-lowering effect was most pronounced for the PECL nanocapsules or nanospheres compared to other two polymers as well as the commercial eye drops, owing to the higher hydrophobicity exhibited by PECL. The hydrophobic character of the polymer allows agglomeration of the nanoparticles in the eye and subsequent prolongation of the drug residence time in the precorneal area. Further, PECL nanocapsules performed better compared to the corresponding nanospheres in that the drug entrapped in the unionized form in the oily core could penetrate better into the cornea (66).

5-Fluorouracil and adriamycin loaded microspheres or poly(lactic acid) and copolymer of lactic/glycolic acid have been prepared using the solvent evaporation method (107,108). The formulations for both the antiproliferative drugs excelled in their in vivo intravitreal kinetics in rabbits compared to their corresponding controls. A 10 μg injection of adriamycin solution led to severe toxic reaction in the retina, while the same amount of drug incorporated in the microspheres substantially decreased the rate of retinal detachment after 4 weeks with no detectable toxic effects. The drug release from 5-FU loaded microspheres extended up to 7 days with no subsequent adverse effects to the ocular tissue.

As shown in Fig. 5, piroxicam loaded in the pectin microspheres (M1, M2) showed faster in vitro dissolution rates compared to the solid micronized drug (109). The precorneal retention of fluorescein-loaded piroxicam microspheres was evaluated in vivo in albino rabbits, and it was observed that an aqueous dispersion of microspheres showed a significantly increased residence time in the eye (2.5 vs. 0.5 h) when compared to a control fluorescein solution. This study also showed significantly improved bioavailability of piroxicam from microspheres in aqueous humor when compared to the commercial piroxicam eyedrops.

In a study involving pilocarpine (110), polyisobutylcyanoacrylate nanocapsules containing 1% pilocarpine were dispersed in an aqueous medium (I) and compared to the same nanocapsule formulation incorporated into a Pluronic® F127 gel delivery system (II) and 1% pilocarpine incorporated into a Pluronic F127 gel containing 5% methyl cellulose (III), by measuring the miotic response in the albino rabbit eye. As shown in Figure 6, polyisobutylcyanoacrylate nanocapsules of pilocarpine dispersed in the Pluronic F127 gel (II) showed extended release of pilocarpine compared to formulations (I) and (III) with respect to the length of miotic response time. As shown in Table 2, statistical analysis indicated a rank

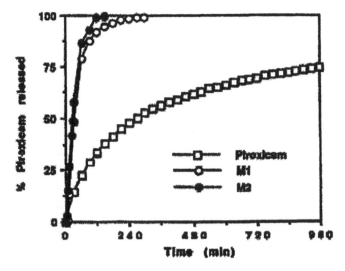

Fig. 5 In vitro release profiles of piroxicam microspheres M1 and M2 compared to the dissolution profile of micronized piroxicam powder. (From Ref. 109.)

PLURONIC® F127-BASED OCULAR DELIVERY SYSTEM OF PILOCARPINE

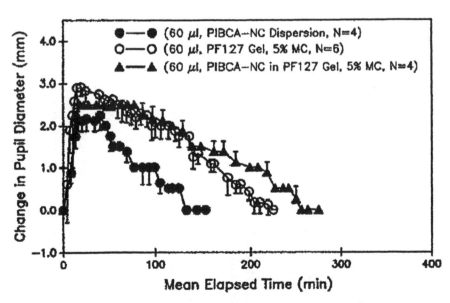

Fig. 6 Miotic response to various formulations of 1% pilocarpine in the albino rabbit eye. (From Ref. 110.)

Table 2 Mitotic Response to Various Pilocarpine Formulations in Albino Rabbit Eye[a]

Treatment (μL) 1% (w/v) pilocarpine (PILO)	Time to peak response (T_p, min)	Duration of mitotic response (min)	Intensity of response (AUC,[b] mm. min)	Peak change in the pupil diameter (I_{max}, mm)	
				Absolute	% change
I					
60 μL, dispersion of PILO-loaded PIBCA-NC (N = 4)	14.13 (0.24)	150.75 (3.11)	167.00 (6.52)	2.13 (0.13)	35.42 (2.08)
III					
60 μL, Pluronic® F127 gel (N = 6), 5% MC	11.58 (1.25)	217.08 (4.61)	374.27 (11.26)	3.00 (0.13)	50.00 (2.15)
II					
60 μL Pluronic® F127 gel (N = 6), 5% MC containing-dispersion of PILO-loaded PIBCA-NC	17.63 (0.55)	259.88 (2.30)	409.16 (3.59)	2.50 (0.00)	41.67 (0.00)
Overall probability (p)	0.0042	<0.0005	<0.0005	<0.0007	<0.0007

[a] Values shown represent means and SEM (in parentheses).
[b] Area under the temporal mitotic response intensity curve.
[c] Vertical lines within a column join data pairs that are not significantly different. All other values within a given column differ significantly ($p < 0.05$).
Source: Ref. 110.

order for both the duration and intensity of miosis as II > III ≫ I, with all differences being significant.

IX. CONCLUSIONS

Particulate systems have the potential to become promising systems for ophthalmic drug delivery. To date, only one microparticulate ophthalmic prescription product, Betoptic® S, has been approved for marketing in the United States. Betoptic S 0.25% is considered to be bioequivalent to Betoptic 0.5% solution. By binding betaxolol to ion exchange resin particles for the Betoptic S formulation, drug release was retarded in the tear and drug bioavailability was enhanced (105). The ocular comfort of betaxolol was also greatly enhanced by reducing the availability of free drug molecules in the precorneal tear film. Thus, microparticulate technology introduces the advantage of superior patient acceptability in combination with extended drug release and improved patient compliance. Particles are suspended in a medium that can be administered topically or intraocularly as an injection. The potential for success of nanoparticles in ophthalmic drug delivery has been demonstrated in a number of studies of either hydrophilic or hydrophobic drugs. Formulation stability, control of particle size, control of the rate of drug release, and large-scale manufacture of sterile preparations are some of the major issues involved in the development of ophthalmic particulate formulations.

REFERENCES

1. Lee, V. H. L., and Robinson, J. R. (1979). Mechanistic and quantitative evaluation of pilocarpine disposition in albino rabbits. *J. Pharm. Sci., 68*:673.
2. Chrai, S. S., and Robinson, J. R. (1984). Ocular evaluation of methylcellulose vehicle in rabbits. *J. Pharm. Sci., 68*:1218.
3. Worakul, N., and Robinson, J. R. (1997). Ocular pharmacokinetics/pharmacodynamics. *Eur. J. Pharm. Biopharm., 44*:71.
4. Barber, R. F., and Shek, P. N. (1993). Liposomes as topical ocular drug delivery system. In: Alain Rolland (ed.), *Pharmaceutical Particulate Carriers*. Marcel Dekker, New York, pp. 1–20.
5. Patton, T. F., and Robinson, J. R. (1975). Ocular evaluation of polyvinyl alcohol vehicle in rabbits. *J. Pharm. Sci., 64*:1312.
6. Saettone, M. F., Giannaccini, B., Teneggi, A., Savigni, P., and Tellini, N. (1982). Vehicle effects on ophthalmic bioavailability: The influence of different polymers on the activity of pilocarpine in rabbit and man. *J. Pharm. Pharmacol., 34*:464.

7.   Allen, T. M., McAllister, L., Mausolf, S., and Gyorffy, E. (1981). Liposome-cell interactions. A study of the interactions of liposomes containing entrapped anti-cancer drugs with the EMT6, S49 and AE1 (transport-deficient) cell lines. *Biochim. Biophys. Acta, 643*:346.

8.   Campbell, P. I. (1983). Toxicity of some charged lipids used in liposome preparations. *Cytobiosis, 37*:21.

9.   Yoshihara, E., and Nakae, T. (1986). Cytolytic activity of liposomes containing stearylamine. *Biochim. Biophys. Acta, 854*:93.

10. Chang, S. C., Bundgaard, H., Buur, A., and Lee, V. H. L. (1987). Improved corneal penetration of timolol by prodrugs as a means to reduce systemic drug load. Invest. *Ophthalmol. Vis. Sci., 28*:487.

11. Lebourlais, C. A., Treupel Acar, L. Rhodes, C. T., Sado, P. A., and Leverage, R. (1995). New ophthalmic drug delivery systems. *Drug. Dev. Ind. Pharm., 21*:19.

12. Bundgaard, H. (1989). Improved ocular delivery of pilocarpine and timolol through prodrugs. 5th Int. Conf. Pharm. Tech. Paris, p. 52.

13. Candida, L., Maria, J. A., Jose, L. V., Francisco, O., Martinez, J., Saavedra, A. S., Jose, C. C. (1992). Reduction of cardiovascular side effects associated with ocular administration of Metipranolol by inclusion in polymeric nanocapsules. *J. Ocul. Pharmacol., 8*:191.

14. Joshi, A. (1994). Microparticulates for ophthalmic drug delivery. *J. Ocul. Pharmacol., 10*:29.

15. Joshi, A. (1996). Microparticulates as an ocular drug delivery system. In: *Ocular Therapeutics and Drug Delivery*, I. K. Reddy (ed.). Technomic, pp. 441–459.

16. Rollot, J. M., Couvreur, P., Roblot Treupe, L., Devissaguet, J. P. H., and Puisieux, F. (1986). Physico-chemical and morphological characterization of polyisobutylcyanoacryate nanocapsules. *J. Pharm. Sci., 75*:361.

17. Schulman, J. A., and Peyman, G. A. (1993). Intracameral, intravitreal, and retinal drug delivery. In: A. K. Mitra (ed.), *Ophthalmic Drug Delivery Systems*. Marcel Dekker, New York, pp. 383–425.

18. Kreuter, J., Tauber, U., and Illi, V. (1979). Distribution and elimination of poly methyl-2-14-(methacrylate) nanoparticle radioactivity after injection in rat and mice. *J. Pharm. Sci., 68*:1443.

19. Lee, V. H. K., Wood, R. W., Kreuter, J., Harima, T., and Robinson, J. R. (1986). Ocular drug delivery of progesterone using nanoparticles. *J. Microen., 3*:213.

20. Gurny, R., Ibrahim, H., Aebi, A., Buri, P., Wilson, C. G., and Washington, N. (1987). Design and evaluation of controlled release systems for the eye. *J. Cont. Rel., 6*:367.

21. Hui, H. W., and Robinson, J. R. (1985). Ocular delivery of progesterone using a bioadhesive polymer. *Int. J. Pharm., 26*:203.

22. Collins, J. A., James, P. M., Levitski, S. A., Brendenburg, C. E., Anderson, R. W., Leonard, F., and Hardway, R. M. (1969). Clinical use in severe combat

casualties. Cyanoacrylate adhesive as topical homeostatic aids. *Surgery,* *65*:260.

23. Cuncha-vaz, J. G. (1997). The blood ocular barriers: past, present and future. *Documenta Ophthalmol., 93*:149.

24. Moritera, T., Ogura, Y., Yoshimura, N., Honda, Y., Wada, R., Hyon, S. H., and Ikada, Y. (1992). Biodegradable microspheres containing adriamycin in the treatment of proliferative vetreonopathy. *Invest Ophth. Vis. Sci., 33*:3125.

25. Khoobehi, B., Stradtmann, M. O., Peyman, G. A., and Aly, O. M. (1991). Clearance of fluorescein incorporated into microspheres from the vitreous after intravitreal injection. *Ophthal. Surg., 21*:175.

26. Khoobehi, B., Stradtmann, M. O., Peyman, G. A., and Aly, O. M. (1990). Clearance of fluorescein incorporated into microspheres from the cornea and aqueous after subjunctival injection. *Ophthal. Surg., 21*:840.

27. Moritera, T., Ogura, Y., Yoshimura, N., Honda, Y., Wada, R., Hyon, S. H., and Ikada, Y. (1991). Microspheres of biodegradable polymers as a drug delivery system in the vitreous. *Invest. Ophth. Vis. Sci., 32*:1785.

28. Martini, B. (1992). Proliferative vitreo-retinal disorders: Experimental models in vivo and in vitro. *Acta Ophthalmol., 201(Suppl.)*:1.

29. Kreuter, J. (1983). Evaluation of nanoparticles as drug delivery systems. I. Preparation methods. *Pharm. Acta. Helv., 58*:196.

30. Fitch, R. M., and Tsai, C. (1970). Polymer colloids: Particle formation in micellar systems. *J. Polymer Sci., Polym. Lett., 8*:703.

31. Fitch, R. M., Prenosil, M. B., and Sprick, K. J. (1993). The mechanism of particle formation in polymer hydrosols. I. Kinetics of aqueous polymerization of methyl methacrylate. *J. Polymer Sci. C, 27*:467.

32. Fitch, R. M. (1993). The homogenous nucleation of polymer colloids. *Br. Poly. J., 5*:467.

33. Kreuter, J. (1992). Nanoparticles-Preparation and applications. In: *Microcapsules and Nanocapsules in Medicine and Pharmacy*, M. Don Brow (ed.). CRC Press Inc., Boca Raton, pp. 126–143.

34. Mezei, M., and Meisner, D. (1993). Liposomes and nanoparticles as ocular drug delivery systems. In: *Biopharmaceutics of Ocular Drug Delivery*. CRC Press, Inc., Boca Raton, pp. 91–101.

35. Harima, T., Kreuter, J., Speiser, P., Boye, T., Gurny, R., and Kubis, A. (1986). Enhancement of miotic response of rabbits with pilocarpine-loaded polybutylcyanoacrylate nanoparticles. *Int. J. Pharm., 33*:187.

36. Kreuter, J. (1978). Nanoparticles and nanocapsules—new dosage forms in the nanometer size range. *Pharm. Acta. Helv., 53*:33.

37. El-Samaligy, M. S., Rhodewald, P., and Mahmoud, H. A. (1986). Polyalkylcyanoacrylate nanocapsules. *J. Pharm. Pharmacol., 38*:216.

38. Krause, H. J., Schwarz, A., and Rohdewald, P. (1986). Interfacial polymerization, a useful method for the preparation of polymethyl cyanoacrylate nanoparticles. *Drug. Dev. Ind. Pharm., 12*:527.

39. Gasco, M. R., and Trotta, M. (1986). Nanoparticles from microemulsions. *Int. J. Pharm., 29*:267.

40. Al Khouri Fallouh, N., Roblot-Treupel, L., Fess, H., Devissaguet, J. P. H., and Puissieux, F. (1986). Development of a new process for the manufacture of polyisobutylcyanoacrylate nanoparticles. *Int. J. Pharm., 28*:125.

41. Marty, J. J., Oppenheim, R. C., and Speiser, P. (1978). Nanoparticles – a new colloidal drug delivery systems. *Pharm. Acta. Helv., 53*:17.

42. Scheffel, U., Rhodes, B. A., Natarajan, T. K., Jr., and Wagner, H. N. (1972). Albumin microspheres for the study of reticuloendothelial system. *J. Nucl. Med., 13*:498.

43. Widder, K., Fluoret, G., and Senyei, A. (1979). Magnetic microspheres: Synthesis of a novel parenteral drug carrier. *J. Pharm. Sci., 68*:79.

44. Kramer, P. A. (1974). Letter: Albumin microspheres as vehicles for achieving specificity in drug delivery. *J. Pharm. Sci., 63*:1646.

45. Gallo, J. M., Hung, C. T., and Perrier, D. G. (1984). Analysis of albumin microsphere preparation. *Int. J. Pharm., 22*:63.

46. Gurny, R., Peppas, N. A., Harrington, D. D., and Banker, G. S. (1981). Development of biodegradable and injectable lattices for the controlled release of potent drugs. *Drug Dev. Ind. Pharm., 7*:1.

47. Chiang, C. H., Tung, S. M., Lu, D. W., and Yeh, M. K. (2001). In vitro and in vivo evaluation of an ocular delivery system of 5-fluorouracil microspheres. *J. Ocul. Pharmacol. Ther., 17*:545.

48. Harper, C. A. 3rd, Khoobehi, B., Peyman, G. A., Gebhardt, B. M., and Dunlap, W. A. (1993–94). Bioavailability of microsphere-entrapped cyclosporine A in the cornea and aqueous of rabbits. *Int. Ophthalmol., 17*:337.

49. De Campos, A. M., Sánchez, A., and Alonso, M. J. (2001). Chitosan nanoparticles: a new vehicle for the improvement of the delivery of drugs to the ocular surface. Application to cyclosporin A. *Int. J. Pharm., 224*:159.

50. Fessi, H., Puisieux, F., Devissaguet, J. P., Ammoury, N., and Benita, S. (1989). Nanocapsule formation by interfacial polymer deposition following solvent displacement. *Int. J. Pharm., 55*:R1.

51. O'Hara, P., and Hickey, A. J. (2000). Respirable PLGA microspheres containing rifampicin for the treatment of tuberculosis: manufacture and characterization. *Pharm. Res., 17*:955.

52. Illum, L., Khan, M. A., Mark, E., and Davis, S. S. (1986). Evaluation of carrier capacity and release characteristics for poly (butyl 2-cyanoacrylate) nanoparticles. *Int. J. Pharm., 30*:17.

53. Kreuter, J., and Zehnder, H. J. (1978). The use of Co-γ-radiation for the production of vaccines. *Radiat. Effects, 35*:161.

54. Rembaum, A., Yen, S. P. S., Cheong, E., Wallace, S., Molday, R. S., Gordon, I. L., and Dreyer, W. J. (1976). Functional polymeric microspheres based on 2-hydroxyethyl methacrylate for immunochemical studies. *Macromolecules, 9*:328.

55. Rembaum, A., Yen, S. P. S., and Molday, R. S. (1979). Synthesis and reaction of hydrophilic functional microspheres for immunological studies. *J. Macromol. Sci. Chem. A, 13*:603.

56. Rembaum, A. (1980). Synthesis, properties, and biomedical applications of hydrophilic, functional, polymeric immunomicrospheres. *Pure Appl. Chem., 52*:1275.

57. Kreuter, J., Liehl, E., Berg, U., Soliva, M., and Speiser, P. P. (1988). Influence of hydrophilicity on the adjuvant effect of particulate polymeric adjuvants. *Vaccine, 6*:253.

58. Ugelstad, J., Rembaum, J. T., Kemshead, K., Mustad, S., Fuderud, S., and Schmid, R. (1984). Preparation and biomedical applications of polymeric particles in microspheres and drug therapy. In: S. S. Davis, L. Illum, J. G. Mcvie, E. Tomlinson (eds.). Elsevier, Amsterdam.

59. Shahar, M., Meshulam, H., and Margel, S. (1986). Synthesis and characterization of microspheres of polystyrene derivatives. *J. Polym. Sci. Chem. Ed., 24*:203.

60. Schwartz, A., and Rembaum, A. (1985). Poly(vinyl pyridine) microspheres. In: K. J. Widder, R. Green (eds.). Academic Press, Orlando.

61. Gurny, R. (1983). Latex systems. In: D. D. Breimer and P. Speiser (eds.). *Topics in Pharmaceutical Sciences.* Elsevier Science Publishers B. V, Amsterdam, pp. 277–288.

62. Wood, R. W., Li, V. H. K., Kreuter, J., and Robinson, J. R. (1985). Ocular disposition of poly-hexyl-2-cyano(3-^{14}C) acrylate nanoparticles in the albino rabbit. *Int. J. Pharm., 23*:175.

63. Das, S. K., Tucker, I. G., Hill, D. J., and Ganguly, N. (1995). Evaluation of poly(isobutylcyanoacrylate) nanoparticles for mucoadhesive ocular drug delivery. I. Effect of formulation variables on physicochemical characteristics of nanoparticles. *Pharm. Res., 12*:534.

64. Zimmer, A., Kreuter, J., and Robinson, J. R. (1991). Studies on the transport pathway of PBCA nanoparticles in ocular tissues. *J. Microen., 8*:497.

65. Losa, C., Marchal-Heussler, L., Orallo, F., Vila Jato, J. L., and Alonso, M. J. (1993). Design of new formulations for topical ocular administration: polymeric nanocapsules containing metipranolol. *Pharm. Res., 10*:80.

66. Marchal-Haussler, L., Fessi, H., Devissaguet, J. P., Hoffman, M., and Maincent, P. (1992). Colloidal drug delivery systems for the eye. A comparison of the efficacy of three different polymers: polyisobutylcyanoacrylate, polylactic-coglycolic acid, poly-epsilon-caprolactone. *Pharm. Sci., 2*:98.

67. Calvo, P., Vila-Jato, J. L., and Alonso, M. J. (1997). Evaluation of cationic polymer-coated nanocapsules as ocular drug carriers. *Int. J. Pharm., 153*:41.

68. Janes, K. A., Calvo, P., and Alonso, M. J. (2001). Polysaccharide colloidal particles as delivery systems for macromolecules. *Adv. Drug Deliv. Rev., 47*:83.

69. Grislain, L., Couvreur, P., Lenaerts, V., Roland, M., Deprez-Decampeneere, D., and Speiser, P. (1983). Pharmacokinetics and distribution of bio-degradable drug carrier. *Int. J. Pharm., 15*:335.

70. Lherm, C., Muller, R. H., Puisieux, F., and Couvreur, P. (1992). Alkyl cyanoacrylate drug carriers: II. Cytotoxicity of cyanoacrylate nanoparticles with different alkyl chain length. *Int. J. Pharm., 84*:13.

71. Lenaerts, V., Couvreur, P., Christiaens-Leyh, D., Joiris, E., Ronald, M., Rollman, B., and Speiser, P. (1984). Degradation of polyisobutylcyanoacrylate nanoparticles. *Biomaterials, 5*:65.

72. Leonard, F., Kulkarni, R. K., Brandes, G., Nelson, J., and Mameron, J. (1966). Synthesis and degradation of poly (alkyl cyanoacrylates). *J. Appl. Polym. Sci., 10*:259.

73. Muller, R. H., Lherm, C., Herbort, J., and Couvreur, P. (1990). In vitro model for the biodegradation of alkyl cyanoacrylate nanoparticles. *Biomaterials, 11*:590.

74. Vezin, W., and Florence, A. (1978). In vitro degradation rates of biodegradable poly-N-alkylcyanoacrylates. *J. Pharm. Pharmacol., 30*:5P.

75. Couvreur, P., Tulkens, P., Roland, M., Trouet, A., and Speiser, P. (1977). Nanocapsules: a new type of lysosomotropic carrier. *FEBS Lett., 84*:323.

76. Davis, S. S., and Illum, L. (1983). The targeting of drugs using polymeric microspheres. *Br. Polym. J., 15*:160.

77. Das, S. K., Tucker, I. G., and Davies, N. M. (1992). A gamma scintigraphic evaluation of the effect of molecular weight of poly(isobutyl cyanoacrylate) Nanoparticles on the precorneal residence in rabbit. *Proc. Int. Symp. Control. Rel. Matter. Controlled Release Society, Inc., 19*:395.

78. Diepold, R., Kreuter, J., Guggenbuhl, P., and Robinson, J. R. (1989). Distribution of poly-hexyl-2-cyano[3-^{14}C]acrylate nanoparticles in healthy and chronically inflamed rabbit eyes. *Int. J. Pharm., 54*:149.

79. Diepold, R., Kreuter, J., Himber, J., Gurny, R., Lee, V. H. L., Robinson, J. R., Saettone, M. F., and Schnaudigel, O. E. (1989). Comparison of different models for the testing of pilocarpine eyedrops using conventional eyedrops as a novel depot formulation (nanoparticles). *Graefe's Arch. Clin. Exp. Ophthalmol., 227*:188.

80. Marchal-Heussler, L., Maincent, P., Hoffman, H., Spittler, J., and Couvreur, P. (1990). Antiglaucomatous activity of betaxolol chlorhydrate sorbed onto different isobutyl cyanoacrylate nanoparticles preparations. *Int. J. Pharm., 58*:115.

81. Fresta, M., Fontana, G., Bucolo, C., Cavallaro, G., Giammona, G., and Puglisi, G. (2001). Ocular tolerability and in vivo bioavailability of poly(ethylene glycol) (PEG)-coated polyethyl-2-cyanoacrylate nanosphere-encapsulated acyclovir. *J. Pharm. Sci., 90*:288.

82. Gurny, R. Preliminary study of prolonged acting drug delivery system for the treatment of glaucoma. *Pharma. Acta. Helv., 56*:130.

83. Gurny, R. Ocular therapy with nanoparticles. In: *Polymeric Nanoparticles and Microspheres*, P. Guiot and P. Couvreur (eds.). CRC Press, Boca Raton, pp. 127–136.

84. Gurny, R., Ibrahim, H., and Buri, P. (1993). The development and use of in situ formed gels, triggered by pH. In: *Biopharmaceutics of Ocular Drug Delivery*, P. Edman (ed.). CRC Press, Boca Raton, pp. 82–89.

85. Weslau, H. (1963). Zur Kenntnis von Acrylsäureenthaltenden Copolymer-dispersionen. II. Die Verdichbarkeit Acrylsäureenthaltender Dispersionen. *Makromol. Chem., 69*:220.

86. Zimmer, A., Mutschler, E., Lambrecht, G., Mayer, D., and Kreuter, J. (1994). Pharmacokinetic and Pharmacodynamic aspects of an ophthalmic pilocarpine nanoparticle-delivery-system. *Pharm. Res., 11*:1435.

87. Losa, C., Calvo, P., Castro, E., Vila-Jato, J. L., and Alonso, M. J. (1991). Improvement of ocular penetration of amikacin sulphate by association to poly(butyl cyanoacrylate) nanoparticles. *J. Pharm. Pharmacol., 43*:548.

88. Vidmar, V., Pepeljnjak, S., and Jalšenjak, I. (1985). The in vivo evaluation of poly(lactic acid) microcapsules of pilocarpine in hydrochloride. *J. Microen., 2*:289.

89. Zimmer, A. K., Chetoni, P., Saettone, M. F. Zerbe, H., and Kreuter, J. (1995). Evaluation of pilocarpine-loaded albumin particles as controlled drug delivery systems for the eye. II. Co-administration with bioadhesive and viscous polymers. *J. Cont. Rel., 33*:31.

90. Ticho, U., Blumenthal, M., Zonis, S., Gal, A., Blank, I., and Mazor, Z. W. (1979). Piloplex, a new long-acting pilocarpine polymer salt. A long-term study. *Br. J. Opthalmol., 63*:48.

91. Ticho, U., Blumenthal, M., Zonis, S., Gal, A., Blank, I., and Mazor, Z. W. (1979). A clinical trial with Piloplex—a new long-acting pilocarpine compound: preliminary report. *Ann. Ophthalmol., 11*:555.

92. Calvo, P., Sánchez, A., Martínez, J., López, M. I., Calonge, M., Pastor, J. C., and Alonso, M. J. (1996). Polyester Nanocapsules as new topical ocular delivery systems for cyclosporin A. *Pharm. Res., 13*:311.

93. Calvo, P., Thomas, C., Alonso, M. J., Vila Jato, J. L., and Robinson, J. R. (1994). Study of the mechanism of interaction of poly(ϵ-caprolactone) nanocapsules with the cornea by confocal laser scanning microscopy. *Int. J. Pharm., 103*:283.

94. Le-Bourlais, C. A., Chevanne, F., Turlin, B., Acar, L., Zia, H., Sado, P. A., Needham, T. E., and Leverge, R. (1997). Effect of cyclosporine A formulations on bovine corneal absorption: ex-vivo study. *J. Microencapsulation, 14*:457.

95. Calvo, P., Alonso, M. J., Vila-Jato, J. L., and Robinson, J. R. (1996). Improved ocular bioavailability of indomethacin by novel ocular drug carriers. *J. Pharm. Pharmacol., 48*:1147.

96. Calvo, P., Vila-Jato, J. L., and Alonso, M. J. (1996). Comparative in vitro evaluation of several colloidal systems, nanoparticles, nanocapsules, and nanoemulsions, as ocular drug carriers. *J. Pharm. Sci., 85*:530.

97. Losa, C., Alonso, M. J., Vila, J. L., Orallo, F., Martinez, J., Saavedra, J. A., and Pastor J. C. (1992). Reduction of cardiovascular side effects associated with ocular administration of metipranolol by inclusion in polymeric nanocapsules. *J. Ocul. Pharmacol., 8*:191.

98. Conti, B., Bucolo, C., Giannavola, C., Puglisi, G., Giunchedi, P., and Conte, U. (1997). Biodegradable microspheres for the intravitreal administration of acyclovir: in vitro in vivo evaluation. *Eur. J. Pharm. Sci., 5*:287.
99. Marchal-Heussler, L., Sirbat, D., Hoffman, M., and Maincent, P. (1993). Poly(ε-caprolactone) nanocapsules in carteolol ophthalmic delivery. *Pharm. Res., 10*:386.
100. Komatsu, A., Ohashi, K., Oba, H., Kakehashi, T., Mizushima, Y., Shirasawa, E., and Horiuchi, M. (1988). Application of lipid microsphere drug delivery system to steroidal ophthalmic preparation. *Jpn. J. Ophthalmol., 32*:41.
101. Kimura, H., Ogura, Y., Moritera, T., Honda, Y., Hyon, S. H., and Ikada, Y. (1992). Biodegradable polymer microspheres for a sustained release of fluconazole in the vitreous. *Invest. Ophthalmol. Vis. Sci. 33*:1013.
102. Joshi, H. N., Stella, V. J., and Topp, E. M. (1992). Drug release from membranes of hyaluronic acid and its esters. *J. Control. Rel., 20*:109.
103. Kyyronen, K., Hume, L., Urtti, A., Topp, E., and Stella, V. (1992). Methylprednisolone esters of hyaluronic acid in ophthalmic drug delivery: In vitro and in vivo release studies. *Int. J. Pharm., 80*:161.
104. Leucuta, S. E. (1989). The kinetics of in vitro release and the pharmacokinetics of miotic response in rabbits of gelatin and albumin microspheres with pilocarpine. *Int. J. Pharm., 54*:71.
105. Genta, I., Conti, B., Perugini, P., Pavanetto, F., Spadaro, A., and Puglisi, G. (1997). Bioadhesive microspheres for ophthalmic administration of acyclovir. *J. Pharm. Pharmacol., 49*:737.
106. Jani, R., Gan, O., Ali, Y., Rodstrom, R., and Hancock, S. (1994). Ion exchange resins for ophthalmic delivery. *J. Ocul. Pharmacol. Ther., 10*:57.
107. Ward, C., and Weck, S. (1990) Dilution and storage of recombinant tissue plasminogen activator (Activase) in balanced salt solutions. *Am. J. Ophthalmol., 109*:98.
108. Becker, G. W., Bowsher, R. R., Mackellar, W. C., Poor, M. L., Tackitt, P. M., and Riggin, R. M. (1987). Chemical, physical and biological characterization of a dimeric form of biosynthetic human growth hormone. *Biotechnol. App. Biochem., 9*:478.
109. Giunchedi, P., Conte, U., Chetoni, P., and Saettone, M. F. (1999). Pectin microspheres as ophthalmic carriers for piroxicam: evaluation in vitro and in vivo in albino rabbits. *Eur. J. Pharm. Sci., 9*:1.
110. Desai, S. D., and Blanchard, J. (2000). Pluronic®F127-based ocular delivery system containing biodegradable polyisobutylcyanoacrylate nanocapsules of pilocarpine. *Drug Deliv., 7*:201.

15

Dendrimers: An Innovative and Enhanced Ocular Drug Delivery System

Jeannette M. Loutsch, Desiree Ong, and James M. Hill
LSU Eye and Vision Center of Excellence, Louisiana State University Health Science Center, New Orleans, Louisiana, U.S.A.

I. INTRODUCTION

Current ocular drug delivery methods include such methods as topical drops, ointments, and therapeutic lenses, soluble ocular drug inserts, collagen shields, liposomes, and transcorneal iontophoresis (reviewed in Refs. 1, 2, 3, 4, and 5, respectively). Topically applied drugs, such as suspensions, ointments, and gels, are seldom maintained at the necessary therapeutic concentration in the target tissues due to rapid tear turnover and drainage, tear dilution, and/or an impermeable corneal surface epithelium. Topical drops, currently the most common form of ocular drug delivery, quickly lose their effectiveness and cannot reach the back of the eye because of their rapid elimination. Reduced ocular bioavailability of the drug, in turn, could result in excessive systemic toxicity, causing unwanted side effects such as uncontrolled growth of nonsusceptible pathogens. Emulsifying the drug in an ointment or viscous solution such as polyvinyl alcohol or methylcellulose can decrease the clearance rate over solutions but decrease vision for a time (1). Other current ocular drug delivery methods are also not devoid of problems; for example, collagen shields reduce visual acuity due to the translucent nature of collagen (3,6). Although advancements have been made in these existing systems, efficient drug delivery to the eye remains problematic.

Dendrimers, synthetic spherical macromolecules named after their characteristic "tree-like" or dendritic branching around a central core, are a new class of polymers. The branching structure makes them a useful vector capable of efficient drug and gene delivery. Their nanoscopic architecture could provide a solution to current ocular drug delivery problems.

II. HISTORICAL BACKGROUND

Many experimental models have suggested that life arose spontaneously; simple inorganic building blocks or monomers combined to form larger, organic clusters with new properties. For years, scientists have attempted to copy the evolutionary process, endeavoring to assemble small, identical subunits into complex macromolecules that could be manipulated to interact with and even mimic life. In this attempt, the first major class of polymers was identified in the 1930s. Staudinger linked identical monomers into a spaghetti-like string called the random-coil polymer. These polymers yielded products such as Styrofoam, polyethylene plastic, nylon, and Plexiglas, known as thermoplastics (7,8). The next decade showed progress in the making of larger molecules that constituted the second class of polymers—the family of cross-linked polymers or thermosets. Flory (9–11) and Stockmayer (12,13) successfully created three-dimensional structures by bridging or "cross-linking" the random-coil polymers at various sites, forming an inflexible molecule. These compounds are insoluble in most liquids due to their rigidity and therefore are used as a component of epoxies, urethanes, fiberglass, resins rubbers, and gels (7,8). The third class of polymers was developed in the 1960s. These randomly branched polymers change the bulk property of a substance such as the differences between low-density polyethylene, which is highly branched, and high-density polyethylene, which is virtually unbranched (8). A change in the properties of these polymers is accomplished by altering the types and combinations of the reagents used in the polymerization process.

The problem with the first three classes of polymers was the difficulty in predicting the precise internal structure of the polymer. In an attempt to further define the submolecular structure, a fourth class of polymers was synthesized. This class was referred to as having a dendritic macromolecular architecture due to the branching structure, similar to that of trees. Tomalia, Vögtle, and Newkome independently reported the synthesis of dendrimers. Buhleier et al. (14) and Newkome et al. (15) developed the first dendritic structures, called cascade molecules and arborols, respectively. Tomalia et al. (16) developed the first dendrimer, named the Starburst^{TM} polyamidoamine (PAMAM) dendrimer because of its dendritic branches and controlled starburst growth. This macromolecule is built on an ammonia core with extending branches of alternating methyl acrylate and ethylene diamine molecules (17). The cascade is continued by adding methyl acrylate moieties onto the reactive ends of the ethylene diamine molecules and then ethylene diamine moieties onto the methyl acrylate. Each addition creates another branched layer, referred to as a generation. Each generation causes an exponential increase in the surface reactive sites that may have functional implications (7).

The prospects for the use of dendrimers were numerous and exciting. Unlike the unpredictable length, size, and shape of the previous classes of polymers, the architecture of these dendritic branched molecules can be controlled. The critical molecular design parameters of size, shape, surface chemistry, flexibility, and topology can be carefully regulated to create the complex molecule. In addition, the dendrimer possesses a remarkably cell-like construction consisting of a low-density core and modifiable internal and external surfaces, making it a perfect container or scaffolding for drugs, DNA, and protein. Dendrimers show great promise for a variety of uses such as drug and gene delivery systems, imaging agents, diagnostic kits, tumor therapy, industrial catalysts, and sensors.

III. CHEMICAL AND PHYSICAL CHARACTERISTICS

A. General Chemical Structure and Synthesis

Dendrimers are composed of concentric, geometrically progressive layers created through radial amplification from a single, central initiator core molecule containing either three or four reactive sites such as ammonia or ethylene diamine. Like the nucleus of the biotic cell, the core contains the basic information of the dendrimer; it defines the final size, shape, multiplicity, and functionality of the entire structure. Starting from the center, each layer stores information, which is transferred to the next outer layer or generation via covalent connections, determining that layer's physical properties (17). This is accomplished by choosing reactants with additional reactive sites. Then through a series of protection/deprotection strategies, all the reactive sites on the core molecules are converted without reacting with the reactive sites of the additional reactants. As these steps are repeated, new generations are added to the dendrimer. The radial transfer of information distinguishes the synthetic dendrimer from the biotic cell that transmits information in a linear fashion using DNA and RNA.

The dendrimer amplification process can be described by the simplified synthesis of the basic PAMAM dendrimer (7,17). The first step adds methanol to the mixture of ammonia (NH_3), the initiator core (I), and methyl acrylate (reactant B), causing a molecule of B to substitute for each of the three hydrogen atoms on I. The second step, ethylene diamine, a primary amine is added to the end of each of the methyl acrylates, completing the first generation of the dendrimer. Each ethylene diamine moiety contains two N-H bonds at the end of each branch of the structure, generating six exposed reactivation sites. The second generation of the dendrimer is created by adding a methyl acrylate moiety at each hydrogen and then an ethylene diamine molecule to the end of the branch, yielding 12 exposed reactive sites (Fig. 1). Thus, with such successive generation, the number of reactive sites increases depending on the substrate added to B. The amplification process can continue for about 9 or 10 generations, when the dendrimer is no longer able to form perfect branches due to steric hindrance (7,17).

Dendrimer molecules can be assembled via two pathways. The original pathway, the divergent process, involves working outward from the initiator molecule with the addition of each generation (17). This method of assembly can create a number of defects within the dendrimer. The defect can be in an individual dendrimer or between dendrimers within the mixture. The intra-

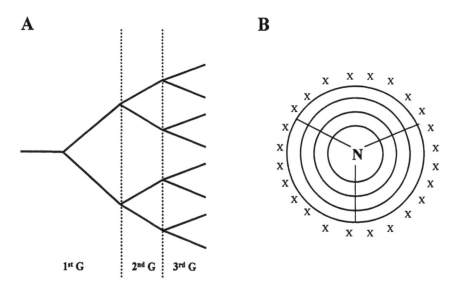

Fig. 1 Schematic drawing of dendrimer structures. Dendrimers are synthesized by two pathways, either the convergent or the divergent pathway. The convergent pathway consists of building the branches prior to addition to the core molecule (A). The divergent pathway consist of building the branches in concentric "layers" (B). Each layer is a generation (G).

dendrimer faults are usually in the branching and are caused by incomplete reactions, branch-juncture fragmentation, or abnormal development or sterically induced stoichiometry. The interdendrimer defects usually arise form the incomplete removal of reagents that may function as a core or dendrimer fragmentation, which may act as an initiator species that can act with other dendrimers (Fig. 2). Optimization of the process and synthesis strategies can eliminate these problems (17). In 1989, Hawker and Fréchet (18) introduced the second pathway, the convergent process, which builds the branch wedge independently and then adds it to the root molecule (Fig. 1). This method allows for using ideal branches because they can be separated from the defective ones. This method may also allow for the creation of dendrimers that have branches with different functions, such as one branch that targets the dendrimer to a cell and a second branch that contains a drug (18). Although this process can generate sufficient dendrimers for the laboratory, it is not conducive to large-scale production (18).

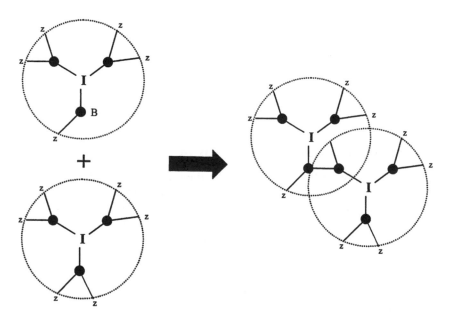

Fig. 2 Defects within dendrimers. Interdendrimer faults can arise form incomplete reactions creating active sites that interact with other dendrimers. The incomplete branching in the top left dendrimer (intradendrimer) has a reactant B, which can react with z from a second dendrimer to interlink the dendrimer structures, creating a defective molecule.

B. Physical Properties

The physical properties of dendrimers depend on the chemical structure/ steric properties of internal and external functional groups. The shape may range from an almost perfect sphere to an ellipsoid to a cylinder-like structure composed of intricately branched "fans" extending out of an elongated base (19). Changes in the core molecule and/or the number of reactive sites present on the core can also influence the shape. Newer dendrimers use phosphorus- or silicone-containing molecules, hydrocarbons, lysine, or thiols as the internal cores (7,17). The dendrimer can also be adjusted based on the selection of reactants. This also can affect the overall size of the dendrimer. Usually size is dependant on the number of generations assembled, but it can also be influenced by the length of the monomers used and the angles between the monomers (7). The average mass of a dendrimer varies from about 500 to 1500 daltons, with the diameter of a spherical dendrimer varying from about 10 Å (first generation) to a maximum of about 130 Å. Each polymerization step increases the diameter by about 10 Å (17).

Dendrimers are relatively stable, covalent macromolecules. They exist independently from each other and from their external environment. As the dendrimer grows, steric congestion eventually prevents further growth. At this point, the dendrimer converts from an open structure to a tight spheroid with open cavities and a dense surface (20). A specific dendrimer's stability depends on the reactivity of the functional groups located on its surface, which can be modified to achieve the necessary level of stability.

C. Dendrimer Core (the "Guest-in-Box System")

Naylor et al. (21) were the first to describe the interior dendrimer space and to demonstrate the large carrying capacity of PAMAM dendrimers. Generations 4 through 7 were capable of encapsulating three times their weight in aspirin. Tomalia and Esfand (19) showed that the dendrimer interior also contains recognition properties specific to the shape and functionality of the guest molecule. The dissolving of water-insoluble molecules, such as ibuprofen, increased in the presence of the dendrimer structure. The ability to encapsulate drugs within the cavities of the dendrimers could result in novel delivery methods.

Jansen et al. (22) reported the synthesis of a "dendrimer box" that is based on a chiral shell of protected amino acids on the dendrimer core. During synthesis of the box, "guest" molecules and small amounts of solvent become trapped within the cavities; the molecules dissolve as they become tightly bound to functional groups on the interior "wall" of the box. Compatible guests such as drugs, DNA, or other small molecules cannot be extracted, and their spontaneous outward diffusion is extremely slow due to the close packing of the shell. Only medium- to high-generation dendrimers possess dense enough shells to capture and retain guests (22). The release of guest molecules can be controlled by changing the pH of the reaction mix (23).

D. Dendrimer Surface

The dendrimer surface ultimately determines the structure's interactions with its environment. The surface serves to protect the internal functional groups via steric interactions, which shield these groups from large molecules while retaining their accessibility and reactivity to small molecules. These interactions also maintain an outside versus inside position with ionic (polar) chain ends containing a high density of positively charged amino groups and a hydrophobic (nonpolar) interior (19). Dendrimer surface properties can be subdivided into endo-receptor properties and exo-receptor properties. Endo-receptor properties are the interior dendritic features such as size, chemical composition, flexibility, and topology, which are responsible for the so-called convergent recognition of guest molecules by the internal dendrimer surface (17). Exo-receptor properties encompass the exterior features, such as shape, reactivity, stoichiometry, flexibility, and fractal character, which similarly govern the divergent recognition of external associator molecules by the external dendrimer surface (17).

The dendrimer surface determines its solubility through chemical recognition of different external reagents/solvents and affects the reactivity of the molecule through the number of reactive surface groups (17). The surface can serve as scaffolding for up to thousands of reactive functional groups such as carbohydrate residues and peptidyl epitopes. Functional groups on the surface of dendrimers show higher chemical reactivity than the same groups attached to other polymer molecules (24). This "charging" allows for important covalent coupling reactions with DNA and other molecules. Furthermore, biologically active molecules, when complexed with dendrimers, tend to retain their maximum activity even when surface groups on the dendrimer are activated for a reaction.

Modifications of the dendrimer surface, specifically the addition of functional groups, occur through the addition of either subnanoscopic or nanoscaled reactants (19). Subnanoscopic reactants can be a variety of small molecules, while nanoscaled reactants are composed of larger molecules such as DNA, antibodies, and proteins that can complex with dendrimers. Scott et al. (25) describe the rapid synthesis of a second-generation dendrimer with primary alcohol groups at the periphery. (The use of modified dendrimers in bioorganic chemistry is reviewed in Ref. 26.)

IV. TISSUE DISTRIBUTION OF DENDRIMERS

For dendrimers to be a viable delivery system for drugs and genes, as well as imaging contrast agents, it must be possible to administer them systemically or orally with reliability. They also must have low cytotoxicity, low immunogenicity, and few adverse side effects.

To determine the potential for dendrimers as drug delivery molecules, Wiwattanapatapee et al. (27) used various [^{125}I]-labeled dendrimers in an ex vivo system, the everted rat intestinal sac model. The distribution of the dendrimers was monitored through the wall of the gut by measuring the radioactivity in the serous fluid and tissues. Anionic PAMAM dendrimers (generation 2.5 and 3.5) had faster, concentration-dependent serosal transfer than cationic PAMAM dendrimers (generation 3 and 4). The anionic PAMAM generation 5.5 and the cationic PAMAM dendrimers had high levels of tissue uptake, thereby slowing the transfer rate (27). These results indicate that these dendrimers have potential as an oral drug delivery system and require an in vivo study.

Sakthivel et al. (28) and Florence et al. (29) gave Sprague-Dawley rats an oral dose of a lipidic peptide dendrimer and monitored tissue distribution. The radiolabeled 2.5 nm dendrimer (generation 4) was given by oral gavage. The first study revealed that the maximum level of the dendrimer was found in the small intestine, with decreasing amounts in the large intestines, blood, and other organs. The amount absorbed by the lymphoid tissue of the intestinal tract was greater than the amount in the nonlymphoid tissues, based on organ weight at 3 and 24 hours (28). In the second study, Peyer's patches were found to absorb more of the dendrimer than normal enterocytes in the small intestine, while the opposite was true in the large intestine, with enterocytes absorbing more (29). The uptake and transport of these lipidic dendrimers was lower than expected based on polystyrene particle data and may indicate that there is an optimum size for dendrimer uptake in the intestines.

Malik et al. (30) investigated the relationship between dendrimer structure and biocompatibility in vitro. Dendrimers with NH_2 termini had a concentration-dependent hemolysis and red cell morphology after 1-hour incubation with rat red blood cell suspension. The PAMAM dendrimers also demonstrated generation-dependent hemolysis. Those with carboxylate termini had no hemolytic or cytotoxicity in cell culture (30). In vivo analysis of cationic and anionic PAMAM dendrimers in the Wistar rat revealed that third- and fourth-generation cationic dendrimers are cleared faster than generations 2.5, 3.5, and 5.5 of the anionic dendrimers. In the case of the anionic dendrimers, the longer clearance times were generation dependent, with the smaller dendrimers remaining in the blood longer (30). The systemic clearance correlated with the increased accumulation of the radiolabeled dendrimer in the liver. However, there was no difference between intravenous and intraperitoneal administration. Dendrimers with low toxicity and carefully tailored surfaces that remain in the circulation with minimal hepatic uptake, especially if they need to reach a target organ, are needed if they are to be used for oral drug delivery. The effect of dendrimer degradation products on tissue also needs to be addressed.

Wiener et al. (31) and Konda et al. (32) adapted dendrimers for use as magnetic resonance (MR) imaging agents. Second- and sixth-generation dendrimers were linked to a chelator that enhanced conventional MR imaging (31). These dendrimers showed enhanced contrast in the heart, liver, kidneys, and blood vessels of Fisher 344 rats. The higher molecular weight dendrimer may aid in the three-dimensional time-of-flight MR angioplasty due to the prolonged clearance time. A fourth-generation dendrimer was linked to folic acid and a chelating agent for use in targeting tumors with folic acid receptor expression (32). Studies in nude mice with ovarian tumors (positive for folic acid receptor expression) showed enhanced contrast 24 hours following administration of the agent while receptor-negative tumors did not. These new contrast agents will aid in the imaging of tumors and normal tissues.

V. THERAPEUTIC USES OF DENDRIMERS

The use of dendrimers in drug and gene therapy is increasing. Table 1 provides a summary of studies that used dendrimers or other small synthetic macromolecules. A discussion of dendrimer-related studies is given below.

A. Dendrimer-Mediated Delivery of Drugs

Studies have shown dendritic drug delivery to tissues to be very promising. Some of the advantages of dendrimers include their capacity to hold a large variety of molecules and to protect these molecules from their surroundings until they are released in a time-dependent, controlled manner. Dendrimers that are synthesized to mimic micelles (hydrophobic inner layer and hydrophilic outer layer) can create a micro-container to transport drugs. The hydroscopic drugs trapped within this space are protected from the environment and have a reduced rate of uptake by the liver and prolonged

Table 1 Use of Nanoparticles, Including Dendrimers, Liposomes, and Micelles, for Drug and Gene Delivery In Vivo and In Vitro

Nanoparticle	Drug/Gene/Virus	Application/Target	Model	Ref.
PAMAM	Epstein-Barr virus plasmid vector	Hepatocellular carcinoma cells	In vitro, cell culture	49
PAMAM	Epstein-Barr virus plasmid vector	Intratumoral injection	In vivo, SCID mice	69
PAMAM	Folate receptor	Ovarian tumors	In vivo, mice	32
PAMAM (G4)	Cisplatin	Cancer chemotherapy	In vivo, mice	40
PAMAM, Linear polyacrylamide polymers, dendron and dendrigraft	Influenza viruses	Block sialic acid receptor and prevent viral attachment	In vitro	35
PAMAM (G0-4)	Biotinylated residues	Pretargeting of cancer cells to allow the increase of radioactivity	In vivo, mouse	70
PAMAM (G2)	Folate residues or methyltrexate	Target tumor cells		71
PAMAM		Inhibit viral challenge in vaginal model of HSV	In vivo, mice	36
PAMAM, liposomes	Normal cystic fibrosis transmembrane regulator gene	Replacement gene therapy	In vitro	61
PAMAM	Cholera toxin	Inhibition of adherence	In vitro	72,73
Poly(D,L-lactide) nanoparticles	Platelet-derived growth factor inhibitor	Prevent restinosis	In vitro and in vivo, rat	74
PAMAM (G5)	IL-10	Cardiac graft rejection	In vivo, mice	53
Poly(lactide-co-glycolide) microspheres	Neurotrophic factors and antimitotic drugs	Blood-brain barrier	In vitro and in vivo	75

PAMAM (G4)	Epidermal growth factor	Target tumor cells for neutron capture therapy	In vitro and in vivo, rats	52
Cationic dendrimer	Folate-conjugated	Folate receptor–mediated gene therapy	In vitro	50
PAMAM	Magnetic resonance imaging contrast agent	Tumor imaging	In vivo	31
PAMAM (G2, G4)	Monoclonal antibody immunoconjugate	Neutron capture therapy	In vivo, mice	51
PAMAM	Antisense oligonucleotide	Gene expression, rescue defective genes	In vitro	46
Polyethyleneimine	Gene and oligonucleotide transfer	Target brain tissue	In vitro and in vivo, mice	76
n-(2-Hydroxypropyl) methacrylamide	Doxorubicin hydrochloride	Chemotherapeutic agent	In vivo, humans	42
PAMAM	Poly(ethylene glycol) grafts and anticancer drugs	Chemotherapeutic agents	In vitro	41
Dendritic unimolecular micelles	Indomethacin	Anti-inflammatory	In vitro	33

systemic half-life (33). The anti-inflammatory drug indomethacin could be incorporated at a rate of nine to ten molecules per micelle, with sustained in vitro release (33).

1. Antibacterials

Dendrimers could assist in counteracting bacterial infections by serving as transport facilitators for antibiotics and antisense nucleotides or by binding to receptors on the bacterial cell, thereby preventing infection. The antisense approach is based on the ability of oligonucleotides to interfere with the biological activity of bacteria by interacting with a necessary protein or hybridizing to the bacterial mRNA. The latter aptameric interaction blocks the synthesis of important bacterial proteins.

Oligonucleotides function at the bacterial ribosome or nucleus and can enter eukaryotic cells via endocytosis. However, the hydrophobic exterior of prokaryotes serves as a barrier to oligonucleotides. Attia et al. (34) reported the use of a small fourth-generation dendrimer combined with ethambutol (a metabolic cell wall inhibitor), which acted as a transport facilitator for oligonucleotides to interact with *Mycobacterium tuberculos* in vitro. Further investigation is needed to determine the effect of the oligonucleotides on treatment of *M. tuberculosis*.

2. Antiviral Agents

Dendrimers can be used to counter viral activity in several different ways. They can be modified with external residues that inhibit virus-host cell interactions (35), act as antivirals themselves (36), or serve as delivery vehicles.

Influenza viruses infect human cells by binding the viral hemagglutinin to the sialic acid receptor on the host cell and then undergoing receptor-mediated endocytosis of the virus into the cell. The influenza virus can modify the antigenicity of the hemagglutinin and therefore can evade neutralizing antibodies as well as antiviral compounds (35). Synthetic dendrimers containing sialic acid moieties on the surface layer can successfully compete with hemagglutinin for the host cell. This interaction can prevent adhesion to the host cell and subsequent infection. These dendrimers are polyvalent inhibitors, meaning that one dendrimer can interact with many hemagglutinin molecules on one virus at one time. This cooperative interaction of individual receptors increases the overall binding affinity. Reuter et al. (35) determined that binding of the influenza virus hemagglutinin and neuraminidase glycoproteins with sialic acid residues attached to a dendrimer resulted in a dose-dependent decrease in influenza infection in vitro.

These dendrimers, which were nontoxic to cells, were the first multivalent sialic acid inhibitor shown to be effective in vitro.

Bourne et al. (36) investigated the potential of five different polylysine PAMAM dendrimers (containing a central benhydrylamine core) as topical microbicides for herpes simplex virus (HSV) types 1 and 2. In vitro studies showed that the dendrimer BRI-2999 could block HSV infection in cytopathic effect (CPE) inhibition assays. In vivo studies in the mouse vaginal model of HSV infection determined that the application of a topical solution of BRI-2999 before viral challenge could significantly reduce the occurrence of disease, with no noticeable signs of toxicity to the mice. The dendrimer prevents normal virus-host cell adhesion/adsorption by complexing with the virus. No effect was seen when the dendrimer was applied after the viral challenge. Further evaluation is needed to determine if these compounds can be used to reduce the spread of sexually transmitted diseases. Additionally, the use of dendrimers has produced promising in vitro inhibitory activity against respiratory syncytial virus. BRI-2999 had potency in the CPE inhibition assay but also had some cytotoxic effects on stationary phase cells (37). In HIV studies, polyanionic dendrimers showed inhibition of HIV replication in MT4 cells (38). The interference came during two phases of the viral life cycle: adsorption and reverse transcription. In vitro efficacy was also seen against cytomegalovirus, HSV-1 and HSV-2, thymidine kinase–deficient HSV-1, vesicular stomatitis virus, yellow fever virus, reovirus type 1, and dengue fever virus (38).

3. Antitumor Drug Therapy

Duncan and Malik (39) use doxorubicin and cisplatin as model drugs to study the potential of dendrimer-anticancer therapeutic agents. They found that these compounds retained biological activity in vitro and may be useful in vivo. PAMAM dendrimers were conjugated to cisplatin to create a dendrimer-platinate molecule that was highly water-soluble and released the drug slowly (40). This compound displayed antitumor activity and was less toxic than cisplatin alone. Kojima et al. (41) report that PAMAM dendrimers with poly(ethylene glycol) grafts possessed a space that could carry anticancer drugs with a biocompatible surface, such as adriamycin and methotrexate. Increasing generations and chain length of the poly(ethylene glycol) grafts allowed for increasing amounts of drugs to be encapsulated within the space. The dendrimer carrying methotrexate released the drug slowly in an aqueous solution but rapidly in an ionic solution (41). Vasey et al. (42) used a polymer linked to doxurubicin (adriamycin) in a phase 1 clinical trial. The drug-polymer complex (PK1) was given to patients with refractory solid tumors such as colorectal, breast, ovary, pancreas, and others. PK1 was found to decrease the nonspecific organ toxicity and side effects to the drug while maintaining antitumor activity without polymer toxicity (42). Although this study did not employ a dendrimer, it demonstrates that polymers could play as significant role in future cancer chemotherapy regimens.

B. Dendrimer-Mediated Gene Therapy for Cancer and Genetic Disease

Gene therapy is an exciting new field focusing on the treatment of illnesses via genetic modification. Conventional medicine often manages to increase the patient's degree of comfort by alleviating the symptoms of the disease while not actually treating the disease. Gene therapy may hold the key to a more permanent solution by seeking to correct the problem at the root of the disease—the defective gene. A reliable gene-delivery vehicle is an indispensable component of gene transfer therapy. Current gene-delivery systems use viruses or liposomes as vectors. However, these vectors have many problems such as immunogenicity or carcinogenicity and potential infectivity (43). The characteristics of the dendrimer (nontoxic, nonimmunogenic, and nonviral) make it a very good candidate for gene therapy. (The use of Starburst^{TM} dendrimers in gene transfer is reviewed in Ref. 44.)

The electrostatic interactions between DNA (negative charge) and the dendrimer (positive charge) yield a complex that forms quickly. The complex is stable over a wide range of pH (45). The DNA condenses when it contacts the polymer, and the degree of condensation is defined by the generation of the dendrimer, the concentration of the DNA, and the DNA : dendrimer charge ratio (46). As the DNA : dendrimer charge ratio increases, so does the biological function of the complex. Electron microscopy shows that DNA complexed with polylysine or whole dendrimer aggregates in solution, whereas DNA complexed with polyethylenimine or fractured dendrimer remains as single discrete units (47). Bielinska et al. (46) and Kukowska-Latallo et al. (45) reported that DNA-dendrimer complexes have a broader concentration range between transfection and cytotoxicity in numerous cell lines.

The efficiency of in vitro transfection increases exponentially with the increase in the generation number of the dendrimer (45). The DNA is protected from nuclease degradation while bound to the dendrimer; however, the DNA is unable to initiate transcription from the promoter. This may be due to the inaccessibility of the promoter to the polymerase enzyme because the secondary and tertiary structure of the DNA is altered when it is complexed with the dendrimer. Elongation of the RNA transcript and translation do not appear to be affected in these molecules (48). Additional in vivo studies are needed to determine cellular localization and transfection efficiency with these dendrimer-DNA complexes.

1. Cancer Gene Therapy

One interesting method for treating certain cancers is to program the tumor cells to self-destruct. This can be achieved by inserting a viral gene, usually herpes simplex virus thymidine kinase (TK), directly into tumor cells, enabling the cells to produce the enzyme. The tumor is then treated with ganciclovir, the substrate of TK, creating the active form of the drug that causes the cancer cells to "commit suicide." Harda et al. (49) transfected human hepatocellular carcinoma cells with an Epstein-Barr virus–based plasmid vector containing the TK gene complexed with either PAMAM dendrimers or cationic liposomes. Addition of therapeutic concentrations of ganciclovir resulted in a significant decrease in the number of viable carcinoma cells in the dendrimer-treated cultures. Carcinoma cells transfected with the liposome vector alone survived the same dose of ganciclovir. The dendrimer-based vectors showed increased efficiency of gene transfer. These results demonstrate the successful use of dendrimers in the transfer of suicide genes in vitro (49).

Dendrimers are being considered for use in targeting therapy to solid organ tumors. Reddy et al. (50) used a folate-targeted, cholesterol-stabilized liposomal vector linked to a sixth-generation dendrimer to target tumor cells. Certain cancer cells over-express folic acid receptor on their surface, making this a viable mechanism for targeting therapeutic and imaging agents to the tumor. The folic acid–linked dendrimer had a higher transfection efficiency compared to the control dendrimer in cell culture (50).

Another method of cancer chemotherapy is to target boron-10, a stable isotope, to the tumor and then activate it by the use of low-energy irradiation, which excites the boron-10 and causes the death of the cancer cell. Barth et al. (51) used boron-10 coupled to a Starburst dendrimer and conjugated to an antibody against mouse B16 melanoma to treat mice with tumors. They found that the immunoconjugate was localized largely in the liver and spleen rather than in the tumor, even though the antibody is very specific for the tumor in vitro (51). This novel approach to targeting and treating tumor cells could be effective if antibody specific for the tumor in vivo can be developed. Yang et al. (52) exploited the fact that gliomas overproduce the epidermal growth factor receptor on the surface of the cancer cell. They linked epidermal growth factor to a boronated fourth-generation Starburst dendrimer and administered it either intravenously or intratumorally to rats with glial tumors. The intratumor injection resulted in 22% and 16% localization in the tumor at 24 and 48 hours, respectively, whereas the intravenous dose showed virtually no localization to the tumor (52). Additionally, the intravenous dose had a greater localization to the liver and spleen than the intratumor injection. These results indicate that intracerebellar injection could be the most effective treatment delivery system in epidermal growth factor receptor–positive tumors.

2. Cardiac Gene Therapy

Qin et al. (53) used plasmid-mediated gene transfer and subsequent expression in a mouse cardiac transplant model to improve graft survival. A plasmid encoding viral interleukin 10 (IL-10) under the control of α-myosin heavy chain promoter (α-MHC-vIL-10) injected into the graft prolonged allograft survival significantly from 13.9 days to 21.4 days. When α-MHC-vIL-10 was complexed with G5EDA dendrimer, a 60-fold decrease in DNA resulted in significantly prolonged graft survival to 38.6 days (53). Increasing the amount and time of immunosuppressive cytokine expression in more tissues allowed for further prolongation of graft survival. This novel method of local immunosuppression could be beneficial to patients undergoing solid organ transplantation.

A concern for dendrimer-mediated therapy is cytotoxicity at the site of the dendrimer localization. Brazeau et al. (54) report that PAMAM dendrimers alone had high myotoxicity in an isolated rat muscle cell. The toxicity decreased when the dendrimer was coupled to a DNA plasmid but not to the level of saline or DNA alone (54). While this is an in vitro system, it is imperative that toxicity studies be examined in vivo.

3. Genetic Disease Therapy

Oligonucleotide therapy has limiting factors that may reduce its usefulness. The majority of these therapies involves the incorporation of antisense oligonucleotide sequences that bind to the mRNA of cells and interfere with protein synthesis. Fomivirsen, and antiviral, is a successful antisense oligonucleotide therapy that is clinically available for the treatment of cytomegalovirus retinitis (55–57). The factors that limit the usefulness of oligonucleotide therapy are degradation, inefficient cellular uptake and intracellular transport, and binding to the RNA target. The use of dendrimers could alleviate these problems by the generation of cell-targeting dendrimers that could deliver the gene to the appropriate cell.

Yoo and Juliano (58) used fifth-generation dendrimers labeled with Oregon green 488 and an oligonucleotide labeled with TAMRA, a red fluorophore to determine localization in transfected HeLa cell by fluorescence microscopy. The oligonucleotide would correct a splicing error in the reporter gene, luciferase, if the transfection was successful and functionally active. They found luciferase activity in the cells as well as the dendrimer and oligonucleotide localized in close proximity to one another. Interestingly, the dendrimers with Oregon green 488 enhanced the delivery of the PAMAM dendrimer-oligonucleotide complex to the cells compared to the unlabeled dendrimer-oligonucleotide complex (58). Helin et al. (59) used FITC-labeled oligodeoxynucleotides (ODN) with and without dendrimers as carriers to determine cellular uptake and intracellular distribution in various cell lines (Table 1). The FITC-ODN had increased cellular fluorescence when complexed with dendrimers. Some cells had perinuclear fluorescence and some cells had intense nuclear staining (59). These studies indicate that oligonucleotide can reach the nucleus, the target for gene therapy. Nilsen et al. (60) suggest that dendrimers can be constructed from nucleic acids for use as a "nucleic acid membrane." This structure could be useful in gene therapy but to date has not been tested.

Cystic fibrosis is a genetic disease caused by a deletion mutation in the cystic fibrosis transmembrane conductance regulator (CFTR) gene that affects the pulmonary system. Patients, mostly children, suffer from respiratory congestion and numerous lung infections. Goncz et al. (61) used dendrimers to deliver a fragment of DNA that could correct the mutated sequence in CFTR. The small single-stranded DNA fragment (488 nucleotides long) was complexed with a Starburst dendrimer and used to transfect primary normal airway epithelial cells (61). The DNA fragment corrected the defective gene in 1 out of 100 cells, a range that could have therapeutic potential. This method of small fragment homologous replacement therapy could be developed into gene therapy strategies for disease caused by site-specific mutations.

C. Additional Therapeutic Uses of Dendrimers

Dendrimers linked with DNA can retain their ability to transfect cells after drying, unlike viral vectors. Bielinska et al. (62) used this novel property of dendrimer-DNA to coat a solid-phase, bioerodable support or to embed the complex in the support. The DNA was a plasmid that expressed either luciferase or green fluorescent protein when transfected into cells. Expression of luciferase or green fluorescent protein was detected following release of the complex from the support or while still attached (62). A membrane that had a dendrimer-DNA complex on the surface was placed on the skin of a hairless mouse. Chloramphenicol transacetylase activity was found in the tissue under the membrane indicating that the DNA was delivered to the skin from the membrane (62).

Kawase et al. (63) created a high-performance, bio-artificial liver support system using fructose-modified dendrimers immobilized on polystyrene

dishes. The modified dishes were capable of increasing the number of hepatocytes attached to the surface, which in turn increased urea synthesis. The
number of cells remained high as the fructose-modified dendrimers appeared
to suppress apoptosis (63). Increasing the generation of the dendrimer led to
increased numbers of hepatocytes adherent to the support system. This may
be a novel way to treat fulminant hepatic failure, similar to renal dialysis.

VI. OCULAR THERAPY

A. Corneal Drug and Gene Delivery

The cornea is composed of epithelial, stromal, and endothelial layers that
provide a barrier to the penetration of most drugs used to treat ocular
disease. As such, the ocular surface presents a challenge for chemotherapy.
The epithelial surface is susceptible to bacterial, fungal, and viral infection
and inflammation, as well as to mechanical injury. The stroma may be
affected by granular or lattice corneal dystrophy, which are diseases that
result in abnormal protein deposits in the stroma caused by autosomal
dominant mutation. The corneal endothelium function to maintain corneal
transparency and normal visual acuity. The endothelial cells cannot regenerate, and therefore corneal transplants are the only way to correct endothelial damage that results in blindness. The ability of dendrimers to be targeted
to specific cell types and to carry drugs or genes could allow for the treatment of these diseases and prevention of corneal graft rejection.

Hudde et al. (64) reported the efficiency of gene transfer to the corneal
endothelium using PAMAM dendrimers in an ex vivo model. The dendrimer was complexed with a plasmid containing a reporter gene, β-galactosi-
dase, in a ratio of 18:1 and incubated with a quarter of a full-thickness
rabbit cornea. The expression of β-galactosidase was assessed after 3 days:
6–10% of the endothelial cells were stained blue (64). The transfection of the
dendrimer-plasmid complex was also determined in human corneas but with
less efficiency ($\sim$ 2% of cells). There was no evidence of cellular toxicity
from the dendrimer. The staining was seen only in the endothelium and
not in the epithelium or stroma in both rabbit and human corneas (64).
In the same study, the introduction and expression of the gene, tumor
necrosis factor receptor fusion protein (TNFR-Ig) was assessed in this ex
vivo system. Tumor necrosis factor (TNF) is produced in high concentrations during transplant rejection and causes severe damage to the graft.
TNFR-Ig could prevent the TNF response and therefore protect the graft.
Rabbit corneas incubated with the dendrimer/plasmid secreted an active
form of TNFR-Ig into the supernatant that inhibited TNF-mediated toxicity in a bioassay (64).

Corneas that will be used for transplantation are stored in a special medium prior to surgery. This corneal storage medium could be modified to contain dendrimers complexed with genes expressing important proteins that could prevent graft rejection. Hudde et al. (64) demonstrated that the dendrimer/TNFR-Ig gene complex transfected into ex vivo corneas produces an active protein that inhibits TNF-mediated cytotoxicity. Qin et al. (53) prolonged cardiac graft survival in mice by giving a dendrimer carrying a plasmid coding for IL-10, an interleukin that enhances immunosuppression and hence improves graft survival. Combinations of these strategies could prolong survival of the transplanted cornea. Dendrimer therapy could also correct hereditary diseases such as lattice corneal dystrophy by introducing the normal gene (i.e., transforming growth factor, β-induced gene) into the endothelial cells so a functioning protein could be expressed. While no ocular dendrimer drug delivery studies have been performed to date, the possibility of dendrimers being used carry drugs to corneal cells should be investigated.

B. Intraocular Drug and Gene Delivery

Treatment of the inner ocular tissues and the posterior region of the eye has posed a significant challenge to ophthalmologists. A major tissue to be targeted is the retina, the transparent tissue lining the back of the eye that is responsible for visual acuity, color discrimination, and peripheral vision. Diseases of the retina include retinitis pigmentosa and macular degeneration; both result in blindness due to the death of retinal cells. Drugs applied to the cornea usually do not reach the back of the eye. Therefore, direct injection of the drugs into the vitreous is required to target the retina. While this method provides adequate drug levels, it is not without significant risk of retinal detachment, endophthalmitis, vitreal hemorrhage, and/or cellular toxicity (65–67). The use of dendrimers to deliver drugs and gene therapy to this area of the eye has great potential.

Urtti et al. (68) investigated the efficacy of in vitro gene delivery in fetal primary human retinal pigment epithelial (RPE) cells using plasmids encoding the reporter gene β-galactosidase or luciferase. The reporter gene plasmids were complexed with either degraded sixth-generation PAMAM dendrimers, cationic lipids, or polyethylene imines (PEI; 25 or 750 kDa) to determine the level of protein expression and cellular toxicity in RPE cells. A degraded dendrimer has several branches removed by boiling in butanol, which does not alter the size and shape but does increase the spaces within the dendrimer and increases the flexibility of the molecule. Naked plasmid DNA was not as effective as complexed DNA in transfecting the RPE cells. When the luciferase plasmid was linked with the dendrimer or

PEI-25, the expression of luciferase was significantly higher than with the other carriers (68). The dendrimer/plasmid and PEI-750/plasmid were also less toxic to the cells than the other vehicles. Although only a small number of RPE cells were transfected, a large amount of protein was expressed from the plasmid (68). This is especially significant with a secreted protein product; a few cells making the protein could secrete enough to counteract the deficiency in all the cells. This method of delivering genes works well in vitro, but additional investigations are needed before the in vivo impact can be determined.

VII. CONCLUSION

The ability of dendrimers to carry drugs and genes may allow for the advancement of drug and gene therapy, not only in ophthalmology, but in other areas of medicine. In the field of ocular drug and gene delivery, the controlled architecture and the nontoxic, nonimmunogenic nature of dendrimers raise the possibility of future replacement of currently problematic delivery systems. The creation of dendrimers that can target specific cells and carry a particular therapy will allow physicians to enhance treatment regimens.

ACKNOWLEDGMENTS

The authors wish to acknowledge Jean Jacobs, Ph.D., Kristina Braud, and Kathy Vu for assistance with this review. None of the authors have any financial or proprietary interest in any of the agents or devices in this review.

REFERENCES

1. Olejnik, O. (1993). Conventional systems in ophthalmic drug delivery. In: A. K. Mitra (ed.), *Ophthalmic Drug Delivery Systems*. Marcel Dekker, Inc., New York, p. 177.
2. Bawa, R. (1993). Ocular insert. In: *Ophthalmic Drug Delivery Systems*. A. K. Mitra (ed.). Marcel Dekker, Inc., New York, p. 223.
3. Hill, J. M., O'Callaghan, R. J., Hobden, J. A., and Kaufman, H. E. (1993). Corneal collagen shields for ocular drug delivery. In: *Ophthalmic Drug Delivery Systems*. A. K. Mitra (ed.). Marcel Dekker, Inc., New York, p. 261.

4. Davies, N. M., Kellaway, I. W., Greaves, J. L., and Wilson, C. G. (1993). Advanced corneal delivery systems: liposomes. In: *Ophthalmic Drug Delivery Systems*. A. K Mitra (ed.). Marcel Dekker, Inc., New York, p. 289.
5. Hill, J. M., O'Callaghan, R. J., and Hobden, J. A. (1993). Ocular iontophoresis. In: *Ophthalmic Drug Delivery Systems*. A. K. Mitra (ed.). Marcel Dekker, Inc., New York, p. 331.
6. Hill, J. M., O'Callaghan, R. J., Hobden, J. A., and Kaufman, H. E. Collagen shields for ocular drug delivery. In: *Ophthalmic Drug Delivery Systems*. M. K. Mitra (ed.). Marcel Dekker, Inc., New York, p. 261.
7. Tomalia, D. A. (1995). Dendrimer molecules. *Sci. Am., 5*:42.
8. Tomalia, D. A., and Brothers, H. M. I. (1998). Regiospecific conjugation to dendritic polymers to produce nanodevices. In: *Biological Molecules in Nanotechnology: The Convergence of Biotechnology, Polymer Chemistry, and Material Science*. International Business Communications, Inc., Southborough, MA, pp. 107–120.
9. Flory, P. J. (1941). Molecular size distribution in three dimensional polymers. I. Gelation. *J. Am. Chem. Soc., 63*:3083–3090.
10. Flory, P. J. (1941). Molecular size distribution in three dimensional polymers. II. Trifunctional branching units. *J. Am. Chem. Soc., 63*:3091–3096.
11. Flory, P. J. (1941). Molecular size distribution in three dimensional polymers. III. Tetrafunctional branching units. *J. Am. Chem. Soc., 63*:3096–3100.
12. Stockmayer, W. H. (1943). Theory of molecular size distribution and gel formation in branched-chain polymers. *J. Chem. Phys., 11*:45–55.
13. Stockmayer, W. H. (1944). Theory of molecular size distribution and gel formation in branched polymers. II. General cross linking. *J. Chem. Phys., 12*:125–131.
14. Buhleier, E., Wehner, W., and Vögtle, F. (1978). "Cascade"- and "nonskid-chain-like" syntheses of molecular cavity topologies. *Synthesis, 55*:155–158.
15. Newkome, G. R., Yao, Z.-Q., Baker, G. R., and Gupta, V. K. (1985). Cascade molecules: A new approach to micelles. A [27]-arborol. *J. Org. Chem., 50*:2003–2004.
16. Tomalia, D. A., Baker, H., Dewald, J., Hall, M., Kallos, G., Roeck, J., Ryder, J., and Smith, P. (1985). A new class of polymers: Starburst-dendritic macromolecules. *Polym. J., 17*:117–132.
17. Tomalia, D. A., Naylor, A. M., and Goddard, W. A. I. (1990). Starburst dendrimers: molecular-level control of size, shape, surface chemistry, topology, and flexibility from atoms to macroscopic matter. *Angew. Chem. Int. Ed. Engl., 29*:138–175.
18. Hawker, C. J., and Fréchet, J. M. J. (1990). Preparation of polymers with controlled molecular architecture. A new convergent approach to dendritic macromolecules. *J. Am. Chem. Soc., 112*:7638–7647.
19. Tomalia, D. A., and Esfand, R. (1997). Dendrons, dendrimers, and dendrigrafts. *Chem. Ind., 6*:416–420.
20. Fréchet, J. M. J. (1994). Functional polymers and dendrimers: Reactivity, molecular architecture, and interfacial energy. *Science, 263*:1710–1715.

21. Naylor, A. M., Goddard III, W. A., Kiefer, G. A., and Tomalia, D. A. (1989). Starburst dendrimers. 5. Molecular shape control. *J. Am. Chem. Soc.,* *111*:2339–2341.

22. Jansen, J. F. G. A., de Brabander-van den Berg, E. M. M., and Meijer, E. W. (1994). Encapsulation of guest molecules into a dendritic box. *Science,* *266*:1226–1229.

23. Stephan, H., Spies, H., Johannsen, B., Kauffmann, C., and Vögtle. (2000). pH-controlled inclusion and release of oxyanions by dendrimers bearing methyl orange moieties. *Org. Lett.,* *2*:2343–2346.

24. Singh, P. (1998). Terminal groups in Starburst dendrimers: activation and reactions with proteins. *Bioconjug. Chem.,* *9*:54.

25. Scott, D. A., Krulle, T. M., Finn, M., and Fleet, G. W. J. (2000). Bis(1,3-dihydroxy-isopropyl)amine (BDI) as an AB4 dendritic building block: rapid synthesis of a second generation dendrimer. *Tetrahedron Lett.,* *41*:3959.

26. Veprek, P., and Jezek, J. (1999). Peptide and glycopeptide dendrimers. Part II. *J. Peptide Sci.,* *5*:203.

27. Wiwattanapatapee, R., Carreno-Gomez, B., Malik, N., and Duncan, R. (2000). Anionic PAMAM dendrimers rapidly cross adult rat intestines in vitro: A potential oral delivery system? *Pharm. Res.,* *17*:991.

28. Sakthivel, T., Toth, I., and Florence, A. T. (1999). Distribution of a lipid 2.5 nm diameter dendrimer carrier after oral administration. *Int. J. Pharm.,* *183*:51.

29. Florence, A. T., Sakthivel, T., and Toth, I. (2000). Oral uptake and translocation of a polylysine dendrimer with a lipid surface. *J. Controlled Release,* *65*:253.

30. Malik, N., Wiwattanapatapee, R., Klopsch, R., Lorenz, K., Frey, H., Weener, J. W., Meijer, E. W., Paulus, W., and Duncan R. (2000). Dendrimers: relationship between structure and biocompatibility in vitro, and preliminary studies on the biodistribution of ^{125}I-labelled polyamidoamine dendrimers in vivo. *J. Controlled Release, 65*:133.

31. Wiener, E. C., Brechbiel, M. W., Brothers, H., Magin, R. L., Gansow, O. A., Tomalia, D. A., and Lauterbur, P. C. (1994). Dendrimer-based metal celates: A new class of magnetic resonance imaging contrast agents. *Magn. Reson. Med., 31*:1.

32. Konda, S. D., Aref, M., Brechbiel, M., and Wiener, E. C. (2000). Development of a tumor-targeting MR contrast agent using the high-affinity folate receptor. *Invest. Radiol., 35*:50.

33. Liu, M., Kono, K., and Fréchet, M. J. (2000). Water-soluble dendritic unimolecular micelles: Their potential as drug delivery agents. *J. Controlled Release, 65*:121.

34. Attia, S. A., Shepherd, V. E., Rosenblatt, M. N., Davidson, M. K., and Hughes, J. A. (1998). Interaction of oligodeoxynucleotides with mycobacteria: Implications for new therapeutic strategies. *Antisense Nucleic Acid Drug Dev., 8*:207.

35. Reuter, J. D., Myc, A., Hayes, M. M., Gan, Z., Roy, R., Qin, D., Yin, R., Piehler, L. T., Esfand, R., Tomalia, D. A., and Baker, J. R. Jr. (1999). Inhibition of viral adhesion and infection by sialic-acid-conjugated dendritic polymers. *Bioconjug. Chem., 10*:271.

36. Bourne, N., Stanberry, L. R., Kern, E. C., Holan, G., Matthews, B., and Bernstein, D. I. (2000). Dendrimers, a new class of candidate topical microbicides with activity against herpes simplex virus infection. *Antimicrob. Agents Chemother., 44*:2471.

37. Barnard, D. L., Sidwell, R. W., Gage, T. L., Okleberry, K. M., Mathews, B., and Holan, G. (1997). Anti-respiratory syncytial virus activity of dendrimer polyanions. *Antiviral Res., 34*:A88.

38. Witvrouw, M., Pannecouque, C., Matthews, B., Schols, D., Andrei, G., Snoeck, R., Neyts, J., Leyssen, P., Desmyter, J., Raff, J., DeClerq, E., and Holan, G. (1999). Dendrimers inhibit the replication of human immunodeficiency virus (HIV) by a dual mechanism of action. *Antiviral Res., 41*:A41.

39. Duncan, R., and Malik, N. (1996). Dendrimers: biocompatibility and potential for delivery of anticancer agents. *Proc. Int. Symp. Control Rel. Bioact. Mater., 23*:105.

40. Malik, N., Evagorou, E. G., and Duncan, R. (1999). Dendrimer-platinate: a novel approach to cancer chemotherapy. *Anticancer Drugs, 10*:767.

41. Kojima, C., Kono, K., Maruyama, K., and Takagishi, T. (2000). Synthesis of polyamidoamine dendrimers having poly(ethylene glycol) grafts and their ability to encapsulate anticancer drugs. *Bioconjugate Chem., 11*:910.

42. Vasey, P. A., Kaye, S. B., Morrison, R., Twelves, C., Wilson, P., Duncan, R., Thomson, A. H., Murray, L. S., Hilditch, T. E., Murray, T., Burtles, S., Fraier, D., Frigerio, E., Cassidy, J., on behalf of the Cancer-Research Campaign Phase I/II Committee. (1999). Phase I clinical and pharmacokinetic study of PK1 [N-(2-hydroxypropyl)methacrylamide copolymer doxorubicin]: first member of a new class of chemotherapeutic agents – drug-polymer conjugates. *Clin. Cancer Res., 5*:83.

43. Cheng, H., Zhou, R., Liu, L., Du B., and Zhou, R. (2000). Cyclic core dendrimer as a new kind of vector for gene transfer into mammalian cells. *Genetica, 108*:53.

44. Kukowska-Latallo, J. F., Bielinska, A. U., Chen, C., Rymaszewski, M., Tomalia, D. A., and Baker, J. R. Jr. (1998). Gene transfer using Starburst™ dendrimers. In *Self-Assembling Complexes for Gene Delivery: From Laboratory to Clinical Trial*. A. V. Kabanov, P. L. Felgner, and L. W. Seymour (eds.). John Wiley & Sons, Ltd., Chichester, p. 240.

45. Kukowska-Latallo, J. F., Bielinska, A. U., Johnson, J., Spindler, R., Tomalia, D. A., and Baker, J. R. Jr. (1996). Efficient transfer of genetic material into mammalian cells using Starburst polyamidoamine dendrimers. *Proc. Natl. Acad. Sci. USA, 93*:4897.

46. Bielinska, A., Kukowska-Latallo, J. F., Johnson, J., Tomalia, D. A., and Baker, J. R. Jr. (1996). Regulation of in vitro gene expression using antisense

oligonucleotides or antisense expression plasmids transfected using starburst PAMAM dendrimers. *Nucleic Acids Res., 24*:2176.

47. Tang, M. X., and Szoka, F. C. (1997). The influence of polymer structure on the interactions of cationic polymers with DNA and morphology of the resulting complexes. *Gene Ther., 4*:823.

48. Bielinska, A. U., Kukowska-Latallo, J. F., and Baker, J. R. Jr. (1997). The interaction of plasmid DNA with polyamidoamine dendrimers: mechanism of complex formation and analysis of alterations induced in nuclease sensitivity and transcriptional activity of the complexed DNA. *Biochim. Biophys. Acta, 1353*:180.

49. Harada, Y., Iwai, M., Tanaka, S., Okanoue, T., Kashima, K., Maruyama-Tabata, H., Hirai, H., Satoh, E., Imanishi, J., and Mazda, O. (2000). Highly efficient suicide gene expression in hepatocellular carcinoma cells by epstein-barr virus-based plasmid vectors combined with polyamidoamine dendrimer. *Cancer Gene Ther., 7*:27.

50. Reddy, J. A., Dean, D., Kennedy, M. D., and Low, P. S. (1999). Optimization of folate-conjugated liposomal vectors for folate receptor-mediated gene therapy. *J. Pharm. Sci., 88*:1112.

51. Barth, R. F., Adams, D. M., Soloway, A. H., Alam, F., and Darby, M. V. (1994). Boronated starburst dendrimer-monoclonal antibody immunoconjugates: evaluation as a potential delivery system for neutron capture therapy. *Bioconjug. Chem., 5*:58.

52. Yang, W., Barth, R. F., Adams, D. M., and Soloway, A. H. (1997). Intratumoral delivery of boronated epidermal growth factor for neutron capture therapy of brain tumors. *Cancer Res., 57*:4333.

53. Qin, L., Pahud, D. R., Ding, Y., Bielinska, A. U., Kukowska-Latallo, J. F., Baker, J. R. Jr., and Bromberg, J. S. (1998). Efficient transfer of genes into murine cardiac grafts by Starburst polyamidoamine dendrimers. *Human Gene Ther., 9*:553.

54. Brazeau, G. A., Attia, S., Poxon, S., and Hughes J. A. (1998). In vitro myotoxicity of selected cationic macromolecules used in non-viral gene delivery. *Pharm. Res., 15*:680.

55. de Smet, M. D., Meenken, C. J., and van den Horn, G. J. (1999). Fomivirsen—a phosphorothioate oligonucleotide for the treatment of CMV retinitis. *Ocul. Immunol. Inflamm., 7*:189.

56. Perry, C. M., and Balfour, J. A. (1999). Fomivirsen. *Drugs, 57*:375.

57. Bochot, A., Couvreur, P., and Fattal, E. Intravitreal administration of antisense oligonucleotides: potential of liposomal delivery. *Prog. Retin. Eye Res., 19*:131.

58. Yoo, H., and Juliano, R. L. (2000). Enhanced delivery of antisense oligonucleotides with fluorophore-conjugated PAMAM dendrimers. *Nucleic Acids Res., 28*:4225.

59. Helin, V., Gottikh, M., Mishal, Z., Subra, F., Malvy, C., and Lavignon, M. (1999). Uptake and intracellular distribution of oligonucleotides vectorized by a PAMAM dendrimer. *Nucleosides Nucleotides, 18*:1721.

60. Nilsen, T. W., Grayzel, J., and Prensky, W. (1997). Dendritic nucleic acid structures. *J. Theor. Biol., 187*:273.

61. Goncz, K. K., Kunzelmann, K., Xu, Z., Gruenert, D. C. (1998). Targeted replacement of normal and mutant CFTR sequences in human airway epithelial cells using DNA fragments. *Hum. Mol. Genet., 7*:1913.

62. Bielinska, A. U., Yen, A., Wu, H. L., Zahos, K. M., Sun, R., Weiner, N. D., Baker, J. R. Jr., and Roessler, B. J. (2000). Application of membrane-based dendrimer/DNA complexes for solid phase transfection in vitro and in vivo. *Biomaterials, 21*:877.

63. Kawase, M., Shiomi, T., Matsui, H., Ouji, Y., Higashiyama, S., Tsutsui, T., and Yagi, K. (2001). Suppression of apoptosis in hepatocytes by fructose-modified dendrimers. *J. Biomed. Mater. Res., 54*:519.

64. Hudde, T., Rayner, S. A., Comer, R. M., Weber, M., Isaacs, J. D., Waldmann, H., Larkin, D. F. P., and George, A. J. T. (1999). Activated polyamidoamine dendrimers, a non-viral vector for gene transfer to the corneal endothelium. *Gene Ther. 6*:939.

65. Henry, K., Cantrill, H., Fletcher, C., Chinnock, B. J., and Balfour, H. H. Jr. (1987). Use of intravitreal ganciclovir (dihydroxy propoxymethyl guanine) for cytomegalovirus retinitis in a patient with AIDS. *Am. J. Ophthalmol., 103*:17.

66. Schwartz, D. M. (1996). New therapies for cytomegalovirus retinitis. *Int. Ophthalmol. Clin., 36*:1.

67. Harris, M. L., and Mathalone, M. B. (1989). Intravitreal ganciclovir in CMV retinitis: Case report. *Br. J. Ophthalmol., 73*:382.

68. Urtti, A., Polansky, J., Lui, G. M., and Szoka, F. C. (2000). Gene delivery and expression in human retinal pigment epithelial cells: effects of synthetic carriers, serum, extracellular matrix, and viral promoters. *J. Drug. Target, 7*:413.

69. Maruyama-Tabata, H., Harada, Y., Matsumura, T., Satoh, E., Cui, F., Iwai, M., Kita, M., Hibi, S., Imanishi, J., Sawada, T., and Mazda, O. (2000). Effective suicide gene therapy in vivo by EBV-based plasmid vector coupled with polyamidoamine dendrimer. *Gene Ther., 7*:53.

70. Wilbur, D. S., Pathare, P. M., Hamlin, D. K., Buhler, K. R., and Vessella, R. L. (1998). Biotin reagents for antibody pretargeting. 3. Synthesis, radioiodination, and evaluation of biotinylated starburst dendrimers. *Bioconjug. Chem., 9*:813.

71. Kono, K., Liu, M., and Frechet, J. M. (1999). Design of dendritic macromolecules containing folate or methotrexate residues. *Bioconjug. Chem., 10*:1115.

72. Thompson, J. P., and Schengrund, C. L. (1998). Inhibition of the adherence of cholera toxin and the heat-labile enterotoxin of *Escherichia coli* to cell surface GM1 by oligosaccharide-derivatized dendrimers. *Biochem. Pharmacol., 56*:591.

73. Thompson, J. P., and Schengrund, C. L. (1997). Oligosaccharide-derivatized dendrimers: Defined multivalent inhibitors of the adherence of the cholera toxin B subunit and the heat labile enterotoxin of E. coli to GM1. *Glycoconj. J., 14*:837.

74. Fishbein, I., Chorny, M., Rabinovich, L., Banai, S., Gati, I., and Golomb, G. (2000). Nanoparticle delivery system of a tyrphostin for the treatment of restenosis. *J. Controlled Release, 65*:221.
75. Benoit, J.-P., Faisant, N., Venier-Julienne, M.-C., and Menei, P. (2000). Development of microspheres for neurological disorders: From basics to clinical applications. *J. Controlled Release, 65*:285.
76. Bousif, O., Lezoulc'h, F., Zanta, M. A., Mergny, M. D., Scherman, D., Demeneix, B., and Behr, J.-P. (1995). A versatile vector for gene and oligonucleotide transfer into cells in culture and in vivo: Polyethylenimine. *Proc. Natl. Acad. Sci. USA, 92*:7297.

16

Ocular Delivery and Therapeutics of Proteins and Peptides

Surajit Dey and Ashim K. Mitra
University of Missouri–Kansas City, Kansas City, Missouri, U.S.A.

Ramesh Krishnamoorthy
Inspire Pharmaceuticals, Durham, North Carolina, U.S.A.

I. INTRODUCTION

Recent advances in molecular biology and biotechnology have resulted in a significant increase in the number of protein and peptide drugs that have been approved for clinical use. Recent use of recombinant DNA technology has enabled us not only to produce these peptides and proteins in large quantities but also to modify these peptides for enhanced therapeutic effect. The application of peptide- and protein-based drugs in the treatment of a variety of ailments has been well documented. Table 1 lists some of the therapeutic agents and their clinical use (1). Along with a wide range of clinical and therapeutic applications, these macromolecular compounds exhibit a wide range of structures and sizes (Table 2).

The barriers associated with the delivery of peptides and proteins as therapeutic agents are primarily associated with their physicochemical and pharmacokinetic properties (size, charge, adsorption characteristics, etc.). Due to their molecular size and hydrophilicity, peptides and proteins do not cross membranes very readily. For these compounds to cross biological membranes readily, the molecular size should be small enough to undergo paracellular transport or be actively transported across the membrane. So far, most proteins have been delivered by invasive routes, such as parenteral administration. Repeated injections, particularly in the treatment of chronic ailments, deter many patients from undergoing intensive therapy. Phlebitis

Table 1 Selected Proteins and Peptides and Their Possible Therapeutic
Applications

Peptide/Protein	Indication
Growth hormone	Increasing the height of children deficient in growth hormone.
Insulin	Lowering blood glucose levels
LHRH	Inducing ovulation in women
TRH	Prolonging infertility and lactation in women
Gastrin antagonists	Reducing secretion of gastric acid
Somatostatin	Reducing bleeding of gastric ulcers
Neurotensin	Inhibiting gastric juice secretion
Nerve growth factor	Simulating nerve growth and repair
β-Endorphin	Relieving pain
Enkephalins	Pain suppressor and reducing inflammation
Cholecystokinin	Suppressing appetite
Salmon calcitonin	Osteoporosis
Bradykinin	Improving peripheral circulation
Angiotensin antagonists	Lowering blood pressure
Tissue plasminogen factors	Dissolving blood clots
Cyclosporin A	Inhibiting function of T lymphocytes
Interferon	Enhancing activity of natural killer cells
Thymopoietin	Selective T-cell–differentiating hormone
Epidermal growth factor	Wound healing
Vasoactive intestinal peptide (VIP)	Inducing relaxation of smooth muscles
Substance P	Reducing inflammation, inducing analgesia
Fibronectin	Helping in wound healing

and tissue irritation are some of the complications of parenteral delivery.
Oral delivery of peptides and proteins has been attempted in the past. The
gastrointestinal tract, which is rich in proteolytic enzymes, digests therapeutic peptides and proteins. Although oral bioavailability of most peptides and
proteins is less than 1%, a few peptides (e.g., cyclosporine) have high bioavailability when administered in a suitable vehicle. Arginine and lysine vasopressin (AVP and LVP) and the synthetic analog 1-deamino-8-D-arginine
vasopressin (DDAVP) are well absorbed following oral administration (3–
5). Numerous attempts have been made to utilize alternative noninvasive
routes for peptide and protein administration (6–10). Numerous approaches
to overcome the problems of low absorption and rapid metabolism of proteins at the site of administration have been pursued. Although buccal (11),
nasal (12–14), transdermal (15,16), tracheal (17), rectal (18), and vaginal (19)
administrations have been attempted, none so far has been found to be

Table 2 Peptide Sizes and Structural Features

Peptide	Size	Structural features
Sandostatin	8 amino acids	One-chain structure
Oxytocin	9 amino acids	Cyclic nanopeptides
Vasopressin	9 amino acids	Cyclic nanopeptides
Desmopressin	9 amino acids	Cyclic nanopeptides
Gonadorelin	10 amino acids	One-chain structure
Tetracosactide	24 amino acids	One-chain structure
Glucagon	29 amino acids	One-chain structure
Calcitonin	32 amino acids	One-chain structure
Corticotrophin	39 amino acids	One-chain structure
Insulin	51 amino acids	Two-chain structure
Aprotinin	6 kDa	Single-chain polypeptide
Interferons	15–30 kDa	Complex structure
Trypsin	24 kDa	Globular (650 amino acids)
Gonadotrophin	30 kDa	Globular ($\alpha\beta$ heterodimer)
Pepsin	35 kDa	Globular
Erythropoietin	38 kDa	Globular (native hormone composed of 165 amino acids)
Streptokinase	46 kDa	—
Urokinase	54 kDa	—
Factor IX	60 kDa	Single chain, NH_2-terminal gla-domain, two EGF domains
Albumin	67 kDa	Oblate ellipsoid (140 × 40 Å) 55% α-helix and 45% random conformation
Tissue plasminogen activator	72 kDa	5 Recurring domains
IgG	150 kDa	Light and dark chains 2 Fab and Fc portion
Factor VIII	330 kDa	One heavy chain (90–220 kDa) and one light chain (76 kDa)

Source: Adapted from Ref. 2.

completely satisfactory. Studies have been carried out to compare the transport barriers of several epithelia. The rank order of intrinsic membrane permeability has been found to be as follows: intestine $\approx$ nasal $\geq$ bronchial $\geq$ tracheal $\geq$ vaginal $\geq$ rectal $>$ corneal $>$ buccal $>$ skin (20).

The ocular route may be considered for systemic delivery of proteins and peptides. This route can be especially beneficial when delivering local therapeutic agents to the anterior segment of the eye.

Several peptides have been shown to traverse the cornea. Moreover, systemic delivery of polypeptide and protein drugs through the ocular route has several advantages:

1. The mode of delivery is convenient, i.e., eye drops.
2. Systemic absorption is extremely rapid.
3. The absorbed peptide can bypass the hepatic circulation and thus avoid first-pass metabolism.
4. The formulation can be designed to prolong drug action and/or reduce drug concentrations to achieve consistent drug action with least side effects.
5. Drug delivery can be controlled precisely.

While this route is well accepted by patients, it yields low systemic bioavailability. Size, charge, and hydrophilic nature of proteins are the primary determinants of their extent of absorption. Because the systemic delivery of peptides depends on their transport and contact time with mucous membrane of the conjunctiva and the nasolacrimal system (21), the following factors need to be considered:

1. The eye drops used must be devoid of any local irritation and/or side effects.
2. Inclusion of permeation enhancers may be necessary when dealing with agents with molecular weight larger than 1000.
3. The absolute quantity of polypeptide that can be instilled in the eye cannot exceed 2.5 mg because the eye cannot tolerate more than $25\,\mu L$ of a 10% (w/v) ophthalmic solution.

Systemic delivery of peptides via the ocular route may exert a local toxic response. This chapter will summarize the work done in this area and will review the experimental methods currently being employed.

II. MECHANISM OF PEPTIDE TRANSPORT

Protein transport across biological membranes depends on a number of physical properties, among which the size and polarity of the compound are most significant. From the changes in permeability coefficients under different experimental conditions, the major pathways of protein permeation can be hypothesized. The kinetic approach provides indirect evidence of the permeability characteristics and can be a powerful tool in deducing pathways.

Electrophysiological measurements and fluorescent confocal microscopy have been used to understand the mechanism of corneal drug permeation (22,23). The latter method provides a sensitive approach to monitoring flux across the corneal tissue and characterizing tissue damage. Confocal microscopy utilizes a laser computer system that permits visualization of a tissue specimen under light microscopy.

Insulin, polylysine, and thyrotropin-releasing hormone have been studied for their corneal permeability behavior using confocal microscopy (24). Based on the results obtained, the movement of these peptides across the cornea appears to be governed by the following factors:

1. A paracellular route is favored irrespective of the charge or size of the peptide.
2. The outermost two cell layers of the corneal epithelium offer the maximum resistance; the intercellular spaces then widen, making the transport across the corneal layer easier.
3. Charge plays an important role in the transport of the small- to medium-sized peptides. The cornea offers greater resistance to negatively charged compounds than it does to positively charged ones.

Minor inflammation of the cornea and calcium chelation may cause a widening of the intercellular spaces, thereby allowing a substantial flux of the peptide compounds. If polypeptide absorption in therapeutic amounts across the cornea is to be achieved, it will be necessary to maintain prolonged contact of the peptide with the corneal surface and also to employ a proper penetration enhancer to potentiate flux across the intercellular spaces.

III. METHODS FOR ENHANCING PEPTIDE AND PROTEIN DELIVERY

Irrespective of the noninvasive route employed to deliver the peptide and protein drugs, some inherent delivery problems must be overcome. Table 3 lists some of the general methods that can be employed to negotiate such formulation difficulties.

Physical methods for increasing absorption such as iontophoresis and phonophoresis have been examined extensively (25–28). Such methods of enhancement are quite complex and may lead to chemical and physical instability of the permeating protein (29–31). Erratic results may also be obtained due to different degrees of surface absorption.

Prolongation of the biological half-life of proteins and enhancement of their systemic bioavailability are also necessary. An attempt has been made by coadministering proteins with known enzyme inhibitors (32). The cova-

Table 3 General Methods for Enhancing Protein Delivery

---

1. By increasing absorption through:
    (a) Application of physical methods like iontophoresis or phonophoresis
    (b) Coadministration with permeation enhancers
    (c) Incorporation into liposomes or other carriers
    (d) Chemical modification of primary structure and development of prodrugs
2. By minimizing metabolism through:
    (a) Covalent attachment to a polymer
    (b) Chemical modification of the primary structure
    (c) Targeting to specific tissues
    (d) Coadministration with an enzyme inhibitor
3. By prolonging blood levels through:
    (a) Use of bioadhesives
    (b) Protection using liposomes, polymers, or other carrier

---

lent attachment of polymers has also been shown to protect a number of proteins from enzymatic hydrolysis (33–37). Thus, azopolymers may be used to deliver proteins orally whereby the system could bypass the digestive enzymes of the small intestine; however, in the flora of the colon the polymer will release the protein. In any event, the problem of low bioavailability still exists, and permeation enhancers may have to be used to overcome this obstacle.

The use of chemical permeation enhancers has been reviewed extensively relative to nasal, oral, and rectal absorption of proteins and peptides (38–41). Three major mechanisms of action are possible for these enhancers: perturbation of membrane integrity, expansion of the paracellular pathway, and increase in the thermodynamic activity of the permeating species.

The following section will briefly discuss the studies performed in other noninvasive routes of protein and peptide delivery, the findings of which may be useful in designing ocular peptide delivery systems.

A. Oral Route

The oral route, though the most convenient, is the least likely to be successful because of extensive degradation of proteins and peptides in the gut. Based on the concentration-dependent absorption of 1-desamino-8-D-arginine-vasopressin (DDAVP), Lundin and Artursson (42) suggested the process to be mediated by passive transport. Other investigators have shown that the permeability of peptides can be enhanced through prodrug modification designed to utilize the peptide transport system of the digestive tract (43–46). Coadministration of enzyme inhibitors may offer some protection in conjunction with a delivery system that can target the protein to the site of optimal absorption (38,47). The incorporation of absorption enhancers to improve the oral bioavailability of proteins has been well documented (48). Lundin et al. (49) showed that sodium taurodihydrofusidate (STDHF) enhanced both the in vitro and in vivo absorption of DDAVP. Schilling and Mitra (50) used the everted gas sac technique to evaluate the optimal site of insulin absorption. The addition of sodium glycocholate and linoleic acid enhanced insulin absorption in the duodenum and jejunum by eight- and threefold, respectively.

B. Nasal Route

The extensive network of blood capillaries underneath the nasal mucosa could provide effective systemic absorption of drugs. The nasal route is capable of providing a rapid absorption with a bioavailability relatively similar to that following subcutaneous injection. Nasal delivery of peptides and proteins has been reviewed (51,52). The polypeptides intended for delivery by this route should be readily soluble in a low mucosal irritant vehicle. It must also be absorbed in effective amounts to make this mode of administration both economical and acceptable (53). This route has been shown to be acceptable for peptides with 10 residues or less (54,55). When the number of amino acids in the peptide approaches 20 or more, satisfactory bioavailability is obtained only with a permeation enhancer (56). The nasal mucosa contains enzymes capable of hydrolyzing peptides such as leucine enkephalin. It appears that the human nasal passage contains a variety of peptidases with wide specificities. The enhancing effect of two enzyme inhibitors, amastatin and bestatin, a mucolytic agent, N-acetyl-L-cysteine, and the permeation enhancers palmitoyl-D,L-carnitine and L-α-lysophosphatidylcholine (LPC) on the nasal absorption of human growth hormone (HGH) was studied by O'Hagan et al. (57). The highest bioavailability relative to the subcutaneous injection was found with amastatin, followed by LPC and palmitoyl-D,L-carnitine. Tengammuay and Mitra (58,59) found that mixed micelles of sodium glycocholate and fatty acids were more effective in enhancing the nasal delivery of peptides than the bile salt itself. Vadnere et al. (60) found that ethylenediaminetetraacetic acid (EDTA) and α-cyclodextrin were capable of increasing the bioavailability of leuprolide when given intranasally.

C. Buccal Route

Delivery of macromolecules through the buccal membrane has also received considerable attention in recent years (61–63). Both keratinized and nonkeratinized mucosae have been used in studying the in vitro rate of penetration of drugs through the buccal tissue. In vivo absorption of peptides/ proteins from the buccal cavity is likely to be influenced by the presence of mucosal secretions and immunological reactions among other factors. Molecular size may not be the limiting factor in the buccal delivery of peptides (64). Gandhi and Robinson (65) reported that amino acid penetrate the buccal membrane by an active process, whereas peptide drugs permeate passively. The buccal cavity exhibits greater proteolytic enzyme activity than the nasal or vaginal mucosa (64). The metabolic activity is shown to reside primarily in the epithelium (67). Aungst and Rogers (8,68) studied a variety of absorption enhancers to determine their effects on buccal absorption and showed that significant changes in the morphology of this mucosal barrier take place following exposure to the absorption enhancers.

D. Pulmonary

Delivery of protein and peptide drugs via the pulmonary route has also received significant attention in recent years. The walls of the alveoli are thinner than the epithelial/mucosal membrane; the surface area of the lung is much greater and the lungs receive the entire blood supply from the heart, all of which work in favor for the absorption of protein drugs more rapidly and to a greater extent. Of course, the lungs are rich in enzymes, and overcoming this barrier is no easy task. Peptide hydrolases, peptidases, and a wide variety of proteinases are present in the lung cells (69). However, some proteinases inhibitors are also present at concentrations varying with the disease state, which might work to prevent the destruction of administered peptides (70). Liposomal delivery of peptide and protein drugs through the pulmonary route have been attempted (71). Molecular modifications have also been undertaken to explore this route of protein and peptide delivery (72).

E. Ocular Route

Lee reviewed the factors affecting corneal drug penetration (73). Rojanasakul et al. showed that polylysine permeated through epithelial surface defects via an intracellular pathway when administered to the eye, whereas insulin predominates in the surface cells of the cornea (23). They noted that there was a significant amount of aminopeptidase activity present in the ocular fluids and tissues. Figure 1 summarizes the results of the metabolism of topically applied enkephalins to the eye (74). Pretreatment with the peptidase inhibitor bestatin had a significant protease inhibitory effect, albeit in the tears only.

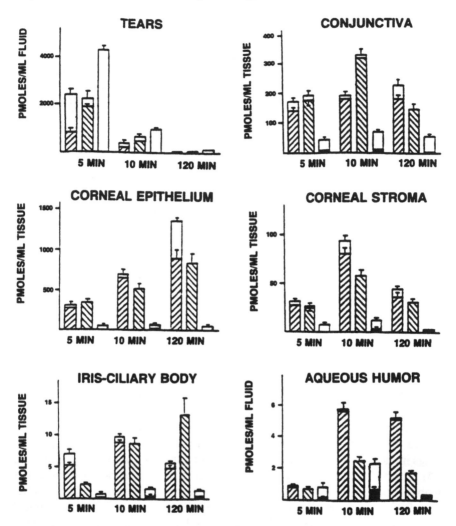

Fig. 1 Concentration of intact (open bar) and degraded (marked bar) leucine enkephalin (///), methionine enkephalin (\\\) or [D-Ala^2]Met-enkephalinamide (filled bar) recovered in each part of the rabbit eye. (From Ref. 74.)

Studies have been conducted with absorption enhancers to improve the delivery of peptides and proteins into the systemic circulation via the ocular route (75–77). Table 4 lists some penetration enhancers that have been used in the ocular delivery of peptide-like drugs. Ocular delivery of insulin to generate a therapeutic glucose-lowering response requires a penetration enhancer (78). Yamamoto et al. (79) reported that the bioavailability

Table 4   Penetration Enhancers Used to Improve Ocular Absorption

Enhancer	Effect
Azone	Threefold increase in cyclosporine absorption
Cetrimide, cytochalasin B	Increased absorption of inulin
EDTA	Threefold increase in glycerol absorption
Taurocholate, taurodeoxycholate	Increased permeation of insulin and FITC-dextran

of insulin could be improved in the following descending order by coadministration of the permeation enhancers: polyoxyethylene-9-lauryl ether > sodium deoxycholate > sodium glycocholate ~ sodium taurocholate.

IV. OCULAR DELIVERY OF PEPTIDE AND PROTEIN DRUGS

Peptides and proteins may be instilled into the eye for local/topical use. Instillation of a topical dose of a drug to the eye leads to absorption of a drug mainly through the conjunctival and corneal epithelia. For drugs meant for topical use, it must be minimally absorbed systemically as it can lead to undesirable side effects. Absorption into the systemic circulation may occur across the conjunctiva and sclera. However, for local delivery the cornea presents a significant barrier to the introcular penetration of peptide drugs in view of their high molecular weight and low lipophilicity. Lee et al. (75) reported that the penetration of inulin through the rabbit cornea was probably occurring via a paracellular route rather than a transcellular route.

Systemic absorption of peptide and protein drugs following topical administration to the eye could occur through contact with the conjunctival and nasal mucosae, the latter occurring as a result of drainage through the nasolacrimal duct. When systemic effects are desired, absorption through the conjunctival and nasal mucosae needs to be maximized. One also must consider other competing processes present in the ocular tissues. Of these processes, absorption by the avascular cornea is important, since a large portion of the drug thus absorbed is distributed to adjacent ocular tissues.

Ahmed and Patton (80) found that noncorneal (scleral) absorption accounted for about 80% absorption of inulin, a highly hydrophilic macromolecule, into the iris-ciliary body. This observation is important, since most therapeutic peptides act locally in the iris-ciliary body, which is contiguous with the sclera. Therefore, macromolecular drug absorption would benefit from scleral absorption.

Beside the transport barrier, another factor severely limiting the ocular absorption of peptide drugs is metabolism by ocular enzymes, specifically peptidases. Endopeptidases, like plasmin and collagenase, and exopeptidases, like aminopeptidases, are present in the ocular fluids and tissues. The endopeptidase levels are usually low unless the eye is inflamed (81,82) or injured (83) and are of little concern relative to the stability of topically applied doses. Lee et al. (74) reported that within 5 minutes postinstillation, about 90% of leucine enkephalin and almost 100% of methionine enkephalin (pentapeptides) was recovered in the rabbit corneal epithelium in a hydrolyzed form. Therefore, aminopeptidase activity must be inhibited to facilitate ocular peptide absorption. Controlling these enzymes in the target tissues may not be practical given the fact that the same enzymes might be necessary for the homeostasis in the eye.

Cyclosporin A has been shown to improve the prognosis for corneal allograft rejection. It was found that when administered by nonocular routes in rabbits, it was detected in the systemic circulation but not in the ocular tissues (20,84,85). Also, topical administration of cyclosporin A did not produce any significant penetration within the eye beyond the cornea or the conjunctiva. This may be because cyclosporin A was bound to corneal and conjunctival epithelial cell membranes. Cyclosporin A eyedrops formulated in absolute ethanol did produce higher levels in intraocular tissues, which may be due to damage to corneal epithelium by alcohol.

Growth factors, especially epidermal growth factor (EGF), have been found to stimulate cell proliferation in the corneal epithelium, thus stimulating epithelialization during wound healing. Growth factors are mostly used in accelerating the wound-healing process, and it would be of great importance in corneal wounds since the cornea is an avascular organ. Many in vitro corneal preparations have been used to demonstrate the wound-healing process. Human EGF promotes endothelial wound healing (84). Many other growth factors also play a major role in corneal wound healing, including transforming growth factor β (TGF-β) (87) and platelet-derived growth factor (PDGF). Basic fibroblast growth factor (bFGF) and insulin-like growth factor I (IGF-I) have been found in higher levels in patients suffering from diabetic retinopathy (88–90). IGF-I and bFGF can also induce fibrovascular changes in the retinal vessels.

A more practical strategy for circumventing the enzymatic barrier would be to administer peptide analogs that are resistant to the principal peptidases but possess equivalent biological activity [D-Ala^2]methionine enkephalinamide (DAMEA), which resists aminopeptidase-mediated cleavage, falls in this category of peptide analogs (74). The permeation and metabolic degradation of DAMEA in the albino rabbit cornea, conjunctiva, and sclera has been studied (91). DAMEA was administered with and without peptidase inhibitors bestatin (aminopeptidase inhibitor) and SCH 39370 (enkephalinase inhibitor). It was found that sclera was the most permeable membrane to DAMEA, while cornea was almost impermeable to DAMEA. Without inhibitors, the permeability coefficients of DAMEA were 2.7×10^{-8} cm/s, 3.1×10^{-6} cm/s, and 12.5×10^{-6} cm/s across the cornea, conjunctiva, and sclera, respectively. When inhibitors were co-administered with DAMEA, the corneal permeability of intact DAMEA increased 15 times, conjunctival permeability increased 5.5 times, while scleral permeability remained practically unaltered.

The corneal and conjunctival penetration of 4-phenylazobenzyloxy-carbonyl-L-Pro-L-Leu-Gly-L-Pro-D-Arg (Pz-peptide) and its effect on the corneal and conjunctival penetration of hydrophilic solutes as well as on the ocular and systemic absorption of topically applied atenolol and propranolol in the rabbit have been evaluated (92). The conjunctiva was 29 times more permeable than the cornea to 3 mM Pz-peptide. Conjunctival Pz-peptide transport was 1.7 times greater in the mucosal-to-serosal than in the opposite direction, whereas corneal Pz-peptide transport showed no directionality. The apparent permeability coefficients of Pz-peptide across the cornea and the conjunctiva increased over the 1–5 mM range, which suggests that Pz-peptide enhanced its own transport across both epithelial tissues. The cornea was more sensitive than the conjunctiva to the penetration-enhancement effect of Pz-peptide. Pz-peptide elevated the corneal transport of mannitol, fluorescein, and FD4 by 50, 57, and 106%, respectively, but it did not affect the conjunctival transport of mannitol and fluorescein. While Pz-peptide enhanced the ocular absorption of topically applied hydrophilic atenolol, it did not affect the ocular absorption of lipophilic propranolol. Interestingly, Pz-peptide did not affect the systemic absorption of either β-adrenergic antagonist. Pz-peptide appeared to facilitate its own penetration across the cornea and the conjunctiva and increase the ocular absorption of topically applied hydrophilic but not lipophilic drugs, while not affecting the systemic absorption of either type of drug.

In addition, the presence of sites beyond the absorbing epithelia that are capable of degrading peptides and protein and the availability of multiple peptidases in a given site further decrease the absorption potential of such compounds. While the ocular route has been widely accepted for the use of topical application, its use in systemic delivery of peptides and proteins will be rather limited.

V. SYSTEMIC ADMINISTRATION OF PEPTIDES AND PROTEINS THROUGH THE OCULAR ROUTE

Systemic absorption of polypeptides and proteins primarily occur through contact with the conjunctival and nasal mucosae. Table 5 lists some of the peptides that could be administered through the ocular route (93). Almost all the studies involving the absorption of peptides and proteins in animal models have been carried out using labeled peptide samples (94–96). Apart from monitoring the blood concentrations for pharmacokinetic evaluation, pharmacodynamic studies have also been extensively pursued. Some of the biological response parameters include reduction in blood sugar by insulin, increase in blood glucose by glucagon, analgesic effects by enkephalins, and increase in blood pressure by vasopressin.

Systemic peptide availability following ocular administration has been related to biological response. The study by Christie and Hanzal (97) showed that insulin instilled into the conjunctiva is absorbed rapidly, giving rise to a fairly constant and consistent lowering of blood sugar levels in rabbits. Another study with somatostatin and its analog revealed that there was an attenuation of the miotic response to noiceptive stimuli by these agents, whereas intracameral injection of 1–50 mg met-enkephalin had no effect on the miotic response (98).

Lee et al. (99) found that enkephalinamide and inulin are absorbed into the blood stream following topical ocular administration, the former to a greater extent than the latter. The authors proposed that depending on the

Table 5 Therapeutically Useful Peptides that Could Be Administered Through the Ocular Route

Peptide	Application
ACTH	Antiallergic, decongestant anti-inflammatory
β-Endorphin	Analgesic
Calcitonin	Paget's disease, hypercalcemia
Glucagon	Hypoglycemic crisis
Insulin	Diabetes mellitus
Leu-enkephalin	Analgesic
Met-enkephalin	Immunostimulant
Oxytocin	Induce uterine contractions
Somatostatin	Attenuate miotic responses
TRH	Diagnosis of thyroid cancer
Vasopressin	Diabetes insipidus
VIP	Secretion of insulin

molecular size, lipophilicity, and susceptibility to proteolysis, other peptides and proteins may also be absorbed to varying extents. Similarly, Chiou and Chuang (94) demonstrated the feasibility of effective systemic delivery of topically instilled peptides in the eye. Their findings suggest that systemic delivery of peptide drugs is superior to the parenteral route, especially when the drug is potent and doses required are low. Enkephalin could effectively be absorbed systemically through the eye with the use of an absorption enhancer (95). This ocular route was found to be superior to administering the peptide by an intravenous route. Similar results have been obtained with other peptides like thyrotropin-releasing hormone (TRH), luteinizing hormone–releasing hormone (LHRH), glucagon, and insulin (94). Spantide, a tachykinin antagonist, is readily taken up into the rabbit eye following topical application. Measurable concentrations of the peptide were observed in the aqueous humor as well as in the general circulation. Similarly, insulin could be absorbed effectively into the systemic circulation through ocular instillation (100). The systemic absorption of 1% insulin through the eyes can be enhanced at least sevenfold when 1% saponin, a surfactant, was added to the solution. This absorption enhancement was not affected by aminopeptidase inhibition. Recently, calcitonin, a polypeptide hormone, was found to be poorly absorbed into the systemic circulation through the ocular rote (101). Inclusion of permeation enhancers like Brij-78 and BL-9 markedly improved its systemic absorption.

In summary, small polypeptides such as TRH (MW 300), enkephalins (MW $\sim$ 600), LHRH (MW 1200), and glucagon (MW 3500) are absorbed to a significant extent through the eyes, almost to the extent of 99% (94). Polypeptides with larger molecular weight such as β-endorphin (MW $\sim$ 5000) and insulin (MW $\sim$ 6000) are also absorbed, but to a much lesser extent. The absorption of such large molecular weight compounds can, however, be improved by simultaneous use of absorption enhancers (78).

VI. ENHANCED SYSTEMIC ABSORPTION WITH PERMEATION ENHANCERS

One of the major problems associated with the ocular delivery of peptide drugs is their poor systemic bioavailability. This may be overcome by using penetration enhancers. Most permeation enhancers need to be evaluated with caution, since most of these agents cause local irritation to the eye. Among them the most effective are Brij-78 and BL-9, because these compounds have been shown to enhance insulin absorption to a significant extent without causing any noticeable irritation (78). Table 6 lists the pene-

Table 6 Effects of Various Permeation Enhancers on Systemic Absorption of Insulin Following Ocular Administration

Permeation enhancer	Concentration of enhancer (%)	Insulin absorption enhanced ($\times$)
Saponin	0.5	4.0
	1.0	7.0
Fusidic acid	0.25	2.3
	0.5	2.7
	1.0	3.9
	2.0	7.5
Polyethylene-9-laurylether (BL-9)	0.25	2.6
	0.5	4.5
	1.0	6.0
	2.0	7.6
Polyethylene-20-stearylether (Brij 78)	0.5	6.8
	1.0	6.3
Polyethylene-20-oleorylether (Brij 99)	0.5	4.0

tration enhancers that have been examined for enhancing insulin absorption by the ocular route and their relative performance (93). Saponin, fusidic acid, and Brij-99 possess high irritation potential and therefore cannot be used. As indicated earlier, the same surfactants are also capable of enhancing the absorption of calcitonin (101).

The permeability barrier of the corner to hydrophilic molecules is presumed to reside in the epithelial layer. The presence of tight junctions render the epithelium almost impermeable to all but the smallest molecules. Grass and Robinson have shown that the aqueous channel of the cornea has a cut-off of around 90 D (102). Other studies have suggested a close relationship between epithelial permeability (or tight junction integrity) and the cell cytoskeleton (103,104). Treatment with cytochalasins or removal of extracellular calcium ions cause opening of tight junctions and increase tight junction permeability (105,106). Cytoskeletal modulators have been explored as corneal penetration enhancers (107,108). The efficacy of EDTA, bile salts, and cytochalasin B (109) in enhancing the ocular permeability of hydrophilic compounds has been examined. Cytochalasin B has the ability to increase corneal permeability with minimum membrane damage, indicating its potential as an ocular penetration enhancer. Further development of novel penetration enhancers with highly specific foci of action, good reversibility, and minimal toxicity is needed for any realistic delivery of peptides and proteins by the ocular route.

VII. CONCLUSIONS

With breakthroughs in biotechnology, newer and more potent peptide and protein drugs are emerging in the market. The majority of these polypeptides require special delivery systems. However, since most of these compounds are very potent, require low doses, and are well absorbed from the mucous membrane, their delivery via the ocular route may be viable. However, one of the principal problems in the ocular delivery of peptide and protein drugs is that of relatively low bioavailability to the ocular tissues. This problem may be circumvented by the use of penetration enhancers. The conjunctival administration of this class of compounds to achieve therapeutic levels in the systemic circulation may well be possible in the near future. We hope that novel drug delivery systems will be developed to deliver potent polypeptide drugs through the ocular route.

REFERENCES

1. Lee, V. H. L. (1987). Ophthalmic delivery of peptides and proteins, *Pharm. Tech.*, *11*:26.
2. Bristow, A. F. (1991).
3. Akerlund, M., Stromberg, P., Forsling, M. L., Melin, P., and Vilhardt, H. (1983). Inhibition of vasopressin effects on the uterus by a synthetic analogue, *Obstet. Gynecol.*, *62*:309.
4. Akerlund, M., Kostrzewska, A., Laudanski, T., Melin, P., and Vilhardt, H. (1983). Vasopressin effects on isolated non-pregnant myometrium and uterine arteries and their inhibition by deamino-ethyl-lysine-vasopressin and deamino-ethyl-oxytocin, *Br. J. Obstet. Gynaecol.*, *90*:732.
5. Vilhardt, H., and Bie, P. (1983). Antidiuretic response in conscious dogs following peroral administration of arginine vasopressin and its analogues, *Eur. J. Pharmacol.*, *93*:201.
6. Tobey, N., Heizer, W., Yeh, R., Huang, T. I., and Hoffner, C. (1985). Human intestinal brush border peptidases, *Gastroenterology*, *88*:913.
7. Ziv, E., Lior, O., and Kidron, M. (1987). Absorption of protein via the intestinal wall, *Biochem. Pharmacol.*, *36*:1035.
8. Aungst, B. J., Rogers, N. J., and Shefter, E. (1988). Comparison of nasal, rectal, buccal, sublingual and intramuscular insulin efficacy and the effects of bile salt absorption promoter, *J. Pharmacol. Exp. Ther.*, *244*:23.
9. Aungst, B. J., and Rogers, N. J. (1988). Site dependence of absorption promoting actions of laureth-9, Na salicylate, Na_2EDTA, and apoprotinin on rectal, nasal and buccal insulin delivery, *Pharm. Res.*, *5*:305.
10. Moore, J. A., Pletcher, S. A., and Ross, M. J. (1986). Absorption enhancement of growth hormone from the gastrointestinal tract of rats, *Int. J. Pharm.*, *34*:35.

11. Anders, R., Merkle, H. P., Schurr, W., and Ziegler, R. (1983). Buccal absorption of protirelin: An effective way to stimulate thyrotropin and prolactin, *J. Pharm. Sci.*, *72*:1481.

12. Salzman, R., Manson, J. E., Griffing, G. T., Kimmerle, R., and Ruderman, N. (1985). Intranasal aerosolized insulin: Mixed meal studies and long term use in Type I diabetes, *N. Engl. J. Med.*, *312*:1078.

13. Moses, A. C., Gordon, G. S., Carey, M. C., and Flier, J. S. (1983). Insulin administration intranasally as an insulin-bile salt aerosol, effectiveness and reproducibility in normal and diabetic subjects, *Diabetes*, *32*:1040.

14. Hirai, S., Ikenaga, T., and Matsuwaza, T. (1978). Nasal absorption of insulin in dogs, *Diabetes*, *27*:296.

15. Siddiqui, O., Sun, Y., Liu, J. C., and Chien, Y. W. (1987). Facilitated transdermal transport of insulin, *J. Pharm. Sci.*, *76*:341.

16. Kari, B. (1986). Control of blood glucose levels in alloxan-diabetic rabbits by iontophoresis of insulin, *Diabetes*, *35*:217.

17. Wigley, F. M., Londono, J.H., Wood, S. H., and Shipp, J. C. (1971). Insulin across respiratory mucosae by aerosol delivery, *Diabetes*, *20*:522.

18. Yamasaki, Y., Shichiri, M., Kawamori, R., Kikuchi, M., and Yagi, T. (1981). The effectiveness of rectal administration of insulin suppository on normal and diabetic subjects, *Diabetes Care*, *4*:454.

19. Fisher, N. F. (1923). The absorption of insulin from the intestine, vagina and scrotal sac, *Am. J. Physiol*, *67*:65.

20. BenEzra, D., Maftzir, G., de Courten, C., and Timonen, P. (1990). Ocular penetration of cyclosporin A. III: The human eye, *Br. J. Ophthalmol.*, *74*:350.

21. Fraunfelder, F. T., and Meyers, S. M. (1987). Systemic side effects from ophthalmic timolol and their prevention, *J. Ocul. Pharmacol.*, *3*:177.

22. Robinson, J. R. (1989). Ocular drug delivery. Mechanism(s) of corneal drug transport and mucoadhesive systems, *S.T.P. Pharma.*, *5*:839.

23. Rojanasakul, Y., Paddock, S. W., and Robinson, J. R. (1990). Confocal laser scanning microscopic examination of transport pathways and barriers of some peptides across the cornea, *Int. J. Pharm.*, *61*:163.

24. Harris, D., and Robinson, J. R. (1990). Bioadhesive polymers in peptide drug delivery, *Biomaterials*, *11*:652.

25. Green, P., Hinz, R., Cullander, C., Yamane, G., and Guy, R. H. (1989). Iontophoretic delivery of amino acids and analogs, *Pharm. Res.*, *6*:S148.

26. Miller, L., Kolaskie, C. J., Smith, G. A., and Riviere, J. (1990). Transdermal iontophoresis of gonadotrophin releasing hormone (LHRH) and two analogues, *J. Pharm. Sci.*, *79*:490.

27. Sun, Y., Xue, H., and Liu, J. C. (1990). A unique iontophoresis system designed for transdermal protein drug delivery, *Pharm. Res.*, *7*:S113.

28. Chien, Y. W., Lelawong, P., Siddiqui, O., Sun, Y., and Shi, W. M. (1990). Facilitated transdermal delivery of therapeutic peptides and proteins by iontophoretic delivery devices, *J. Controlled Rel.*, *7*:1.

29. Dill, K. A. (1990). Dominant forces in protein folding, *Biochemistry*, *29*:7133.

30. Creighton, T. E. (1990). Protein folding, *Biochem. J.*, *270*:1.

31. Horbett, T. A., and Brash, J. L. (1987). Proteins at interfaces: Current issues and future prospects. In: *Proteins at Interfaces: Physicochemical and Biochemical Studies.* T. A. Horbett and J. L. Brash, (eds.). American Chemical Society, Washington, DC, Chap. 1.

32. Okumura, K., Kiyohara, Y., Komade, F., Mishima, Y., and Fuwa, T. (1990). Protease inhibitor potentiates the healing effect of epidermal growth factor in wounded or burned skin, *J. Controlled Rel., 13*:310.

33. Katre, N. V., Knauf, M. J., and Laird, W. J. (1987). Chemical modification of recombinant interleukin 2 by polyethylene glycol increase its potency in the murine Meth A sarcoma model, *Proc. Natl. Acad. Sci. USA, 84*:1487.

34. Yoshihiro, I., Casolaro, M., Kono, K., and Imanishi, Y. (1989). An insulin releasing system that is responsible to glucose, *J. Controlled Rel., 10*:195.

35. Hori, T., Komada, F., Iwakawa, S., Seino, Y., and Okumura, K. (1989). Enhanced bioavailability of subcutaneously injected insulin coadministered with collagen in rats and humans, *Pharm. Res., 6*:813.

36. Fuertges, F., and Abuchowski, A. (1990). The clinical efficacy of poly(ethylene glycol)-modified proteins. *J. Controlled Rel., 11*:139.

37. Saffran, M., Kumar, G. S., Neckers, D. C., Pena, J., Jones, R. H., and Field, J. (1990). Biodegradable copolymer coating for oral delivery of peptide drugs, *Biochem. Soc. Trans., 18*:752.

38. Lee, V. H. L. (1990). Protease inhibitors and penetration enhancers as approaches to modify peptide absorption, *J. Controlled Rel., 13*:213.

39. Lee, V. H. L., and Yamamoto, A. (1990). Penetration and enzymatic barriers to peptide and protein absorption, *Adv. Drug. Deliv. Rev., 4*:171.

40. De Boer, A. G., Van Hoogdalem, E. J., Heijligers-Feigen, C. D., Verhoef, J. C., and Breimer, D. D. (1990). Rectal absorption enhancement of peptide drugs, *J. Controlled Rel., 13*:241.

41. Pontiroli, A. E. (1990). Intranasal administration of calcitonin and of other peptides: Studies with different promoters, *J. Controlled Rel., 13*:247.

42. Lundin, S., and Atursson, P. (1990). Absorption of vasopressin analogue, 1-desamino-8-D-arginine-vasopressin (dDAVP), in human intestinal epithelial cell line, CaCO-2, *Int. J. Pharm., 64*:181.

43. Amidon, G. L., Sinko, P. J., Hu, M., and Leesman, G. D. (1989). Absorption of difficult drug molecules: Carrier mediated transport of peptides and peptide analogues. In: *Novel Drug Delivery and Therapeutic Application.* L. F. Presscot and W. S. Ninmo (eds.). Wiley, New York, Chap. 5.

44. Sinko, P. J., Hu, M., and Amidon, G. L. (1987). Carrier mediated transport of amino acids, small peptides and their drug analogs, *J. Controlled Ref., 6*:115.

45. Hu, M., Subramaniam, P., Mosberg, H. I., and Amidon, G. L. (1989). Use of the peptide carrier system to improve the intestinal absorption of L-α-methyl-dopa: Carrier kinetics, intestinal permeabilities and in vitro hydrolysis of dipeptidyl derivatives of L-α-methyldopa, *Pharma. Res., 6*:66.

46. Friedman, D. I., and Amidon, G. L. (1990). Characterization of the intestinal transport parameters for small peptide drugs, *J. Controlled Rel., 13*:141.

47. Ungell, A., and Andreasson, A. (1990). The effect of enzymatic inhibition versus increased paracellular transport of vasopressin peptides, *J. Controlled Rel., 13*:313.

48. Drewe, J., Vonderscher, J., Hornung, K., Munzer, J., Reinhardt, J., Kissel, T., and Beglinger, C. (1990). Enhancement of oral absorption of somatostatin analog Sandostatin in man. *J. Controlled Rel., 13*:315.

49. Lundin, S., Pantzar, N., Hedin, I., and Westron, B. R. (1990). Intestinal absorption by sodium taurodihydrofusidate of a peptide hormone analogue (dDAVP) and a macromolecule (BSA) in vitro and in vivo, *Int. J. Pharm., 59*:263.

50. Schilling, R. J., and Mitra, A. K. (1990). Intestinal mucosal transport of insulin, *Int. J. Pharm., 62*:53.

51. Su, K. S. E. (1991). Nasal route delivery of peptide and protein drug delivery. In: *Peptide and Protein Drug Delivery*. V. H. L. Lee (ed.). Marcel Dekker, New York, Chap. 13.

52. Harris, A. S. (1986). Biopharmaceutical aspects of the intranasal administration of peptides. In: *Delivery Systems for Peptide Drugs*. S. S. David, I. Illum, and E. Tomlinson (eds.). Plenum Press, New York, p. 191.

53. Sandow, J., and Petri, W. (1985). Intranasal administration of peptides, biological activity and therapeutic efficacy. In: *Transnasal Systemic Medications*. Y. W. Chien (ed.). Elsevier, New York, Chap. 7.

54. Solbach, H. G., and Wiegelmann, W. (1973). Intranasal application of luteinizing hormone releasing hormone, *Lancet, 1*:1259.

55. Dashe, A. M., Kleeman, C. R., Czarczkes, J. W., Rubinoff, H., and Spears, I. (1964). Synthetic vasopressin nasal spray in the treatment of diabetes insipidus. *JAMA, 190*:113.

56. Flier, J. S., Moses, A. C., Gordon, G. S., and Silver, R. S. (1985). Intranasal administration of insulin efficacy and mechanism. In: *Transnasal Systemic Medications*. Y. W. Chien (ed.). Elsevier, New York, Chap. 9.

57. O'Hagan, D. T., Critchley, H., Farraj, N. F., Fisher, A. N., Hohansen, B. R., David, S. S., and Illum, L. (1990). Nasal absorption enhancers for synthetic human growth hormone in rats, *Pharm. Res., 7*:772.

58. Tengamnuay, P., and Mitra, A. K. (1990). Bile salt-fatty acid mixed micelles as nasal absorption promoters of peptides. I. Effects of ionic strength, adjuvant composition and lipid structure on the nasal absorption of [D-Arg^2]kyotrophin, *Pharm. Res., 7*:127.

59. Tengamnuay, P., and Mitra, A. K. (1990). Bile salt-fatty acid mixed micelles as nasal absorption promoters of peptides. II. In vivo nasal absorption of insulin in rats and effects of mixed micelles on the morphological integrity of the nasal mucosa, *Pharm. Res., 7*:370.

60. Vadnere, M., Adjei, A., Doyle, R., and Johnson, E. (1990). Evaluation of alternative routes for delivery of leuprolide, *J. Controlled Rel., 13*:322.

61. Merkle, H. P., Anders, R., Sandow, J., and Schurr, W. (1985). Self adhesive patches for buccal delivery of peptides, *Proc. Int. Symp. Controlled Rel. Bioact. Mater., 12*:85.

62. Squier, C. A., and Hall, B. K. (1985). The permeability of skin and oral mucosa to water and horseradish peroxidase as related to the thickness of the permeability barrier, *J. Invest. Dermatol., 84*:176.

63. Yokosuka, T., Omori, Y., Hirata, Y., and Hirai, S. (1977). Nasal and sublingual administration of insulin in man, *J. Jpn. Diabetic Soc., 20*:146.

64. Tolo, K., and Jonsen, J. (1975). In vitro penetration of tritiated dextrans through rabbit oral mucosa, *Arch. Oral Biol., 20*:419.

65. Gandhi, R. B., and Robinson, J. R. (1990). Mechanism of transport of charged compounds across rabbit buccal mucosa, *Pharm. Res., 7*:S116.

66. Dodda-Kashi, S., and Lee, V. H. L. (1986). Enkephalin hydrolysis in homogenates of various absorptive mucosae of the albino rabbit: Similarities in rate and involvement of aminopeptidases, *Life Sci., 38*:2019.

67. Garren, K. W., and Repta, A. J. (1988). Buccal absorption. III. Simultaneous diffusion and metabolism of an aminopeptidase substrate in the hamster cheek pouch, *Pharm. Res., 6*:966.

68. Aungst, B. J., and Rogers, N. J. (1989). Comparison of the effects of various transmucosal absorption promoters on buccal insulin delivery, *Int. J. Pharm., 53*:277.

69. Crooks, P. (1990). Lung peptidases and their activities. Presented at Respiratory Drug Delivery II, Keystone, Colorado.

70. Schankar, L. S., Mitchel, E. W., and Brown, R. A. (1986). Species comparison of drug absorption from the lung after aerosol inhalation or intratracheal injection, *Drug Metab. Dispos., 14*:79.

71. Maruyama, K., Homberg, E., Kennel, S. J., Klibanov, A., Forchlin, V. P., and Huang, L. (1990). Characterization of in vivo immunoliposome targeting to pulmonary endothelium, *J. Pharm. Sci., 79*:978.

72. O'Donnell, M. (1990). Novel approaches to the development of peptide bronchodilator drugs. Presented at Respiratory Drug Delivery II, Keystone, Colorado.

73. Lee, V. H. L. (1990). Mechanisms and facilitations of corneal drug penetration, *J. Controlled Rel., 11*:79.

74. Lee, V. H. L., Carson, L. W., Dodda-Kashi, S., and Stratford, R. E. (1986). Metabolic permeation barriers to the ocular absorption of topically applied enkephalins in albino rabbits, *J. Ocul. Physiol., 2*:345.

75. Lee, V. H. L., Carson, L. W., and Takemoto, K. A. (1986). Macromolecular drug absorption in the albino rabbit eye, *Int. J. Pharm., 29*:43.

76. Newton, C., Gebhardt, B. M., and Kaufman, H. E. (1988). Topically applied cyclosporine in zone prolongs corneal allograft survival, *Invest. Ophthalmol. Vis. Sci., 29*:208.

77. Morimoto, K., Nakai, T., and Morisaka, K. (1987). Evaluation of permeability enhancement of hydrophilic compounds and macromolecular compounds by bile salts through rabbit corneas in vitro, *J. Pharm. Pharmacol., 39*:124.

78. Chiou, G. C., and Ching, Y. C. (1989). Improvement of systemic absorption of insulin through the eyes with absorption enhancers, *J. Pharm. Sci., 78*:815.

79. Yamamoto, A., Luo, A. M., Dodda-Kashi, S., and Lee, V. H. L. (1989). The ocular route for the systemic insulin delivery in the albino rabbit, *J. Pharm. Exp. Ther., 249*:249.

80. Ahmed, I., and Patton, T. F. (1985). Importance of the noncorneal absorption route in topical ophthalmic drug delivery, *Invest. Ophthalmol. Vis. Sci., 26*:584.

81. Pandolfi, M., Astedt, B., and Dyster-Aas, K. (1972). Release of fibrinolytic enzymes from the human cornea, *Acta. Ophthalmol., 50*:199.

82. Berman, M., Manseau, E., Law, M., and Aiken, D. (1983). Ulceration is correlated with degradation of fibrin and fibronectin at the corneal surface, *Invest. Ophthalmol. Vis. Sci., 24*:1358.

83. Hayasaka, S., and Hayasaka, I. (1979). Cathepsin B and collagenolytic cathepsin in the aqueous humor of patients with Bechet's disease, *Albrecht v. Graefes Arch. Klin. Exp. Ophthal., 206*:103.

84. BenEzra, D., and Maftzir, G. (1990). Ocular penetration of cyclosporin A. The rabbit eye, *Invest. Ophthalmol. Vis. Sci., 31*:1362.

85. BenEzra, D., and Maftzir, G. (1990). Ocular penetration of cyclosporine A in the rat eye, *Arch. Ophthalmol., 108*:584.

86. Hoppenreijs, V. P., Pels, E., Vrensen, G. F., Oosting, J., and Treffers, W. F. (1992). Effects of human epidermal growth factor on endothelial wound healing of human corneas, *Invest. Ophthalmol. Vis. Sci., 33*:1946.

87. Pasquale, L. R., Dorman-Pease, M. E., Lutty, G. A., Quigley, H. A., and Jampel, H. D. (1993). Immunolocalization of TGF-beta 1, TGF-beta 2, and TGF-beta 3 in the anterior segment of the human eye, *Invest. Ophthalmol. Vis. Sci., 34*:23.

88. Grant, M. B., Caballero, S., and Millard, W. J. (1993). Inhibition of IGF-I and b-FGF stimulated growth of human retinal endothelial cells by the somatostatin analogue, octreotide: a potential treatment for ocular neovascularization, *Regul. Pept., 48*:267.

89. Grant, M. B., Mames, R. N., Fitzgerald, C., Ellis, E. A., Caballero, S., Chegini, N., and Guy, J. (1993). Insulin-like growth factor I as an angiogenic agent. In vivo and in vitro studies, *Ann. NY Acad. Sci., 692*:230.

90. Grant, M. B., Mames, R. N., Fitzgerald, C., Ellis, E. A., Aboufriekha, M., and Guy, J. (1993). Insulin-like growth factor I acts as an angiogenic agent in rabbit cornea and retina: Comparative studies with basic fibroblast growth factor, *Diabetologia, 36*:282.

91. Hamalainen, K. M., Ranta, V. P., Auriola, S., and Urtti, A. (2000). Enzymatic and permeation barrier of [D-Ala(2)]-Met-enkephalinamide in the anterior membranes of the albino rabbit eye, *Eur. J. Pharm. Sci., 9*:265.

92. Chung, Y. B., Han, K., Nishiura, A., and Lee, V. H. (1998). Ocular absorption of Pz-peptide and its effect on the ocular and systemic pharmacokinetics of topically applied drugs in the rabbit, *Pharm. Res., 15*:1882.

93. Chiou, G. C. (1991). Systemic delivery of polypeptide drugs through ocular route, *Ann. Rev. Pharmacol. Toxicol., 31*:457.

94. Chiou, G. C., and Chuang, C. Y. (1988). Systemic delivery of polypeptides with molecular weights between 300 and 3500 through the eye, *J. Ocul. Pharmacol., 4*:165.

95. Chiou, G. C., Chuang, C. Y., and Chang, M. S. (1988). Systemic delivery of enkephalin peptide through eyes, *Life Sci., 43*:509.

96. Chiou, G. C., and Chuang, C. Y. (1988). Treatment of hypoglycemia with glucagon eye drops, *J. Ocul. Pharmacol., 4*:179.

97. Christie, C. D., and Hanzal, R. F. (1931). Insulin absorptin by the conjunctival membranes in rabbits, *J. Clin. Invest., 10*:787.

98. Stjernschantz, J., Sears, M. L., and Oksala, O. (1985). Effects of somatostatin, a somatostatin analog, neurotensin, and metenkephalin in the eye with special reference to the irritative response, *J. Ocul. Pharmacol., 1*:59.

99. Lee, V. H. L., Carson, L. W., Dodda-Kashi, S. D., and Stratford, R. E. Jr. (1988). Systemic absorption of ocularly administered enkephalinamide and inulin in the albino rabbit: Extent, pathways and vehicle effects, *J. Pharm. Sci., 77*:838.

100. Chiou, G. C., Chuang, C. Y., and Chang, M. S. (1989). Systemic delivery of insulin through eyes to lower the glucose concentration, *J. Ocul. Pharmacol., 5*:81.

101. Li, B. H. P., and Chiou, G. C. Y. (1992). Systemic administration of calcitonin through ocular route, *Life Sci., 50*:349.

102. Grass, G. M., and Robinson, J. R. (1988). Mechanisms of corneal drug penetration I: In vivo and in vitro kinetics, *J. Pharm. Sci. 77*:3.

103. Meza, I., Ibarra, G., Sabanero, M., and Cereijido, M. (1980). Occluding junctions and cytoskeletal components in cultures transporting epithelium, *J. Cell Biol., 87*:746.

104. Madara, J. L., Barenberg, D., and Carlson, S. (1986). Effects of cytochalasin D on occluding junctions of intestinal absorptive cells. Further evidence that the cytoskeleton may influence paracellular permeability and junctional charge selectivity, *J. Cell Biol., 102*:2125.

105. Bentzel, C. J., Hainau, B., Ho, S., Hui, S. W., Edelman, A., Anagnostopoulos, T., and Benedetti, E. L. (1980). Cytoplasmin regulation of tight junction permeability: effect of plant cytokinins, *Am. J. Physiol., 239*:C75.

106. Martinez-Palomo, A., Meza, I., Beaty, G., and Cereijido, M. (1980). Experimental modulation of occluding junctions in a cultured epithelium, *J. Cell Biol., 87*:736.

107. Aldridge, D. C., Armstrong, J. J., Speake, R. N., and Turner, W. B. (1967). The cytochalasins, a new class of biologically active mold metabolites, *Chem. Commun., 1*:26.

108. Rothweiler, W., and Tamm, C. (1966). Isolation and structure of phomin, *Experientia, 22*:750.

109. Binder, M., and Tamm, C. (1973). The cytochalasins: A new class of biologically active microbial metabolites, *Agnew. Chem. Int. Edit., 12*:370.

17
Retinal Disease Models for Development of Drug and Gene Therapies

Leena Pitkänen
University of Kuopio and Kuopio University Hospital, Kuopio, Finland

Lotta Salminen
University of Tampere and Tampere University Hospital, Tampere, Finland

Arto Urtti
University of Kuopio, Kuopio, Finland

I. INTRODUCTION

In humans the retina is the innermost layer of the eye, which consists of retinal pigment epithelium (RPE) and neural retina. The neural retina has several layers and various cell types, which are illustrated in Figure 1. RPE is a single layer of hexagonal cells that maintains the homeostasis of neural retina. It has essential biochemical, physiological, physical, and optical functions in maintaining the visual system, including phagocytosis of rod outer segments, transport of substances between photoreceptors and choriocapillaries, and uptake and conversion of the retinoids, which are needed in visual cycle. Together with endothelial cell linings of retinal capillaries, RPE forms the blood-retinal barrier. The neural retina is a complicated and delicate multilayer. The thickness of neural retina varies from 0.4 mm near the optic nerve to about 0.1 mm anteriorly at the ora serrata. The photoreceptors are the light-sensing part of retina. The electric impulses are amplified and integrated by bipolar, horizontal, amacrine, and ganglion cells. The principal glial cell of the retina is the Müller cell. The bipolar cells

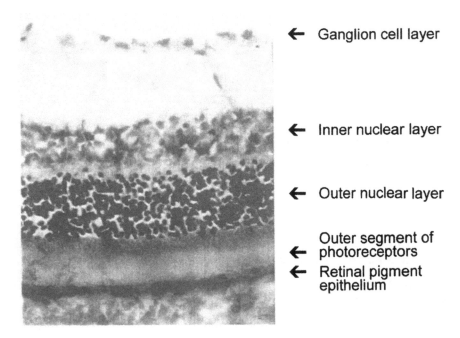

← Ganglion cell layer

← Inner nuclear layer

← Outer nuclear layer

← Outer segment of
   photoreceptors
← Retinal pigment
   epithelium

Fig. 1 Light photomicrograph of a rat retinal section. The inner nuclear layer includes the nuclei of bipolar, amacrine, horizontal, and Müller cells. The nuclei of rods and cones are in the outer nuclear layer.

are the first and ganglion cells the second neuron of the visual pathway from photoreceptors to brain. Macula is the central part of retina located temporally of optic nerve head between the upper and lower temporal vessels. Fovea is the central, approximately 1.5 mm wide sloping part of macula. Visual acuity is decreased quickly in the paramacular areas. Of the photoreceptors, the cones take care of photoptic and color vision and are located mainly in the macula. Rods are the main photoreceptor type in the periphery; they are specialized to scotopic vision.

The human retina may be affected by many vascular diseases such as occlusions, vasculitis, and anomalies. Retinopathy of prematurity (ROP) is a retinal disease affecting premature children, where the growth of developing retinal vasculature is interrupted. Diabetic retinopathy is a common cause of blindness, while arteriosclerosis, hypertension, and other cardiovascular diseases may cause changes in the retinal vasculature. Neovascularization is also associated in macular degeneration.

In retinal detachment, fluid is collected in the potential space between the neural retina and RPE. In rhegmatogenous detachment, the fluid comes from the vitreous cavity through a retinal hole or tear. Extravasation may originate from choroid or retina and results in secondary retinal detachment. Retinal detachment caused by the traction of fibrous bands in vitreous is called traction retinal detachment. Traumas, intraocular inflammations, retinal or vitreal degeneration, or vitreal bleeding are etiological factors of retinal detachment. Proliferative vitreoretinopathy (PVR) is found in about 5% of retinal detachments. It is characterized by the formation of vitreal, epiretinal, or subretinal membranes after retinal reattachment surgery or ocular trauma. In some cases the membranes cause traction and distortion of retina. Severe postoperative PVR is the most common cause of failed retinal detachment surgery.

Retinoblastoma is a malignant retinal tumor with an incidence of about 1 : 20,000. The genetic abnormality of this disease located to 13q14. Both genes in this locus must be abnormal before this malignancy develops. In the nonhereditary form, mutation occurs only in the retinal cells. In the hereditary form the patient has inherited the first mutation from his or her parents, and 90% of these patients develop a clinical retinoblastoma.

In this chapter we present some recent development in the retinal disease models of animals. Models of retinal degeneration, proliferative diseases, and neovascularization are presented. These models are important tools in current research, since various growth factors, gene therapies, and transplantation strategies have demonstrated possibilities for treating severe retinal diseases.

II. RETINAL DEGENERATION—GENETIC MODELS

Retinal degeneration leads to impaired function of the photoreceptors and consequently gradual loss of vision., Many types of degeneration are based on genetic factors, e.g., retinitis pigmentosa, a common term for various mutations causing retinal degeneration. In addition to genetic factors, environmental factors (e.g., light exposure) may lead to retinal degeneration. Macular degeneration is the most common type of retinal degeneration, being the leading cause of vision loss in the industrial world. In the following sections we present some genetic and environmental animal models of retinal degeneration.

A. Natural Mutation Mouse Models

The naturally occurring mouse rd (retinal degeneration) and rds (retinal degeneration slow) photoreceptor dystrophies are recessively inherited. The mice have defects in the cGMP phosphodiesterase beta subunit gene

(1,2) and in the peripherin gene (3,4). The rd mouse is a model of retinitis pigmentosa in which a mutation of a rod-specific photophodiesterase leads to the rapid loss of photoreceptors during early postnatal life. Very little is known about the associated changes in the inner retinal neurons. Bipolar and horizontal cells of the rd mouse retina undergo dramatic morphological changes accompanying photoreceptor loss, demonstrating a dependence of second-order neurons on photoreceptors (5).

The rds phenotype is considered to be an appropriate model for peripherin 2/rds-mediated retinitis pigmentosa. Peripherin 2 glycoprotein is needed for the formation of photoreceptor outer discs. The photoreceptor cell is the primary site of the genetic defect that results in retinal dystrophy in the rds mouse model (6).

The protective effect of a number of survival factors on degenerating photoreceptors in mutant mice with naturally occurring inherited retinal degenerations, including retinal degeneration (rd/rd), retinal degeneration slow (rds/rds), nervous (nr/nr), and Purkinje cell degeneration (pcd/pcd), in three different forms of mutant rhodopsin transgenic mice and in light damage in albino mice were examined by La Vail et al. (7). The slowing of degeneration in the rd/rd and Q344ter (a naturally occurring stop codon mutation that removes the last five amino acids of rhodopsin) mutant mice demonstrated that intraocularly injected survival factors can protect photoreceptors from degenerating. Importantly, these animal models have the same or similar genetic defects as those in human inherited retinal degenerations (7). Such models have also been used to improve the condition of photoreceptors by adeno-associated virus-mediated peripherin 2 gene therapy (8). The outcome of the gene therapy was dependent on the timing of the therapy (9).

B. Transgenic Mouse Models

To generate transgenic animals, whole genes are injected into a fertilized egg pronucleus. The genes associate randomly into the genome, and their expression is controlled by their own regulatory sequences. Due to the complexity of the photoreceptor biology, several genes can be used to generate transgenic mouse models of retinal degeneration.

The VPP mouse carries three mutations (P23H, V20G, P27L) near the N-terminus of opsin, the apoprotein of rhodopsin, the rod photopigment. These animals have slowly progressive degeneration of the rod photoreceptors and subsequent changes in retinal function. These changes mimic autosomal dominant retinitis pigmentosa of humans, which results from a point mutation (P23H) in opsin (10). The rate of photoreceptor degeneration in VPP mice seems to be adversely affected by the existence of the albino phenotype (11). Light deprivation affects the rate of degeneration in pigmented transgenic VPP mice (12).

To establish a transgenic mouse line with a mutated mouse opsin gene in addition to the endogenous opsin gene, a mutated mouse opsin gene was introduced into the germ line of a normal mouse. Simultaneous expression of mutated and normal opsin genes induces a slow degeneration of both rod and cone photoreceptors. The time course mimics the course of human autosomal dominant retinitis pigmentosa (13).

The biochemical, morphological, and physiological analyses of a transgenic mouse model for retinal degeneration slow (RDS) retinitis pigmentosa have been carried out. RDS retinitis pigmentosa is caused by a substitution of proline 216 to leucine (P216L) in rds/peripherin. The phenotype in P216L-transgenic mice probably caused by a combination of two genetic mechanisms: a dominant effect of the P216 substituted protein and a reduction in the concentration of normal rds/peripherin. The expression of the normal and mutant genes is similar to that predicted for humans with RDS-mediated autosomal-dominant retinitis pigmentosa. These mice may be used as an animal model for this disease (14).

The W70A transgenic mouse carries a point mutation (W70A) in the gene that encodes for the gamma-subunit of rod cGMP phosphodiesterase. This mouse represents a new model of stationary nyctalopia that can be recognized by its unusual ERG (electroretinogram) features (15).

Another transgenic mouse model with defective expression of the alpha subunit of the rod cGMP-gated channel was reported recently (16). Expression was reduced by antisense RNA. The low expression of the rod cGMP-gated channel causes a disease model that can be used to test therapies designed to slow down or cure retinal degenerations (16).

Mice (Pdegtm1/Pdegtm1) that are homozygous for a mutant allele of the gamma subunit of retinal cyclic guanosine monophosphate phosphodiesterase (PDE gamma) have a severe photoreceptor degeneration. Interestingly, the transgene that encodes the BCL2 protein was introduced by mating into the mutant background. Antiapoptotic transgene BCL2 delayed temporarily the degeneration of photoreceptors in this murine model of retinal degeneration (17).

C. Knockout Mouse Models

Knockout mutation is created by transferring a gene that is inactivated by mutation to pluripotent embryonal stem cells. They often find their copy in the genome and settle beside it and then change places by recombination. The cells with wanted recombination are transferred to blastocysts to produce chimeric animals. Homozygous animals with the mutation can be produced by mating.

A retinitis pigmentosa GTPase regulator-deficient mouse model for X-linked retinitis pigmentosa has been created by gene knockout. In the mutant mice, cone photoreceptors exhibit ectopic localization of cone opsins. Rod photoreceptors have a reduced level of rhodopsin, and subsequently photoreceptors degenerate (18).

Likewise, rhodopsin knockout (opsin−/−) mice have been generated as an animal model of retinitis pigmentosa. In that case a gene encoding ciliary neurotrophic factor (CNTF) was delivered subretinally with adeno-associated virus-vector. CNTF gene therapy delayed the death of photoreceptors (19).

Homozygous rhodopsin knockout (Rho−/−) mice have a mutation in exon 2 of the rhodopsin gene. They show a complete absence of functional rhodopsin and do not build rod outer segments. The Rho(−/−) mice can serve during postnatal weeks 4–6 as a model for pure cone function (20). These mice do not elaborate rod outer segments, and the photoreceptors are lost in 3 months. No rod ERG response is seen in 8-week-old animals. In contrast, Rho+/− animals retain most of their photoreceptors, although the inner and outer segments of the cells display some structural disorganization. These animals may be a useful genetic background on which other mutant opsin transgenes can be expressed. (21).

Knockout mice with arrestin gene defect have been generated. Excessive light accelerated the cell death in pigmented arrestin knockout mice. Human patients with mutations leading to nonfunctional arrestin and rhodopsin kinase have Oguchi disease. This disease is a form of stationary night blindness (22).

D. Rat Models

The Royal College of Surgeons (RCS) rat is the first animal model with inherited retinal degeneration. Although the genetic defect is actually not known, the RCS rat is widely used as a model of photoreceptor degeneration with relevance to retinitis pigmentosa and hereditary retinal dystrophies (23,24). Experiments with RCS rats have been used to demonstrate the beneficial effects of growth factors (like basic fibroblast growth factor, bFGF) on retinal degeneration (25).

Adenovirus-mediated gene transfer has been used to develop a rat model for photoreceptor degeneration. Recombinant adenovirus-mediated downregulation of cathepsin S (CatS) in the retinal pigment epithelium and/or neural retina was achieved. These results demonstrate that the transient modulation of gene expression in RPE cells induced changes in the retina.

Despite the low expression of endogenous CatS in RPE cells, this enzyme appears to play an important role in the maintenance of normal retinal function (26).

Transgenic rat P23H have been used as a model of autosomal dominant retinitis pigmentosa. Substitution of proline by histidine in position 23 in rhodopsin (P23H) is the most common human mutation in RP in the United States, with a prevalance of 15%. Several sublines of this strain have been developed. These lines have a similar genotype, but the rate of retinal degeneration varies. In line 1, almost complete degeneration is seen in 2 months, but in line 2 similar degeneration develops in one year. Similarly, there are many sublines of transgenic rats that carry a rhodopsin mutation S334ter with different rates of retinal degeneration. Ribozyme-directed cleavage of mutant mRNAs slows the rate of photoreceptor degeneration in this rat model (27). D-*cis*-Diltiazem did not rescue photoreceptors of Pro23His rhodopsin mutation line 1 rats treated according to the protocol used in rd mouse (28). Extended photoreceptor viability by light stress has been detected in RCS rats but not in opsin P23H mutant rats (29). The photoreceptors of transgenic rats expressing either a P23H or an S334ter rhodopsin mutation were protected from apoptosis by recombinant adeno-associated virus-mediated production of fibroblast growth factors fgf-2, fgf-5, and fgf-18 (30,31), while lens epithelium-derived growth factor promoted photoreceptor survival in light-damaged and RCS rats, but not in P23H rats (32).

In addition to biochemical measures, these disease state models can be monitored on the basis of retinal morphology (number of outer nuclear layers) and ERG (a and b waves).

E. Cat Models

Abyssinian cats with recessively inherited rod-cone degeneration have been introduced (33). Photoreceptor allografts were examined to determine the viability and influence of such transplants on the host retina of the cats. Also, clinical and pathological features, light and electron microscopy, and the electrophysiology of an autosomal dominant, early-onset feline model of rod/cone dysplasia (Rdy cats) have been documented (34–36). The immunohistochemical changes in the retina and photoreceptor cell death of this model have also been studied (37).

F. Transgenic Pig Model

Transgenic pigs that express a mutated rhodopsin gene (Pro347Leu) were generated (38). These transgenic pigs provide a large animal model to study the protracted phase of cone degeneration in retinitis pigmentosa and for preclinical treatment trials.

G. Dog Models

Canine rcd1 model of retinitis pigmentosa is caused by a null mutation in the PDE6B gene. Treatment of rcd1-affected dogs with D-*cis*-diltiazem did not modify the photoreceptor disease (39).

Rod-cone dysplasia types 1 (rcd1; Irish setter) and 2 (red2; collie) in dogs are early-onset forms of progressive retinal atrophy, which serve as models of retinitis pigmentosa in humans (40).

Swedish Briard dogs have a very slowly progressive retinal dystrophy that is inherited in an autosomal recessive manner. The lipid and fatty acid compositions of plasma, retina, and retinal pigment epithelium were analyzed in this model (41). These studies provide evidence for yet another animal model of inherited retinal degeneration with a defect in retinal polyunsaturated fatty acid metabolism. The fatty acid pattern in affected dogs resembles that in the retina in n-3 fatty acid deficiency.

III. RETINAL DEGENERATION—LIGHT-INDUCED MODELS

Retinal damage by light has two distinct action spectra. One peaks in the ultraviolet A (UVA) and the other in the midvisible wavelength. It was shown in the Long Evans rat that UVA and green light can produce histologically dissimilar types of damage. UVA light in particular produces severe retinal damage at low irradiation levels (42).

Albino rats were continuously exposed to blue light for 1–7 days. Continuous exposure of albino rats to moderate blue light for 2–5 days selectively eliminated most of the photoreceptors while leaving the RPE intact (43).

Monocularly aphakic gray squirrels were exposed for 10 minutes to monochromatic near-ultraviolet radiation to determine if their yellow pigmented lens protected retinal tissue from photochemical damage. In aphakic eyes the retinas revealed irreversible lesions to the photoreceptors. Eyes exposed to ultraviolet radiation with their lenses intact were devoid of significant retinal lesions. This study represents a model system for studying the potential damaging effects of near-UV radiation to the aphakic eyes of humans (44).

Constant fluorescent light can also be used to generate light-induced degeneration model. Albino rats of the F344 strain were exposed to 1 or 2 weeks of constant light, either with or without intravitreal or subretinal bFGF solution injected 2 days before the start of light exposure. Constant light exposure causes a decrease in the thickness of the outer nuclear layer and blocks ERG responses. The results indicated that the photoreceptor rescue activity of bFGF is not restricted to inherited retinal dystrophy in the rat. The light damage is an excellent model for studying the normal function of bFGF and its survival-promoting activity (45). It has been shown that, in the retina, basic fibroblast growth factor delays photoreceptor degeneration in Royal College of Surgeons rats with inherited retinal dystrophy. bFGF also reduces or prevents the rapid photoreceptor degeneration produced by constant light in the rat. This light-damage model was used to assess the survival-promoting activity in vivo of a number of growth factors and other molecules. Photoreceptors can be significantly protected from the damaging effects of light by intravitreal injection of eight different growth factors, cytokines, and neurotrophins. They act through several distinct receptor families. In addition to basic fibroblast growth factor, effective photoreceptor rescue was obtained with brain-derived neurotrophic factor, ciliary neurotrophic factor, interleukin 1 beta, and acidic fibroblast growth factor. Less activity was seen with neurotrophin 3, insulin-like growth factor II, and tumor necrosis factor alpha, while nerve growth factor, epidermal growth factor, platelet-derived growth factor, insulin, insulin-like growth factor I, heparin, and laminin did not show any protection (25).

IV. PROLIFERATIVE VITREORETINOPATHY

Proliferative vitreoretinopathy (PVR) is found in about 5% of retinal detachments. The cellular evens of PVR include migration of glial cells, pigment epithelial cells, and fibrocytes into the vitreous cavity, where they proliferate and transform and dedifferentiate. The cells may interact with endogenous membranous components of the vitreous. This leads to the formation of vitreal, epiretinal, and subretinal membranes and traction retinal detachment (47). Severe postoperative PVR is the most common cause of failed retinal detachment surgery. Animal models of PVR are based on environmental injuries.

A. Cell Injection

Injury can be caused by intraocular injection of fibroblasts into rabbit eye. This was used as a model to test treatment of PVR by gene therapy. A classification of severity of PVR in this model has been published (48–50).

The extent of PVR by cells that do or do not express the receptors for platelet-derived growth factor (PDGF) was investigated. Mouse embryo fibroblasts was derived from PDGF receptor knock-out embryos. They do not express PDGF receptors and induced PVR poorly when injected into the eyes of rabbits. PDGF made an important contribution to the development of PVR in this animal model. Furthermore, there was a marked difference between the two receptors from PDGF. PDGF α receptor was capable of inducing PVR (51).

B. Dispase

PVR can be induced by injecting dispase intravitreally to rabbits (Dutch belted, New Zealand white). Proliferative vitreoretinopathy developed in response to subretinal or intravitreal dispase, with or without retinal break. Severity of PVR was correlated with increasing doses of dispase. The dispase model of PVR is easy to perform, and it permits a clear view of the retina. This model showed a high success rate in development of PVR (52), and intravitreally administered prinomastat decreased development of PVR in this experimental model (53).

C. Combined Models

A proliferative vitreoretinopathy model was generated in albino rabbits by combing some factors that probably cause the disease. The eyes were injected with platelet-rich plasma, and in addition they underwent cryotherapy or vitrectomy or both procedures. Total retinal detachment and giant holes were obtained more often in experimental eyes than in controls. Microscopic investigation showed intravitreal or preretinal proliferation of fibroblast-like cells (54).

Another combination model involves retinotomy with removal of vitreous, cryotherapy, and platelet-rich plasm injection. This is an efficient model of PVR: retinal detachments were produced in 100% of rabbit eyes (55).

In a similar model (56) combined therapy of systemic methylprednisolone, sodium diclofenac, and colchicine was combined with topical atropine, adrenaline, and dexamethasone phosphate. The therapies were useful in treating experimental PVR.

D. Laser

Laser-induced retinal injury can be used to provoke PVR formation. For example, pigmented rabbits underwent argon laser panretinal photocoagulation in one eye. Then cultured fibroblasts were implanted into the intact vitreous of both eyes. More severe PVR developed in the eye with prior panretinal photocoagulation than in the controls (57).

E. Other Models

Platelet-rich plasma causes PVR after injection into the vitreous in rabbit eyes (59). It contributed more effectively to the development of an experimental porcine PVR than PDGF. The efficacy depends on the platelet concentration of the plasma. It seems that other growth factors and plasma components may interact synergistically with PDGF in the pathogenesis of PVR (58).

V. NEOVASCULARIZATION

Neovascularization is involved in various diseases (e.g., cancer, psoriasis), and the mechanism of angiogenesis has intensely been studied. Neovascularization complicates the treatment of many retinal diseases, and, therefore, appropriate animal models are needed.

A. Laser-Induced Neovascularization

Subretinal neovascularization (NV) can be induced by intense laser photocoagulation in monkey eyes (60). In pigs, the laser-induced branch of retinal venous obstruction with rose bengal develops neovascularization of the optic nerve head and retina (612). This process was assisted by photodynamic thrombosis. A model of retinal ischemia and associated NV established by venous thrombosis was produced. After anesthesia, eyes of pigmented rats received an intraperitoneal injection of sodium fluorescein prior to laser treatment. With a blue-green argon laser, selected venous sites next to the optic nerve head were photocoagulated (64).

B. Angiogenic Factor

Several ocular NV models are based on exposing the retina to excess of angiogenic compounds. The effect of increased vascular endothelial growth factor (VEGF) expression in the retina was investigated using transgenic mice in which bovine rhodopsin promoter is coupled with the gene for human VEGF. This study demonstrated that overexpression of VEGF in the retina was sufficient to cause intraretinal and subretinal NV and provided a valuable new animal model (62).

Controlled-release systems have been developed in order to provide a long-term supply of angiogenic factors to the retina at defined levels. Ethylene–vinyl acetate copolymer pellets release VEGF slowly into the vitreous cavity of rabbits and primates. This induces neovascularization. Sustained intravitreal release of VEGF caused widespread retinal vascular dilation and breakdown of the blood-retinal barrier. Retinal NV seems to require persistent high levels of VEGF at the retinal surface. This can be achieved in rabbits more easily than in primates (63).

In alternative controlled-release models, subretinal implantation of bFGF-impregnated gelatin microspheres is used to induce subretinal neovascularization in the rabbit (65).

C. Ischemia

Relative hypoxia triggers formation of neovessels in the retina. When one-week-old C57BL/6J mice were exposed to 75% oxygen for 5 days and then to room air, the retinal neovascularization occurs between postnatal days 17 and 21. This model can then be used to study the therapeutic strategies (66). In a similar ischemia-induced ocular neovascularization model, the expression of Flk-1 and neuropilin-1 was restricted on neovascularized vessels, suggesting that these molecules may play important roles in retinal NV (67).

NV studies with ischemic models suggest that PaO_2 fluctuation is more important than extended hyperoxia for retinal neovascular response in rats (68). Indeed, a cycled hypoxia/hyperoxia (10–50% O_2) protocol followed by normoxia (20% O_2) has been used as a retinal model of retinopathy of prematurity to induce neovascularization in rat pups (69,70).

The time course and degree of proliferative vascular response after hyperoxic insult were examined in dogs after oxygen-induced retinopathy. In the neonatal dog, revascularization after hyperoxic insult involves a period of marked vasoproliferation peaking 3–10 days after a return to room air. Oxygen-induced changes in the extravascular milieu probably affect the pattern of reforming vasculature and possibly restrict the growth anteriorly (71).

D. Genetic Models

NV of the RPE occurs earlier in a line of P23H mutant rhodopsin transgenic mice than in most other mice and rats. The temporal course of RPE NV in P23H mice was compared with that of two other retinal degeneration mutants with a similar time course of photoreceptor cell loss. The findings suggest that the P23H mutant rhodopsin transgenic mouse may be a useful model for studying the regulation of NV in the outer retina (72).

E. Other Models

NH4Cl gavage in the neonatal rat produced a metabolic acidosis–induced retinopathy that may be a model for retinopathy of prematurity. Acidosis is induced by high-dose acetazolamide. Independently of hyperoxemia or hypoxemia, the treatment is associated with preretinal neovascularization in the neonatal rat (73).

A consistent model of preretinal NV in the rabbit was developed by partially digesting the posterior virtreous with repeated injection of hyaluronidase. Then 250,000 homologous dermal fibroblasts were injected intravitreally (74). Neovascular events observed in this model agree with those previously described for diabetic retinopathy and retinopathy of prematurity in humans (75).

REFERENCES

1. Bowes, C., Li, T., Danciger, M., Bacter, L. C., Applebury, M. L., and Farber, D. B. (1990). Retinal degeneration in the rd mouse is caused by a defect in the beta subunit of rod cGMP-phosphodiesterase, *Nature, 347*:677.
2. Pittler, S. J., and Baehr, W. (1991). Identification of a nonsense mutation in the rod photoreceptor cGMP phosphodiesterase beta-subunit gene of the rd mouse, *Proc. Natl. Acad. Sci., 88*:8322.
3. Travis, G. H., Sutcliffe, J. G., and Bok, D. (1991). The retinal degeneration slow (rds) gene product is a photoreceptor disc membrane-associated glycoprotein, *Neuron, 6*:61.
4. Connell, G., Bascom, R., Molday, L., Reid, D., McInnes, R. R., and Molday, R. S. (1991). Photoreceptor peripherin is the normal product of the gene responsible for retinal degeneration in the rds mouse, *Proc. Natl. Acad. Sci., 88*:723.
5. Strettoi, E., and Pignatelli, V. (2000). Modifications of retinal neurons in a mouse model of retinitis pigmentosa, *Proc. Natl. Acad. Sci., 97*:11020.
6. Li, L., Sheedlo, H. J., and Turner, J. E. (1993). Retinal pigment epithelial cell transplants in retinal degeneration slow mice do not rescue photoreceptor cells, *Invest. Ophthalmol. Vis. Sci., 34*:2141.
7. LaVail, M. M., Yasumura, D., Matthes, M. T., Lau-Villacorta, C., Unoki, K., Sung, C. H., and Steinberg, R. H. (1998). Protection of mouse photoreceptors by survival factors in retinal degenerations, *Invest. Ophthalmol. Vis. Sci., 39*:592.
8. Ali, R. R., Sarra, G. M., Stephens, C., Alwis, M. D., Bainbridge, J. W., Munro, P. M., Fauser, S., Reichel, M. B., Kinnon, C., Hunt, D. M., Bhattacharya, S. S., and Thrasher, A. J. (2000). Restoration of photoreceptor ultrastructure and function in retinal degeneration slow mice by gene therapy, *Nat. Genet., 25*:306.

9. Sarra, G. M., Stephens, C., de Alwis, M., Bainbridge, J. W., Smith, A. J., Thrasher, A. J., and Ali, R. R. (2001). Gene replacement, therapy in the retinal degeneration slow (rds) mouse: the effect on retinal degeneration following partial transduction of the retina, *Hum. Mol. Genet., 10*:2353.

10. Wu, T. H., Ting, T. D., Okajima, T. I., Pepperberg, D. R., Ho, Y. K., Ripps, H., and Naash, M. I. (1998). Opsin localization and rhodopsin photochemistry in a transgenic mouse model of retinitis pigmentosa, *Neuroscience, 87*:709.

11. Naash, M. I., Ripps, H., Li, S., Goto, Y., and Peachey, N. S. (1996). Polygenic disease and retinitis pigmentosa: albinism exacerbates photoreceptor degeneration induced by the expression of a mutant opsin in transgenic mice, *J. Neurosci., 16*:7853.

12. Naash, M. L., Peachey, N. S., Li, Z. Y., Gryczan, C. C., Goto, Y., Blanks, J., Milam, A. H., and Ripps, H. (1996). Light-induced acceleration of photoreceptor degeneration in transgenic mice expressing mutant rhodopsin, *Invest. Ophthalmol. Vis. Sci., 370*:775.

13. Naash, M. I., Hollyfield, J. G., al-Ubaidi, M. R., and Baehr, W. (1993). Simulation of human autosomal dominant retinitis pigmentosa in transgenic mice expressing a mutated murine opsin gene, *Proc. Natl. Acad. Sci., 90*:5499.

14. Kedzierski, W., Lloyd, M., Birch, D. G., Bok, D., and Travis, G. H. (1997). Generation and analysis of transgenic mice expressing P216L-substituted rds/peripherin in rod photoreceptors, *Invest. Ophthalmol. Vis. Sci., 38*:498.

15. Salchow, D. J., Gouras, P., Doi, K., Goff, S. P., Schwinger, E., and Tsang, S. H. (1999). A point mutation (W70A) in the rod PDE-gamma gene desensitizing and delaying murine rod photoreceptors, *Invest. Ophthalmol. Vis. Sci., 40*:3262.

16. Leconte, L., and Barnstable, C. J. (2000). Impairment of rod cGMP-gated channel alpha-subunit expression leads to photoreceptor and bipolar cell degeneration, *Invest. Ophthalmol. Vis. Sci., 41*:917.

17. Tsang, S. H., Chen, J., Kjeldbye, H., Li, W. S., Simon, M. I., Gouras, P., and Goff, S. P. (1997). Retarding photoreceptor degeneration in Pdegtm1/Pdegtm1 mice by an apoptosis suppressor gene, *Invest. Ophthalmol. Vis. Sci., 38*:943.

18. Hong, D. H., Pawlyk, B. S., Shang, J., Sandberg, M. A., Berson, E. L., and Li, T. (2000). A retinitis pigmentosa GTPase regulator (RPGR)-deficient mouse model for X-linked retinitis pigmentosa (RP3), *Proc. Natl. Acad. Sci., 97*:3649.

19. Liang, F. Q., Dejneka, N. S., Cohen, D. R. Krasnoperova, N. V., Lem, J., Maguire, A. M., Dudus, L., Fisher, K. J., and Bennett, J. (2001). AAV-mediated delivery of ciliary neurotrophic factor prolongs photoreceptor survival in the rhodopsin knockout mouse, *Mol. Ther., 3*:241.

20. Jaissle, G. B., May, C. A., Reinhard, J., Kohler, K., Fauser, S., Lutjen-Drecoll, E., Zrenner, E., and Seeliger, M. W. (2001). Evaluation of the rhodopsin knockout mouse as a model of pure cone function, *Invest. Ophthalmol. Vis. Sci., 42*:506.

21. Humphries, M. M., Rancourt, D., Farrar, G. J., Kenna, P., Hazel, M., Bush, R. A., Sieving, P. A., Sheils, D. M., McNally, N., Creighton, P., Erven, A., Boros, A., Gulya, K., Capecchi, M. R., and Humphries, P. (1997). Retinopathy induced in mice by targeted disruption of the rhodopsin gene, *Nat. Genet., 15*:216.

22. Chen, J., Simon, M. I., Matthes, M. T., Yasumura, D., and LaVail, M. M. (1999). Increased susceptibility to light damage in an arrestin knockout mouse model of Oguchi disease (stationary night blindness), *Invest. Ophthalmol. Vis. Sci., 40*:2978.

23. Yu, D. Y., Cringle, S. J., Sue, E. N., and Yu, P. K. (2000). Intraretinal oxygen levels before and after photoreceptor loss in the RCS rat, *Invest. Ophthalmol. Vis. Sci., 41*:3999.

24. Strauss, O., Stumpff, F., Mergler, S., Wienrich, M., and Wiederholt, M. (1998). The Royal College of Surgeons rat: An animal model for inherited retinal degeneration with a still unknown genetic defect, *Acta Anat., 162*:101.

25. LaVail, M. M., Unoki, K., Yasumura, D., Matthes, M. T., Yancopoulos, G. D., and Steinberg, R. H. (1992). Multiple growth factors, cytokines, and neurotrophins rescue photoreceptors from the damaging effects of constant light, *Proc. Natl. Acad. Sci., 89*:11249.

26. Lai, C. M., Shen, W. Y., Constable, I., and Rakoczy, P. E. (2000). The use of adenovirus-mediated gene transfer to develop a rat model for photoreceptor degeneration, *Invest. Ophthalmol. Vis. Sci., 41*:580.

27. Lewin, A. S., Drenser, K. A., Hauswirth, W. W., Nishikawa, S., Yasumura, D., Flannery, J. G., and LaVail, M. M. (1998). Ribozyme rescue of photoreceptor cells in a transgenic rat model of autosomal dominant retinitis pigmentosa, *Nat. Med., 4*:967.

28. Bush, R. A., Kononen, L., Machida, S., and Sieving, P. A. (2000). The effect of calcium channel blocker diltiazem on photoreceptor degeneration in the rhodopsin Pro213His rat, *Invest. Ophthalmol. Vis. Sci., 41*:2697.

29. Nir, I., Harrison, J. M., Liu, C., and Wen, R. (2001). Extended photoreceptor viability by light stress in the CS rats but not in the opsin P23H mutant rats, *Invest. Ophthalmol. Vis. Sci., 42*:842.

30. Green, E. S., Rendahl, K. G., Zhou, S., Ladner, M., Coyne, M., Srivastava, R., Manning, W. C., and Flannery, J. G. (2001). Two animal models of retinal degeneration are rescued by recombinant adeno-associated virus-mediated production of fgf-5 and fgf-18, *Mol. Ther., 3*:507.

31. Lau, D., McGee, L. H., Zhou, S., Rendahl, K. G., Manning, W. C., Escobedo, J. A., and Flannery, J. G. (2000). Retinal degeneration is slowed in transgenic rats by AAV-dilated delivery of FGF-2, *Invest. Ophthalmol. Vis. Sci., 41*:3622.

32. Machida, S., Chaudhry, P., Shinohara, T., Singh, D. P., Reddy, V. N., Chylack, L. T. Jr, Sieving, P. A., and Bush, R. A. (2001). Lens epithelium-derived growth factor promotes photoreceptor survival in light-damaged and RCS rats, *Invest. Ophthalmol. Vis. Sci. 42*:1087.

33. Ivert, L., Gouras, P., Naeser, P., and Narfstrom, K. (1998). Photoreceptor allografts in a feline model of retinal degeneration, *Graefes Arch. Clin. Exp. Ophthalmol., 236*:844.

34. Curtis, R., Barnett, K. C., and Leon, A. (1987). An early-onset retinal dystrophy with dominant inheritance in the Abyssinian cat. Clinical and pathological findings, *Invest. Ophthalmol. Vis. Sci., 28*:131.

35. Leon, A., and Curtis, R. (1990). Autosomal dominant rod-cone dysplasia in the Rdy cat. 1. Light and electron microscopic findings, *Exp. Eye Res., 51*:361.

36. Leon, A., Hussain, A. A., and Curtis, R. (1991). Autosomal dominant rod-cone dysplasia in the Rdy cat. 2. Electrophysiological findings, *Exp. Eye Res., 53*:489.

37. Chong, N. H., Alexander, R. A., Barnett, K. C., Bird, A. C., and Luthert, P. J. (1999). An immunohistochemical study of an autosomal dominant feline rod/cone dysplasia (Rdy cats), *Exp. Eye Res., 68*:51.

38. Petters, R. M., Alexander, C. A., Wells, K. D., Collins, E. B., Sommer, J. R., Blanton, M. R., Rojas, G., Hao, Y., Flowers, W. L., Banin, E., Cideciyan, A. V., Jacobson, S. G., and Wong, F. (1997). Genetically engineered large animal model for studying cone photoreceptor survival and degeneration in retinitis pigmentosa, *Nat. Biotechnol., 15*:965.

39. Pearce-Kelling, S. E., Aleman, T. S., Nickle, A., Laties, A. M., Aguirre, G. D., Jacobson, S. G., and Acland, G. M. (2001). Calcium channel blocker D-cis-diltiazem does not slow retinal degeneration in the PDE6B mutant rcd1 canine model of retinitis pigmentosa, *Mol. Vis., 7*:42.

40. Wang, W., Acland, G. M., Ray, K., and Aguirre, G. D. (1999). Evaluation of cGMP-phosphodiesterase (PDE) subunits causal association with rod-cone dysplasia 2 (rcd2), a canine model of abnormal retinal cGMP metabolism, *Exp. Eye Res., 69*:445.

41. Anderson, R. E., Maude, M. B., Narfstrom, K., and Nilsson, S. E. (1997). Lipids of plasma, retina, and retinal pigment epithelium in Swedish briard dogs with a slowly progressive retinal dystrophy, *Exp. Eye Res., 64*:181.

42. Rapp, L. M., Tolman, B. L., and Dhindsa, H. S. (1990). Separate mechanisms for retinal damage by ultraviolet-A and mid-visible light, *Invest. Ophthalmol. Vis. Sci., 31*:1186.

43. Seiler, M. J., Liu, O. L., Cooper, N. G., Callahan, T. L., Petry, H. M., and Aramant, R. B. (2000). Selective photoreceptor damage in albino rats using continuous blue light. A protocol useful for retinal degeneration and transplantation research, *Graefes Arch. Clin. Exp. Ophthalmol., 238*:59.

44. Collier, R. J., Waldron, W. R., and Zigman, S. (1989). Temporal sequence of changes to the gray squirrel retina after near-UV exposure, *Invest. Ophthalmol. Vis. Sci., 30*:631.

45. Faktorovich, E. G., Steinberg, R. H., Yasumura, D., Matthes, M. T., and LaVail, M. M. (1992). Basic fibroblast growth factor and local injury protect photoreceptors from light damage in the rat, *J. Neurosci., 12*:3554.

46. Organisciak, D. T., Darrow, R. M., Barsalou, L., Darrow, R. A., Kutty, R. K., Kutty, G., and Wiggert, B. (1998). Light history and age-related changes in retinal light damage, *Invest. Ophthalmol. Vis. Sci., 39*:1107.

47. Berman, E. R. (1991). *Biochemistry of the Eye*. Plenum Press, New York.

48. Hida, T., Chandler, D. B., and Sheta, S. M. (1987). Classification of the stages of proliferative vitreoretinopathy in a refined experimental model in the rabbit eye, *Graefes Arch. Clin. Exp. Ophthalmol., 225*:303.

49. Murata, T., Kimura, H., Sakamoto, T., Osusky, R., Spee, C., Stout, T. J., Hinton, D. R., and Ryan, S. J. (1997). Ocular gene therapy: experimental studies and clinical possibilities, *Ophthalmic Res., 29*:242.

50. Fastenberg, D. M., Diddie, K. R., Dorey, K., and Ryan, S. J. (1982). The role of cellular proliferation in an experimental model of massive periretinal proliferation, *Am. J. Ophthalmol., 93*:565.

51. Andrews, A., Balciunaite, E., Leong, F. L., Tallquist, M., Soriano, P., Refojo, M., and Kazlauskas, A. (1999). Platelet-derived growth factor plays a key role in proliferative vitreoretinopathy, *Invest. Ophthalmol. Vis. Sci., 40*:2683.

52. Frenzel, E. M., Neely, K. A., Walsh, A. W., Cameron, J. D., and Gregerson, D. S. (1998). A new model of proliferative vitreoretinopathy, *Invest. Ophthalmol. Vis. Sci., 39*:2157.

53. Ozerdem, U., Mach-Hofacre, B., Cheng, L., Chaidhawangul, S., Keefe, McDermott, C. D., Bergeron-Lyn, G., Appelt, K., and Freeman, W. R. (2000). The effect of prinomastat (AG3340), a potent inhibitor of matrix metalloproteinases, on a subacute model of proliferative vitreoretinopathy, *Curr. Eye Res., 20*:447.

54. Pinon, R. M., Pastor, J. C., Saornil, M. A., Goldaracena, M. B., Layana, A. G., Gayoso, M. J., and Guisasola, J. (1992). Intravitreal and subretinal proliferation induced by platelet-rich plasma injection in rabbits, *Curr. Eye. Res., 11*:1047

55. Goldaracena, M. B., Garcia-Layana, A., Pastor, J. C., Saornil, M. A., de la Fuente, F., and Gayoso, M. J. (1997). The role of retinotomy in an experimental rabbit model of proliferative vitreoretinopathy, *Curr. Eye Res. 16*:422.

56. Pastor, J. C., Rodriguez, E., Marcos, M. A., and Lopez, M. I. (2000). Combined pharmacologic therapy in a rabbit model of proliferative vitreoretinopathy (PVR), *Ophthalmic Res., 32*:25.

57. Algvere, P. V., Hallnas, K., Dafgard, E., and Hoog, A. (1990). Panretinal photocoagulation aggravates experimental proliferative vitreoretinopathy, *Graefes Arch. Clin. Exp. Ophthalmol., 228*:461.

58. Garcia-Layana, A., Pastor, J. C. Saornil, M. A., and Gonzalez, G. (1997). Porcine model of proliferative vitreoretinopathy with platelets, *Curr. Eye Res., 16*:556.

59. Baudouin, C., Khosravi, E., Pisella, P. J., Ettaiche, M., and Elena, P. P. (1998). Inflammation measurement and immunocharacterization of cell proliferation in an experimental model of proliferative vitreoretinopathy, *Ophthalmic Res., 30*:340.

60. Ishibashi, T., Inomata, H., Sakamoto, T., and Ryan, S. J. (1995). Pericytes of newly formed vessels in experimental subretinal neovascularization, *Arch. Ophthalmol., 113*:227.

61. Danis, R. P., Yang, Y., Massicotte, S. J., and Bold, H. C. (1993). Preretinal and optic nerve head neovascularization induced by photodynamic venous thrombosis in domestic pigs, *Arch. Ophthalmol., 111*:539.

62. Okamoto, N., Tobe, T., Hackett, S. F., Ozaki, H., Vinores, M. A., LaRochelle, W., Zack, D. J., and Campochiaro, P. A. (1997). Transgenic mice with increased expression on vascular endothelial growth factor in the retina: A new model of intraretinal and subretinal neovascularization, *Am. J. Pathol., 151*:281.

63. Ozaki, H., Hayashi, H., Vinores, S. A., Moromizato, Y., Campochiaro, P. A., and Oshima, K. (1997). Intravitreal sustained release of VEGF causes retinal neovascularization in rabbits and breakdown of the blood-retinal barrier in rabbits and primates, *Exp. Eye Res., 64*:505.

64. Saito, Y., Park, L., Skolik, S. A., Alfaro, D. V., Chaudhry, N. A., Barnstable, C. J., and Liggett, P. E. (1997). Experimental preretinal neovascularization by laser-induced venous thrombosis in rats, *Curr. Eye Res., 16*:26.

65. Kimura, H., Sakamoto, T., Hinton, D. R., Spee, C., Ogura, Y., Tabata, Y., Ikada, Y., and Ryan, S. J. (1995). A new model of subretinal neovascularization in the rabbit. *Invest. Ophthalmol. Vis. Sci., 36*:2110.

66. Smith, L. E., Wesolowski, E., McLellan, A., Kostyk, S. K., D'Amato, R., Sullivan, R., and D'Amore, P. A. (1994). Oxygen-induced retinopathy in the mouse, *Invest. Ophthalmol. Vis. Sci. 35*:101.

67. Ishihama, H., Ohbayashi, M., Kurosawa, N., Kitsukawa, T., Matsuura, O., Miyake, Y., and Muramatsu, T. (2001). Colocalization of neuropilin-1 and Flk-1 in retinal neovascularization in a mouse model of retinopathy, *Invest. Ophthalmol. Vis. Sci., 42*:1172.

68. Penn, J. S., Henry, M. M., Wall, P. T., and Tolman, B. L. (1995). The range of PaO_2 variation determines the severity of oxygen-induced retinopathy in newborn rats, *Invest. Ophthalmol. Vis. Sci., 36*:2063.

69. Lukiw, W. J, Gordon, W. C., Rogaev, E. I., Thompson, H. and Bazan, N. G. (2001). Presenilin-2 (PS2) expression up-regulation in a model of retinopathy of prematurity and pathoangiogenesis, *Neuroreport 12*:53.

70. Zhang, S., Leske, D. A., and Holmes, J. M. (2000). Neovascularization grading methods in a rat model of retinopathy of prematurity, *Invest. Ophthalmol. Vis. Sci., 41*:887.

71. McLeod, D. S., Crone, S. N., and Lutty, G. A. (1996). Vasoproliferation in the neonatal dog model of oxygen-induced retinopathy, *Invest. Ophthalmol. Vis. Sci., 37*:1322.

72. Nishikawa, S., and LaVail, M. M. (1998). Neovascularization of the RPE: temporal differences in mice with rod photoreceptor gene defects, *Exp. Eye Res., 67*:509.

73. Zhang, S., Leske, D. A., Lanier, W. L., Berkowitz, B. A., and Holmes, J. M. (2001). Preretinal neovascularization associated with acetazolamide-induced systemic acidosis in the neonatal rat, *Invest. Ophthalmol. Vis. Sci., 42*:1066.

74. Antoszyk, A. N., Gottlieb, J. L., Casey, R. C., Hatchell, D. L., and Machemer, R. (1991). An experimental model of preretinal neovascularization in the rabbit, *Invest. Ophthalmol. Vis. Sci., 32*:46.

75. de Juan, E. Jr., Humayun, M. S., Hatchell, D. L., and Wilson, D. (1989). Histopathology of experimental preretinal neovascularization, *Invest. Ophthalmol. Vis. Sci., 30*:1495.

18

New Experimental Therapeutic Approaches for Degenerative Diseases of the Retina

Joyce Tombran-Tink
University of Missouri–Kansas City, Kansas City, Missouri, U.S.A.

I. INTRODUCTION

The eye is made up of highly specialized and complex groups of tissues that are important to vision. Visual impairment can result from severe damage to the cornea, lens, nerve tissue of the eye, optic nerve, retina, or the brain. Central visual disturbances usually involve macular atrophy and change in the vitreous and aqueous humor, complications that often lead to a complete loss of vision. While cataracts and corneal opacity account for most cases of blindness in developing countries, degenerative diseases of the retina are the leading cause of blindness in the Western world.

Retinal degenerative diseases are etiologically complex disorders that, for the most part, lack appropriate animal models, which are essential to elucidate the progression of the disease or to test the efficacy of many promising pharmacological agents. In this regard, the development of effective treatments for most forms of retinal degeneration has been slow, and the intervention strategies currently available are aimed at preserving vision only and not reversing the process of the disease. With the recent explosion of sophisticated molecular technologies, the genetic and biochemical bases of many retinal diseases are being better defined. This knowledge will accelerate experimental studies and facilitate the emergence of novel therapies for ocular pathologies.

The objectives of this chapter are: (a) to describe the clinically relevant innovations for managing degenerative diseases of the retina, (b) to understand the biology, development, and unique characteristics of each approach, (c) to discuss the clinical potential and limitations associated with the developing therapeutics, and (d) to examine modifications that may potentiate the therapeutic benefit of each application. A critical evaluation of basic and clinical research in the area of retinal and stem cell transplantation, retinal prosthesis, viral and nonviral DNA-based therapies, and the use of soluble neurotrophic factors in managing retinal diseases will be provided. These innovations are still in their infancy but promise enormous therapeutic benefits to blind individuals. However, because they are still being defined, a true comparison between them is clearly beyond the scope of this chapter. Before discussing developing therapeutics in the eye, it will be pertinent to review a few relatively, well-defined degenerations of the retina that are leading causes of blindness.

II. DEGENERATIVE DISEASES OF THE RETINA

Diseases that affect the center of the retina are commonly categorized as retinal degenerations. The death of photoreceptor cells, the light-sensitive neurons of the retina, is the hallmark of these disorders. Loss of function of the retinal pigment epithelium (RPE) and increased neovascularization are often complicating factors in advanced stages of many retinal diseases. While a relatively significant body of information is available for some forms of retinal degeneration, knowledge about specific mechanisms that cause the death of photoreceptor cells is still obscure and hinders the progress of developing effective treatments. One feature that further complicates diagnosis and treatment is the high level of genetic heterogeneity associated with inherited retinal diseases. For example, more than 150 mutations have been identified in rhodopsin- and peripherin-linked retinitis pigmentosa. In addition, the cellular diversity in ocular tissues allows a single pathology to be associated with the dysfunction of more than one cell type. This contributes to the disease progression and interferes with diagnosis in advanced cases. In these conditions, end-stage pathologies are complex and often involve multiple genes, many mutations, several dysfunctional cell types, and the interruption of many biochemical pathways. Thus, it is virtually impossible for any single mutation-based or cell-based treatment to emerge as an effective cure for late-state retinal degenerations. In this regard, multimodal approaches and adjuvant therapies may prove to be more effective in clinical attempts to impede the loss of vision in advanced retinal pathologies. The genetic information currently available for retinitis pigmentosa (RP), one of the better-characterized eye diseases, has been useful in developing excellent natural and transgenic RP models for preclinical testing and for developing pharmaceutics. Progress, however, is slowed for other degenerative diseases leading to blindness, such as macular degeneration, because of their less well-defined etiologies and lack of appropriate animal models. Careful characterization of the genetic and biochemical basis of these degenerations is essential for developing better animal models to study disease progression and to evaluate new treatments.

A. Macular Degeneration

The two most common degenerative diseases of the retina are macular degeneration and retinitis pigmentosa. In both diseases, degeneration of photoreceptor cells is the underlying cause of the pathology. Dysfunction of the RPE cells and choroidal neovascularization are also major contributing factors in the development of macular degeneration.

Diseases that are grouped as macular degenerations affect central vision. Damage to the macular region is the primary cause for the loss of vision. Symptoms include blurred vision, distortion of lines and shapes, blind spots, reading difficulties, and an inability to recognize faces. Peripheral vision is not severely affected in these individuals. There are two groups of macular degeneration: age-related macular degeneration (AMD) and juvenile inherited macular degeneration. AMD affects more than 700,000 Americans each year and approximately 30 million individuals worldwide. It is the leading cause of irreversible blindness in the Western world in individuals over the age of 50. The disease affects the center of the retina and is related to aging, light iris color, prolonged exposure to sunlight, smoking, and a family history. Aging mechanisms are the main factors associated with degeneration of the RPE and photoreceptor cells and the subsequent progression of AMD. Loss of RPE cell function compromises the blood-retinal barrier, resulting in additional macula edema and further degeneration of the few surviving photoreceptor cells. A loss of photoreceptor function results in the inability of the retina to convert light stimulus to electrical signals.

Two forms of AMD are identified: wet and dry. In wet AMD, blood vessels in the choroid undergo abnormal growth and invade the subretinal space located in the retina and the choroid. The disease is referred to as "wet" because the blood vessels leak their contents into the retina. The accumulation of fluid in the macula region subsequently leads to damage of the retina. Leakage, bleeding, and scarring from choroidal neovascularization eventually result in irreversible blindness. Ninety percent of individuals with the wet form of AMD suffer severe visual loss (1–4).

Unfortunately, no curative treatments are currently available for wet AMD. A new photodynamic therapy has shown potential to delay the progression of the disease with early diagnosis. In this treatment, the drug visudyne (verteporfin) is activated by laser light after intravenous injection. At best, however, laser-activated treatments can only delay visual loss, not reverse the condition, restore vision, or prevent a loss of vision (5–8).

The dry form of AMD is milder and more common. It accounts for approximately 90% of all AMD cases. It is not usually associated with abnormal growth of blood vessels and fluid leakage in the retina but, rather, with aging, yellow spots called drusen. Drusen accumulate in a scattered pattern in the affected retina region and interfere with the function of photoreceptor and RPE cells (9). There is still no effective FDA-approved treatment for dry AMD. Fortunately, visual acuity is not severely affected in dry AMD, and the disease progression is relatively slow as compared to wet AMD.

A small percentage of individuals have a genetic predisposition to macular degeneration. This form of retinal degeneration is called juvenile inherited macular degeneration and is diagnosed at a very young age. Two examples of this disorder are vitelliform dystrophy, an autosomal dominant disorder, and Stargardt disease, an autosomal recessive condition (10,11).

When developing a therapeutic approach for macular degeneration, numerous factors are taken into consideration:

1. Limiting further degeneration of the retina
2. Promoting survival of existing photoreceptors
3. Replacing photoreceptors that have degenerated
4. Restoring functional synaptic connections between the photoreceptors and inner neural retinal cells to maintain the appropriate retinal circuitry
5. Replacing dysfunctional RPE cells
6. Regulating choroidal neovascularization
7. Repairing Bruch's membrane
8. Eliminating negative effects of surgical procedures and spontaneous biochemical changes
9. Restoring vision
10. Preventing recurrence of the condition.

B. Retinitis Pigmentosa

The term retinitis pigmentosa describes a group of inherited eye diseases associated with the dysfunction of rods and cones, often characterized by night blindness. The disease affects 4 million individuals worldwide and is the leading cause of inherited blindness. RP is usually characterized by an early onset and is diagnosed in children and early adolescents. Patients with RP present with varying symptoms, such as diminished night vision (nyctalopia) and a gradual loss of peripheral vision. Central vision disturbances are not generally evident until the later stages of the disease. In RP, the affected photoreceptor cells are predominantly the light-sensitive rods. Individuals suffering from RP experience peripheral field constriction and a diminishing ability to see in dim light.

The first signs of RP are marked by attenuation of retinal arterioles and scattered brown-pigmented granules around the atrophied area. As the disease progresses, degeneration of the RPE, choriocapillaries, and photoreceptor outersegments occurs. Metabolic by-products, such as lipofuscin, accumulate and subsequently interfere with the visual transduction cascade. Changes in the RPE cells compromise the integrity of the blood-retinal barrier, and, as a consequence, subretinal leakage and macular edema ensue.

Dozens of mutations have been identified with RP in at least 10 different genes, including the genes for rhodopsin and peripherin. Given the genetic complexity of this disease, it is not surprising that research has not yet resulted in a successful mutation-based therapy for the condition. To date, there is still no effective cure for any form of retinitis pigmentosa. RP will likely benefit the most from innovative DNA-based therapies due to the current genetic information and excellent RP animal models available for this disease (12–15).

Usher syndrome is another type of retinitis pigmentosa. It is a recessively inherited condition accompanied by a loss of hearing. This condition accounts for approximately 6% of hearing impairment in deaf individuals. Sufferers may experience both a severe loss of vision and loss of hearing, a situation that increases social isolation of these individuals as auditory and visual communication progressively decreases (16).

C. Leber Congenital Amaurosis

RP is just one type of inherited disease that affects the retina. Leber congenital amaurosis (LCA) is an early-onset form of retinal degeneration characterized by severe blindness from birth or early childhood. Individuals with LCA have no detectable electroretinogram measurements because the retina is unable to respond to light (17). Only recently, a mutation in a gene called RPE65 was identified as the cause of a specific form of LCA (18). RPE65 is a product of the RPE cells and supports the function of photoreceptor cells. The gene is involved in the biochemical cascade of phototransduction and is important in converting light to neural signals. Since the LCA mutation was defined, many experiments to replace the function of the mutated RPE65 gene have been carried out in animal models. These show promise in restoring some level of vision in individuals suffering from LCA.

Other less well-defined inherited diseases that result in degeneration of the retina include:

1. Choroideremia, a disease with symptoms similar to RP but which is also accompanied by degeneration of the choroid
2. Gyrate atrophy, a retinal disease with RP-like symptoms, cataract formation, and loss of peripheral vision
3. Bardet-Biedl syndrome, a form of RP with the additional complications of mental retardation, obesity, and kidney disorders
4. Refsum syndrome, a complex disease manifesting many RP symptoms, as well as hearing impairment, neurological problems, abnormalities in red blood cells, and skin disorders
5. Bassen-Kornzweig syndrome, which involves RP complications and accompanying neurological disturbances

There are no effective treatments for any of the RP or RP-like diseases. Vitamin A supplements have been successful in slowing the progression of RP without reversing the condition. The use of vitamin A, however, has not gained wide acceptance as a treatment for retinitis pigmentosa. At the present time, advanced stages of retinal degenerations are irreparable by current pharmacological interventions. Patients suffering from advanced retinal degeneration may benefit the most from developing technologies in molecular medicine where the benefits outweigh the risks of the treatment. For the remainder of this chapter, a few of the more innovative approaches in the management of ocular diseases will be discussed, with emphasis on their relevance in treating degenerative diseases of the retina.

III. NEW THERAPEUTIC METHODS FOR RETINAL DISEASES

A. Retinal Transplants

Human retinal transplants are in the early stages of development as a therapeutic approach to retinal degenerations. The objective of this strategy is to improve vision by replacing the lost function of retinal cells. Since degeneration of the RPE and photoreceptor cells is the underlying cause of several retinal diseases, transplants of the neural retina, RPE, iris pigment epithelium (IPE), and photoreceptor cells are currently being evaluated for their potential to integrate into the retina and to permanently substitute for the function of cells they are replacing (19–25). The technology has received intense criticism as being unrealistic in its effort to improve vision. At the same time, however, it has stimulated a rapid increase in experimental studies, with both retinal and stem cells transplants. The results obtained from animal models and clinical trials of blind individuals are promising and show potential for retinal transplants as an intervention strategy that can improve and stabilize vision.

1. Animal Studies

a. RPE Transplant. An animal model of hereditary retinal degeneration, often used to study the effects of transplants in the eyes, is the Royal College of Surgeons (RCS) rats. These animals suffer from a well-characterized, early-onset form of photoreceptor cell degeneration. One of the earliest indications that grafts of human fetal RPE cells are capable of rescuing photoreceptor degeneration in RCS rats was found in a report by Little and coworkers (26). In the study, sheets of healthy fetal human RPE cells were transplanted into the subretinal space of dystrophic RCS rats that have been immunosuppressed with cyclosporine. The thickness of the outer nuclear layer (ONL), which contains the photoreceptor cells, was measured 4 weeks after transplantation. A fourfold increase in thickness of the ONL, in the area where the grafts were placed, was observed after the transplant period. Furthermore, the protected cells in the ONL were morphologically similar to their normal counterparts in healthy retinas. ONL thickness remained unchanged in areas of the retina distant from the site of transplant or in the retina of sham injected controls. This preliminary study indicates that transplanted RPE cells are capable of rescuing a significant percentage of photoreceptors from degenerating.

One question raised by many researchers in the ophthalmic field is: Are the rescued photoreceptor cells functional? Results from a follow-up study suggested that morphological as well as functional rescue of photoreceptor cells can be achieved with RPE transplants (27). Data from the study showed that a progressive central to peripheral loss of visual responsiveness occurs in pigmented dystrophic RCS rats. Recordings of single and multiunit receptive fields across the surface of the superior colliculus were used to determine the changes in visual responsiveness in the rat retinas. The potential of RPE transplants to slow down progressive loss of vision was subsequently tested in these animals by subretinal injections of healthy RPE cells into the eyes of the dystrophic RCS rats. Recordings taken 85–108 days after the transplantation procedure indicated that photoreceptor rescue occurred in the region of the graft and that the progressive central to peripheral loss of visual responsiveness in the animals was delayed by the healthy donor RPE cells. Many RPE transplant studies have now been carried out in a number of animal models, and most have confirmed the clinical potential of RPE transplants to integrate into the retina, to rescue photoreceptor cells, and to improve vision.

   b. Cograft Transplant: RPE-Retina Complex.   For transplant procedures to become clinically feasible, it is important that the transplanted tissue provide long-term benefits to blind individuals. In a study that examined the long-term survival of retinal transplants, Sharma and coworkers observed that neuronal components of retinal grafts did not survive as well as glial cells after transplant (28). They proposed that photoreceptors require contact and trophic support of the adjacent RPE cells to survive over an extended period of time. Cotransplantation of these two tissues, therefore, may be clinically more advantageous in promoting tissue survival and retina repair for diseases in which both the RPE and photoreceptor cells have degenerated. This hypothesis was supported by a recent study, which showed healthy morphology and normal cell function of RPE-retina cografts after successful transplant into the subretinal space of albino RCS rats (29). Morphological and biochemical evaluations of the transplanted tissue suggest that the photoreceptor cells in the cografts were well differentiated and capable of normal visual function (Fig. 1).

   In support of the cograft study, another group demonstrated the beneficial effects of RPE-retina cografts on photoreceptor cell morphology and function in a study using a large number of dystrophic RCS rats (30). Recordings in the superior colliculus, from areas of the retina restricted to the site of transplant, indicated that visually evoked responses were restored in the brain after cograft integration into the retina. These preliminary results are encouraging and could have only been possible if normal retinal circuitry was established by functional photoreceptor connections within the cografts.

   c. IPE Transplant.   The need for readily available tissue alternatives that can promote photoreceptor survival has led many laboratories to examine the transplant effects of the IPE in the retina. Several clinically appealing features are associated with the use of IPE transplants for retinal degenerations. These features include: (a) the IPE contains pigmented cells of the same embryological origin as the RPE cells; (b) IPE cells have a high transdifferentiation potential; (c) they can be obtained with relative ease by peripheral iridectomy; and, perhaps the most advantageous aspect of this approach, (d) the promise of functionally autologous IPE transplants in patients with retinal degeneration.

   A few studies have now demonstrated the clinical potential of IPE transplants for retinal diseases. In one of the initial experiments, IPE cells, obtained by iridectomy from Long-Evans rats, were transplanted into the choroid and subretinal space of RCS rats. The beneficial effects of the allografts were evaluated 6 months after the procedure using computer-assisted morphometric and microscopic analyses. In the transplanted rat retinas, a remarkable effect on photoreceptor survival was observed even though a high percentage of the grafted IPE cells were located in the choroid. The rescue appeared to be specific as photoreceptors were absent in the nontransplanted group (31,32). These results confirmed earlier reports suggesting that the IPE cells are capable of delaying photoreceptor degeneration (22,35), and this may be a useful alternative approach to retinal transplants (Fig. 2).

d. Autologous IPE Transplant.   Recently, the successful transplantation of autologous IPE cells in animals has made the use of IPE cells for retinal degeneration even more clinically appealing. In a study carried out with a group of 25 rabbits, autologous IPE cells were harvested by iridectomy from one eye of each rabbit and transplanted into the subretinal space of the contralateral eye. After a transplant period of 5 months, the presence of healthy IPE was observed in the rabbit's retina by light and electron microscopic examination. The IPE grafts formed a polarized monolayer above the retinal pigment epithelium and projected microvillous processes towards the photoreceptor cells. Furthermore, they appeared to be involved in the process of phagocytosis of shed photoreceptor outer segments, a biological activity associated with the RPE and one that is important to outersegment renewal. The lack of immunological side effects with the IPE transplants is of significant clinical importance (33). In addition to the experiments with rabbits, successful transplant of autologous IPE was also shown in monkey retinas. Monkey IPE cells, obtained by peripheral iridectomy, were first cultured with autologous serum and labeled with DIL prior to the experimental procedure. Labeled autologous IPE cells were subsequently transplanted into the monkey's submacular region, and the eyes were observed regularly by fluorescein angiography and fundus examination. Analysis of histological preparations, indicated that autologous IPE was present in the submacular region and that these appeared to interact with the RPE cells. Their presence was determined by the intense fluorescence of Dil-labeled IPE cells in the region. The transplanted cells stayed in the area for at least 6 months after the experiment and did not mount an immunological response in the animals (35) (Fig. 3). Autologous IPE transplants may, therefore, prove to be of significant therapeutic benefit in the treatment of retinal diseases because they are easy to obtain, are capable of RPE function, and do not promote host-graft rejection.

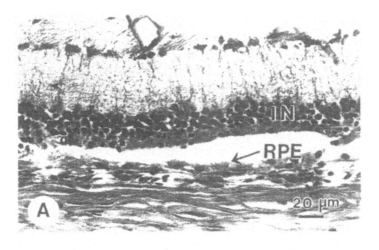

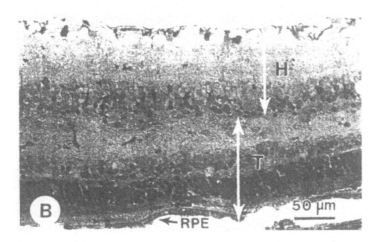

Figure 1 Albino RCS rat retinal degeneration model. This rat has a genetic defect in the RPE and needs both photoreceptors and RPE replaced. The transplants presented in B and C were achieved by transplanting sheets of fetal neural retina together with its RPE. (A) Recipient RCS rat retina, close to the transplant, age 3 months. The photoreceptor layer is almost completely degenerated, and the inner nuclear layer (IN) is immediately adjacent to the defective RPE. (Hematoxylin-Eosin staining.) (B) Reconstructed area of RCS host retina (H) by a transplant (T) of neural retina and RPE. Note the good integration between host and retinal transplant. (Toluidine blue staining.) Donor age E20, host age at time of transplantation, 2.2 months; age at time of death, 3.9 months. (From Ref. 29.)

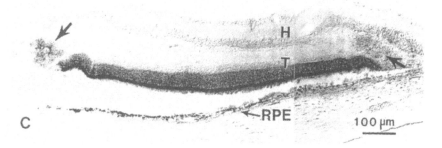

Figure 1 (C) Overview of a co-transplant. The transplanted pigmented RPE sheet can easily be seen because of the albino host. The parallel photoreceptor layer of the transplant in contact with the supporting RPE sheet shows strong immunoreactivity for the phototransduction protein rod α-transducin. Note that the photoreceptors in rosettes (arrows) at the edges of the transplant show only weak staining. (No stain in the host retina.) Host age at time of transplantation, 1.8 months; age at time of death, 3.2 months. The spaces in the section are tissue processing artifacts. (From Ref. 29.)

e. Genetically Modified Transplant. Trophic factors, released in a sustained manner by transplanted RPE cells, are known to influence the progression of hereditary retinal degeneration in the RCS rats. Examples of these are: basic fibroblast growth factor (bFGF), glial-derived neurotrophic factor (GDNF), and ciliary neurotrophic factor (CNTF), all of which have been reported to promoted photoreceptor survival and delay the progression of retinal degenerations (34).

An interesting variation in autologous IPE transplants involves the genetic engineering of IPE cells to secrete high levels of specific cytokines or growth factors, above their endogeneous levels, before transplanting them into the retina. In a study designed to test whether genetically modified cells were more potent in promoting photoreceptor survival, IPE cells were transfected with the bFGF cDNA, which was cloned into the high-expression vector pCXN2 and subsequently transplanted into the subretinal space of dystrophic RCS rats. An increase in the expression of bFGF in the retina was observed as expected, and this level correlated with prolonged photoreceptor survival as compared to the control experiments (35). The increased beneficial effects on photoreceptor cells were attributed to the soluble trophic factor secreted by the IPE cells. Genetically engineered transplants may have an advantage in prolonging cell survival by transferring therapeutic genes that have the potential to augment the intrinsic pharmacological efficacy of the transplanted cells. Gene transfer approaches for retinal degenerative diseases are discussed in more detail in Sec. III.D.

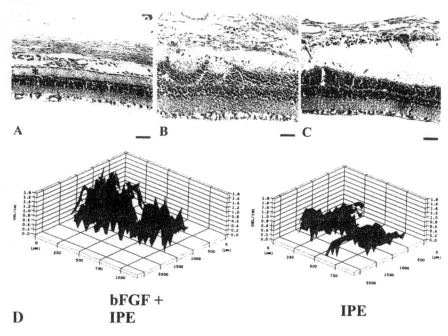

Figure 2 (A) IPE or bFGF transfected IPE cells were transplanted into the subretinal space of 21-day-old RCS rat eyes. Eyes were enucleated at 30 days after transplantation. (A) RCS rat retina; (B) IPE-transplanted retina; (C) bFGF-IPE transplanted retina. Asterisk and arrows indicate debris and transplanted bFGF-IPE, respectively. Bar = 50 μm. (D) Thickness of outer nuclear layer in bFGF-IPE or IPE transplanted retina. (Courtesy of Dr. Toshiaki Aloe, Tohoku University, Sendai, Japan.)

2. Clinical Trials

a. Human RPE Transplant. The success of the RPE and IPE transplants in animal models has prompted several pilot studies in AMD and RP patients. A surgical team of ophthalmologists at the Johns Hopkins Medical Institute recently attempted a Phase 1 clinical trial aimed at restoring vision with fetal human neural retinal transplants (36). Patients selected for the transplant had advanced cases of retinitis pigmentosa and neovascular age-related macular degeneration. The objective of the pilot study was to determine the safety of the surgical procedure, the patient's tolerance for the grafted tissue, and the visual outcome. The procedure involved surgically grafting small healthy fragments of fetal human neural retina sheets into the subretinal space of eight patients with RP and one with AMD. Recipients of the allografts were not given postoperative systemic immunosuppressive drugs. Several criteria were used to assess visual improvement after the procedure. These included, pre- and postoperative fundus photography, flourescein angiography, scanning laser ophthalmoscope (SLO), macular microperimetry, electroretinogram (ERG) recordings, and visual function testing. Safety of the procedure was demonstrated in all nine subjects, and graft-versus-host complications were not severe in any of the patients involved in the clinical trial. An improvement in light sensitivity was recorded for three of the patients in the study. However, any positive changes in the quality of vision were short-lived and disappeared a few months after the transplant procedure. Only one individual in the group, an RP patient, developed new blood vessels at the graft site. It was difficult to determine a statistically significant effect of the transplants from this initial trial since only a small cohort was tested. However, a high tolerance for grafte retinal tissue in humans was clearly demonstrated. The procedure is still in its experimental stages, but with careful modifications in surgical procedures and types of tissue selected for transplant, it may prove to be a feasible biopharmaceutic approach for preventing the loss of vision caused by degeneration of key retinal cells (36).

Adjuvant therapy using RPE transplants is another approach currently being evaluated in retinal disorders requiring surgical removal of neovascular membranes. Surgical removal of choroidal neovascular membranes is a technique used to slow down the progression of degeneration in the retina, but it can also result in a loss of RPE cells and subsequent disruption of the blood-retinal barrier. Under those conditions, vision is further compromised by additional leakage and bleeding from the choroidal blood vessels into the retinal tissue. Prior to the Johns Hopkins study, a research team from Sweden reported that disruption of the blood-retinal barrier in advanced AMD cases is highly likely to increase allograft rejection. They showed in their preliminary study that subretinal human RPE transplants were rejected in 75% of the recipients treated. Tissue rejection appeared to occur sooner (within 3 months after transplant procedures) in all cases of neovascular AMD where the blood-retinal barrier was disrupted by surgical removal of neovascular membranes. Long-term tolerance (6–20 months) of the grafted tissue was only seen in AMD patients with intact blood-retinal barrier function (37). In 1994, the same group reported that RPE transplants were well tolerated in the fovea or parafoveal regions of AMD recipients who were subjected to surgical removal of subretinal neovascular membranes. While macular edema was observed, the fetal human RPE cells survived and were capable of replacing lost RPE cells and repairing the damage caused to the retina by surgical intervention (19). While these studies were preliminary, adjuvant transplant therapy is an interesting concept worthy of more research effort. It is possible that administration of

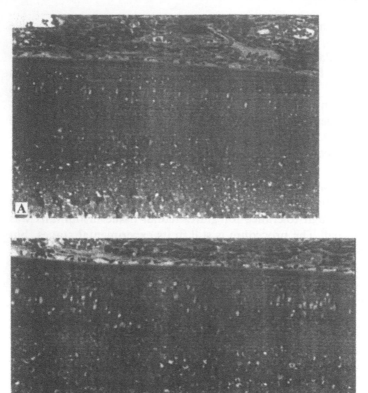

Figure 3   (A) Control: normal monkey retina; (B) autologous IPE transplant: light microscopic examination. (Courtesy of Dr. Toshiaki Aloe, Tohoku University, Sendai, Japan.)

immunosuppressive drugs after removal of CNV membranes may increase the adjuvant potential of RPE grafts.

   b. Human IPE Transplant.   The clinical efficacy of autologous IPE to improve vision after subretinal removal of neovascular membranes was evaluated in AMD patients as well. Evidence accumulated from animal studies indicated that iris pigment epithelium is easy to isolate, can integrate into the retina and substitute for RPE function, and is not associated with graft-versus-host complications. For these reasons, a pilot

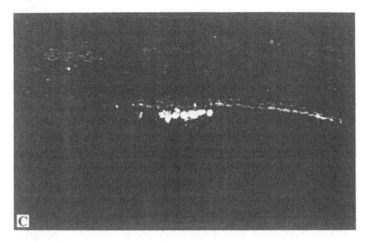

Figure 3 (C) Autologous Dil-labeled IPE transplant seen in cryostat section. Intensely fluorescent IPE cells are seen between the photoreceptors and RPE layers. (Courtesy of Dr. Tokashi Aloe, Tohoku University, Sendai, Japan.)

study was conducted using human autologous IPE to improve vision. A cohort of 20 who had neovascular membranes removed was used in this clinical trial. The transplant procedure was successful, and visual improvement was recorded for 5 patients. Thirteen individuals showed stable visual acuity, and 2 of the 20 patients experienced reduced vision with the autologous IPE transplants. Rejection of the graft and other immunologically related complications were not observed in any of the AMD recipients (38). The clinical trial points to the use of IPE transplants as a more feasible treatment option than RPE cells for retinal degenerations or for those conditions associated with a loss of RPE cells after surgery.

So far, the therapeutic efficacy of retinal transplants to improve and maintain vision remains nebulous. A significant sustained positive effect on visual function has not yet been demonstrated by any single transplantion procedure. The results from animal and human studies indicate a reasonable degree of success in graft tolerance, tissue integration, and function of the transplanted tissue, but the data are still inconclusive and the procedure is open for debate. Although these findings are promising for future efforts in the field, several technical and biological concerns still need to be addressed for the procedure to emerge as a successful and clinically relevant therapeutic approach for retinal degenerative diseases (20,23,36,39,40). Some of these concerns include:

1. Choice of tissue: As yet, retinal tissue from other species cannot be used for human transplantation purposes. Finding suitable

human alternatives that are easily accessible and functional limits current efforts in the field. Human fetal retina tissue is, perhaps, the most successful transplant treatment option for improving human vision. The cells from these tissues are not well differentiated and may contain stem cell populations with high survival potential in the eye. However, there is much controversy over the use of human fetal tissue for clinical applications, even though they may provide the best therapeutic outcomes. Adult neurons, on the other hand, are highly differentiated, do not survive as well as fetal neurons after transplant, and are not easily accessible. Autologous iris pigment epithelium has now emerged as a very attractive alternative treatment approach for retinal degenerations, but more clinical trials using this tissue need to be carried out. Neuronal cell lines may have potential because they are easy to culture and manipulate, but their high tumorigenic potential eliminates them as a viable transplant option at this time.

2. Surgical and mechanical considerations: During surgical implantation, tissues are directly grafted into the subretinal space through a small retinotomy made in a posterior incision of the sclera, underlying choroid, and peripheral retina. Retinal detachment and damage to the lens and vitreous can occur during this procedure. Severe visual loss or other ocular complications can result from the surgery. In this regard, the technique used should allow for retinal reattachment in the area of transplant in a relatively short period and small peripheral excisions that can heal without suturing. Transplantation procedures are also often followed by ocular infection, vasculitis, inflammation, and hemorrhaging in the eye (20). If substrates are used during the procedure, as shown in some animal models, they should be nontoxic, improve site-specific integration, and facilitate correct orientation of the transplants. Thickness, degradability, malleability, and permeability of the substrates are some features that affect the success of the transplant. For example, rigid substrates can introduce tears in the host tissue, leading to excessive bleeding or retinal detachment. Thin biodegradable sheets of polyglycolic and polylactic acid are reported to be optimal substrates for RPE grafts in rat retinas. They degrade easily, leaving well-established sheets of RPE cells in the correct orientation in the host retina. Transplant procedures, therefore, should seek to minimize the risk of retinal detachment, ocular injuries, or other complications that could have severe negative effect on vision.

3. Graft rejection: Rejection of grafted tissue accounts for a significant percentage of unsuccessful retinal transplants. Loss of integrity of the RPE-retina complex and the blood-retinal barrier contributes to the rejection of transplants in the retina. It is believed that nonclassical mechanisms of tissue rejection may be operative in the retina, even though this tissue is considered an immunologically privileged site. In severe retinal degenerations, however, the retina may lose its immune protective status and elicit a strong response to allogeneic transplants, with the risks being higher in older patients. Immunosuppressive therapy for nonneuronal allografts is essential but is not a requirement for neural tissues. Where autologous transplants are not possible, the use of immunosuppressive drugs in cases of severe retinal degenerations may be essential to provide increased tissue tolerance.

4. Functional retinal circuitry: Proper host integration and orientation of transplants into target retinal sites are key factors in predicting the efficacy of the transplant procedure. Improvement in vision depends on correctly integrated grafts that develop normal retinal lamination and functional synapses with the host retina. Pigmented epithelial cells are polar in nature, with specific apical and basal characteristics that are important to their function of phagocytosis and trophic influence. Transplanted dissociated RPE cells often integrate randomly into the host retina with little structural or functional polarity. They frequently wander into the subretinal space where their proliferation can promote retinal detachment or inhibit visual transduction processes. Where degeneration of the retina is localized, transplantation procedures must be refined to promote tissue integration with correct orientation and rapid reestablishment of the host retina to achieve positive visual outcome. It is difficult to determine the success of transplant integration in humans without histopathological information. So far, integration of grafted tissue and restoration of retinal circuitry have only been examined and confirmed in histological preparations of animal retinas. For morphological and histochemical evaluations, the eyes are monitored ophthalmoscopically after the transplant procedure and eyes are enucleated at various time points. Integration of tissue and expression of biological test markers are visible in the preparations using light microscopy and immunocytochemistry techniques. Lack of this information results in somewhat speculative data regarding morphological

and functional connections of human retinal transplant. Visual improvement correlates of type, site, and number of transplants, as well as sham effects on vision, are useful in determining the success of the technology.

5. Trophic influence: Growth factors, upregulated after mechanical stress to ocular tissues, have resulted in a temporary delay of retinal degenerations and a positive, transient effect on vision. In this regard, surgically induced trophic influence may account for differentiation and survival of the grafts and does not accurately reflect the clinical efficacy of the transplanted tissue. In addition, these factors may also promote neovascularization, leading to complications that further compromise vision and reduce the beneficial effects of the transplant. Therefore, appropriate measures must be taken to evaluate the secondary effects of trophic factors, induced by surgical manipulation, to obtain conclusive results to validate the efficacy of a specific transplant approach.

6. Visual improvement and stabilization: Transplanted tissues must have the ability to improve vision. Grafts must integrate, restore retinal circuitry, and perform functions required for long-term visual therapy. Morphological or biochemical alterations in the phenotype of the grafted cells can hinder the therapeutic effects of the transplant on vision recovery. Long-term survival of the grafted tissue must be ensured to maintain stabilized vision.

B. Stem Cell Transplant

Stem cells are precursor cells that can give rise to different types of tissue in an animal if placed in the right microenvironment. They have the potential to undergo symmetrical as well as asymmetrical cell division. In symmetrical division, both daughter cells retain stem cell characteristics. In asymmetrical division, a daughter cell can either maintain the stem cell identity or initiate specific differentiation processes. The latter feature is of particular interest in the field of clinical medicine as the cells could be exploited to differentiate into a specific target cell type.

In humans, stem cells have an intrinsic potential to differentiate into any of the 210 tissues making up the body. Their potential to supply human tissue is limitless and is a clinically attractive feature for tissue-replacement therapy. Research in human developmental biology has led scientists to isolate these precursor cells to study their multipotent characteristics and application to replacing lost or nonfunctional tissues in the body. Although stem cell transplantation studies in animal models have been in progress for many years, it only has been recently that their application in human diseases has been investigated.

In November 1998, Thomas and Shamblott (41,42) led the pioneering field of utilizing human embryonic stem cells for clinical applications. Their work was conducted independently using private funds because the cells used in their studies were isolated from the inner cell mass of human blastocysts stage embryos. Five immortalized cell lines were developed from the blastocysts, each with the potential to propagate indefinitely or differentiate into any adult human cell. The cell lines met the requirements to be classified as human embryonic stem cells. Since then, over 50 stem cell populations have been isolated from the human blastocysts with the potential to develop into useful cell lines.

Scientists have been encouraged by this breakthrough despite the contoversy surrounding the use of fetal tissue for developing biopharmaceuticals. The ethical dilemma stemming from embryonic stem cell study has led researchers to focus on identifying similar precursor cells in adult human tissues. Stem cell research initiatives now include the use of embryonic stem cells (ES), embryonic germ cells (EG), as well as fetal and adult stem cells. In 1999, adult neural stem cells were isolated and shown to have the potential to differentiate in several blood cell lines. These lines can grow indefinitely as precursors in the lab for all other human cells (43) and may prove to be a feasible option for fetal-derived stem cell populations.

The use of stem cells for tissue replacement or gene transfer in medicine is unlimited and offers hope for repopulating a tissue with cells that have degenerated or are dysfunctional. For example, blood stem cells from the umbilical cord show success in treatments for life-threatening diseases such as leukemia or aplastic anemia (44–46). Human bone marrow cells can be induced to differentiate into heart muscle cells, and this transdifferentiation potential of marrow cells is significant for developing new treatments for millions suffering from heart diseases (47). Stem cell transplant studies are also underway to boost a patient's immune response to infection (48).

The molecular mechanisms that drive stem cell plasticity are not clear. It is obvious, though, that mechanisms must exist to balance the self-renewal and differentiation capacities of stem cells. Molecular technologies, such as cDNA subtraction hybridization and microarray-based transcription profiling, are now available and will allow us to dissect these intricate regenerative and differentiation processes in stem cells. In fact, several conserved subsets of stem cell genes have been identified by these technologies, and they are believed to be involved with proliferative and differentiation mechanisms (49). Structural and functional characterization of these genes will increase our knowledge of how stem cells function and, perhaps, how they can be generated from differentiated tissue.

Stem cell transplantation presents unprecedented opportunities for medical advances in several life-threatening human diseases. It has the potential to treat disorders such as heart disease, diabetes, and many types of cancer. The possible use of adult stem cells to replace degenerating or lost cells in the central nervous system could revolutionize neurobiology. Neurodegenerative diseases, such as Parkinson's disease, Alzheimer's disease, amyotrophic lateral sclerosis (ALS), and retinal pathologies, are prime candidates for treatment approaches involving stem cells (50).

1. Stem Cells in the Retina

It has been generally accepted that the mature mammalian retina lacks regenerative capacity. Contrary to this belief, several laboratories have now reported that stem cell populations are present in the adult vertebrate retina and that these cells can give rise to almost all of the cell types found in the retina. Cell fate–determination studies indicate several fundamental principles associated with progression from progenitor to a specific adult retinal cell. One emerging consensus model suggests that postmitotic retinal neurons are produced during embryological development from a pool of cycling progenitors in a process that is highly organized. Both intrinsic and extrinsic regulators are believed to control cell fate choices during neurogenesis. The model proposes that progenitor retinal cells advance through intrinsically determined states, during which time they are exposed to extrinsic cell fate modifiers that influence the cells decision to differentiate into morphologically and biochemically distinct cell types (51). Events that trigger mitotically active progenitor cells to acquire cell-specific traits will remain an area of debate until currently available molecular tools are able to construct seminal renewal and differentiation pathways in stem cell function.

Studies identifying progenitor cells in the adult mammalian eye show that they exhibit properties that classify them as stem cells. They are multipotent and have self-renewing properties. They have the capacity to differentiate into several retinal specific cell types, including rod photoreceptors, bipolar neurons, and Müller glia. Quiescent cells in the pigmented ciliary margin of the adult mouse eye can clonally proliferate in vitro and form neural spheres in the presence of fibroblast growth factor 2 (FGF2). The resulting differentiated cells express molecular markers corresponding to the specific adult retinal cell type (52,53). In chicken, fish, and amphibians, a zone of mitotically active proliferating cells is found in the peripheral margin of the retina. These cells incorporate the thymidine analog BrdU and express the cell cycle regulator proliferating cell nuclear antigen (PCNA), indications of their proliferative capacity. The proliferating cells also express homeodomain transcription factors, Pax6 and Chx-10, molecular marker molecules expressed in multipotent progenitor cells. Dissociated embryonic avian retina cells reaggregate in rotating cultures and form cellular spheres with well-stratified retinal layers, a phenomenon that indicates the presence of stem cell populations. The resulting differentiated cells express markers typical of their adult counterpart in the retina (54–58). These discoveries are biomedically relevant to transplantation strategies, in which retinal precursor cells are essential to replace degenerating retinal cells. Macular degeneration and retinitis pigmentosa are two diseases that could benefit from these findings.

2. Stem Cell Transplant Therapy in the Retina

With this recent knowledge, stem cell populations, derived from a number of human organs, are being evaluated for their pluripotency in models of ocular diseases. Already the transplantation of adult rat hippocampus-derived neural stem cells (AHPCs), into ischemic retina has proven to be successful. In this exciting study, AHPCs were shown to have the capacity to differentiate into cells with retina-specific characteristics. When hippocampal stem cells were injected into the eyes of adult rats subjected to ischemic reperfusion injury, the cells were shown to integrate well into the injured host retinas and expressed morphological and biochemical characteristics of specific retinal cell types, as observed in histochemical preparations (59). A similar experiment was performed to test the plasticity of retrovirally engineered AHPCs in the retina of adult and newborn rat eye. Integration into the host retina was seen 4 weeks after intravitreal injection of the genetically modified AHPCs. The cells developed characteristics of photoreceptors, Müllers, amacrine, bipolar, horizontal, and astroglia at the site of injection and were found in the correct spatial orientation in the retinal layer. They expressed some, but not all, of the features of the specific adult retinal cell, possibly because of the absence of early developmental cues of retinal neurogenesis (60). Long-term therapeutic benefits of stem cells were also shown for other eye tissues. For example, success in ocular surface reconstruction and corneal wound healing was observed after limbal stem cell allotransplants and amniotic membrane transplants in patients with limbal stem cell deficiency or corneal damage (61,62).

There are limitations, however, to the use of stem cells for clinical applications. One major disadvantage is that stem cells tend to spontaneously differentiate in culture and lose their multipotent characteristics. A homogeneous population of stem cells is difficult to maintain in vitro. Cultures often contain multiple cell types because of spontaneous differentiation in many biochemical directions. Some labs have transfected selection markers, such as the gene for green fluorescent protein (GFP), into cultured stem cells as an effective way to ensure that only undifferentiated cells expressing the marker will be selected for transplantation studies. Undifferentiated cells are easily identified with this approach, as only the spontaneously differentiated cells will downregulate the fluorescent marker molecule (63). These investigations offer unique conceptual and therapeutic perspectives that can be developed clinically as alternate approaches to interrupt the pathological consequences of genetic or acquired insults to the retina.

C. Retinal Prosthesis

The goal of retinal prosthesis is to restore vision by using highly sophisticated, miniaturized electronic devices (64–78). In the normal retina, the function of the photoreceptors is to initiate a neural signal in response to light. The neural signal stimulates synapsing bipolar and horizontal cells and is transmitted through the retina and output ganglion cells to the optic nerve for interpretation in the brain. In retinal diseases in which photoreceptor function is lost, the retina becomes insensitive to light and visual signals cannot be transmitted. For this reason, RP patients may still suffer from blindness despite an intact optic nerve connection to the brain. In the early stages of many degenerative retinal diseases, the inner retinal layer is often spared, leaving healthy ganglion cells connected to the brain through the optic nerve. Retinal prostheses are constructed to take advantage of these intact neural connections. The electronic devices respond to light and generate signals that electronically stimulate the spared ganglion cells, thereby activating the visual system. In this regard, the technology aims to replace the function of the photoreceptor cells that have degenerated. Two types of retinal prosthetic devices, subretinal and the epiretinal implants, have shown relative success as surgical implants capable of transmitting neural signals. A brief overview of the potential of these implants is presented below.

1. Subretinal Implant

Subretinal prosthetics are surgically implanted in the subretinal space located between the RPE and photoreceptor cells. In this location, it is hoped that current generated by the implant in response to light stimulation will alter the membrane potential of healthy inner retinal neurons and subsequently activate the visual system. The aim of this treatment is to mimic photoreceptor cell function in the visual transduction cascade.

Early efforts to use subretinal implants for this purpose have not shown significant success because of technical and microsurgical limitations associated with the technology. Stability and biocompatibility of the implants in the retina have also been factors limiting the development of successful retinal prosthesis technology. In efforts to minimize these limitations, semiconductor technology consisting of thousands of silicon microphotodiode arrays has been introduced as a new subretinal prosthetic approach (64,68–71,73,74). Chow and coworkers (74) were able to show reasonable success using semiconductor-based photodiodes to perform photoreceptor function. In their initial studies, the device was surgically implanted into the subretinal space of rabbits through a posterior retinotomy. The array was placed in close proximity to surviving horizontal and bipolar cells in the retina and was sensitive to both visible and infrared light. No external power supply was used with the device. Infrared stimuli were used to distinguish between implant- and native photoreceptor–mediated response. Recordings and histological examination of the retina indicated that the implants maintained a stable, functional position in the subretinal space. Data obtained from electrophysiological recordings showed that the microphotodiode arrays generated current in response to light, and this was transmitted through the output ganglion cells to the brain. A major setback to the study was the significant degeneration of retinal cells in the area of the implant. This was due to the fact that nutrients from the choriocapillaris were unable to reach the retina because of the nonpermeable nature of the gold electrode–based implant. The remainder of the retina architecture remained intact, and other side effects were not promoted by the implants. The construction of devices that would minimize blockage of nutrients to the retina is a current focus in the field.

2. Epiretinal Implant

Efforts to develop an independently functioning epiretinal device for patients with outer retina degeneration are also promising for restoring simple basic visual perception (67,72,75–78). It is a similar concept to the subretinal prosthesis. Epiretinal devices are constructed, however, to utilize the output capacity of spared ganglion cells to transmit the signals they generate to activate the visual system. They are designed to rest on the inner surface of the retina rather than being implanted in the subretinal space, where they can utilize the functional output potential of the ganglion cells and optic nerve to stimulate the visual cortex (Fig. 4).

The advantage of the epiretinal approach over subretinal implants is that the ganglion cells can be easily stimulated because of their accessibility in the inner surface of the retina. These implants have shown success in an

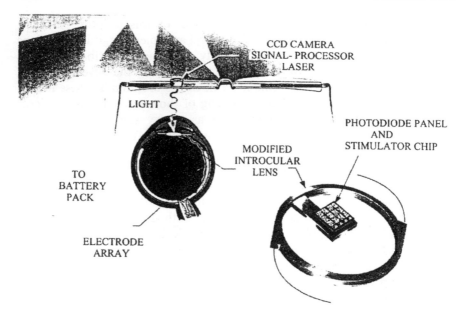

Figure 4 Patients with retinitis pigmentosa and macular degeneration become blind when the rods and cones degenerate and no longer convert incoming light into electrical impulses. While other parts of the retina remain healthy, the brain stops receiving impulses required to provide vision. The retinal prosthesis is designed to bypass the lost rods and cones and directly stimulate the surviving ganglion cells that are connected to the brain through the optic nerve. Specially designed glasses capture the visual scene and transmit this information into the eye through an invisible laser beam. The laser strikes a solar panel (photodiode array) located within the pupil to generate internal power. An ultra-thin electrode array carries the power to the retinal surface, where it stimulates the ganglion cells. (Courtesy of Dr. Joseph F. Rizzo, Harvard University, USA.)

initial study that used flat platinum microelectrode arrays, embedded in a thin film of polyimide, as implants. The device was stabilized onto the inner retina surface of cat eyes using cyanoacrylate adhesive. Recordings of neuronal activities in the visual cortex indicated electrical responses to retinal stimulation experiments. Neither retinal detachment nor intraocular inflammatory responses were observed after prolonged periods of implantation (75). The retina microelectronic prosthetic field has expanded considerably in the last 5 years. Initial studies are exciting, and even though ambitious, the method is proving to be a feasible approach to restoring vision. Several types of retinal prosthesis have now been used to electrically stimulate the visual system to produce flashes of visual perception in blind individuals.

The technology is available for modification and microfabrication of less complex, sophisticated devices that promise hope for mechanically restoring vision. The challenges, however, that face the technology are numerous and formidable. Major obstacles facing the visual prosthesis technology include (65–68,71,77):

1. Establishing a functional connection between the implant, the neural retina and the brain
2. Detachment of the retina during microsurgical implantation
3. Inflammatory reactions of the retina against the implanted devices
4. Ocular infection following implantation procedures
5. Rejection of the electronic device
6. Wiring the retinal surface and maintaining mechanical stability of an epiretinal or subretinal implant
7. Epiretinal devices may stimulate formation of retinal surface membranes, which, in turn, could dislodge the implant and create an electrical resistance between the electrodes and the target output cell
8. Subretinal implants could stimulate the RPE cells to migrate into the retina, causing fibrosis, or impede the transport of nutrients and trophic factors from the choriocapillaris to the retina, resulting in further degeneration of the retina
9. Surviving photoreceptor cells could degenerate at the site of subretinal implants because the devices may block choroidal circulation to the outer retina.

It is possible that photoreceptor function could be replaced by retinal prosthesis? Could microelectronic devices establish a long-term functional connection between the inner retina and the brain? Could vision be restored to the blind? The preliminary studies have suggested that the use of retinal prosthesis to restore visual loss is possible if the mechanical and surgical limitations are reduced, precise electrical stimulation and integration with the brain are achieved, and long-term biocompatibility of the implants with the retina is attained. At the present time, however, the clinical usefulness of visual microelectronic prosthesis still remains at a conceptual level.

D. Gene Therapy

Millions of years of evolution have been dedicated to the development of efficient viral delivery systems for transfer of genes within and across species. Viruses have developed highly sophisticated mechanisms for cellular tropism and nuclear targeting. In the host cell they replicate by using the host transcription and translation machinery to express, replicate, package, and release their genetic material to infect surrounding tissues. Many viruses have developed strategies to recombine with and stably integrate their genetic material into the host genome. Others do not integrate into the host DNA but replicate their genetic material as episomes.

These viral properties have specific advantages in gene therapy, and considerable interest has been expressed in utilizing the natural biological properties of viruses in molecular medicine. The groundbreaking discovery by Hershey and Chase in 1952 (79) that DNA is the genetic material, followed by the elucidation of the double helix and the genetic code (80,81), were keys to the subsequent characterization of viral and cellular genomes. These discoveries led to an increased understanding of the genetic disposition of many human diseases and an explosion in gene identification and characterization. The genetic basis of many human diseases will continue to expand with the completion of the Human Genome Project and, with it, a rapid increase in the formulation of novel therapeutic approaches for many diseases.

Several DNA-based therapies, using both viral and nonviral delivery systems, have been developed and show varying degrees of success in clinical trials. These represent a significant percentage of current strategies in clinical trials, especially in the area of cancers. It is interesting to read the earlier literature on the possible application of gene therapy in humans and the potential problems arising from the technology. For example, it was initially thought that the success of gene therapy would be dependent on its potential to correct the genetic defect in every cell associated with a particular disease. This assumption is no longer valid, as studies have now shown that even transient expression of some therapeutic genes in a small percentage of target cells is sufficient to slow the progression of a disease. Many concerns still surround the technology, and many questions still remain unanswered, but there is great optimism for the future of DNA-based therapies, especially for diseases that are currently incurable. In this section, I will present an overview of gene therapy applications, with emphasis on this approach as a practical treatment modality for retinal degenerations.

1. Gene Therapy Applications

Each individual carries a number of defective genes unknown to the carrier unless the disease symptoms are expressed. This is because each of us carries two copies of nearly all genes—one inherited from our mother and the other from our father. The exception to this are genes located on the Y chromosome, found only in males. In many cases if we carry only one defective copy of a gene, the other, normal copy will assume the function of its defective counterpart, and its expression alone will be sufficient to mask the symptoms of the diseases. Such a gene and the associated disease are referred to as "recessive." An individual carrying such a gene is considered a "carrier." The disease phenotype will only develop if both copies of the gene are defective in the same individual. The gene for sickle cell anemia is an example of a recessive gene. The disease affects the normal function of the red blood cells and is inherited as an autosomal recessive trait. In other cases, a single defective copy of a gene alone can cause expression of the disease phenotype. These genes are referred to as "dominant." An example of such a disease is Huntington's disease, which is inherited as an autosomal dominant disease affecting the nervous system.

Not all defective genes produce harmful effects. The environment in which a gene operates contributes to its function. Some defective genes may actually provide us with a selective advantage of survival in a particular environment. For example, if both copies of the sickle cell gene are defective in a person, a defective blood protein is produced and that individual will suffer from the disease. If only one copy of the gene is defective, the individual is a carrier of the disease but does not express the disease symptoms. A remarkable feature of the sickle cell gene is that a person carrying one defective copy is resistant to infection by malaria parasites and, therefore, possesses a distinct survival advantage in environments where malaria is endemic.

Approximately 1 in 10 individuals has or will develop an inherited genetic disorder. Some diseases are caused by more than one defective gene, while others are the result of a single defective gene. Hundreds of specific disease conditions caused by mutations in only one gene have been identified. These are referred to as single gene disorders, or monogenic diseases, and are currently the best targets for gene therapy. Cystic fibrosis is a monogenic disease in which a mutation in a single gene results in the disease phenotype. Other diseases, such as retinitis pigmentosa, a retinal degenerative disease causing blindness, are complex and are associated with genetic defects in a number of genes. These are referred to as polygenic disorders. Replacement of a single defective gene that contributes to this phenotype may not necessarily result in curing the disease but may slow down its progression.

Theoretically, if defective genes are prevented from producing defective proteins and a normal functioning protein can be put back into the tissue, a disease phenotype should be reversed or the disease progression slowed. This very simplistic assumption is the basis of gene therapy—the introduction of genetic material into an affected cell to correct an existing disorder or to introduce a new function into cells with resulting therapeutic benefits.

A disease may result from the production of a defective protein or the overexpression, underproduction, or absence of a normal protein. Of all the therapies currently on the horizon, perhaps the most tantalizing of them are ones that will repair a single mutated gene or that will replace its defective function. A target cell could also be provided with a new function that allows it to fight off a disease or infection. The goal of gene therapy is not only to introduce a therapeutic gene into diseased tissue, but also to control its level of expression with a precision not likely to be achieved using other methods and to cure or retard the progression of the disease after a single administration of the gene. Current applications of gene transfer technology aim to:

1. Replace the defective gene in recessive diseases
2. Inactivate a gene in dominant diseases
3. Express a cell rescue factor
4. Express a protein that will inhibit the progression of a disease
5. Augment or downregulate the activity of an existing gene
6. Transfer "suicide" or "toxic" genes that mediate apoptotic events that will selectively kill unwanted proliferating cells
7. Modulate the immune system in an effort to ward off the disease
8. Transfer drug-resistant genes
9. Confer sensitivity to an inert prodrug
10. Interrupt the life cycle of an infectious disease

At the present time, gene therapy approaches will probably be most successful in diseases where patients are unable to synthesize a specific protein and where the target gene is introduced into a single organ. If the target tissue is somatic, the effects that result from the gene transfer intervention will only occur in the individual undergoing the therapy. In contrast, germ line therapy will not only affect the individual being treated, but will also be evident in the offspring of that person. Germ line gene therapy has the potential to eliminate many crippling hereditary disorders, however, it is ethically unacceptable at this stage and may not be attempted until the hurdles of somatic gene manipulations have been successfully dealt with. While many limitations exist for gene therapy, a wide range of human diseases, both familial and nonfamilial, are good candidates for this approach.

2. The Retina as a Candidate Tissue for Gene Therapy

Ophthalmic involvement in the genetic basis of retinal disease has increasingly advanced due to the recent explosion in biotechnology. Ocular pathologies have been recognized for centuries, but many are now being reclassified as their genetic etiologies undergo intense investigation at the molecular level. This increases the potential for developing new DNA-based treatments for inherited and acquired eye diseases.

The etiologies of blinding diseases, such as AMD, are often obscured by secondary complications and therefore diagnosed at a late stage when adjacent ocular tissues are also affected. The impact of gene transfer intervention may be significant in the management of such diseases as we continue to understand early promoting mechanisms underlying their progression. Prerequisites for effective DNA-based intervention in the eye include:

1. Knowledge of the etiology of the disease
2. Characterization of the gene(s) associated with the disease
3. Effective delivery of the therapeutic gene
4. Low toxicity and immunological tolerance of the gene transfer vector
5. Targeting transgenes to the specific affected area in the eye
6. Expression of the delivered gene at a therapeutic level
7. Long-term gene expression for reversing or correcting the disease

Diseases of the retina are good targets for gene transfer approaches. Visual function hinges on two critical layers of the retina: the outer nulcear layer, which contains the photoreceptor cells, and the retinal pigment epithelium, which lies adjacent to the photoreceptors. The relationships between the RPE and photoreceptor cells is critical not only to normal function but also to the pathology of several blinding hereditary diseases, including retinitis pigmentosa, Leber's congenital amaurosis, and macular degeneration.

Delivery of a therapeutic product to the RPE and photoreceptor cells is likely to be most successful if the delivery system is designed to target those specific cells. Because of the many compartments and structural complexity of the eye, it is easy for innoculated material to get trapped and diffused in any of the eye spaces and cell layers, reducing the availability of the transgene to target sites. In addition, the expression of certain genes is controlled through spatial and temporal regulation. Administration of high vector titers is, therefore, necessary to achieve reasonable levels of gene expression at the target site for attenuation of the disease. Attempts are currently underway to minimize widespread effects of an exogenous gene by using tissue- or cell-specific promoters to achieve regionally restricted gene transfer.

Some of the most widely used vectors in ocular gene delivery include the retrovirus, the adenovirus, and adeno-associated viruses. The choice of viral vectors, the design of efficient delivery systems, and the development of well-characterized animal models of retinal diseases are key elements for gene therapy to be successful in ocular pathologies.

3. Viral Vectors

Advances in genetic engineering and recombinant DNA technology have made it possible to use viruses as clinical tools to transfer therapeutic genes to treat human diseases. Viruses have developed effective mechanisms that promote their survival and replication in a host cell. These intrinsic mechanisms allows them to (a) evade host immune surveillance, (b) attach to the cell membrane, invade the cell, and enter the nucleus, and (c) direct the host cell replication machinery to allow viral multiplication. They are armed with features that meet gene therapy criteria. Research in the development of gene transfer vectors has, thus, focused on the use of these viral properties to facilitate the delivery of therapeutic genes to the nucleus of the cell where the genes can be amplified and expressed.

Hundreds of viruses have been identified and their genome and structure well characterized. This knowledge has allowed researchers to select those viruses with high tropism and low toxicity for the use in gene therapy. Many viruses, however, can only infect a limited number of cell types. Some viruses are pathogenic and will elicit a strong host immune response due to the production of viral proteins required for infectivity, major disadvantages to current gene therapy protocols. Other criteria essential to using a viral-based delivery system for therapeutic DNA include:

1. Stable gene transfer and expression
2. Long-term gene expression where a therapeutic product is needed to attenuate the disease
3. The use of replication-deficient viral vectors
4. Minimal intrinsic toxicity of the input vector and other associated pharmacological toxicity
5. High efficiency of transfection—a critical number of the transgene must enter a sufficient number of affected cells to elicit a significant biological response
6. Optimization of the delivery system to limit reinoculation
7. Use of vectors that do not result in insertional mutagenesis by activating oncogenes or by inactivating of other essential genes

Genetic engineering designs to improve the safety and efficiency of viral gene transfer aim to manipulate the host immune system to reduce immunological response to viral proteins, minimize infection by impairing the viral replication machinery to limit the viral particle to a single infectious cycle, and modify viral tropism and increase viral target specificity by altering viral envelope proteins. Designing second-generation viruses with decreased pathogenicity and high infectivity will increase the success of gene therapy in biomedical research.

A recombinant viral vector can be constructed by cutting the viral DNA and the gene of interest at specific sites with a restriction enzyme. The cut pieces are subsequently ligated with a DNA ligase to create a recombinant vector. Before the cutting and ligation procedure, the viral genome is first modified to remove key regulatory genes. This will render the virus replication deficient once it infects a host cell and create enough space for ligation of the new gene. Other accessory genes may be removed from the viral DNA to make the vector less immunogenic. Transfection of the recombinant viral genome into *trans*-complementing cells lines, stably transformed with the deleted regulatory coding cassettes from the viral genome, allows for replication and packaging of the recombinant viral DNA in vitro. Administration of a titer of recombinant virus obtained by this method should result in viral infection of the target tissue and expression of the inserted gene without viral replication or production of infectious progeny viruses in vivo (Fig. 5) (82,83).

a. Retrovirus. Retroviruses are RNA viruses that infect a wide variety of eukaryotic cells. The retroviral genome codes for three core genes—gag, pol, and env—which are flanked on either side by a long-term repeat (LTR) sequence (Fig. 6). The gag gene, located in the 5' region of the genome, encodes the viral core proteins. The pol gene is the second gene in the cassette and codes for three products: reverse transcriptase (RT), which allows the viral RNA to be transcribed into DNA after entry into a host cell; viral integrase (Int), which facilitates integration of viral DNA into the host DNA; and viral protease, which acts on the viral core proteins. The env gene is 3' of the pol gene and encodes the glycosylated viral envelope proteins, which determine the tropism of the virus.

The LTRs flank both ends of the genome and contain *cis*-acting sequences that regulate viral replication, transcription, and integration into the host genome. A packaging signal, which facilitates assembly of viral particles, is found immediately 3' of the 5' LTR. When a retrovirus infects a cell, its RNA is reversed-transcribed into DNA by RT. The DNA subsequently integrates into the host chromosome as a provirus and directs the synthesis of viral proteins by the host transcription and translation machinery. While most retroviruses are nonpathogenic, a few have been known to cause cancer. For example, the Rous sarcoma virus causes tumors of the connective tissue in chickens. The tumorigenic properties of these viruses have been associated with accessory genes called oncogenes.

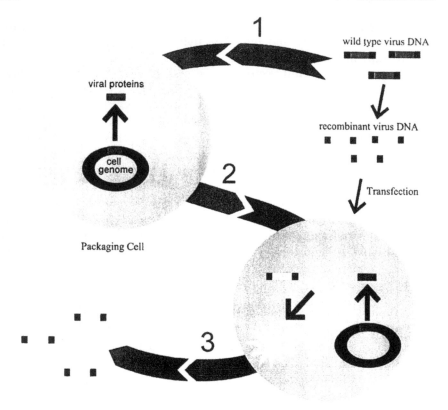

Figure 5   Viral packaging: (1) transfection of the vital genome into the packaging cell to produce viral proteins; (2) transfection of recombinant viral DNA into the *trans* complementing packaging cell line and replication of the viral DNA; (3) release of infectious particles.

The most common retroviral vector used for gene transfer is the Moloney murine leukemia virus (MoMuLV). The viral genome is modified by deleting the three core genes—gag, pol, and env—before recombination with the target gene. The deleted segment of the viral genome is then replaced with the therapeutic gene of interest, and the recombinant vector can be grown to therapeutic titers by transfecting it into a suitable packaging cell line that has been stably transformed with the deleted viral core gene cassette. Replication and viral assembly proceed similar to infection with a wild-type virus (84–86). Recombinant viruses maintain their high targeting efficiency and stably integrate into the host genome. While long-

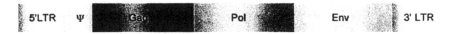

Figure 6 Schematic representation of a basic retrovirus genome showing the age, pol, and env genes, which are flanked by the long-terminal repeats (LTR). A packaging signal (ψ) is located next to the 5' LTR.

term gene expression is increased with stable integration, the potential risk of activating protooncogenes or inactivating essential host genes at the site of host genome integration are concerns when using this vector is gene therapy approaches.

New engineering technologies are being developed to modify the tropism of retroviruses by altering the envelope proteins. Such modifications are designed to facilitate the cell-specific targeting by the virus. Retroviruses, however, do not infect postmitotic cells. They require the active process of mitosis for entry into the nucleus, a feature that does not make them a suitable delivery system for post-mitotic tissues. The use of retroviral vectors in gene transfer therapies is also limited because of the size of the transgene insert that they can package and the low viral titers obtained in vitro. Currently, therapeutic genes larger than 9–10 kb cannot be stably cloned into the retroviral genome (Table 1). In addition to these limitations, murine retroviruses are sensitive to inactivation by the human complement lysis–mediated pathway. Current research to minimize this sensitivity is focused on the use of human packaging cells lines or modification of the viral envelope proteins to produce complement-resistant retroviral pseudotypes. Despite these constraints, retroviruses are still the most widely used vectors in current gene delivery systems and account for approximately 40% of all gene therapy–related clinical trials. Stable expression of many therapeutic genes delivered by retroviruses has been observed for periods of over one year.

Several studies have shown a clinical potential of retroviruses as a gene delivery vehicle in the eye. In one report, modified retroviruses encoding either a urokinase-type plasminogen activator (u-PA) or a tissue-type plasminogen activator (t-PA) gene was successfully transfected into human RPE cell cultures. Ten weeks after infection, transfected cells were co-cultured with umbilical vein endothelial cells (HUVECs) and their effects on cell proliferation and wound healing assessed. Both transgenes were observed to express large amounts of biologically active products in the RPE cells. The expression of u-PA promoted HUVEC cell proliferation and wound healing, while t-PA or the control, noninfected RPE cells in nonconfluent cultures had no significant effect. Other retroviral constructs, designed to carry an internal opsin promoter fragment, were able to specifically direct

Table 1 Comparison of Vectors for Gene Therapy

	Structure	Advantages	Disadvantages
Viral vectors			
Retrovirus	Enveloped Genome size ~ 10 kb	Moderate gene transfer efficiency Long-term gene expression	Integrates into host DNA titer ~ 10^8–10^9 Insertional mutagenesis Infect replicating cells only Insert capacity ~ 9–10 kb
Adenovirus	Nonenveloped Genome size ~ 36 kb	High gene transfer efficiency Infects quiescent and replicating cells High titer ~ 10^{11}–10^{12} kb	Nonintegrating Transient expression Immunogenic Insert capacity < 7 kb
Adeno-associated virus (AAV)	Nonenveloped Genome size ~ 4.7 kb	High gene transfer efficiency Infects quiescent and replicating cells Long-term gene expression	Integrates into host DNA Insertional mutagenesis titer ~ 10^9–10^{10} Contamination with helper virus Insert capacity ~ 4.5 kb
Herpes simplex virus (HSV)	Enveloped Genome size ~ 152 kb	Large insert capacity ~ 150 kb Infects quiescent cells	Nonintegrating titer ~ 10^8–10^9
Non viral vectors			
Liposome		Nonreplicating Accommodate large therapeutic genes	Low gene transfer efficiency
DNA complexes or naked DNA			Low gene transfer efficiency

gene expression in retinal photoreceptor cells after transduction of the cells (87,88). The use of retroviruses to transfer genes that modify the angiogenic potential of RPE cells or to rescue degenerating photoreceptor cells shows potential for gene therapeutic applications in retinal diseases associated with these processes.

Retrovirus-mediated transfer of "suicide genes" has also been tested in several ocular disease models to determine transduction efficiency of the virus and feasibility of this approach as a treatment strategy. In one study, an animal model that developed posterior capsule opacification (PCO) was used to test the effect of the suicide gene, HSV-tk, and the subsequent sensitivity of the transduced cells to ganciclovir (GCV). PCO is a major complication of cataract surgery and develops from hyperplasia of the lens epithelium following phacoemulsification. Retrovirus-mediated transfer of the suicide gene, herpes simplex virus thymidine kinase (HSV-tk), into rabbit lens epithelial cells resulted in efficient transduction of the gene after in vitro and in vivo administration. While the transduced cells were reported to be sensitive to GCV treatment after transduction, capsule opacification was not attenuated. The study, however, shows promise for the use of retroviruses to transfect lens epithelial cells. In this case, modification of the vector to increase sensitivity to GCV may be required for successful alleviation of PCO (89).

A similar experiment was performed in vitro using human RPE cells (HRPE), a major component of the membranes found in proliferative vitreoretinopathy (PVR). In PVR, the RPE cells, fibroblasts, and other proliferating cells form contractile membranes in the vitreous cavity of the eye, which result in traction retinal detachment. The study was aimed to test the transduction efficiency of HSV-tk recombinant retroviral vector and the bystander effect after treatment with GCV as a possible treatment strategy for PVR. Stable transfection of HRPE and fibroblast cells and a strong bystander effect after GCV treatment were reported in vitro (90). Transduction of the cells in experimental PVR-induced rabbits was lower compared to the number of cells transduced in vitro, but a strong bystander effect was observed for HSV-tk–positive cells along with a significant reduction in the severity of PVR in the animals (91,92). Human and rabbit keratinocytes were also stably transduced by retroviral-mediated transfer of HSV-tk gene in a study that tested the efficacy of this treatment in corneal wound healing after superficial keratectomy. Topical application of supernatant containing the vector was administered after superfiical stromal keratectomy in rabbits. Transduction of the rabbit keratinocytes was confirmed, with an efficiency of approximately 20–40%. Corneal stromal haze and scarring were significantly reduced after postoperative application of topical GCV (93).

Polycations, such as polybrene and protamine sulfate, were reported to significantly improve the transduction efficiency of the gene transfer into keratocytes (93).

Other genes have been successfully transferred by retroviruses into cells that are involved with retinal neovascularization. For example, retroviral-mediated transfer of tissue inhibitor of metalloproteinase-2 (TIMP-2) into bovine choroidal cells resulted in the production of biologically active TIMP-2 and a subsequent increase in angiogenic response to VEGF (94,95). Adjuvant anti-angiogenic gene transfer in diabetic retinopathy, a major cause of acquired blindness associated with retinal neovascularization and subsequent traction retinal detachment, into photocoagulation sites of the retina shows feasibility for retroviral-mediated gene therapy in this disorder (96). While photocoagulation therapy delays visual loss, it does not prevent progression to blindness. These innovative approaches indicate the versatile potential of retrovirus-mediated gene transfer to attenuate PVR, to modulate corneal wound-healing mechanisms, and as possible treatments for choroidal and retinal neovascularization.

b. Adenovirus.   Increased clinical interest has focused on adenoviruses as vectors for gene transfer because of their broad host range infectivity in both postmitotic and proliferating cells. Forty-seven different serotypes of human adenoviruses have been identified with a range of primary target site of infection, including the respiratory epithelium, eye, gastrointestinal, and urinary tract cells. Adenoviruses are currently the viral gene delivery vehicle of choice for many retinal disease–related protocols.

Structurally, adenoviruses are not bound by an envelope like the retroviruses. They are encapsulated by a protein shell, which forms an icosahedral capsid structure around the DNA inner core. The capsid contains three groups of proteins: (a) the hexons, which are structural proteins that associate as trimers called hexomers (trimeric hexons arrange on the planes of the icosahedral structure of the virus); (b) the pentons, which associate as pentomers and penton complexes to form the 12 vertices of the icosahedrons; (c) the fibers, which assemble as trimeric fibers and associate with the penton vertices to form protruding spikes. The penton and fiber subunits constitute the infection machinery of the adenovirus. The protruding trimeric fibers mediate the initial attachment of the virus to cell surface receptors. Subsequent internalization of the virus is mediated by its pentameric base and the integrins on the cell surface (97). A new class of artificial, silk-like fibrous material is being evaluated in efforts to improve adenoviral tropism.

The adenovirus genome is a single linear double-stranded DNA molecule approximately 36 kb in length. The genome is divided into two functional noncontiguous, overlapping domains, which contain early (E1A, E1B, E2, E3, E4) and late (L1–L5) expressed genes. The regions are so defined because of the onset time of transcription of the viral genes after entry of the viral DNA into the host cell nucleus. The early and late genes are flanked by inverted terminal repeats (ITRs) that are important to replication of the viral genome and an encapsidation signal, located adjacent to the 5′ ITR, that is essential for viral packaging (98). Deletion of nonessential viral genes, such as the E1 genes, generates a replication-deficient viral vector into which a passenger gene can be inserted. The size of foreign DNA that can be packaged by the virus after E1 deletion is approximately 7.8 kb. The small DNA packaging size of the virus limits its use as vector for the transfer of larger therapeutic genes. E1 genes are the first to be transcribed upon entry of the viral DNA into the nucleus because their products are essential to initiate expression of other key viral replication genes. Deletion of the E1 gene cassette, therefore, interrupts the virus infectious cycle by disabling the replication, assembly, and packaging machinery of the virus. Furthermore, modification to the viral genome limits the recombinant vector to one cycle of infection. Using recombinant DNA technology, the deleted viral function can be rescued by transfecting the modified recombinant vector into transformed E1 complementing packaging cells that constitutively express E1 gene products. The recombinant replication-deficient virus can then be grown and concentrated to the high titers required for therapeutic doses. After transfection into the target host cell, replication of the adenovirus DNA is independent of the host cell replication. The viral DNA rarely integrates into the host genome and resides as an episome in the nucleus, a feature that makes adenoviruses a safe gene transfer vector because oncogene activation and gene toxicity are minimized. Transgene expression usually occurs within 24 hours of inoculation and can be determined by assays, such as polymerase chain reaction (PCR), ELISA, Western, and Northern blotting technology (99,100).

The clinical advantages that makes this an attractive vehicle for gene transfer include the relative ease with which the viral genome can be manipulated to generate stable recombinants, low pathogenicity, and generation of high viral titers in vitro. Major concerns that limit the use of adenovirus-based vectors include transient gene expression, limited size of the transgene insert, and immunogenicity. Thus far, gene delivery using retroviruses has proven to be very efficient, but long-term gene expression is relatively poor (Table 1) and is often caused by the pathology at the site of gene transfer, which could promote the loss of transduced cells in the region. Repeated administration of the recombinant vector is not advisable because of the high immunogenicity of the viral proteins. Therefore, improvements in vector design to produce less immunogenic, second-generation adenoviruses or ones that can evade the host immune response will be significant advancements in the use of this vector in broad-scale gene therapy.

Adenoviral vectors can infect a few retinal cells, including RPE. They have not been reported to be infectious agents for normal mature photoreceptor cells but successfully transduce developing or degenerating photoreceptor neurons. Adenoviruses are widely used in gene therapy protocols in animal models of retinal degenerations. For example, a recombinant adenovirus carrying the wild-type β subunit of the cGMP gene has shown efficiency of transfection and transient rescue of degenerating photoreceptors in the rd mice. Protection of RPE cells against hemoglobin toxicity has also been observed after infection with an adenoviral vector encoding the human heme oxygenase (HO-1) gene. Heme oxygenase is an antioxident produced by RPE cells. Transfected RPE cells overexpressed the HO-1 gene product more than threefold compared to nontransfected cells and showed increased survival rates (93%) compared to controls (65–75%) when challenged with hemoglobin (101). Adenovirus-mediated transfer of HO-1 may be of clinical relevance in retinal pathologies requiring cellular antioxidant defense mechanisms.

In addition, adenoviral-mediated transfer of genes encoding trophic factors has proved to be a useful strategy in promoting photoreceptor survival. Limitations of intraocular administration with therapeutic doses of soluble trophic factors are often associated with the pharmacokinetics of the gene product and the need for multiple injections for effective long-term beneficial changes to the retina. In this regard, transfer of neuroprotective and antiangiogenic genes into the retina may be a more efficient approach than direct injection of some soluble survival factors into the eye (102,103). We have identified a 50 kDa neurotrophic protein, pigment epithelium-derived factor (PEDF), secreted by RPE cells, which is widely shown to have neuroprotective and antiangiogenic activities (102,104,105). Injections with the soluble protein have shown enormous therapeutic potential of PEDF to inhibit neovascularization and promote photoreceptor survival. However, a single administration of adenoviral-mediated transfer of the PEDF gene in the eye has shown promise for the use of this approach in retinal degenerations (106). In a recent study, a recombinant adenoviral vector encoding the PEDF gene was injected into the vitreous of a mouse angiogensis model, in which choroidal neovascularization was promoted by laser-induced rupture of Bruch's membrane. A significant correlation between increased expression of the PEDF gene and reduction in choroidal neovascularization was observed after transfection with the recombinant adenovirus. Similar results were obtained with the PEDF gene in two other mouse models of retinal neovascularizations: (a) transgenic mice that overexpress vascular endothelial growth factor (VEGF) in photoreceptor cells, and (b) mice with oxygen-induced ischemic retinopathy. In both cases, increased intraocular expression of PEDF, after transduction with the recombinant vector, resulted in statistically significant inhibition of retinal neovascularization when compared to mice injected with null vectors. Adenovirus-mediated transfer of the VEGF receptor shows a similar reduction in the growth of choroidal blood vessels in the retina. The recombinant virus was constructed with the human VEGF receptor, flt-1, which was fused to the Fc portion of IgG (Adflt-ExR vector). Subsequent transfection of Adflt-ExR into pigmented rats, in which subretinal neovascularization (SNR) was induced by intense photocoagulation of the retina, resulted in the inhibition of SNR with hybrid flt-1 soluble receptor overexpression in the subretinal space. The inhibition of neovascularization in the eye by transfer of PEDF and the soluble VEGF receptor genes represents new advances in the treatment of blinding diseases associated with apoptotic and angiogenic mechanisms (107).

Adenoviral-mediated transfer of other neurotrophic genes also demonstrates neuroprotective effects in the retina. Transfection with an adenovirus encoding ciliary neurotrophic factor (CNTF), in retinal degeneration slow (rds/rds) or rd mice, resulted in constitutive expression of the CNTF transgene. Promotion of photoreceptor outersegment formation, increased expression of rhodopsin photopigment, decreased apoptotic events, and an increase in the amplitude of a- and b-waves of scotopic electroretinograms were some of the effects of the overexpressed CNTF transgene (108,109). Similarly, administration of adenoviral vectors carrying βPDE, basic fibroblast growth factor (bFGF), or the bcl-2 gene has shown success of the approach as a therapeutic strategy to slow the course of retinal degeneration (110–113). Modifications in the adenovirus genome to create second-generation constructs appear to enhance the effectiveness of the virus in ocular gene therapy. In one modification, the vector was constructed by deleting all of the essential viral genes, resulting in an encapsidated adenovirus mini-chromosome (EAM), which only contained the ITRs for replication and the encapsidation signal necessary for packaging. EAM-mediated delivery of βPDE not only effectively transduced retinal cells in the rd mice, it also promoted prolonged transgene expression, increased survival of photoreceptors, and resulted in decreased toxicity when compared to the first-generation viruses (114). Design of second-generation viruses with low toxicity, effective gene transfer mechanisms, and long-term transgene expression capabilities will be advantageous to the future of this vector in ocular gene therapy.

In addition to transfection of photoreceptor and RPE cells with adenoviral vectors, retinal ganglion cells (RGCs), corneal epithelium, and conjunctival epithelium are also target tissues into which therapeutic genes can be transferred with recombinant adenovirus. In an RGC model of degeneration, approximately 80% of RGCs could be induced to undergo apoptosis and degenerate following intraorbital transection of the optic nerve. A single dose of adenovirus encoding brain-derived neurotrophic factor (Ad-BDNF) coinjected with a free radical scavenger, N-tert-butyl-(2-sulfophenyl)-nitrone (S-PBN), resulted in the survival of 63% axotomized RGCs, indicating the clinical usefulness of the approach for treating RGCs following optic nerve transection (115,116). Similar strategies were tested in the management of corneal and conjunctival abnormalities. Adenovirus type 5 (Ad 5) vector is reported to successfully deliver the reporter lacZ gene to these tissues in humans and rats. Maximum lacZ expression occurred 2–7 days after inoculation. Moreover, the nonspecific upregulation of the inflammatory cytokines IL-6, IL-8, and ICAM-1 in the tissues, induced by Ad5 infection, was suppressed with betamethasone, thereby allowing longer-term transgene expression (117). Some groups have found that other combinations, such as coinjection of E1-deleted AV vectors carrying the lacZ reporter gene with a modified adenovirus encoding a secreted immunomodulatory molecule (CTLA4-Ig), could significantly reduce the immunological consequences of gene transfer with adenoviruses and, thus, promote prolonged transgene expression (118,119).

Corneal opacity, a condition associated with the expression of TGF-β, is another serious cause of visual loss. The accessibility of the cornea has encouraged many in the field to turn to gene therapy alternatives to reduce this condition. An example of the potential usefulness of gene therapy approach for treating corneal opacity is shown in a study that used an adenoviral vector encoding a fusion gene containing the human type II TGF-β receptor and the Fc fragment of human IgG (AdTbeta-ExR). Transfection with the recombinant vector has proven successful in the expression of a soluble TGF-β receptor in Balb/c mice (120). High levels of the soluble receptor were found in serum and ocular fluids for at least 10 days after AdTbeta-ExR injection into the femoral muscle of the animals. Furthermore, the overexpression of soluble TGF-β receptor inhibited TGF-β signaling and may have resulted in the reduced corneal opacity observed in mice subjected to silver nitrate-induced corneal injury. Angiogensis and edema were also reduced in the injured corneas

Corneal opacity, a condition associated with the expression of TGF-β, is another serious cause of visual loss. the accessibility of the cornea has encouraged many in the field to turn to gene therapy alternatives to reduce this condition. An example of the potential usefulness of gene therapy approach for treating corneal opacity is sown in a study that used an adenoviral vector encoding a fusion gene containing the human type II TGF-β receptor and the Fc fragment of human IgG (AdTbeta-ExR). Transfection with the recombinant vector has proven successful in the expression of a soluble TGF-β receptor in Balb/c mice (120). High levels of the soluble receptor were fond in serum and ocular fluids for at least 10 days after AdTbeta-EXR injection into the femoral muscle of the animals. Furthermore, the overexpression of soluble TGF-β receptor inhibited TGF-β signalling and may have resulted in the reduced corneal opacity observed i mice subjected to silver nitrate–induced corneal injury. Angiogenesis and edema were also reduced in the injured corneas with the overexpression of TGF-β. Taken together, the results from these experiments suggest that adenoviral-mediated delivery of therapeutic genes is a useful approach to attenuate visual loss.

c. Adeno-Associated Viruses. Adeno-associated viruses (AAVs) have no known pathogenic effects in humans. It is estimated that 80% of the population develop antibodies to these viruses. AAVs have a wide host range, a high transduction frequency, and they preferentially integrate into the human genome on chromosome 19q13.4. They do not require host cell replication for integration. The AAV rep and cap gene cassettes are deleted before packaging a passenger gene. However, the target gene capacity of AAVs is limited to approximately 4.8 kb (Table 1). AAVs induce less host immune response than adenoviruses because a large percentage of their genome is deleted to accommodate the transgene. Thus, few viral proteins are expressed in vivo. The viruses are naturally replication incompetent and usually require the gene function of a coinfected adenovirus of herpes simplex, as well as *trans*-complementation of the deleted rep and cap genes to generate viral progeny. Production of high AAV titers is difficult to obtain and toxicity to the host is increased because of the contaminating helper virus (121,122). While this is a potentially powerful gene transfer vehicle, the transgene capacity is a limiting feature in the widespread utility of AAVs in gene transfer approaches.

Until recently, transduction of normal, mature photoreceptor cells has been inefficient and limited by toxicity and host immune response directed against viral proteins. AAV transduction appears to obviate some of these problems, but their use is constrained because of passenger gene size limitation and low titer. Efficient transduction using recombinant AAVs, however, has been achieved in all retinal layers, the pigment epithelium, and the optic nerve. Stable transgene expression, lower cytopathology, and reduced immunogenicity have been reported after transduction with the recombinant virus in some retinal studies (123–129).

In one protocol, the AAV has shown considerable potential as an effective system for delivering a functional active therapeutic gene in the treatment of Leber's congenital amaurosis (LCA). LCA is a clinically severe retinal degeneration causing near total blindness in children. It is associated with a mutation in the RPE65 gene. In a breakthrough study, a recombinant AAV vector encoding the RPE65 gene was used to test the effectiveness of wide-type RPE65 in a spontaneously occurring RPE65 canine model. The dogs suffer from an early onset of visual dysfunction similar to that seen in humans affected with LCA. Intraocular innoculations with the recombinant AAV-RPE65 construct resulted in effective transduction and expression of the wild-type RPE65 gene product. Gene expression of the wild-type protein correlated with a significant improvement in visual acuity in the transfected animals (130). AAV transfer of another gene, CNTF, was shown to improve photoreceptor function in a rhodopsin knockout mouse model for retinitis pigmentosa. After transfection into the subretinal space, long-term expression of the biologically active, secreted CNTF resulted in prolonged survival of photoreceptors in the rhodopsin knockout (131). In the retinal degeneration slow (rds) mice, another mouse model for RP, the wild-type peripherin-2 gene (Prph2), transferred by an AAV vector, promoted ultrastructure stabilization of the photoreceptor layer in the retina. Prph2 is a photoreceptor-specific membrane glycoprotein found in the rims of the cell's outer segment discs. These discs contain photopigments essential for photon capture during visual transduction. Prph forms a complex with the rom-1 gene product in the outersegments. The complex is essential to induce stable generation of outer segments and formation of new stacks of discs. During the study, it was noted that Prph2 transgene overexpression was associated with the reestablishment of complex ultrastructure in the photoreceptor layer. This subsequently led to an electrophysiological correction of the outer nuclear layer of the Prph2 transfected retinas (132). Efficient transduction and long-term gene expression of the wild-type βPDE were also reported to preserve photoreceptor cells after AAV transduction in the retina (133). The results, although preliminary, suggest that AAV is another potentially useful vector for transferring therapeutic genes to the human retina.

d. Herpes Simplex Virus. Herpes simplex viruses (HSVs) are large DNA pathogens that infect approximately 60–90% of the world's population. The co-evolution of this virus with humans is due, in part, to its ability to evade host immune surveillance. It establishes a latent infection in its host, a condition that allows the virus to remain unnoticed. These viruses are predominantly neurotrophic pathogens that can infect both quiescent and proliferating cells, an important feature in gene therapy protocols for central nervous system (CNS) disorders. HSVs have the potential to establish a lifetime latent infection in cells of the nervous system.

Acute infection or reactivation of latent HSV elicits a strong immune response from the host, often leading to corneal blindness or fatal sporadic encephalitis. Chronic episodes of reactivation of latent HSV result in stromal keratitis and scarring corneal blindness. The viral genome encodes 81 known genes, 38 of which are important to in vitro viral replication. During the construction of a recombinant vector, several of the immediate early genes are deleted to accommodate a passenger gene of > 150 kb (134). Tropism, latent infective activity, large transgene capacity, and the ability to evade the host immune system are some desirable features in the use of this vector for gene therapy (Table 1).

Gene transfer experiments into the cornea, subconjunctiva and anterior chamber of the mouse eye with HSV-1 indicate that the virus is an effective gene delivery vehicle in the eye (135,136). The efficiency of HSV-mediated transfer of the lacZ gene was also tested in monkey eyes, human trabecular meshwork, and human ciliary muscle cells. Gene transfer was reported to be successful after determination of the β-galactosidase activity in the infected tissues. However, significant inflammation, mild vitritis, and retinitis were observed in the eye after infection. Transgene delivery and expression in RPE cells, optic nerve, retinal ganglion cells, and the iris epithelium were also reported with HSV (137). The possibilities for HSV as a gene delivery vehicle in retinal degenerative diseases are enormous because the virus has a large gene transfer capacity and can infect a wide range of retinal cells. However, its potential will only be fully realized with modifications that will decrease the vector's immunogenicity and reduce packaging instability of the target gene.

The above-described four viruses are currently the most advanced gene delivery system in clinical protocols, but others, including the lentivirus and human immunodeficiency viruses (HIVs), are being approached as possibilities for gene transfer therapy (138–143). They are endowed with features that could be advantageous to the gene therapy approach. Engineering second-generation viruses with predictable biological properties and reduced immunogenicity or developing chimeric vectors that combine the advantageous properties of several delivery systems will enhance the use of gene therapy and provide flexibility in the treatment of many diseases.

4. Non Viral Vectors

One of the greatest concerns that researchers are faced with in gene therapy is the safety of viral vectors as gene delivery vehicles. Consequently, considerable effort has been devoted to evaluating and designing alternative strategies for gene delivery. Nonviral approaches that are currently in development take into consideration the size of the therapeutic gene to be delivered, targeting specificity, immunogenicity, and toxicity.

a. Naked DNA. Perhaps the simplest nonviral gene delivery system in use today is the transfer of naked DNA directly into cells. The overall efficiency of this method, however, is very poor when compared to viral gene transfer. Without mechanical or chemical help, naked DNA will not enter cells rapidly, and once inside, the nucleic acid is exposed and susceptible to enzymatic degradation. In addition, plasmid DNA carrying therapeutic gene does not usually integrate into the host genome, and gene expression is transient in those cells that are successfully transfected. In spite of these limitations, surprisingly high levels of gene expression have been obtained in a few accessible tissues, such as skin and muscle, using plasmid DNA. In such cases, treatment is carried out by directly injecting the plasmid DNA into the tissue because the DNA is vulnerable to degradation in body fluids. So far, the method is safe and nontoxic, but it lacks the ability to transduce a large number of cells and requires surgical procedures to access internal tissues.

An improved strategy for delivery nucleic acid directly into cells is by high velocity bombardment of the cells with DNA attached to gold particles using a "gene gun" approach. Microparticle bombardment has shown some impressive results in focal delivery of naked DNA to corneal cells with little damage or irritation to the tissue (144). It is a method that is being developed for more widespread use and may be a solution to some of the problems encountered with viral vectors. Most gene transfer studies in the eye are carried out using viral vector, but plasmid delivery of a few therapeutic genes, such as tissue plasminogen activator and IFN-α, has been tested and shows potential benefits in treating corneal-related pathologies (145–157). A few studies have also reported successful gene expression in the retina using plasmid DNA. In one case it was demonstrated that condensed plasmids containing the human fibroblast growth factor genes were able to transduce a small population of choroidal and RPE cells after subretinal injections into RCS rat eyes. FGF gene expression in those tissues consequently resulted in a delay in photoreceptor degeneration (148). While the current methods of delivering naked DNA are still very inefficient, the eye is in a prime location to benefit from improvements in mechanical delivery strategies that increase the therapeutic index of this approach.

b. Liposomes. Liposomes are probably the most widely known nonviral vectors used to transfer DNA into cells. The strategy involves encapsulation of plasmid DNA in lipid complexes that are capable of fusing with the cell membrane and delivering the therapeutic genes intracellularly. Initially, this approach has encountered difficulties because classical liposomes are negatively charged lipids that do not interact spontaneously with DNA. Charge limitations and the need to separate DNA-liposome complexes after delivery have led to the development of positively charged cationic lipids. These interact with DNA more readily and have proven to be valuable tools that can compact and deliver DNA across the cell membrane with greater efficacy (149–170). Cationic liposomes are typically formulated using a positively charged lipid and a co-lipid that will stabilize the DNA complex. A commonly used formulation is a mixture of a cytofectin with a neutral lipid component such as DOPE. This combination can be formulated into unilammellar vesicles by several methods, including reverse phase evaporation and microfluidization. Stable complexes are formed when DNA is combined with the vesicles. The DNA is subsequently condensed in the vesicles, forming nanometric particles that are referred to as lipoplexes. These complexes protect the DNA, interact with cell surface proteoglycans, and enter the cell by endocytosis (170) (Fig. 7).

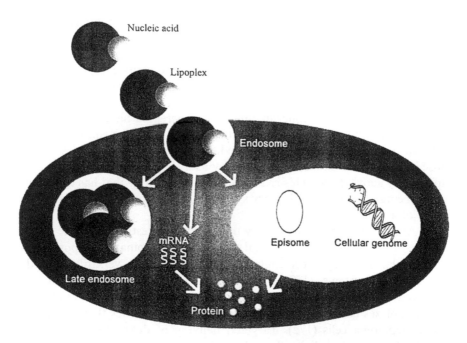

Figure 7 Liposome-mediated transfer of nucleic acid. The nucleic acid is condensed in the liposome to form lipoplexes. These enter the cell by endocytosis. The majority of lipoplexes are trapped in late endosome. A small percentage can either be released into the cytoplasm (mRNA), where they are functional, or traffic non-specifically to the nucleus, where they may form episomes.

Currently, no more than 30 genes transfer–competent cationic liposomes have been developed and are commercially available. Perhaps the most widely used formulations are DOTAP and DOTMA, the latter of which is sold as Lipofectin, an in vitro transfecting agent.

A disadvantage of current methods of liposome-mediated gene transfer is due to the large percentage of the DNA-bound complexes trapped in late endosomes, where they undergo enzymatic degradation and are no longer therapeutically useful. Only a small percentage of the bound nucleic acid escapes systemic inactivation and endosome entrapment. Those that manage to escape face yet another hurdle of getting to the nucleus and maintaining their functional integrity. As with viral delivery, in vitro effectiveness of liposome-mediated gene transfer is often misleading and is a poor guide for clinical efficacy. Conventional liposome formulations lack cell specificity and can take hours for uptake into the cell. They are highly susceptible to inactivation by a number of serum proteins that bind and cause membrane destabilization, a major obstacle for systemic administration of liposomes. A current research focus in the pharmaceutical industry is the development of sterically stable liposome formulations that are resistant to serum disruption and that will not aggregate prior to delivery. One modification currently in development uses conventional liposome lipid membranes to covalently attach polymers such as polyethylene glycol (PEG-lipid) to create stealth liposomes (152,155,156,162,169). Properly formulated polymer-grafted liposomes are shown to be sterically stabilized compounds that have long residence times in circulation, increased biodistribution, and reduction in uptake by cells of the reticuloendothelial system. Other clinically advantageous features of pegylated liposome pharmacokinetics include dose independence and increased efficacy as a slow release system for therapeutically active drugs. This is a fascinating technology that has the potential of being a tailor-made delivery system that will improve the therapeutic index of a number of drugs.

Another modification strategy under active investigation is the manufacture of ligand-targeted liposomal drugs using combinatorial approaches. Such molecular conjugates could potentially be more versatile than the conventional systems (159–164). In a recent study, transfection was observed to be increased in hepatoma cells after the administration of modified lipoplexes containing triantennary galactosyl residues that specifically target hepatoma cells (172). Targeted delivery of doxorubicin to human umbilical vein endothelial cells and subsequent decrease in the survival of the cells were also achieved with immunoliposomes that were conjugated to a monoclonal antibody against E-selectin, a surface marker of HUVECs (173). While targeting will increase transfection efficiency to specific tissues, it does not address problems of DNA release encountered in the endosomes.

Some researchers have shown that the association of amphiphilic peptides, such as GALA, a pH-sensitive peptide, with cationic liposomes can induce fusion and permeabilization at acidic pH values and improve release of the DNA from endosomes. The peptides induce osmotic swelling and subsequent rupture of the endosomal membranes so that the DNA can escape easily (174). These new modifications, however, are not without problems. Competition between ligand-mediated processes and nonspecific interactions with the cell membrane can hinder the efficacy of gene delivery and must be resolved before ligand-modified liposomes are of clinical relevance.

In addition to engineering modifications that result in specific cell targeting and more efficient DNA release, mechanisms that will increase nucleic acid condensation and promote nuclear targeting are promising areas of research that will improve liposome-mediated gene delivery. Modifications using DOTAP liposome-protamine sulfate-DNA (LPD) formulations are shown to produce denser particles when bound to DNA and result in consistently higher gene expression levels (175,176). Complexes formed with polycations are also observed to be much smaller than those formed with liposomes alone and have increased resistance to nuclease degradation. Smaller-size complexes may allow for higher levels of gene expression because of increased cellular internalization. An interesting variation to this hybrid concept is the use of UV-irradiated Japanese Sendai virus (HVJ)-cationic liposome to facilitate nuclear targeting. The binding of high mobility group 1 protein (HMG-1) increase the potency of the complex and enhances nuclear targeting and stability of the DNA after delivery into the nuclear envelope. The success of HVJ-liposome complexes in cancer applications is thought to result from the ability of the complex to bypass the endocytosis process, thereby minimizing the difficulties encountered when the DNA is released from the endosomes (171). The development of "synthetic chemical viruses" that are capable of (a) extended blood circulation, (b) increased DNA microparticle condensation, (c) improved cellular uptake, (d) flexible tropism, (e) escaping enzymatic degradation, and (f) nuclear targeting is an attractive challenge in the area of biopharmaceutics. If realized, such compounds have enormous potential in gene therapy protocols and may surpass the clinical usefulness of viral vectors.

Liposome-based techniques have been optimized to successfully transfer functional genes into human primary RPE cells. In one study, differences in the efficiency of transfection were observed between the types of liposomes used in the assay. Nontoxic transfer was achieved after each liposome treatment, but the Tfx-50 formulation showed the most significant results when compared to transfection of the RPE cells with other liposome variations, including lipofectin, lipofectamine, Cellfectin, and DMRIE-C (177). A fascinating variation of gene transfer by liposomes was achieved by a group of researchers who used liposome eye drops to transfer rat retinal ganglion cells. Transfection was reported to be efficient and nontoxic to ocular tissues. This approach represents an interesting development in non-surgical gene delivery for retinal diseases (178). The use of another liposome method, hemagglutinating virus of Japan liposomes, was tested for efficacy in delivering tissue inhibitor of metalloproteinase-3 gene into rat RPE cells. Not only was the transfection successful, but expression of the introduced gene inhibited the development of experimental choroidal neovascularization induced by laser photocoagulation after transfection of the tissue (179). These are only a few examples showing the feasibility of using, nonviral, nontoxic synthetic DNA-complexing derivatives to transfer therapeutic genes to the retina.

The development of innovative nonviral delivery system is still in its infancy, but many advantages are associated with their use in gene transfer applications: (a) they can package and deliver a transgene of any size; (b) packaging cell lines are not required to generate high titers; (c) they are nonpathogenic and cannot replicate; (d) immunogenicity, toxicity, and inflammation are minimized with their use; and (e) they can become completely synthetic. While these are safe gene delivery systems, the disadvantages currently lie in their overall inefficiency of transfection and their inability to achieve cell-specific and nuclear targeting. Modifications that improve these features will allow synthetic polymer-based gene vectors to be the candidates of choice for pharmacological intervention in many diseases.

5.   Gene Knockdown Therapy

a. Antisense Drugs.   Antisense technology is a novel gene delivery method that is increasingly applied to knock down the expression of a specific target gene for therapeutic purposes or to study the function of that gene. The fundamental principle of the antisense approach is to silence a gene using a short synthetic DNA or RNA sequence that is homologous to that contained within the target gene. Antisense oligodeoxynucleotides (ODNs) are synthesized in the opposite direction of the known complementary DNA sequence and are designed to hybridize specifically with their target sequences to interrupt the production of the corresponding protein. Almost all human diseases are associated with a dysfunctional protein. While most conventional drugs are designed to inhibit the disease-causing activity of a dysfunctional protein, antisense molecules are designed to inhibit the production of the protein. In principle, gene silencing may be accomplished at the genetic level by inhibiting biological events, such as transcription, translation, or gene splicing (180–183). During the inhibition of transcription events, ODNs bind to double-stranded DNA to induce the formation of a short triple-helical structure. This structure is mediated by Hoogsteen hydrogen bonds and sterically hinders the transcription of a specific mRNA. In addition, translation of RNA species can be interrupted by binding of ODNs to tRNA or pre-RNA to prevent their transport from the nucleus or by directly interacting with target mRNA molecule after transcription. In cases where inhibition occurs after the transcript is matured, antisense binding to RNA is intended to block ribosomal assembly or ribosomal sliding along the mRNA during translation of the protein. ODNs can also be of therapeutic value if they are designed to target the intron-exon junctions of premature RNA. In this regard, they prevent splicing events that are essential for maturation of the RNA transcript. Three regions of the RNA that are considered the best targets when designing ODNs are the 5' Cap region, the AUG translational initiation codon, and the 3' untranslated region.

The concept of disabling the function of a mRNA by hybridization of antisense reagents is a simple one, but, like other gene-based therapies, the technology has encountered difficulties in the past. The technical problems experienced in the early pioneering stages of antisense technology are only now being elucidated and are the focus of active study. From these analyses, several features are apparent in the design of effective antisense molecules: determining the length of sequence with the greatest activity and specificity; cellular uptake; specific targeting of the ODN; antisense stability; and toxicity. Other factors that have influenced the effectiveness of antisense molecules are frequency of protein turnover, the intracellular environment of the cell, and the extent of longevity of ODNs after administration.

Gene knockdown practices are still under development and will require significant modifications before being clinically acceptable as a therapeutic modality. Introducing variations in antisense chemistry by subtle changes in the phosphate or sugar moieties of the nucleic acid backbone is one method that shows success in minimizing nuclease degradation of the molecules. Replacing a nonbridging oxygen with a sulfur atom in the phosphodiester bond between nucleotides on the phosphate backbone generates a phosphorothioate linkage, which is reported to be one of the most successful modification of antisense oligonucleotides to date (184,195). Phosphorothioate compounds have shown efficacy in delivery and are less vulnerable to intracellular nuclease degradation. A disadvantage of their use, however, is that the constructs are chiral and form a racemix mixture of ODN species that exhibit both desirable and undesirable properties in vivo (186). Some ODNs are reported to be toxic, while others show nonspecific affinity for proteins (1987). The technical progress in chemical modification of antisense has recently shifted from the first-generation phosphodiester oligonucleotides, which are still nuclease sensitive, to the more nuclease-resistant chimeric compounds that contain methoxyethyl modifications at the end of the ODNs. The development of oligonucleotide conjugates with cell-penetrating and nuclear-targeting peptides and colloidal antisense carriers that protect against degradation is emerging rapidly and will significantly improve cellular uptake, stability, subcellular trafficking, and increased in vivo activity (188–192). Over 200 patents disclose antisense sequences with therapeutic utility in the treatment of human diseases. It is a powerful tool with exceptional clinical value and is being exploited to identify gene function and validate new drug targets.

Formivirsen (ISIS 2922) is the first antisense oligonucleotide drug approved for the treatment of cytomegalovirus (CMV)–induced retinitis. The 21-phosphorothioate oligonucleotide inhibits viral replication in the human eye by binding to complementary sequences of early mRNA CMV viral transcripts. In preliminary clinical trials, the progression of CMV retinitis in AIDS patients is significantly delayed after intravitreal administration of formivirsen. Drug-clearance studies show that formivirsen exhibits first-order kinetics with a half-life of 62 hours in rabbits and 78 hours in monkey. A mild and transient inflammatory response and increase in intraocular pressure are observed after treatment with formivirsen. These appear to be resolved spontaneously or reversed with topical steroid treatment (193–196).

Diseases characterized by retinal neovascularization are among the principal candidates for antisense treatment. The use of antisense oligonucleotide against vascular endothelial growth factor (VEGF) has shown promising results for the treatment of proliferative retinopathy. After intraocular administration in a murine model of retinal neovascularization, phosphorothioate antisense molecules reduced VEGF protein synthesis and the growth of new blood vessels in a dosage-dependent manner. The study shows the therapeutic potential of ODNs in ischemia-induced proliferative retinopathies (197). Proliferative vitreoretinopathy (PVR) is an ocular disorder often associated with proliferating RPE cells. Antisense knockdown of c-myc, a protein active in the mitogenic pathway, inhibits the proliferation of human retinal pigment epithelial cells, suggesting that c-myc ODNs may be an exciting perspective in the treatment of PVR (198).

Retinal ganglion cell death is associated with increased expression of the Bax protein after transection of the optic nerve. A phosphorothioate Bax antisense oligonucleotide was reported to show therapeutic utility in preserving ganglion cell following axotomy. Bax expression was reduced and the number of surviving neurons increased after treatment with Bax ODNs. This represents a novel approach for neurodegeneration due to optic nerve injury (199). The use of ODNs to silence the expression of another retinal gene GLAST, a glial glutamate transporter, showed significant changes in normal retinal transmission and indicates the importance of GLAST in maintaining retinal function (200). Similarly, an antisense compound generated against the trkB receptor mRNA for brain-derived neurotrophic factor (BDNF) alters the neurochemical phenotype of retinal neurons (201). BDNF and its receptor are important to survival and differentiation of the retina and are potentially useful targets in retinal degenerative diseases. Antisense targeting of fibronectin transcripts was also shown to reduce the expression of fibronectin in retinal vascular cells (202). The use of antisense oligonucleotides in these studies reflects the significance of the technology in understanding the function and regulation of a specific protein and the potential therapeutic benefits for antisense-based ocular therapies.

b. Ribozymes. Ribozymes are naturally occurring catalytic RNA and a new class of genetic tools used to inhibit gene expression. Designer ribozymes are chemically designed to recognize and bind specific RNA through complementary base-pair hybridization. Their value in human therapeutics is dependent on their ability to distinguish between mutant and wild-type RNA species and to act as molecular scissors to digest or edit the target RNA in a way that will prevent translation of the corresponding protein (203–205). There are developed as an alternate approach to antisense drugs. Analysis of the physical, biochemical, and biological properties of naturally occurring ribozymes has allowed researchers to classify them according to their various catalytic functions:

1. Hammerhead ribozymes: These are approximately 30 nucleotides long and the smallest ribozymes identified. They are found in many viral DNA and are capable of site-specific cleavage of a phosphodiester bond. Hammerhead ribozymes have been extensively studied, and many have been synthesized against RNA targets. In recent years they have emerged as a potentially effective therapeutic measure in models of retinitis pigmentosa. In areas of the brain, hammerhead ribozymes have been directed against the amyloid peptide precursor (B-APP), which is associated with the pathogenesis of Alzheimer's disease. Others, such as angiozyme, have been synthesized against angiogenic processes involved in the progression of tumor metastasis.
2. Group 1 and Group 11 intron ribozymes: These species can self-splice, digest, and ligate phosphodiester bonds. They are found in lower eukaryotes and some bacteria. Group 1 intron ribozymes mediate *trans*-splicing of RNA targets and is considered a useful genetic tool in repairing mutations in defective genes.

    3.   Ribonuclease P: Cleaves phosphodiester bonds of tRNA precursor molecules.

The catalytic activity of these molecules make them particularly interesting in the treatment of dominantly inherited diseases. In autosomal dominant retinitis pigmentosa (ADRP), a substitution of histidine for proline occurs at codon 23 in the rhodopsin gene. This mutation is referred to as P23H and is responsible for the synthesis of a mutant gene product that results in the death of photoreceptor cells (206). Because the field is relatively new, only a few studies have been carried out in the retina to test the therapeutic effect of ribozymes in ocular diseases. One research team has now shown that in vivo expression and activity of hairpin and hammerhead ribozymes can be achieved in a transgenic rat model of ADRP. Efficient transduction and stable expression of the ribozymes were accomplished using an adeno-associated virus that contained a rod opsin promoter. The results suggested that the expressed ribozymes discriminated between wild-type and mutant rhodopsin RNA and specifically destroyed the P23H mutant specie. As a result, translation of the P23H protein was inhibited and progression of photoreceptor degeneration in ADRP model was significantly slowed down (206–212). Combining the advantages of current gene delivery strategies with catalytic ribozymes has broad therapeutic implications for dominantly expressed retinal diseases where the disease is already in progression.

E. Neurotrophic Factors

The neurotrophic approach to treating retinal diseases is of therapeutic relevance in ophthalmology because trophic factors target apoptotic mechanisms that are independent of the genetic mutation(s) for the disease. Treatment with soluble neurotrophic factors has been shown to prevent the death of retinal neurons in complex or difficult-to-treat ocular diseases where the etiologies are not completely defined or where mutations in several genes are associated with the progression of the disease. The method of delivering highly concentrated amounts of trophic factors to the eye is straightforward and relatively simple to perform and bypasses the need for complex viral or non viral delivery systems. Subretinal or intravitreal injections are common routes of delivery to the affected area. Preparative amounts of neurotrophic proteins can be easily purified from recombinant expression systems, and combinations of several therapeutic proteins can be administered simultaneously to the area of pathology. Another clinically appealing feature of this approach is that the therapeutic efficacy of soluble trophic factors is not hindered by the immunologic and toxic limitations that are usually associated with vector-mediated delivery of DNA.

Designing an effective treatment protocol, however, is based on adequate knowledge of the pharmacokinetics of the trophic factor in a biological system and establishing its ability to function in a physiological environment. A limitation associated with the use of trophic factors in retinal diseases is the need for multiple treatments to significantly effect reversal of the pathology. Unless these agents are administered topically to the eye or packaged in a slow-release system, the method, while safe, is not convenient for long-term management of retinal diseases.

One endogenous neurotrophic factor, which we have isolated and characterized in our laboratory, is a 50 kDa protein, pigment epithelum-derived factor (PEDF) (103,213), so named because it was initially isolated from the retinal pigment epithelium. Functionally, there is a striking association between PEDF, or the lack thereof, and biological processes involving survival and death of retinal cells as well as angiogenic mechanisms in the eye (35,215–219,229). The PEDF gene is well characterized and is classified as a serine protease inhibitor because of its structural and sequence homology with members of this group of genes (104,227). In addition, PEDF maps to human chromosome 17p13.3 and is tightly linked to an autosomal dominant retinitis pigmentosa locus in that region of the chromosome. Several polymorphisms have been identified in the gene, but none has shown a direct correlation between PEDF and specific retinal pathologies (220–224). However, in vivo and in vitro studies with the soluble protein consistently demonstrate the neuroprotective and antiangiogenic activities of PEDF, suggesting a promising future for this protein as a therapeutic that can circumvent the effects of specific mutations or chemical stimulators that cause the death of visual cells.

We first identified the PEDF protein in the conditioned medium of primary cultures of fetal human RPE cell and in the interphotoreceptor matrix (IPM) located between the RPE and neural retina (103,213,225,226). The protein is expressed in high concentration in fetal and young adult RPE cells but appears to be severely downregulated in senescing RPE cultures, a finding that suggests that it may play a role in age-related retinal dysfunctions. In one of the first studies, we showed that PEDF inhibits the growth of a human retinoblastoma cell line (Y79) by inducing differentiation of the tumor cells into a phenotype that is reminiscent of matured neurons. In nontreated cultures, the Y79 cells grow as clusters in suspension and do not spontaneously attach or differentiate. Treatment of these cells with a small dose of PEDF is effective in promoting extensive neurite outgrowths from the tumor cells, upregulating neurofilament proteins and neuron-specific enolase, and promoting connections between the growing neurites of newly differentiated cells (Fig. 8). Approximately 90% of the cultures attach and differentiate on poly-D-

Figure 8 PEDF induces differentiation in human Y79 retinoblastoma cells. (Left) Proliferating nontreated cells are rounded in appearance. (Right) Cells treated with 50 ng/mL PEDF. Treated cells are nonproliferating, project long neurites, and stain positive for the neurofilament protein.

lysine–coated surfaces and maintain their differentiated phenotype for longer than 4 weeks in culture after a single PEDF treatment. This period is extended by additional doses of PEDF to the cultures. From these initial results, PEDF is implicated as a useful therapeutic for reducing ocular tumor progression and prevent degeneration, associated with the growing tumor, in the surrounding retinal tissue.

A role for PEDF in angiogenesis emerged when Dawson and colleagues provided convincing evidence that PEDF, in addition to its neurotrophic activity, functions as an angiogenic inhibitor (214). They showed that PEDF inhibited the formation of new blood vessels in a rat model of corneal neovascularization and also prevented the migration of endothelial cells in a dose-dependant manner. The group also reported that PEDF inhibited endothelial cell migration even in the presence of such angiogenic stimulators as bFGF, VEGF, interleukin-8, aFGF, and lyopohosphatic acid. Furthermore, when tested against other antiangiogenic agents, such as angiostatin and endostatin, its efficacy was slightly more potent than those inhibitors. In support of their study, we showed higher concentrations of PEDF in the vitreous of patients with avascular proliferative vitreal retinopathy and diabetic retinopathy when compared to patients with retinal pathologies associated with increased angiogenic activity (228). Based on the clinical data, as well as vivo studies using animal models, it appears that the concentration of PEDF in the eye is important to the vascular state of ocular tissues. These results have stirred much interest in the ophthalmic field and have encouraged several groups to exploit the therapeutic potential of PEDF in ocular diseases, such as age-related macular degeneration, where both cell death and increased angiogenesis contribute to severe visual loss.

In several modes of induced retinal degeneration, convincing evidence that photoreceptor cells survive in the presence of PEDF has been provided. In an in vitro model of retinal damage, a large percentage of retinal neurons undergo apoptosis and die after exposure to hydrogen peroxide (H_2O_2) (215–217). Hydrogen peroxide is a reactive oxygen species (ROS) found in elevated concentration in light-damaged retinas. It is believed that ROS contribute to degenerative and aging processes in the eye. To test the protective effects of PEDF in H_2O_2-damaged eyes, rat retinal cultures were treated with PEDF before they were exposed to H_2O_2. In the presence of PEDF, apoptotic mechanisms that led to cell death were inhibited, and approximately 60% of the cells that would have otherwise degenerated survived. Furthermore, a high percentage of the treated cells were rhodopsin positive and, therefore, highly likely to be rod photoreceptors. In vivo, the retina can also be damaged by exposure to constant light, in part because of the generation of reactive oxygen species in a high-lipid-content region of the retina. Photoreceptor degeneration is visible as early as the third day of light exposure in the rat. In a study aimed at testing the effect of PEDF in light-damaged rat eyes, we found that a single intravitreal injection of PEDF, prior to chronic light exposure, was potent enough to inhibit the light damage effects on photoreceptor. This was clearly seen in histological preparations of the treated retina and electrophysical measurements of the nuclei in the outer nuclear layer (ONL) (Fig. 9).

In a similar study, photoreceptor survival with PEDF treatment was examined in two mutant mice types, homozygous retinal degeneration (rd/rd) and retinal degeneration slow (rds/rds), in which photoreceptor loss is a hallmark of the mutations. Intravitreal injections of PEDF resulted in a transient but significant delay in the death of photoreceptors in both mutants (229). The efficacy of PEDF was also assessed in an embryonic *Xenopus* model of retinal degeneration (218). In this model, mechanical removal of the RPE cells from the *Xenopus* retina results in a distortion of photoreceptor ultrastructure and disruption of outersegment formation,

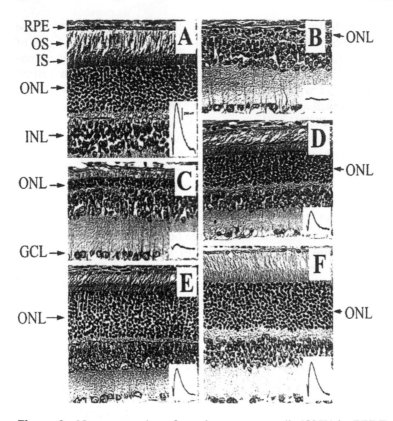

RPE →
OS →
IS →

ONL →

INL →

ONL →

GCL →

ONL →

← ONL

← ONL

← ONL

Figure 9   Neuroprotection of rat photoreceptor cells (ONL) by PEDF after 7 days exposure to constant light. Severe damage to photoreceptor cells (ONL) is seen after light exposure. (A) Unexposed normal rat retina; (B) retinal exposed to 7 days constant light. (C–F) Cross section of rat retina exposed to 7 days of constant light after injections with PEDF, bFGF, or both: (C) PBS; (D) 1 μg PEDF; (E) 1 μg bFGF; (F) 1 μg bFGF + 1 μg PEDF; (inset) electroretinograms (ERG) B-waves amplitudes of the retina with each treatment. RPE, Retinal pigment epithelial cells; OS, photoreceptor outersegment; IS photoreceptor inner segment; ONL, outer nuclear layer; INL, inner nuclear layer; GCL, ganglion cell layer. (Courtesy of Dr. James McGinnis and Wei Cao, Dean McGee Eye, Oklahoma, USA.)

a condition that eventually leads to the death of photoreceptors. In this study it was found that administration of PEDF to the retina after RPE detachment promoted features such as reorganization of the outersegments, increased opsin synthesis by the photoreceptors, and a general correction of the ONL ultrastructure. Moreover, the activity of PEDF in RPE detached retinas was blocked by a neutralizing polyclonal antibody to the 50 kDa native protein, suggesting that the rescuing effect was specific.

From these findings it appears that the course of photoreceptor degeneration can be altered by neuroprotective agents, like PEDF, which can prevent pathomorphological and apoptotic effects of neurodegenerative promoters. Other trophic factors, such as bFGF, CNTF, and BDNF have shown similar results in promoting photoreceptor survival in naturally occurring inherited retinal degeneration models with genetic defects similar to those in human inherited retinal degeneration (230). Survival factors are, therefore, particularly attractive therapeutic tools that may prove to be increasingly important in treating retinal degenerations if long-term, sustained delivery to the affected area is to be maintained.

REFERENCES

1. Adler, R., Curcio, C., Hicks, D., Price, D., and Wong, F. (1999). Cell death in age-related macular degeneration. *Mol. Vis.,* 5:31.
2. Votruba, M., and Gregor, Z. (2001). Neovascular age-related macular degeneration: present and future treatment options. *Eye,* 15(Pt 3):424–429.
3. Sickenberg, M. (2001). Early detection, diagnosis and management of choroidal neovascularization in age-related macular degeneration: the role of ophthalmologists. *Ophthalmologica,* 215(4):247–253.
4. Rubin, G. S. (2001). Vision rehabilitation for patients with age-related macular degeneration. *Eye,* 15(Pt 3):430–435.
5. Harding, S. (2001). Photodynamic therapy in the treatment of subfoveal choroidal neovascularization. *Eye,* 15(Pt 3):407–412.
6. Schmidt-Erfurth U., and Hasan, T. (2000). Mechanisms of action of photodynamic therapy with verteporfin for the treatment of age-related macular degeneration. *Surv. Ophthalmol.,* 45(3):195–214.
7. Verma, L., Das, T., Binder, S., Heriot, W. J., Kirchhof, B., Venkatesh, P., Krebs, I., Stolba, U., Jahn, C., Feichtinger, H., Kellner, L., Krugluger, H., Pawelka, I., Frohner, U., Kruger, A., Li, W., and Tewari, H. K. (2000). New approaches in the management of choroidal neovascular membrane in age-related macular degeneration. *Indian J. Ophthalmol.,* 48(4):263–278.
8. Ho, Ac. (1999). Laser treatment in eyes with drusen. *Curr. Opin. Ophthalmol.,* 10(3):204–208.
9. Hageman, G. S., and Mullins, R. F. (1999). Molecular composition of drusen as related to substructural phenotype. *Mol. Vis.,* 5:28.
10. Blodi, C. F., and Stone, E. M. (1990). Best's vitelliform dystrophy. *Ophthal. Paediatr. Genet.,* 11(1):49–59.
11. Bither, P. P., and Berns, L. A. (1988). Stargardt's disease: a review of the literature. *J. Am. Optom. Assoc.,* 59(2):106–111.

12. Phelan, J. K., and Bok, D. (2000). A brief review of retinitis pigmentosa and the identified retinitis pigmentosa genes. *Mol. Vis., 6*:116–124.

13. Baumgartner, W. A. (2000). Etiology, pathogenesis, and experimental treatment of retinitis pigmentosa. *Med. Hypotheses, 54*(5):814–824.

14. van Soest, S., Westerveld, A., de Jong, P. T., Bleeker-Wagemakers, E. M., and Bergen, A. A. (1999). Retinitis pigmentosa: defined from a molecular point of view. *Surv. Ophthalmol., 43*(4):321–334.

15. Shastry, B. S. (2000). Hereditary degenerative retinopathies: optimism for somatic gene therapy. *IUBMB Life, 49*(6):479–484.

16. Eudy, J. D., and Sumegi, J. (1999). Molecular genetics of Usher syndrome. *Cell Mol. Life Sci., 56*(3–4):258–267.

17. Perrault, I., Rozet, J. M., Gerber, S., Ghazi, I., Leowski, C., Ducroq, D., Souied, E., Dufier, J. L., Munnich, A., and Kaplan, J. (1999). Leber congenital amaurosis. *Mol. Genet. Metab., 68*(2):200–208.

18. Harris, E. W. (2001). Leber's congenital amaurosis and RPE65. *Int. Ophthalmol. Clin., 41*(1):73–82.

19. Algvere, P. V., Berglin, L., Gouras, P., and Shen, Y. (1994). Transplantation of fetal retinal pigment epithelium in age-related macular degeneration with subfoveal neovascularization. *Graefes Arch. Clin. Exp. Ophthalmol., 232*:707–716.

20. Mohand-Said, S., Hicks, D., Dreyfus, H., and Sashel, J. A. (2000). Selective transplantation of rods delays cone loss in a retinitis pigmentosa model. *Arch. Ophthalmol., 118*:807–811.

21. Sheedlo, H. J., Li, L., and Turner, J. E. (1991). Photoreceptor cell rescue at early and late RPE-cell transplantation periods during retinal disease in RCS dystrophic rats. *J. Neural Transplant Plast., 2*:55–63.

22. Rezai, K. A., Kohen, L., Wiedemann, P., and Heimann, K. (1997). Iris pigment epithelium transplantation. *Graefes Arch. Clin. Exp. Ophthalmol., 235*:558–562.

23. Bhatt, N. S., Newsome, D. A., and Fenech, T. (1994). Experimental transplantation of human retinal pigment epithelial cells on collagen substrates. *Am. J. Ophthalmol., 117*:214–221.

24. Jiang, L. Q., Jorquera, M., and Streilein, J. W. (1993). Subretinal space and vitreous cavity as immunological privileged sites for retinal allografts. *Invest. Ophthalmol. Vis. Sci., 34*:3347–3354.

25. Mohand-Said, S., Hicks, D., Dreyfus, H., and Sashel, J. A. (2000). Selective transplantation of rods delays cone loss in a retinitis pigmentosa model. *Arch. Ophthalmol., 118*:807–811.

26. Little, C. W., Castillo, B., DiLoreto, D. A., Cox, C., Wyatt, J., del Cerro, C., and del Cerro, M. (1996). Transplantation of human fetal retinal pigment epithelium rescues photoreceptor cells from degeneration in the Royal College of Surgeons on rat retina. *Invest. Ophthalmol. Vis. Sci., 37*(1):204–211.

27. Sauve, Y., Klassen, H., Whiteley, S. J., and Lund, R. D. (1998). Visual field loss in RCS rats and the effect of RPE cell transplantation. *Exp. Neurol., 152*(2):243–250.

28. Sharma, R. K., Bergstrom, A., Zucker, C. L., Adolph, A. R., and Ehringer, B. (2000). Survival of long-term retinal cell transplants. *Acta. Ophthalmol. Scand., 78*:396–402.

29. Aramant, R. B., Seiler, M. J., and Ball, S. L. (1999). Successful cotransplantation of intact sheets of fetal retinal with retinal pigment epithelium. *Invest. Ophthalmol. Vis. Sci., 40*:1557–1564.

30. Woch, G., Aramant, R. B., Seiler, M. J., Sagdullaev, B. T., and McCall, M. A. (2001). Retinal transplants restore visually evoked responses in rats with photoreceptor degeneration. *Invest. Ophthalmol. Vis. Sci., 42*(7):1669–1676.

31. Schraermeyer, U., Kayatz, P., Thumann, G., Luther, T. T., Szurman, P., Kociok, N., and Bartz-Schmidt, K. U. (2000). Transplantation of iris pigment epithelium into the choroid slows down the degeneration of photoreceptors in the RCS rat. *Graefes Arch. Clin. Exp. Ophthalmol., 238*(12):979–984.

32. Schraermeyer, U., Kociok, N., and Heimann, K. (1999). Rescue effect of IPE transplants in RCS rats: short-term results. *Invest. Ophthalmol. Vis. Sci., 40*(7):1545–1556.

33. Thumann, G., Bartz-Schmidt, K. U., El Bakri, H., Schraermeyer, U., Spee, C., Cui, J. Z., Hinton, D. R., Ryan, S. J., and Heimann, K. (1999). Transplantation of autologous iris pigment epithelium to the subretinal space in rabbits. *Transplantation, 68*(2):195–201.

34. Carwile, M. E., Culbert, R. B., Sturdivant, R. L., and Kraft, T. W. (1998). Rod outer segment maintenance is enhanced in the presence of bFGF, CNTF and GDNF. *Exp. Eye Res., 66*(6):791–805.

35. Abe, T., Tomita, H., Kano, T., Yoshida, M., Ohashi, T., Nakamura, Y., Nishikawa, S., and Tamai, M. (2000). Autologous Iris pigment epithelial cell transplantation in monkey subretinal region. *Curr. Eye Res., 20*:268–275.

36. Humayun, M. S., de Juan, E., del Cerro, M., Dagnelie, G., Radner, W., Sadda, S. R., and del Cerro, C. (2000). Human neural retinal transplantation. *Invest. Ophthalmol. Vis. Sci., 41*:3100–3106.

37. Algvere, P. V., Gouras, P., and Dafgard Kopp, E. (1999). Long-term outcome of RPE allografts in non-immunosuppressed patients with AMD. *Eur. J. Ophthalmol., 9*(3):217–230.

38. Thumann, G., Aisenbrey, S., Schraermeyer, U., Laufaut, B., Esser, P., Walter, P., and Bartz-Schmidt, K. U. (2000). Transplantation of autologous iris pigment epithelium after removal of choroidal neovascular membranes. *Arch. Ophthalmol., 118*(10):1350–1355.

39. Bhatt, N. S., Newsome, Da., and French, T. (1994). Experimental transplantation of human retinal pigment epithelial cells on collagen substrates. *Am. J. Ophthalmol., 117*:214–221.

40. Fang, S. R., Kaplan, H. J., Del Piore, L. V., Liu, Y., Wang, X., Hornbect, R., Landgraf, M., Mason, G., and Silverman, M. S. (1993). Development of a surgical procedure and instrument for transplantation of extended gelatin sheets to the subretinal space. *Invest. Ophthalmol. Vis. Sci., 34*:1093.

41. Thomas, J. A., Itskovitz-Eldor, J., Shapiro, S. S., Waknitz, M. A., Swiergiel, J. J., Marshall, V. S., and Jones, J. M. (1998). Embryonic stem cell lines derived from human blastocysts. *Science, 282*:1145–1147.

42. Shamblott, M. J., Axeman, J., Wang, S., Bugg, E. M., Littlefield, J. W., Donovan, P. J., Blumenthal, P. D., Huggins, G. R., and Gearhart, J. D. (1998). Derivation of pluripotent system cells from cultured human primordial germ cells. *Proc. Natl. Acad. Sci. USA, 95*:13726–13731.

43. Bjornson, C. R., Rietze, R. L., Reynolds, B. A., Magli, M. C., Vescovi, A. L. (1999). Turning brain into blood: a hematopoietic fate adopted by adult neural stem cells in vivo. *Science, 283*(5401):534–537.

44. Joshi, S. S., Tarantolo, S. R., Kuszynski, C. A., and Kessinger, A. (2000). Antitumor therapeutic potential of activated human umbilical cord blood cells against leukemia and breast cancer. *Clin. Cancer Res., 6*(11):4351–4358.

45. Gluckman, E. (2000). Current status of umbilical cord blood hematopoietic stem cell transplantation. *Exp. Hematol., 28*(11):1197–1205.

46. Howery, R. P., Martin, P. L., Driscoll, T., Szabolcs, P., Kelly, T., Shpall, E. J., Bearman, S. I., Slat-Vasquez, V., Rubinstein, P., Stevens, C. E., and Kurtzberg, J. (2000). Graft-versus-leukemia-induced complete remission following unrelated umbilical cord blood transplantation for acute leukemia. *Bone Marrow Transplant, 26*(11):1251–1254.

47. Orlic, D., Kajstura, J., Chimenti, S., Jakoniuk, I., Anderson, S. M., Li, B., Pikel, J., McKay, R., Nadal-Ginard, B., Bodine, D. M., Leri, A., and Anversa, P. (2001). Bone marrow cells regenerate infarcted myocardium. *Nature, 410*(6829):701–705.

48. Brown, J. M., Weissman, I. L., and Shizuru, J. A. (2001). Immunity to infections following hematopoietic cell transplantation. *Curr. Opin. Immunol., 13*(4):451–457.

49. Terskikh, A. V., Easterday, M. C., Li, L., Hood, L., Kornblum, H. I., Geschwind, D. H., and Weissman, I. L. (2001). From hematopoiesis to neuropoiesis: evidence of overlapping genetic programs. *Proc. Natl. Acad. Sci. USA, 98*(14):7934–7939.

50. Gokhan, S., and Mehler, M. F. (2001). Basic and clinical neuroscience applications of embryonic stem cells. *Anat. Rec., 265*(3):142–156.

51. Livesey, F. J., and Cepko, C. L. (2001). Vertebrate neural cell-fate determination: lessons from the retina. *Nat. Rev. Neurosci., 2*(2):109–118.

52. Tropepe, V., Coles, B. L., Chiasson, B. J., Horsford, D. J., Elia, A. J., McInnes, R. R., and van der Kooy, D. (2000). Retinal stem cells in the adult mammalian eye. *Science, 287*(5460):2032–2036.

53. Ahmed, I., Tang, L., and Pham, H. (2000). Identification of neural progenitors in the adult mammalian eye. *Biochem. Biophys. Res. Commun., 270*(2):517–521.

54. Henderson, T. R., Coster, D. J., and Williams, K. A. (2001). The long term outcome of limbal allografts: the search for surviving cells. *Br. J. Ophthalmol., 85*(5):604–609.

55. Perron, M., and Harris, W. A. (2000). Retinal stem cells in vertebrates. *Bioessays, 22*(8):685–688.

56. Tamalu, F., Chiba, C., Ishida, A. T., and Saito, T. (2000). Functional differentiation of ganglion cells from multipotent progenitor cells in sliced retinal of adult goldfish. *J. Comp. Neurol., 419*(3):297–305.

57. Layer, P. G., Rothermel, A., and Willbold, E. (2001). From stem cells towards neural layers: a lesson from re-aggregated embryonic retinal cells. *Neuroreport, 12*(7):A39–46.

58. Otteson, D. C., D. Costa, A. R., Hitchcock, P. F. (2001). Putative stem cells and the lineage of rod photoreceptors in the mature retina of the goldfish. *Dev. Biol., 232*(1):62–76.

59. Kurimoto, Y., Shibuki, H., Kaneko, Y., Ichikawa, M., Kurokawa, T., Takahashi, M., and Yoshimura, N. (2001). Transplantation if adult rat hippocampus-derived neural stem cells into retina injured by transient ischemia. *Neurosci Lett., 306*(1–2):57–60.

60. Takahashi, M., Palmer, T. D., Takahashi, J., and Gage, F. H. (1998). Widespread integration and survival of adult-derived neural progenitor cells in the developing optic retina. *Molec. Cell Neurosci., 12*(6):340–348.

61. Henderson, T. R., Coster, D. J., and Williams, K. A. (2001). The long term outcome of limbal allografts: the search for surviving cells. *Br. J. Ophthalmol., 85*(5):604–609.

62. Anderson, D. F., Ellies, P., Pires, R. T., and Tseng, S. C. (2001). Amniotic membrane transplantation for partial limbal stem cell deficiency. *Br. J. Ophthalmol., 85*(5):567–575.

63. Eiges, R., Schuldiner, M., Drukker, M., Yanuka, O., Itskovitz-Eldor, J., and Benvenisty, N. (2001). Establishment of human embryonic stem cell-transfected clones carrying a marker for undifferentiated cells. *Curr. Biol., 11*(7):514–518.

64. Chow, A. Y. (1993). Electrical stimulation of the rabbit retinal with subretinal electrodes and high density microphotodiode array implants. *Invest. Ophthalmol. Vis. Sci., 34*:835.

65. Rizo, J. F. 3rd, Wyatt, J., Humayun, M., de Juan, E., Liu, W., Chow, A., Eckmiller, R., Zrenner, E., Yagi, T., and Abrams, G. (2001). Retinal prosthesis: an encouraging first decade with major challenges ahead. *Opthalmology, 108*(1):13–14.

66. Rizzo, J. F., and Wyatt, J. (1997). Prospects for a visual prosthesis. *Neuroscientists, 3*:251–262.

67. Eckmiller, R. (1997). Learning retina transplants with epiretinal contacts. *Ophthalmol. Res., 9*:281–289.

68. Peyman, G., Chow, A. Y., Liang, C., Chow, V. Y., Perlman, J. I., and Peachey, N. S. (1998). Subretinal semiconductor microphotodiode array. *Ophthalmic Surg. Lasers, 29*(3):234–241.

69. Chow, A. Y., and Chow V. Y. (1997). Subretinal electrical stimulation of the rabbit retina. *Neurosci. Lett. 255*:13–16.

70. Zrenner, E., Stett, A., Weiss, S., Aramant, R. B., Guenther, E., Kohler, K., Miliczek, K. D., Seiler, M. J. and Haemmerle, H. (1999). Can subretinal microphotodiodes successfully replace degenerated photoreceptors? *Vision Res., 39*(15):2555–2567.

71. Peachey, N. S., and Chow, A. Y. (1999). Subretinal implantation of semiconductor-based photodiodes: progress and challenges. *J. Rehabil. Res. Dev., 36*(4):371–376.

72. Humayun, M. S., de Juan, G., Dagnelie, R. G., Greenberg, R. H., Propst, D. H., and Phillips, (1996). Visual perception elicited by electrical stimulation of the retina in blind humans. *Arch. Ophthalmol., 114*:40–46.

73. Zrenner, E., Miliczek, D. K., Gabel, V. P., Graf, H. G., Guenther, E., Haemmerle, H., Hoefflinger, B., Kohler, K., Nish, W., Schubert, M., Stett, A., and Weiss, (1997). The development of subretinal microphotodiodes for replacement of degenerated photoreceptors. *Ophthalmic Res., 29*:269–280.

74. Chow, A. Y., Pardue, M. T., Chow, V. Y., Peyman, G. A., Liang, C., Perlman, J. I., and Peachey, N. S. (2001). Implantation of silicon chip microphotodiode arrays into the cat subretinal space. *IEEE Trans. Neural Syst. Rehabil. Eng., 9*(1):86–95.

75. Hesse, L., Schanze, T., Wilms, M., and Eger, M. (2000). Implantation of retina stimulation electrodes and recording of electrical stimulation responses in the visual cortex of the cat. *Graefes Arch. Clin. Exp. Ophthalmol., 238*(10):840–845.

76. Walter, P., Szurman, P., Vobig, M., Berk, H., Ludtke-Handjery, H. C., Richter, H., Mittermayer, C., Heimann, K., and Sellhaus, B. (1999). Successful long-term implantation of electrically inactive epiretinal microelectrode arrays in rabbits. *Retina, 19*(6):546–542.

77. Nadig, M. N. (1999). Development of a silicone retinal implant: cortical evoked potentials following focal stimulation of the rabbit retina with light and electricity. *Clin. Neurophysiol., 110*(9):1545–1553.

78. Grumet, A. E., Wyatt, J. L. Jr, and Rizzo, J. F. 3rd. (2000). Multi-electrode stimulation and recording in the isolated retina. *J. Neurosci. Methods, 101*(1):31–42.

79. Hershey, A. D., and Chase, M. (1952). Independent functions of viral proteins and nucleic acid in growth of bacteriophage. *J. Gen. Physiol., 36*:39–56.

80. Watson, J. D., and Crick, F. H. C. (1953). Molecular structure of nucleic acids: a structure for deoxyribose nucleic acid. *Nature, 171*:737–738.

81. Crick, F. H. C., Barnett, L., Brenner, S., and Watts-Tobin, R. J. (1961). General nature of the genetic code for proteins. *Nature, 192*:1227–1232.

82. Danos, O., and Mulligan, R. C. (1988). Safe and efficient generation of recombinant retroviruses with amphotropic and ecotropic host ranges. *PNAS, 85*:6460–6464.

83. Markowitz, D., Goff, S., and Bank, A. (1988). A safe packaging line for gene transfer: separating viral genes on two different plasmids. *J. Virol. 62*:1120–1124.

84. Cone, R. D., and Mulligan, R. C. (1992). High-efficiency gene transfer into mammalian cells: generation of helper-free recombinant retrovirus with broad mammalian host range. *Biotechnology, 24*:420–424.
85. Coffin, J. M. (1996). Retroviridae: the viruses and their replication. In: *Fields Virology* (B. N. Fields, D. M. Knippe, and P. Howley, eds.). Lippincott-Raven, Philadelphia, pp. 1767–1840.
86. Battini, J. L., Heard, J. M., and Danos, O. (1992). Receptor choice determinants in the envelope glycoproteins of amphotropic, xenotropic, and polytropic murine leukemia viruses. *J. Virol, 66*:1468–1475.
87. Sakamoto, T., Spee, C., Scuric, Z., Gordon, E. M., Hinton, D. R., Anderson, W. F., and Ryan, S. J. (1998). Ability of retroviral transduction to modify the angiogenic characteristics of RPE cells. *Graefes Arch. Clin. Exp. Opthalmol., 236*(3):220–229.
88. Kido, M., Rich, K. A., Yang, G., Barron, E., Kohn, D. B., al-Ubaidi, M. R., Blanks, J. C., and Lang, G. (1996). Use of retroviral vector with an internal opsin promoter to direct gene expression to retinal photoreceptor cells. *Curr. Eye Res., 15*(8):833–844.
89. Couderec, B. C., de Neuville, S., Douin-Echinard, V., Serres, B., Manenti, S., Darbon, J. M., and Malecaze, F. (1999). Retrovirus-mediated transfer of a suicide gene into lens epithelial cells in vitro and in an experimental model of posterior capsule opacification. *Curr. Eye Res., 19*(6):472–482.
90. Schubert, C. A., Kimura, H., Spee, C., Hinton, D. R., Gordon, E. M., Anderson, W. F., and Ryan, S. J. (1997). Retrovirus-mediated transfer of the suicide gene into retinal pigment epithelial cells in vitro. *Curr. Eye Res., 16*(7):656–665.
91. Kimura, H., Sakamoto, T., Cardillo, J. A., Spee, C., Hinton, D. R, Gordon, E. M., Anderson, W. F., and Ryan, S. J. (1996). Retrovirus-mediated suicide gene transduction in the vitreous cavity of the eye: feasibility in prevention of proliferative vitreoretinopathy. *Hum. Gene Ther., 1*:7(7):799–808.
92. Sakamoto, T., Kimura, H., Scuric, Z., Spee, C., Gordon, E. M., Hinton, D. R., Anderson, W. F., and Ryan, S. J. (1995). Inhibition of experimental proliferative vitreoretinopathy by retroviral vector-mediated transfer of suicide gene. Can proliferative vitreoretinopathy be a target of gene therapy? *Ophthalmology, 102*(10):1417–1424.
93. Seitz, B., Baktanian, E., Gordon, E. M., Anderson, W. F., LaBreed, L., and McDonnell, P. J. (1998). Retroviral vector-mediated gene transfer into keratocytes: in vitro effects of polybrene and protamine sulfate. *Graefes Arch. Clin. Exp. Ophthalmol., 236*(8):602–612.
94. Bradshaw, J. J., Obritsch, W. F., Cho, B. J., Gregerson, D. S., and Holland, E. J. (1999). Ex vivo transduction of corneal epithelial progenitor cells using a retroviral vector. *Invest. Ophthalmol. Vis. Sci., 40*(1):230–235.
95. Murata, T., Cui, J., Taba, K. E., Oh, J. Y., Spee, C., Hinton, D. R., and Ryan, S. J. (2000). The possibility of gene therapy for the treatment of choroidal neovascularization. *Ophthalmology, 107*(7):1364–1373.

96. Murata, T., Hoffman, S., Ishibashi, T., Spee, C., Gordon, E. M., Anderson, W. F., Hinton, D. R., and Ryan, S. J. (1998). Retrovirus-mediated gene transfer targeted to retinal photocoagulation sites. *Diabetologia, 41*(5):500–506.

97. vanRaaij, M. J., Mitraki, A., Lavigne, G., and Cusack, S. (1999). A triple ?-spiral in the adenovirus fibre shaft reveals a new structural motif for a fibrous protein. *Nature 401*:935–938.

98. Shenk, T. (1996). Adenoviridae. The viruses and their replication. In: *Fields Virology* (B. N. Fields, D. M. Knippe, and P. Howley, eds.). Lippincot-Raven, Philadelphia, pp. 2111–2148.

99. Stratford-Perricaudet, L. D., Makeh, I., Perricaudet, M., and Briand, P. (1992). Wide-spread long-term gene transfer to mouse skeletal muscles and heart. *J. Clin. Invest., 90*:626–630.

100. Bett, A. J., Haddara, W., Prevec, L., and Graham, F. L. (1994). An efficient and flexible system for construction of adenovirus vectors with insertions of deletions in early regions 1 and 3. *PNAS, 91*:8802–8806.

101. Abraham, N. G., Da Silva, J. L., Dunn, M. W., Kigasawa, K., and Shibahara, S. (1998). Retinal pigment epithelial cell-based gene therapy against hemoglobin toxicity. *Int. J. Mol. Med., 1*(4):657–663.

102. Verma, L., Das, T., Binder, S., Heriot, W. J., Kirchhof, B., Venkatesh, P., Krebs, I., Stobla, U., Jahn, C., Feichtinger, H., Kellner, L., Krugluger, H., Pawelka, I., Frohner, U., Druger, A., Li, W., and Tewari, H. K. (2000). New approaches in the management of choroidal neovascular membrane in age-related macular degeneration. *Indian J. Ophthalmol., 48*:263–278.

103. Tombran-Tink, J., Chader, G. G., and Johnson, L. V. (1991). PEDF: a pigment epithelium-derived factor with potent neuronal differentiative activity. *Exp. Eye Res., 53*(3):411–414.

104. Steele, F. R., Chader, G. J., Johnson, L. V., and Tombran-Tink, J. (1993). Pigment epithelium-derived factor: neurotrophic activity and identification as a member of the serine protease inhibitor gene family. *Proc. Natl. Acad. Sci., 15*;90(4):1526–1530.

105. Dawson, D. W., Volpert, O. V., Gillis, P., Crawford, S. E., Xu, H., Benedict, W., and Bouck, N. P. (1999). Pigment epithelium-derived factor: a potent inhibitor of angiogenesis. *Science, 9*;285(5425):245–248.

106. Mori, K., Duh, E., Gehlbah, P., Ando, A., Takahashi, K., Pearlman, J., Mori, K., Yang, H. S., Zack, D. J., Ettyreddy, D., Brough, D. E., Wei, L. L., and Campochiaro, P. A. (2001). Pigment epithelium-derived factor inhibits retinal and choroidal neovascularization. *J. Cell Physiol., 188*(2):253–263.

107. Honda, M., Sakamoto, T., Ishibashi, T., Inomata, H., and Ueno, H. (2000). Experimental subretinal neovascularization is inhibited by adenovirus-mediated soluble VEGF/flt-1 receptor gene transfection: a role of VEGF and possible treatment for SRN in age-related macular degeneration. *Gene Ther., 7*(11):978–985.

108. Cayouette, M., and Gravel, C. (1997). Adenovirus-mediated gene transfer of ciliary neurotrophic factor can prevent photoreceptor degeneration in the retinal degeneration (rd) mouse. *Hum. Gene Ther., 8*(4):423–430.

109. Cayouette, M., Behn, D., Sendtner, M., Lachapelle, P., and Gravel, C. (1998). Intraocular gene transfer of ciliary neurotrophic factor prevents death and increases responsiveness of rod photoreceptors in the retinal degeneration slow mouse. *J. Neurosci., 18*(22):9282–9293.

110. Bennett, J., Pakola, S., Zeng, Y., and Maguire, A. (1996). Humoral response after administration of E1-deleted adenoviruses: immune privilege of the subretinal space. *Hum. Gene Ther., 7*(14):1763–1769.

111. Bennett, J., Tanabe, T., Sun, D., Zeng, Y., Kjeldbye, H., Gouras, P., and Maguire, A. M. (1996). Photoreceptor cell rescue in retinal degeneration (rd) mice by in vivo gene therapy. *Nat. Med. 2*(6):649–654.

112. Akimoto, M., Miyatake, S., Kogishi, J., Hangai, M., Okazaki, K., Takahashi, J. C., Saiki, M., Iwaki, M., and Honda, Y. (1999). Adenovirally expressed basis fibroblast growth factor rescues photoreceptor cells in RCS rats. *Invest. Ophthalmol. Vis. Sci., 40*(2):273–279.

113. Bennett, J., Zehng, Y., Bajwa, R., Klatt, L., Li, Y., and Maguire, A. M. (1998). Adenovirus-mediated delivery of rhodopsin-promoted bc1-2 results in a delay in photoreceptor cell death in the rd/rd mouse.

114. Kumar-Singh, R., and Farber, D. B. (1998). Encapsidated adenovirus minichromosome-mediated delivery of genes to the retina: application to the rescue of photoreceptor degeneration. *Hum. Mol. Genet., 7*(12):1893–1900.

115. Isenmann, S., Klocker, N., Gravel, C., and Bahr, M. (1998). Short communication: protection of axotomized retinal ganglion cells by adenovirally delivered BDNF in vivo. *Eur. J. Neurosci., 10*(8):2751–2756.

116. Weise, J., Isenmann, S., Klocker, N., Kugler, S., Hirsch, S., Gravel, C., and Bahr, M. (2000). Adenovirus-mediated expression of ciliary neurotrophic factor (CNTF) rescues axotomized rat retinal ganglion cells but does not support axonal regeneration in vivo. *Neurobiol. Dis., 7*(3):212–223.

117. Tsubota, K., Inoue, H., Ando, K., Ono, M., Yoshino, K., and Saito, I. (1998). Adenovirus-mediated gene transfer to the ocular surface epithelium. *Exp. Eye Res., 67*(5):531–538.

118. Ali, R. R., Reichel, M. B., Byrnes, A. P., Stephens, C. J., Thrasher, A. J., Baker, D., Hunt, D. M., and Bhattacharya, S. S. (1998). Co-injection of adenovirus expressing CTLA4-Ig prolongs adenovirally mediated lacZ reporter gene expression in the mouse retina. *Gene Ther., 5*(11):1561–1565.

119. Reichel, M. B., Ali, R. R., Thrasher, A. J., Hunt, D. M., Bhattacharya, S. S., and Baker, D. (1998). Immune response limit adenovirally mediated gene expression in the adult mouse eye. *Gene Ther., 5*(8):1038–1046.

120. Sakamoto, T., Ueno, H., Sonoda, K., Hisatomi, T., Shimizu, K., Ohashi, H., Inomata, H. (2000). Blockage of TGF-beta by in vivo gene transfer of a soluble TGF-beta type II receptor in the muscle inhibits corneal opacification, edema and angiogenesis. *Gene Ther., 7*(22):1915–1924.

121. Berns, K. L. (1996). Parvoviridae: the viruses and their replication. In: *Fields Virology* (B. N. Fields, D. M. Knippe, and P. Howley, eds.). Lippincot-Raven, Philadelphia, pp. 2173–2196.

122. McKeon, C., and Samulski, R. J. (1996). NIDDK Workshop on AAV Vectors: Gene Transfer into Quiescent Cells. *Hum. Gene Ther., 7*:1615–1619.

123. Ali, R. R., Reichel, M. B., Thrasher, A. J., Levinsky, R. J., Kinnon, C., Kanuga, N., Hunt, D. M., and Bhattacharya, S. S. (1996). Gene transfer into the mouse retina mediated by an adeno-associated viral vector. *Hum. Mol. Genet., 5*(5):591–594.

124. Flannery, J. G., Zolotukhin, S., Vaquero, M. I., LaVail, M. M., Muzyczka, N., and Hauswirth, W. W. (1997). Efficient photoreceptor-targeted gene expression in vivo by recombinant adeno-associated virus. *Proc. Natl. Acad. Sci. USA, 94*(13):6916–6921.

125. Grant, C. A., Ponnazhagan, S., Wang, X. S., Srivastava, A., and Li, T. (1997). Evaluation of recombinant adeno-associated virus as a gene transfer vector for the retina. *Curr. Eye Res., 16*(9):949–956.

126. Lai, Y. K., Rakoczy, P., Constable, I., and Rolling, F. (1998). Adeno-associated virus-mediated gene transfer into human retinal pigment epithelium cells. *Aust. NZ J. Ophthalmol.,* Suppl 1:S77–79.

127. Guy, J., Qi, X., Muzyczka, N., and Hauswirth, W. W. (1999). Reporter expression persists 1 year after adeno-associated virus-mediated gene transfer to the optic nerve. *Arch. Ophthalmol., 117*(7):929–937.

128. Dreyer, E. B., Vorwerk, C. K., Zurakowski, D., Simon, P. D., and Bennett, J. (1999). Infection with adeno-associated virus may protect against excitotoxicity. *Neuroreport, 10*(14):2887–2890.

129. Bennett, J., Maguire, A. M., Cideciyan, A. V., Schnell, M., Glover, E., Anand, V., Aleman, T. S., Chirmule, N., Gupta, A. R., Huang, Y., Gao, G. P., Nyberg, W. C., Tazelaar, J., Hughes, J., Wilson, J. M., and Jacobson, S. G. (1999). Stable transgene expression in rod photoreceptors after recombinant adeno-associated virus-mediated gene transfer to monkey retina. *Proc. Natl. Acad. Sci. USA, 96*(17):9920–9925.

130. Acland, G. M., Aguirre, G. D., Ray, J., Zhang, Q., Aleman, T. S., Cideciyan, A. V., Pearce-Kelling, S. E., Anand, V., Zeng, Y., Maguire, A. M., Jacobson, S. G., Hauswirth, W. W., and Bennett, J. (2001). Gene therapy restores vision in a canine model of childhood blindness. *Nat. Genet., 28*(1):92–95.

131. Liang, F. Q., Dejneka, N. S., Cohen, D. R., Krasnoperova, N. V., Lem, J., Maguire, A. M., Dudus, L., Fisher, K. J., and Bennett, J. (2001). AAV-mediated delivery of ciliary neurotrophic factor prolongs photoreceptor survival in the rhodopsin knockout mouse. *Mol. Ther., 3*(2):241–248.

132. Ali, R. R., Sarra, G. M., Stephens, C., Alwis, M. D., Bainbridge, J. W., Munro, P. M., Fauser, S., Reichel, M. B., Kinnon, C., Hunt, D. M., Bhattacharya, S. S., and Thrasher, A. J. (2000). Restoration of photoreceptor ultrastructure and function in retinal degeneration slow mice by gene therapy. *Nat. Genet., 25*(3):245–246.

133. Jomary, C., Vincent, K. A., Grist, J., Neal, M. J., and Jones, S. E. (1997). Rescue of photoreceptor function by AAV-mediated gene transfer in a mouse mode of inherited retinal degeneration. *Gene Ther., 4*(7):683–690.

134. Glorioso, J. C., DeLuca, N. A., and Fink, D. J. (1995). Development and application of herpes simplex virus vectors for human gene therapy. *An. Rev. Microbiol., 49*:675–710.

135. Rodahl, E., and Haarr, L. (2000). A herpes simplex virus type I vector as marker for retrograde neuronal tracing: characterization of lacZ transcription and localization of labeled neuronal cells in sensory and autonomic ganglia after inoculation of the anterior segment of the eye. *Exp. Eye Res., 71*(5):495–501.

136. Hudde, T., Rayner, S. A., De Alwis, M., Thrasher, A. J., Smith, J., Coffin, R. S., George, A. J., and Larkin, D. F. (2000). Adeno-associated and herpes simplex viruses as vectors for gene transfer to the corneal endothelium. *Cornea, 19*(3):369–373.

137. Spencer, B., Agarwala, S., Miskulin, M., Smith, M., and Brandt, C. R. (2000). Herpes simplex virus-mediated gene delivery to the rodent visual system. *Invest. Ophthalmol. Vis. Sci., 41*(6):1392–1401.

138. Wang, X., Appukuttan, B., Ott, S., Patel, R., Irvine, J., Song, J., Park, J. H., Smith, R., and Stout, J. T. (2000). Efficient and sustained transgene expression in human corneal cells mediated by a lentiviral vector. *Gene Ther., 7*(3):196–200.

139. Galileo, D. S., Hunter, K., and Smith, S. B. (1999). Stable and efficient gene transfer into the mutant retinal pigment epithelial cells of mitf(vit) mouse using a lentiviral vector. *Curr. Eye Res., 18*(2):135–142.

140. Yang, M., Wang, X. G., Stout, J. T., Chen, P., Hjelmeland, L. M., Appukuttan, B., and Fong, H. K. (2000). Expression of a recombinant human RGR opsin in lentivirus-transduced cultured cells. *Mol. Vis., 6*:237–242.

141. Takahashi, M., Miyoshi, H., Verma, I. M., and Gage, F. H. (1999). Rescue from photoreceptor degeneration in the rd mouse by human immunodeficiency virus-mediated gene transfer. *J. Virol., 73*(9):7812–7816.

142. Miyoshi, H., Takahashi, M., Gage, F. H., and Verma, I. M. (1997). Stable and efficient gene transfer into the retina using an HIV-based lentiviral vector. *Proc. Natl. Acad. Sci. USA, 94*(19):10319–10323.

143. Sikorski, R., and Peters, R. (1998). Gene therapy. Treating with HIV. *Science, 282*(5393):1438.

144. Tanelian, D. L., Barry, M. A., Johnston, S. A., Le, T., and Smith, G. (1997). Controlled gene gun delivery and expression of DNA within the cornea. *Biotechniques, 23*(3):484–488.

145. Sakamota, T., Oshima, Y., Nakagawa, K., Ishibashi, T., Inomata, H., and Sueishi, K. (1999). Target gene transfer of tissue plasminogen activator to cornea by electric pulse inhibits intracameral fibrin formation and corneal cloudiness. *Hum. Gene Ther., 10*(15):2551–2557.

146. Oshima, Y., Sakamoto, T., Yamanaka, I., Nishi, T., Ishibashi, T., and Inomata, H. (1998). Targeted gene transfer to corneal endothelium in vivo by electric pulse. *Gene Ther.*, *5*(10):1347–1354.

147. Noisakran, S. J., and Carr, D. J. (2000). Therapeutic efficacy of DNA encoding IFN-alpha1 against corneal HSV-1 infection. *Curr. Eye Res.*, *20*(5):405–412.

148. Neuner-Jehl, M., Berghe, L. V., Bonnel, S., Uteza, Y., Benmezaine, F., Rouillot, J. S., Marchant, D., Kobetz, A., Dufier, J. L., Menasche, M., and Abitbol, M. (2000). Ocular cell transfection with human basic fibroblast growth factor gene delays photoreceptor cell degeneration in RCS rats. *Hum. Gene Ther.*, *11*(13):1875–1890.

149. Farhood, H., Gao, X., and Son, K. (1994). Cationic liposome for direct gene transfer in therapy of cancer and other diseases. *Ann. NY Acad. Sci.*, *716*:23–34.

150. Felgner, P. L., Tsai, Y. J., Sukhu, L., Wheeler, C. J., Manthorpe, M., Marshall, J., and Cheng, S. H. (1995). Improved cationic lipid formulations for in vivo gene therapy. *Ann. NY Acad. Sci.*, *772*:126–139.

151. Bedu-Addo, F. K., Tang, P., Xu, Y., and Huang, L. (1996). Interaction of poly-ethyleneglycol-phospholipid conjugates with cholesterol-phosphatidyl-choline mixtures: sterically stabilized liposome formulations. *Pharmacol. Res.*, *13*:718–724.

152. Singh, M., Ferdous, A. J., Kanikkannan, N., and Faulkner, G. (2001). Stealth monensin immunoliposomes as potentiator of immunotoxins in vitro. *Eur. J. Pharm. Biopharm.*, *52*(1):13–20.

153. Gabizon, A. (1993). Tailoring liposomes for cancer drug delivery: from the bench to the clinic. *A. Biol. Clin. (Paris)*, *51*(9):811–813.

154. Needham, D., McIntosh, T. J., and Lasic, D. D. (1992). Repulsive interactions and mechanical stability of polymer-grafted lipid membranes. *Biochim. Acta*, *1108*(1):40–48.

155. Allen, T. M., and Hansen, C. (1991). Pharmacokinetics of stealth versus conventional liposomes: effect of dose. *Biochim. Biophys. Acta*, *1068*(2):133–141.

156. Allen, T. M., Mehra, T., Hansen, C., and Chin, Y. C. (1992). Stealth liposomes: an improved sustained release system for 1-beta-D-arabinofuranosyl-cytosine. *Cancer Res.*, *52*(9):2431–2439.

157. Gabizon, A., and Martin, F. (1997). Polyethylene glycol-coated (pegylated) liposomal doxorubicin. Rationale for use in solid tumors. *Suppl 4*:15–21.

158. Newman, M. S., Colbern, G. T., Working, P. K., Engbers, C., and Amantea, M. A. (1999). Comparative pharmacokinetics, tissue distribution, and therapeutic effectiveness of cisplatin encapsulated in long-circulating, pegylated liposomes (SPI-077) in tumor-bearing mice. *Cancer Chemother. Pharmacol.*, *43*(6):524.

159. Coa, Y., and Suresh, M. R. (2000). Bispecific Mab aided liposomal drug delivery. *J. Drug Target*, *8*(4):257–266.

160. Cristiano, R. J., and Roth, J. A. (1995). Molecular conjugates: a targeted gene delivery vector for molecular medicine. *J. Mol. Med.*, *73*(10):479–486.

161. Gabizon, A. A. (2001). Pegylated liposomal doxorubicin: metamorphosis of an old drug into a new form of chemotherapy. *Cancer Invest., 19*(4):424–436.

162. Gabizon, A. A. (2001). Stealth liposomes and tumor targeting: one step further in the quest for the magic bullet. *Clin. Cancer Res., 7*(2):223–225.

163. Ishida, T., Iden, D. L., and Allen, T. M. (1999). A combinatorial approach to producing sterically stabilized (Stealth) immunoliposomal drugs. *FEBS Lett., 460*(1):129–133.

164. Riveria, E., Valero, V., Syrewicz, L., Rahman, Z., Esteva, F. L., Theriault, R. L., Rosales, M. M., Booser, D., Murray, J. L., Bast, R. C. Jr, and Hortobagyi, G. N. (2001). Phase I study of stealth liposomal doxorubicin in combination with gemcitabine in the treatment of patients with metastatic breast cancer. *J. Clin. Oncol., 19*(6):1716–1722.

165. Schatzlein, A. G. (2001). Non-viral vectors in cancer gene therapy: principles and progress. *Anticancer Drugs, 12*(4):275–304.

166. Shimada, K., Matsuo, S., Sadzuka, Y., Miyagishima, A., Nozawa, Y., Hirota, S., and Sonobe, T. (2000). Determination of incorporated amounts of poly(ethylene glycol)-derivatized lipids in liposomes for the physicochemical characterization of stealth liposomes. *Int. J. Pharm., 203*(1–2):255–263.

167. Singh, M., Ferdous, A. J., Kanikkannan, N., and Faulkner, G. (2001). Stealth monensin immunoliposomes as potentiator of immunotoxins in vitro. *Eur. J. Pharm. Biopharm., 52*(1):13–20.

168. Takeuchi, H., Kojima, H., Yamamoto, H., and Kawashima, Y. (2001). Evaluation of circulation profiles of liposomes coated with hydrophilic polymers having different molecular weights in rats. *J. Control. Release, 75*(1–2):83–91.

169. Vaage, J., Donovan, D., Wipff, E., Abra, R., Colbern, G., Uster, P., and Working, P. (1999). Therapy of a xenografted human colonic carcinoma using cisplatin or doxorubicin encapsulated in long-circulating pegylated stealth liposomes. *Int. J. Cancer, 80*(1):134–137.

170. Miller, A. D. (1999). *Non-Viral Delivery Systems for Gene Therapy in Understanding Gene Therapy. Bios Scientific Publisher*, pp. 43–60.

171. Yonemitsu, Y., Alton, E. W. F . W., Komori, K., Yoshizumi, T., Sugimachi, K., and Kaneda, Y. (1998). HVJ (Sendai virus) liposome-mediated gene transfer: current status and future perspective. *Int. J. Oncol., 12*:1277–1285.

172. Remy, J. S., Kichler, A., Mordvinov, V., Schuber, F., and Behr, J. P. (1995). Targeted gene transfer into hepatoma cells with lipopolyamine-condensed DNA particles presenting galactose ligands: a stage toward artificial viruses. *Proc. Natl. Acad. Sci. USA, 92*(5):1744–1748.

173. Spragg, D. D., Alford, D. R., Greferath, R., Larsen, C. E., Lee, K. D., Gurtner, G. C., Cybulsky, M. I., Tosi, P. F., Nicolau, C., and Gimbrone, M. A. Jr. (1997). Immunotargeting of liposomes to activated vascular endothelial cells: a strategy for site-selective delivery in the cardiovascular system. *Proc. Natl. Acad. Sci. USA, 94*(16):8795–8800.

174. Simoes, S., Slepushkin, V., Gaspar, R., de Lima, M. C., and Duzgunes, N. (1998). Gene delivery by negatively charges ternary complexes of DNA, cationic liposomes and transferrin of fusigenic peptides. *Gene Ther.* 5(7):955–964.

175. Li, S., and Huang, L. (1997). In vivo gene transfer via intravenous administration of cationic lipid-protamine-DNA (LPD) complexes. *Gene Ther.*, 4(9):891–900.

176. Li, S., Rizzo, M. A., Bhattachrya, S., and Huang, L. (1998). Characterization of cationic lipid-protamine-DNA (LPD) complexes for intravenous gene delivery. *Gene Ther.*, 5(7):930–937.

177. Abul-Hassan, K., Walmsley, R., and Boulton, M. (2000). Optimization of non-viral gene transfer to human primary retinal pigment epithelial cells. *Curr. Eye Res.*, 20(5):361–366.

178. Matsuo, T., Masuda, I., Yasuda, T., and Matsuo, N. (1996). Gene transfer to the retina of rat by liposome eye drops. *Biochem. Biophys. Res. Commun.*, 219(3):947–950.

179. Takahashi, T., Nakamura, T., Hayashi, A., Kamei, M., Nakabayashi, M., Okada, A. A., Tomita, N., Kaneda, Y., and Tano, Y. (2000). Inhibition of experimental choroidal neovascularization by overexpression of tissue inhibitor of metalloproteinases-3 in retinal pigment epithelium cells. *Am. J. Ophthalmol.*, 130(6):774–781.

180. Zamecnik, P. C., and Stephenson, M. L. (1978). Inhibition of Rous sarcoma virus replication and cell transformation by a specific oligodeoxynucleotides. *Journal*, 75(1):280–284.

181. Crooke, S. T., and Lebleu, B. (1993). *Antisense Research and Applications*. *CRC Press*, Boca Raton, FL.

182. Agrawal, S. (1996). Antisense oligonucleotides: towards clinical trials. *Trends Biotechnol.*, 14(10):376–387.

183. Crooke, S. T. (1998). An overview of progress in antisense therapeutics. *Antisense Nucleic Acid Drug Dev.*, 8(2):115–122.

184. Matsukura, M., Shinozuka, K., Zon, G., Mitsuya, H., Reitz, M., Cohen, J. S., and Broder, S. (1987). Phosphorothioate analogs of oligodeoxynucleotides: inhibitors of replication and cytopathic effects of human immunodeficiency virus. *Proc. Natl. Acad. Sci. USA*, 84(21):7706–7710.

185. Stein, C. A., Subasinghe, C., Shinozuka, K., and Cohen, J. S. (1988). Physicochemical properties of phosphorothioate oligodeoxynucleotides. *Nucleic Acids Res.*, 16(8):3209–3221.

186. LaPlanche, L. A., James, T. L., Powell, C., Wilson, W. D., Uznanski, B., Stec, W. J., Summers, M. F., and Zon, G. (1996). Phosphorothioate-modified oligodeoxyribonucleotides, III. NMR and UV spectroscopic studies of the Rp-Rp, Sp-SP, and Rp-Sp duplexes, [d(GGSAATTCC)]2, derived from diastereomeric O-ethyl phosphorothioates. *Nucleic Acids Res.*, 14(22):9081–9093.

187. Srinivasan, S. K., and Iversen, P. (1995). Review of in vivo pharmacokinetics and toxicology of phosphorothioate oligonucleotides. *J. Clin. Lab. Anal.*, 9(2):129–137.

188. Stepkowski, S. M. (2000). Development of antisense oligodeoxynucleotides for transplantation. *Curr. Opin. Mol. Ther., 2*(3):304–317.

189. Sohail, M., and Southern, E. M. (2000). Hybridization of antisense reagents to RNA. *Curr. Opin. Mol. Ther., 2*(3):264–271.

190. Srinivasan, S. K., and Iversen, P. (1995). Review of in vivo pharmacokinetics and toxicology of phosphorothioate oligonucleotides. *J. Clin. Lab. Anal., 9*(2):129–137.

191. Lambert, G., Fattal, E., and Couvreur, P. (2001). Nanoparticulate systems for the delivery of antisense oligonucleotides. *Adv. Drug Deliv. Rev., 47*(1):99–112.

192. Lebedeva, I., and Stein, C. A. (2001). Antisense oligonucleotides: promise and reality. *Annu. Rev. Pharmacol. Toxicol., 41*:403–419.

193. de Smet, M. D., Meenken, C. J., and van den Horn, G. J. (1999). Fomivirsen—a phosphorothioate oligonucleotide for the treatment of CMV retinitis. *Ocul. Immunol. Inflamm., 7*(3–4):189–198.

194. Flores-Aguilar, M., Besen, G., Vuong, C., Tatebayashi, M., Munguia, D., Gangan, P., Wiley, C. A., and Freeman, W. R. (1997). Evaluation of retinal toxicity and efficacy of anti-cytomegalovirus and anti-herpes simplex virus antiviral phosphorothioate oligonucleotides ISIS 2922 and ISIS 4015. *J. Infect. Dis., 175*(6):1308–1316.

195. Perry, C. M., and Balfour, J. A. (1999). Fomivirsen. *Drugs, 57*(3):375–380.

196. Detrick, B., Nagineni, C. N., Grillone, L. R., Anderson, K. P., Henry, S. P., and Hooks, J. J. (2001). Inhibition of human cytomegalovirus replication in a human retinal epithelial cell model by antisense oligonucleotides. *Invest. Ophthalmol. Vis. Sci., 42*(1):163–169.

197. Robinson, G. S., Pierce, E. A., Rook, S. L., Foley, E., Webb, R., and Smith, L. E. (1996). Oligodeoxynucleotides inhibit retinal neovascularization in a murine model of proliferative retinopathy. *Proc. Natl. Acad. Sci. USA, 93*(10):4851–4856.

198. Capeans, C., Pineiro, A., Dominguez, F., Loidi, L., Buceta, M., Carneiro, C., Garcia-Caballero, T., and Sanchez-Salorio, M. (1998). A c-myc antisense oligonucleotide inhibits human retinal pigment epithelial cell proliferation. *Exp. Eye Res., 66*(5):581–589.

199. Isenmann, S., Engel, S., Gillardon, F., and Bahr, M. (1999). Bax antisense oligonucleotides reduce axotomy-induced retinal ganglion cell death in vivo by reduction of Bax protein expression. *Cell Death Differ., 6*(7):673–682.

200. Barnett, N. L., and Pow, D. V. (2000). Antisense knockdown of GLAST, a glial glutamate transporter, compromises retinal function. *Invest. Ophthalmol. Vis. Sci., 41*(2):585–591.

201. Rickman, D. W., and Rickman, C. B. (1996). Suppression of trkB expression by antisense oligonucleotides alters a neuronal phenotype in the rod pathway of the developing rat retina. *Proc. Natl. Acad. Sci. USA, 93*(22):12564–12569.

202. Roy, S., Zhang, K., Roth, T., Vinogradov, S., Kao, R. S., and Kabanov, A. (1999). Reduction of fibronectin expression by intravitreal administration of antisense oligonucleotides. *Nat. Biotechnol., 17*(5):476–479.

203. Goodchild, J. (2000). Hammerhead ribozymes: biochemical and chemical considerations. *Curr. Opin. Mol. Ther.*, *2*(3):272–281.

204. Kiehntopf, M., Esquival, E. L., Brach, M. A., and Herrmann, F. (1995). Ribozymes: biology, biochemistry, and implications for clinical medicine. *J. Mol. Med.*, *73*(2):65–71.

205. Michel F., and Ferat, J. L. (1995). Structure and activities of group II introns. *Annu. Rev. Biochem.*, *64*:435–461.

206. Lewin, A. S., Drenser, K. A., Hauswirth, W. W., Nishikawa, S., Yasumura, D., Flannery, J. G., and LaVail, M. M. (1998). Ribozyme rescue of photoreceptor cells in a transgenic rat model of autosomal dominant retinitis pigmentosa. *Nat. Med.*, *4*(8):967–971.

207. Hauswirth, W. W., and Lewin, A. S. (2000). Ribozyme uses in retinal gene therapy. *Prog. Retin. Eye Res.*, *19*(6):689–710.

208. Shaw, L. C., Skold, A., Wong, F., Petters, R., Hauswirth, W. W., and Lewin, A. S. (2001). An allele-specific hammerhead ribozyme gene therapy for a porcine model of autosomal dominant retinitis pigmentosa. *Mol. Vis.*, *26*(7):6–13.

209. LaVail, M. M., Yasumura, D., Matthes, M. T., Drenser, K. A., Flannery, J. G., Lewin, A. S., and Hauswirth, W. W. (2000). Ribozyme rescue of photoreceptor cells in P23H transgenic rats: long-term survival and late-state therapy. *Proc. Natl. Acad. Sci. USA*, *97*(21):11488–11493.

210. Hauswirth, W. W., LaVail, M. M., Flannery, J. G., and Lewin, A. S. (2000). Ribozyme gene therapy for autosomal dominant retinal disease. *Clin. Chem. Lab. Med.*, *38*(2):147–153.

211. Shaw, L. C., Whalen, P. O., Drenser, K. A., Yan, W., Hauswirth, W. W., and Lewin, A. S. (2000). Ribozymes in treatment of inherited retinal disease. *Methods Enzymol.*, *316*:761–776.

212. Drenser, K. A., Timmers, A. M., Hauswirth, W. W., and Lewin, A. S. (1998). Ribozyme-targeted destruction of RNA associated with autosomal-dominant retinitis pigmentosa. *Invest. Ophthalmol. Vis. Sci.*, *39*(5):681–689.

213. Tombran-Tink, J., and Johnson, L. V. (1989). Neuronal differentiation of retinoblastoma cells induced by medium conditioned by human RPE cells. *Invest. Opthalmol. Vis. Sci.*, *30*:1700–1707.

214. Dawson, D. W., Volpert, O. V., Gillis, P., Crawford, S. E., Xu, H., Benedict, W., and Bouck, N. P. (1999). Pigment epithelium-derived factor: a potent inhibitor of angiogenesis. *Science*, *285*(5425):245–248.

215. McGinnis, J. G., Chen, W., Tombran-Tink, J., Mrazek, D. A., Lerious, V., and Cao, W. (1999). Retinal neurons in primary cell culture: inhibition of apoptosis by pigment epithelial derived factor (PEDF). In: *Retinal Degenerative Diseases and Experimental Therapy*, Kluwer Academic/Plenum Publishers, New York, pp. 527–537.

216. Cao, W., Tombran-Tink, J., Chen, W., Mrazek, D., Elias, R., and McGinnis, J. F. (1999). Pigment Epithelium-Derived Factor protects cultured retinal neurons against hydrogen peroxide-induced cell death. *J. Neurosci. Res.*, *57*(6):789–800.

217. Cao, W., Tombran-Tink, J., Elias, R., Sezates, Mrazek, D., and McGinnis, J. F. (2001). In vivo protection of photoreceptors from light damage by pigment epithelium-derived factor. *Invest. Ophthalmol. Vis. Sci., 42*:1646–1652.

218. Jablonski, M. M., Tombran-Tink, J., Mrazek, D. A., and Iannaccone, A. (2000). Pigment Epithelium-Derived Factor supports normal development of photoreceptor neurons and opsin expression after retinal pigment epithelium removal. *J. Neurosci., 20*(19):7149–7157.

219. Jablonski, M. M., Tombran-Tink, J., Mrazek, D. A., and Iannaccone, A. (2001). Pigment Epithelium-Derived Factor supports normal Muller cell development and Glutamine synthetase expression after removal of the retinal pigment epithelium. *Glia., 35*:14–25.

220. Tombran-Tink, J., Pawar, H., Swaroop, A., and Chader, G. J. (1994). Localization of the gene for pigment epithelium-derived factor to chromosome 17p13.1 and expression in cultured retinoblastoma cells. *Genomics, 19*:266–272.

221. Goliath, R., Tombran-Tink, J., Chader, G. J., Ramser, R., and Greenberg, J. (1996). The gene for PEDF, a retinal growth factor is a prime candidate for retinitis pigmentosa and is tightly linked to the RP13 locus on chromosome 17p13.3. *Mol. Vis., 2*:5.

222. Tombran-Tink, J., Chader, G., and Koenekoop, R. (1997). Molecular analysis of the human PEDF gene, a candidate gene for retinal degeneration: localization to 17p13.3. *Degen. Retin. Dis., 3*:245–254.

223. Greenberg, J., Goliath, R., Tombran-Tink, J., Chader, G. J., and Ramesar, R. (1997). Growth factors in the retina: pigment epithelium-derived factor (PEDF) now fine mapped to 17p13.3 and tightly linked to the RP13 locus. *Degen. Retin. Dis., 3*:291–294.

224. Koenekoop, R. K., Loyer, M., Pina, A. L., Davidson, J., Robitaille, J., Maumenee, I., and Tombran-Tink, J. (1999). Four polymorphic variations in the PEDF gene identified during the mutation screening of patients with leber congenital amaurosis. *Mol. Vis., 5*:10.

225. Tombran-Tink, J., Shivaram, S. M., Chader, G. J., Johnson, L. V., and Bok, D. (1995). Expression, secretion and age-related downregulation of pigment epithelium-derived factor, a serpin with neurotrophic activity. *J. Neurosci., 15*(7):4992–5003.

226. Tombran-Tink, J., Li, A., Johnson, M. A., Johnson, L. V., and Chader, G. J. (1992). Neurotrophic activity of interphotoreceptor matrix on human Y79 retinoblastoma cells. *J. Comp. Neurol., 317*:175–186.

227. Tombran-Tink, J., Mazaruk, K., Chung, D., Linker, T., Chader, G. J., and Rodriguez, I. (1996). Organization, evolutionary conservation, expression and unusual Alu density of the human gene for pigment epithelium-derived factor, a unique neurotrophic serpin. *Mol. Vis., 2*:11.

228. Ogata, N., Tombran-Tink, J., Nishikawa, M., Nishimura, T., Mitsuma, Y., Sakamoto, T., and Matsumura, M. (2001). Pigment Epithelium-derived factor in the vitreous is low in diabetic retinopathy and high in rhegmatogenous retinal detachment. *Am. J. Ophthalmol., 132*(3):378–382.

229. Cayouette, M., Smith, S. B., Becerra, S. P., and Gravel, C. (1999). Pigment epithelium-derived factor delays the death of photoreceptors in mouse models of inherited retinal degenerations. *Neurobiol. Dis., 6*:523–532.
230. LaVail, M. M., Yasumura, D., Mathes, M. T., Lau-Villacorta, C., Unoki, K., Sung, C. H., and Steinberg, R. H. (1998). Protection of mouse photoreceptors by survival factors in retinal degenerations. *Invest. Ophthalmol. Vis. Sci., 39*:592–602.

19
Gene, Oligonucleotide, and Ribozyme Therapy in the Eye

Sudip K. Das
Idaho State University, Pocatello, Idaho, U.S.A.

Keith J. Miller
Bristol-Myers Squibb Company, Pennington, New Jersey, U.S.A.

I. INTRODUCTION

Both antisense oligonucleotide as well as gene therapy aim at the transfer of genetic material to the target cells for preventing or altering a particular disease process. In gene therapy a good gene is inserted into the cell to repair or replace the faulty gene to produce health-giving proteins, while an oligonucleotide can block the disease-causing protein. With the advances in the identification of the major genes responsible for causing various diseases, an increased focus on the use of therapeutic genes and oligonucleotides has developed, including treatments for ocular diseases. Inherited retinal degeneration is one of the most common causes of blindness in the western world, for which there is no therapy at all. The most researched form of inherited retinal degeneration is retinitis pigmentosa (RP; damage to photoreceptors of the retina by a single abnormal gene) with an occurrence up to 1:3000. A number of important developments have been reported in last few years in identifying genetic defects in RP. Gene and oligonucleotide therapy has been successfully applied in retinal diseases, including the introduction of the antisense oligonucleotide Vitravene® for cytomegalovirus (CMV) retinitis in patients with acquired immunodeficiency syndrome (AIDS) and other immuno suppressed states. Thus, an important milestone in antisense therapy for the eye has been reached. In this chapter we will discuss the principles of gene, oligonucleotide, and ribozyme therapy with an emphasis on delivery of these drugs to the eye.

II. GENE THERAPY

The goal of gene therapy is to replace the defective or missing gene in a human cell to correct its malfunction. The most extensively studied disease in which gene therapy has been attempted is cystic fibrosis; treatment involves the replacement of the mutant cystic fibrosis transmembrane conductance regulator (CFTR) gene (1). The main principle of gene therapy involves transfection of cells with nonresident genes to accomplish in situ (a) removal of a mutant gene and replacing it with a normal gene, (b) correction of a mutant gene by site-directed recombination, and (c) improvement of a gene function to enable production of sufficient levels of product to supplement or replace normal expression (2,3). The progress of gene therapy, based on systemic delivery, has been slowed recently by reports of adverse events, including the death of a patient (4). On the other hand, a recent study showed the efficacy of a gene therapy product that encodes clotting factor VIII in two hemophilia patients who had no spontaneous bleeding episodes for nearly one year (5).

The eye is an attractive target for gene therapy because of its accessibility and its immune privilege. In ophthalmology, the concept of gene therapy has attracted interest for a number of retinal diseases, including retinitis pigmentosa, age-related macular degeneration, and proliferative vitreoretinopathy (6). In retinal disorders, specific genetic defects have been found in 20 of the 87 mapped genes causing genetic eye disorders, and most of the genetic defects result from single gene defects that are both highly disabling and potentially correctable (7). The clinical transplantation of retinal pigmental epithelium with fetal RPE cells in the subretinal space of patients with age-related macular degeneration could cause cystoid-like macular edema due to slow graft rejection (8). Therefore, in vivo administration of gene therapy drugs has high potential in treating those diseases. The current status of gene therapy in the eye is restricted to somatic gene therapy (the gene is introduced to somatic cells) performed by in vivo gene transfer (administration of genes locally or systemically).

Early studies with gene therapy involved bombardment of cells ex vivo with naked DNA. However, that process had several limitations, including nonapplicability in clinical medicine and the absence of prolonged gene expression in the target tissue. With the advances of molecular biology and virology and better understanding of viral genome, it is now possible to investigate a number of viral vectors for gene therapy. Hauswirth and

Beaufrere have listed four basic prerequisites that should be fulfilled for ocular gene therapy (9):

1. An efficient and nontoxic gene delivery technique should be available.
2. The genetic basis of the disease should be characterized so that an appropriate therapeutic approach can be taken.
3. Expression of the therapeutic gene needs to be properly controlled in terms of the types of cells that do or do not support expression.
4. An experimental animal model of the disease should be available for preclinical testing of therapy.

Since the systemic delivery of genes does not reach, to a satisfactory level, the ocular tissues, most gene therapy agents (except for gene delivery to surface corneal epithelium) need to be administered through intravitreal or intracameral injection. Because the flow of fluids in the eye is from posterior to anterior segment, the delivery of therapeutic agent in the vitreal chamber leads to distribution of the drug in the anterior cell linings and also the general circulation in addition to distribution in the vitreal cell linings.

A. Viral-Vector–Mediated Gene Therapy

Gene delivery is the main obstacle preventing the full exploitation of the genetic information at our disposal in this postgenomic era (10). The size, charge, surface properties, and interaction with blood components determine the distribution of a colloidal system or macromolecule in the body (11). Due to the large size of DNA, it does not diffuse well through the endothelium, keratinized tissues, and specialized barriers in the body. The availability of large DNA to specified tissues is dependent mainly on the blood flow. Moreover, those drugs administered through intravascular routes are cleared from the body by first-pass effect and by the mononuclear phagocyte system. In addition, due to enzymatic action, DNA is prone to degradation and fragmentation within a short time after vascular administration. Therefore systemic gene delivery to achieve sufficient concentration in ocular tissues is extremely difficult. Normally two types of gene delivery techniques are used in in vivo gene therapy: viral-mediated and non–viral-mediated. Due to the natural ability to infect cells efficiently, a number of viruses, such as adenovirus, retrovirus, adeno-associated virus and herpesvirus, have been widely studied for their ability to deliver genes to specific tissues (12). Most viruses used in gene therapy are inactivated at the

DNA replication level so they do not multiply outside the specific laboratory cell lines.

The hypothesis that genetic disorders can be treated using viral-mediated gene transfer became reality in 1990, with the first phase I gene therapy clinical trial for the treatment of adenosine deaminase (ADA) deficiency (13). Also in 1990, retroviral-mediated gene therapy was conducted in patients with melanoma with success (14). A comparison of the viral vectors for gene delivery is illustrated, with an emphasis on ocular targets, in Table 1. Of the gene transfer protocols listed, by viral vectors as well as by number of patients in clinical trials, retroviral vectors account for the largest number (38.3% by protocols and 51% by number of patients). This is followed by adenovirus (25.6% by protocols and 18% by number of patients), poxvirus (6.4% by protocols and 2.6% by number of patients), adeno-associated virus (1.9% by protocols and 1% by number of patients), and herpes simplex virus (0.6% by protocols and 0.6% by number of patients) (15).

B. Retrovirus in Gene Therapy

A retrovirus is a positive strand, diploid, RNA virus that replicates through a DNA intermediate (18). On infecting a cell, the RNA genome is copied onto double-stranded DNA, which is integrated into the genome of the infected cells. Murine leukemia virus (MLV) is the recombinant retrovirus most widely used for gene delivery. For delivery, the plasmid carrying the cloned gene is transfected into mouse cells that express the genes of the retrovirus; also, the envelope protein of the MLV is changed so that it infects human cells. Retroviruses can infect a wide variety of cells in a number of species at a very slow rate, only a few copies of the retrovirus integrating per genome. However, retroviruses can only infect actively dividing cells (19), as the breakdown of nuclear membrane is essential for the transport of preintegration complex to the nucleoplasm. Therefore the lack of infecting ability of retroviruses precludes their use in nondividing cells like neuronal or some ocular tissues. Although the chance of mutagenesis is small, the retroviruses can be carcinogenic as they integrate themselves in the genome of the infected cells. A retrovirus binds to a new host cell by virtue of the interaction of the Env glycoprotein (one of the three basic polyproteins that retroviral genome codes for) with an appropriate cellular receptor. This interaction triggers a series of events that ultimately lead to the fusion of the lipid envelope surrounding the virus with the target cell membrane. In addition to the limitation of foreign sequences in the viral genome, the stability of engineered vectors could also be a concern.

C. Adenovirus in Gene Therapy

Human adenoviruses are a group of large, nonenveloped, double-stranded DNA viruses that have been isolated from respiratory tract infections, conjunctivitis, and infant diarrhea (20,21). The pathology is primarily from inflammation and loss of infected epithelial cells (22). Adenoviruses replicate in two main phases: early and late. In the early phase, the viruses adsorb and penetrate (via receptor-mediated endocytosis), followed by transcription and translation of an early set of genes. By removing the early region genes it is possible to make the adenoviruses replication defective. The late phase consists of the onset of DNA replication followed by expression of viral genes and assembly of virions (23). These viruses are fairly stable and responsive to purification and concentration by cesium chloride density centrifugation and stored frozen until use. The DNA of adenoviruses rarely integrates to the target genome and is therefore gradually lost after cell division and thus is not oncogenic in humans. Their genome is completely defined and modified, and recombinant viruses can be produced in large quantities at a high concentration without compromising their ability to infect cells (24,25). Moreover, adenoviruses can infect a wide variety of cells and have a broad host range. However, they are highly immunogenic and could originate inflammatory and toxic reactions in the host (26). Life-long treatment of genetic disorders requires periodic virus administration, which is contraindicated due to humoral immune response. The route of administration has significant effect on transduction, being highest in the immediate vicinity of the administration. In spite of several disadvantages, adenoviruses are preferred over the retroviruses for gene therapy mainly due to; (1) high titer values, (2) incorporation of bigger DNA molecule, maximum of 7–8 kb, possibly involving the complete deletion of the viral genome.

D. Adeno-Associated Virus Vector

Adeno-associated virus (AAV) is a small, DNA-containing virus that belongs to the family Parvoviridae. It obtained its name because once it was mistakenly identified as an adenovirus and was found to be dependent on adenovirus for its replication (27). AAV has not been associated with any disease, but it has been isolated in humans in association with adenoviruses. For replication, it requires co-infection with either an adenovirus or herpes simplex virus as a helper virus (28). However, it replicates in many cell lines with wide cell and tissue specificity (29) provided the appropriate helper virus is present. Moreover, it can infect nondividing cells (30) and has a property of site-specific integration of its genome (31). However, recombi-

Table 1 Comparison of Viral Vectors for Gene Delivery

Vectors	Characteristics	Ocular target	Disadvantages
Retroviruses	Relatively high titers (10^6–10^7 cfu/mL) Stable gene expression Integrate to host genome No toxic effects on infected cells Only infect dividing cells Insert capacity in the virion is in the range of 10 kb	Does not infect nondividing cells	Random insertion of viral genome may possibly lead to mutagenesis Possibility of replication competent virus formation by homologous recombination
Adenoviruses	Very high titers (10^{10} pfu/mL) Transiently high levels of gene expression Do not integrate to host genome They can also infect nondividing cells Large DNA inserts can be accommodated in the vector (7–8 kb)	Corneal endothelium Corneal epithelium Iris Müller cells Retinal pigmental epithelium Photoreceptor Trabecular meshwork	Not suitable for long-term expression due to the lack of integration into host genome Host immune response Complicated vector genome
Lentiviruses	Stable gene expression Can infect nondividing cells Total insert capacity in the virion in the range of 10 kb Can be pseudotyped with retroviral or VSV G envelopes leading to broad tropism	Photoreceptor Retinal pigmental epithelium	Possible proviral insertional mutagenesis in target cells Serum conversion to HIV-1 Presence of HIV-1 accessory proteins may represent hazard in humans, in spite of lack of HIV-1 infection

Adeno-associated viruses	Difficult to obtain high titers	Photoreceptor	Limited capacity for foreign genes
	Wide range of cells can be infected, including ones that do not divide	Retinal pigmental epithelium	Requires helper adeno- or herpesvirus for replication
	Insert capacity is limited, 4.1–4.9 kb		Lack of specific integration for recombinant adeno-associated vectors (vira)
	Ability of the virus to establish latent infection by viral genome integration into cell genome		lined rod cell function for a minimum of 8 months after single
	Nonpathogenic, nontoxic		

Source: Refs. 16, 17.

nant adeno-associated viruses do not share the integration site specificity of wild-type AAV. Site-specific integration is especially advantageous as it reduces the risks of transformation of the target cell through insertional mutagenesis. The virus particles are heat stable and resistant to a variety of chemicals such as chloroform and alcohol. The specific advantages of using AAV—the lack of need for integration specificity in recombinant AAV and its ability to infect nondividing cells—has made this vector very popular for gene delivery. The main problem of AAV in gene therapy lies in accommodating large foreign genes, the maximum range being 4.1–4.9 kb (32) that can be replaced completely by the gene of interest, thus totally avoiding any immunity problem associated with viral proteins upon transduction of the target cell.

E.   Lentivirus

Due to the fact that lentivirus vectors are based on HIV or SIV (human and simian immunodeficiency viruses), a big hurdle in using these vectors for gene delivery involves deleting substantial segments of HIV genome. Moreover, since the integration of HIV-based vectors appears to be random, there is a possibility of integration-induced mutagenesis.

F.   Current Status of Viral-Vector–Mediated Gene Therapy in the Eye

Adenoviral vectors are able to enter a number of retinal tissues, including retinal pigment epithelium, but they do not efficiently transduce mature wild-type photoreceptors. Recombinant adenovirus carrying wild-type cDNA has been used for transient rescue of degenerating photoreceptors in the rd mouse. However, one of the major problems is the inflammatory response caused by adenovirus (Ad5)-mediated gene transfer. Hoffman et al. studied the cell-mediated immune response and stability of intraocular transgene expression after adenovirus-mediated gene delivery (33). It has been demonstrated that with the replication-deficient recombinant adenovirus, vectors based on adenovirus type 5 can be used for direct gene transfer to conjunctival and corneal epithelium in vitro and in vivo (34). However there was nonspecific upregulation of inflammatory cytokines IL-6 and IL-8 in conjunctival epithelium that was suppressed by betamethasone. Adenoviral vector–mediated transfer of the gene for catalase, the reactive oxygen species scavenger that suppresses experimental optic neuritis, to the optic nerve in animals with experimental optic neuritis showed significant reduction of demyelination and disruption of the blood-brain barrier (35). Another problem with recombinant adenovirus is that transduction of cells by adenovirus vectors results in only short-term transgene expression. Long-term effects can be obtained with transplantation of cornea infected ex vivo with adenoviral vectors (36). Based on the fact that glaucomatous neurons die by apoptotic cell death, the use of gene therapy agents targeted to the ganglion cells via intravitreal or via brain delivery has been found to be promising. Delivery of adenoviral vectors with the gene encoding for brain-derived neurotropic factor (BDNF) to Müller cells of rats with axotomized retinal ganglion cells (RGC) caused temporary prolongation of the life of the cells (37).

Recombinant adeno-associated virus (rAAV) slowly integrates at random chromosomal sites over a period of weeks or months, which leads to long-term photoreceptor transduction, in rodents, of about 1.5 years. Unlike recombinant adenovirus, rAAV is able to transduce normal photoreceptor as well as retinal pigmental epithelium and retinal ganglion cells. A drawback to rAAV is that it takes about 3–5 weeks before full rAAV gene expression is noticed in rodent photoreceptors. rAAV have been used to deliver the gene expressing neurturin (a potential neuronal survival factor in central and peripheral nervous system) in vitro in retinal cells and in vivo for intraocular delivery in mice (38). rAAV-mediated gene transfer of basic fibroblast growth factor (FGF-2) in transgenic rat model of RP has shown promise as a therapy for retinal degeneration (39). Lentivirus vectors containing the glycoprotein of vesicular stomatitis virus have been successfully tested in rat retinas. A number of studies have been reported with lentiviral vectors, mostly in rodents. In view of the potential of lentivirus and rAAV in retinal gene therapy, more studies are necessary using these vectors.

Herpes virus vectors that have tissue-specific integration with high expression and large payload of foreign gene can be used to deliver gene therapy products to nondividing cells in the eye. Liu et al. (40) studied the delivery of ribonucleotide reductase mutant (hrR3) expressing the *E. coli* lacZ gene in primate ocular tissues. Transgene expression was detected in retinal pigmented epithelium cells and sporadic retinal ganglion cells in primate eyes receiving virus intracamerally and intravitreally, respectively. Although replacement of a normal copy of the gene is one of the approaches of gene therapy, in many conditions that are autosomal dominant, producing a normal copy of the gene would not correct the problem. Rather, a replication-competent, virulent, ribonuclease reductase–deficient herpes simplex virus can provide the means to deliver therapeutic polypeptides (like growth factors, neutrophins, and cytokines) in a continuous manner to the cells (41).

Retinitis pigmentosa refers to a number of related inherited retinal diseases with an incidence of 1 in 3000. An understanding of the genetic causes of retinitis pigmentosa could lead to delivery of specific genes in

RP. A number of retinal diseases in humans affect preferentially one region of retina, commonly either fovea or peripheral retina, and gradually progress to entire retina (42). The diseases include retinitis pigmentosa, gyrate atrophy, choroideremia and rod-cone dystrophy. A recent study by Bernstein and Wong showed that regional gene expression likely plays a significant but nonexclusive role in the development of regional retinal disease (43). Retinal degeneration in the mouse due to high levels of visible light has been shown to be dependent on the activation of transcription factor AP-1 leading to apoptotic cell death of photoreceptors (44). Grimm et al. showed that expression of *c-fos* and *c-jun* mRNA is transiently induced by exposure to damaging light (45). As only the caspase-1 (apoptosis-related genes) expression is upregulated, it could be possible that a gene that downregulates caspase-1 could be helpful in progression of light-induced degeneration.

A recent report suggests that retroviral vectors can also be used in ex vivo transfer of β-galactosidase gene transduced to human retinal pigment epithelial cells and transplanted under the rabbit retina. RPE cells at the site of transplantation formed a monolayer and expressed β-galactosidase for 14 days (46). This concept could be applied to gene therapy in choroidal neovascularization, which is responsible for most cases of severe visual loss in age-related macular degeneration.

As far as the foreseeable future, there is no universal vector that can be used for gene therapy. More clinical studies are needed to establish the delivery of gene therapy products.

G. Nonviral Vectors in Gene Therapy

Although viral vectors have been proven to be very effective in gene therapy, there are a number of drawbacks associated with them. Nonviral gene delivery systems consist of a therapeutic gene and a synthetic gene delivery system. The main functions of the synthetic carrier are to protect the therapeutic gene from premature degradation and deliver the gene to the nucleus of the target cell. Nonviral approaches to gene therapy have three key elements: (a) a gene that codes for a specific therapeutic protein, (b) a gene carrier system that is targeted to a specific tissue or cells, and (c) a plasmid-based gene expression system that can modulate the duration and expression levels of the therapeutic protein. The subcellular delivery of DNA can occur in five steps (47): membrane binding, internalization, endosomal release, nuclear localization, and decomplexation (Fig. 1). The transport of transfected DNA from the cytosol to the nucleus is the most crucial point in successful gene transfer (48). It was also reported that nondividing cells are poorly transfectable by nonviral gene transfer

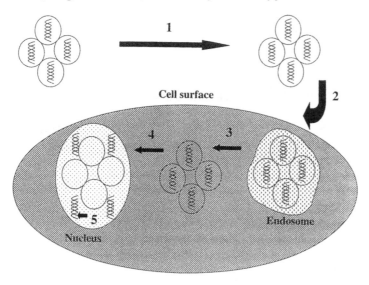

Figure 1 Subcellular gene delivery using nonviral techniques.

systems, and based on the fact that DNA particles are bigger than 24 nm, it is postulated that the nuclear uptake occurs preferentially in those cells that are beginning mitosis consequent to breakdown of the nuclear membrane. Upon entering the cell, the genetic information is transcribed and translated to a therapeutic protein that can produce a systemic effect, a cell surface effect, and/or an intracellular effect (Fig. 2). The gene expression can be modulated so that the therapeutic protein is secreted out of the cell or stays inside the cell. Other applications of gene delivery involve the creation of DNA vaccines. The nonviral vectors have gained popularity mainly because (49):

1. They are nonimmunogenic (this may be a major advantage over the viral vectors in the eye, where the blood-retinal barrier is compromised in a number of diseases and during retinal surgery) (50).
2. They can be designed based on thoroughly characterized chemical agents, and thus their physical interactions with the cells are reproducible.
3. They can be designed based on the size of the DNA to be transported.
4. Large-scale production of plasmid DNA and transfection agents is rather inexpensive and they can be produced in large quantity.
5. Testing of synthetic materials is less laborious.

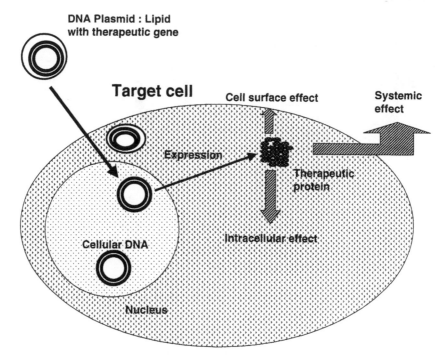

Figure 2 Effects following gene transfer in cells.

6. Normally the synthetic carriers are degraded in the body without causing any toxic effect.

At the same time, nonviral vectors are associated with the major disadvantage of lower efficiency than viral vectors in gene transfer and their transient gene expression. Although nonviral gene delivery has aroused general research interest in recent years, the literature suggests that application of nonviral gene delivery to ocular tissues is limited. This may be due to the fact that gene delivery in the ocular tissues needs efficient gene expression that has not yet been achieved. For example, human retinal pigment epithelial cells have phagocytic activity and can internalize fairly large ($2\,\mu m$) particles (51). The internalization is probably not the major obstacle, but the escape of DNA from the endosomes or DNA entry into the nucleus may be the major rate-limiting step (52). The serum components adhering to the complexes may cause degradation of the complexes or prevent escape of DNA from the endosomes (53). In the remainder of this chapter we will briefly overview the techniques of nonviral gene delivery with emphasis on ocular delivery.

1. Naked DNA

Researchers became interested in naked or free DNA because DNA itself is only weakly immunogenic and nonimmunogenic carriers could be delivered safely. Although there are a number of techniques available for preparation of purified plasmid DNA, there is no standardized method and most of the techniques are proprietary. In addition, polymeric DNA is highly negatively charged and can bind with a variety of agents by electrostatic and hydrophobic forces (54). Endotoxin and protein removal becomes difficult at times (55). Naked DNA is useful in delivering the gene of interest to muscle cells (56) directly or to tumors (57), where they induce transgene expression. A gene for a particular protein is often ligated to a specifically designed plasmid (circular duplex DNA that is replicated extrachromosomally in bacteria and sometimes in cells of other organisms). About 1–10 mg of purified plasmid can be separated from 1 L of bacterial broth. While the general DNA interaction is dependent on the primary, secondary, or tertiary structure of DNA, the gene expression is dependent on the primary structure and the sequence of ligation of DNA into the plasmid (58). Vacik et al. (59) reported an interesting model whereby transcription factors bind to the DNA in the cytoplasm to create a protein-DNA complex that can enter the nucleus using the protein import mechanism. Therefore, by using DNA elements containing binding sites for transcription factors expressed in unique cell types, it is possible to create plasmids that target the nucleus in a cell-specific manner (59). A recent study with supercoiled plasmid DNA injected into the cytoplasm of human corneal cells and keratocytes showed that primary, nontransformed human corneal epithelial cells and keratocytes display sequence-specific nuclear import of plasmid DNA in the absence of mitosis. The small sequence that mediates nuclear localization of plasmids is active in both microinjection and cationic liposome-transfected cells. It was suggested that the inclusion of DNA sequence into non-viral vectors should improve the efficiency of ocular gene transfer in vivo (60).

Nonviral vector-mediated transfections are classified under two subheadings: techniques suitable for in vitro transfection only and techniques suitable for both in vitro and in vivo. Techniques for in vitro transfections in cells involve calcium phosphate transfection, microinjection of plasmid DNA into the cell nucleus, and electroporation, which involves application of high voltage to a mixture of DNA and cells, forcing the DNA to move through the pores formed. These techniques have been discussed elsewhere and will not be discussed here as there is limited application in in vivo systems.

2. Gene Gun

Gene gun transfer of DNA has been successfully used in plant, microbial, and mammalian cells (61). In addition to the advantage of nonimmunogenicity, it also provides good in vivo gene transfer efficiency and focal gene delivery. The process involves penetration of gold-coated DNA particles into the target organ using an electric arc generated by high-voltage discharge that accelerates DNA-coated particles to high velocity (62). Plasmid DNA encoding nontoxic green fluorescent protein was delivered in rabbit cornea, and there was no evidence of corneal or ocular damage (63). It has also been shown that the ballistic transfer of genes for IL-4 and CTLA-4 in orthotopic corneal grafting in BALB/c mice caused prolonged gene expression for 5 days (64). In vitro, gene expressing cornea specific keratin 12 protein in T antigen transformed rabbit corneal epithelium (65). Since the target tissue is to be surgically exposed, this technique can be applied to the surface of the eye only.

3. Liposomes

Liposomes are spherical particles composed of a lipid bilayer membrane that encapsulates a part of the solvent. Depending on the nature of the concentric layers, they are designated SUV (small unilamellar vesicle; $0.02-0.2\,\mu m$), LUV (large unilamellar vesicle; $0.1-0.5\,\mu m$), and LMV (large multilamellar vesicle, $0.1-10\,\mu m$). The surface characteristics of liposomes can be made neutral, negative, or positively charged depending on the nature of the ligands on the surface. A number of lipids have been studied for delivery of gene therapy products, but no single type has been identified as the most suitable for all types of gene delivery (66). The use of plasmid-based gene expression is limited by their size (about 3000 kDa), hydrophilicity, and a large negative surface charge (-30 to -70 mV) (67). These properties influence the distribution in the tissues, cellular uptake, and intracellular trafficking of gene therapy drugs (68). It is now accepted that cationic lipids are necessary for development of a liposomal formulation for gene therapy because the negative charge is a hindrance to cell membrane transport (69,70). The nature of the hydrophilic and hydrophobic parts and the linkers plays an important role, although the structure-function relationships have not been established. On the other hand, cationic lipids (Table 2) cannot form liposomes alone and are normally accompanied by a neutral lipid or a lipid-like compound, such as DOPE (dioleyl phosphatidylethanolamine) (71) or cholesterol. It has been shown that polycations that bind to the negatively charged surface of the mammalian cell membranes can cause charge neutralization, cell distortion, lysis, and agglutination (72). They can also cause immune system stimulation (73) and can bind to the cell nuclei

Table 2 Commonly Used Cationic Lipids

Abbreviated name	Chemical name
BGTC	Bis-guanidinium-tren-cholesterol
DC-Chol	3 β-[N-(N',N'-Dimethylaminoethane)carbamoyl] cholesterol
DMRIE	1,2-Dimyristoyloxypropyl-3-dimethylhydroxyethylammonium bromide
DODAB	Dioctadecyldimethylammonium bromide
DODAC	Dioleoyldimethylammonium chloride
DOGS	Dioctadecylamidoglycospermine
DORI	1,2-Dioleoyloxypropyl-3-dimethylhydroxyethylammonium bromide
DOSPA	2,3-Dioleoyloxy-N-[2-sperminecarboxamido)ethyl]-N,N-dimethyl-1-propanaminium
DOSPER	1,3-Dioleoyloxy-2 (6-carboxy spermyl) propylamide-4-acetate
DOTAP	1,2-Dioleoyloxy-3-(trimethylammonio)propane
DOTIM	1-[2-(Oleoyloxy)-ethyl]-2-oleoyl-3-(2-hydroxyethyl) imidazolinium chloride
DOTMA	N-[1-(2,3-Dioleoyloxy)propyl]-N,N,N-trimethylammonium chloride
DPPES	Dipalmytoylphosphatidylethanolamidospermine
EDMPC	1,2-Dimyristoyl-sn-glycero-3-ethylphosphocholine chloride
ELMPC	1,2-Dilauroyl-sn-glycero-3-ethylphosphocholine chloride
EOMPC	1,2-Dioleoyl-sn-glycero-3-ethylphosphocholine chloride
GAP-DLRIE	($\pm$)-N-(3-Aminopropyl)-N,N-dimethyl-2,3-bis(dodecyloxy)-1-propanaminium bromide
SAINT-n	A series of dialkyl pyridinium–alkyl halides

and internal membranes, interfering with the enzyme and cellular function (74). Synthetic cationic phosphonolipids that are very similar to their natural counterparts may have lesser toxicity towards normal cells (75). Synthetic polymers together with lipids have been found to be very effective in transfection compared to lipid-DNA alone. Commercially available lipid-based transfection agents have been reviewed in a recent publication (76). Polylysine Lipofectamine complexes have been found to be two to three times more effective in luciferase expression than Lipofectamine alone (77), with low molecular weight poly(L-lysine) being most effective. Block copolymer micelles consisting of polyoxyethylene chains, being hydrophilic, are considered a suitable vehicle for delivery of DNA. The biodistribution of intravenously administered cationic liposome–plasmid DNA complexes is not suitable because those complexes exhibiting strong zeta potential are rapidly cleared from the circulation (78).

Although liposomal gene delivery has been widely reviewed (79), there are only a few ocular gene transfer studies using liposomes. Matsuo et al. (80) demonstrated that instillation of liposomal eye drops of an expression plasmid vector for β-galactosidase could transfer the gene to the retinal ganglion cells of rat without causing any inflammation (80). A recent study comparing liposome, calcium phosphate–, and DEAE dextran–based delivery of firefly luciferase cDNA to human primary retinal pigment epithelial cells in vitro shows that calcium phosphate and DEAE dextran techniques failed to transfect the vector and led to high cytotoxicity, while liposome-based methods successfully transferred the vectors to the RPE cells. The efficiency varied for different liposomes: Tfx-50 > Lipofectin > Lipofectamine > Cellfectin > DMRIE-C (81). Cytomegalovirus-promoted LacZ genes and nonhistone nuclear protein, high mobility group 1 (HMG1), were coencapsulated in liposomes, and the liposomes were then coated with the envelope of inactivated hemagglutinating Sendai virus by fusion (HVJ liposome) for in vivo transfer and expression of a reporter gene into adult mammalian retina (82). A large array of literature suggests that there is no universal delivery system that can be proposed for delivery of DNA-lipid complexes, while it is a fact that cationic lipids affect the observable DNA expression. Lipid-DNA complexes are referred to as "lipoplex," polymer-DNA complexes as "polyplex," and liposome-polymer-DNA complexes as "lipopolyplex."

Lipoproteins that form natural biological emulsions have been proposed as carriers for gene transfer. Very-low-density lipoproteins (VLDL), low-density lipoproteins (LDL), and high-density lipoproteins (HDL) are now being considered potential delivery vehicles for gene transfer (83).

4. Peptides

A number of membrane-active peptides including bacterial proteins, pH-specific fusogenic, or lytic peptides have been studied for improvement of polycationic-DNA based transfection. Peptides can act in two ways: (a) anionic peptides prevent DNA degradation in endosomes by buffering the endosomal compartment; (b) cationic peptides bind to the DNA favoring endocytosis. A series of natural or synthetic membrane-destabilizing peptides have been identified as suitable for gene therapy (84). Peptides from viral sequences such as the N-terminus of influenza virus hemagglutinin HA-2, the N-terminus of rhinovirus HRV2 VP-1 protein, and other synthetic and natural sequences of amphipathic peptides have been found to increase transfection efficiency due to membrane- or vesicle-destabilizing activity (85). The presence of endoosmolytic peptides significantly improves the cytoplasmic delivery. Two such peptides have been tested for their ability to deliver the β-galactosidase reporter gene to the corneal endothelial cells of rabbit, pig, and human. Approximately 30% of corneal endothelial cells were transfected with the integrin-binding moiety of the toxin from the American pit viper (86).

5. Polylysine and Polyethylenimine

Poly(L-lysine) and polyethylenimine (PE) have linear and branched structures, respectively. Polylysine-DNA complexes have been found to possess good transfection ability at a high polycation:DNA ratio that is toxic to normal cells. The complexes can be delivered efficiently to the internal vesicles of the cell, but most often this does not improve the transfection rate, possibly due to the fact that a membrane in the cell separates the complexes. Chloroquine or glycerol often improves the transfection by causing lysosomal breakdown (87). PE contains ethyleneimine as the repeating units. A large number of amino group nitrogens gives it a highly cationic charge. Approximately 20% of amino nitrogens are protonated under normal physiological conditions, therefore, it has a better buffer capacity than polylysine over the entire physiological pH range (88). A possible explanation for the higher gene transfer efficiency of PE is that the buffering of endosomes through PE provokes an enormous amount of proton accumulation followed by passive chloride influx. Such events could cause osmotic swelling and subsequent endosome disruption and escape of contents of the endosome (89). RPE, which is involved in age-related macular degeneration, is considered a potential gene therapy target because of its high intrinsic phagocytic function in vivo. It was reported that human RPE cell uptake and expression of green fluorescent protein and neomycin-resistant gene was significantly enhanced using polyplex. Although there was a rapid decline in gene expression over 2 weeks, stable integration occurs at low frequency (90). Toxicity data on polycations suggest that many polymers used for transfections are most effective at concentrations that are just subtoxic, and the cellular uptake of the complexes may be mediated by membrane destabilization (91). Although polylysine could cause aggregation of erythrocytes at low doses and a wide variety of polycations have been reported to be cytotoxic (92) or have other adverse effects in culture in vivo, there is lack of information on all cationic polymers used in gene therapy.

6. Dendrimers

Dendrimers are fractal polymers. Their formation begins with a core molecule with at least three chemically reactive chains. Further polymerization occurs at the end of the chains to produce a spherical branched polymer. They terminate at charged and uncharged amino groups and bind to the negatively charged DNA (93). On internalization, the dendrimers buffer the endosomal environment and inhibit pH-dependent lysosomal nucleases. The efficiency of the dendrimers can be increased severalfold by heat treatment in water or isobutanol, which trims away parts of the molecule and makes it more flexible (94). Dendrimers have been found to possess low cytotoxicity in vitro and in vivo (95). Polyamidoamine dendrimers are a new class of nonviral agents that have been used for ex vivo gene transfer to corneal epithelium. Whole thickness of rabbit or human corneas was transfected with activated dendrimers and plasmids containing lacZ or TNFR-Ig genes. The expression was restricted to endothelium for 3 days (96). Dendrimers could be used as a potential delivery system for gene therapy in the eye to prevent allograft rejection or in the treatment of other disorders of corneal endothelium. Recently Urtti et al. (97) studied the delivery of plasmids encoding β-galactosidase (pCMVnLacZ) and luciferase (pCLuc4, pRSVLuc, pSV2Luc) in human retinal pigment epithelial cells, and they found that polyamidoamine starburst dendrimers and high molecular weight polyethylenimine produce better transgene expression than cationic lipids (DOTAP), despite the low percentage of transfected cells. It was also shown that dendrimers and polyethylenimine combinations produce less cellular toxicity in retinal pigment epithelial cell transfection.

7. Formulation Aspects of Nonviral Gene Delivery Products

A number of nonviral agents have been developed in recent years, but a major limitation is the remarkable instability of the formulations (98). A recent review by Pogocki and Schoneich discussed the factors affecting the chemical stability of nucleic acid–derived drugs (99). Normally the solutions of the carrier and the DNA are mixed to form a nonuniform mixture and administered. However, the transfection rate depends greatly on the physicochemical properties of the DNA-carrier complex (100). An ideal formulation would be a stable and transportable lyophilized powder or a frozen sample that can be easily reconstituted into a homogenous isotonic solution for ready administration. It was reported that agitation and freeze-thaw process in shipping and storage of lipid-DNA complexes could significantly reduce the transfection rates, slow freezing being more detrimental than quick freezing, while some sugars are able to retain transfection capability and complex size during the freeze-thaw process (101,102). It is believed that the same concept of "preferential exclusion" as applicable in frozen protein formulations is also applicable in DNA-carrier complexes (103).

III. OLIGONUCLEOTIDES

Oligonucleotide (ON) therapy is based on the principle of blocking the synthesis of cellular proteins by interfering with either the transcription of DNA to mRNA or the translation of mRNA to proteins. The expression of a specific gene blocked on the translation level by a complementary oligonucleotide using Watson-Crick hybridization to targeted mRNA is called an antisense oligonucleotide. Among several mechanisms by which antisense molecules disrupt gene expression and inhibit protein synthesis, the ribonuclease H mechanisms is the most important. Ribonuclease H (RNaseH), an enzyme present in most cells, recognizes the DNA-RNA or RNA-RNA duplex and disrupts the base pairing by digesting the RNA part of the double helix, rendering the digested mRNA incapable of translation. When the single-stranded complementary DNA binds to portions of DNA and forms a triple helix and inhibits protein synthesis, it is called the triplex approach. The functions of different oligonucleotides are depicted in Figure 3. Some researchers believe that the triplex approach is not a true antisense approach. In August 1998, Vitravene™ (fomivirsen

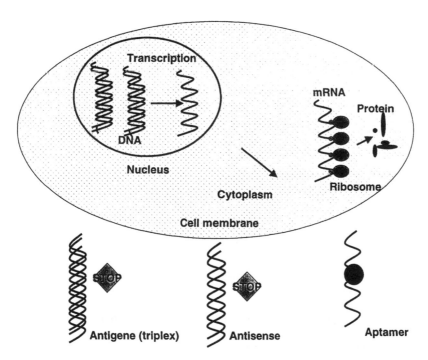

Figure 3 Functions of oligonucleotides.

sodium intravitreal injectable, ISIS 2922) became the world's first antisense compound to be approved for marketing in the United States for cytomegalovirus retinitis (CMVR). CMVR occurs in an estimated 4–7% of AIDS patients, with the incidence increasing as immunosuppression (decreased CD4 count) becomes more severe. Fomivirsen sodium is a phosphorothioate oligonucleotide, 21 nucleotides in length, with the following sequence: 5'-GCG TTT GCT CTT CTT GCG-3'. Studies demonstrate that human retinal pigment epithelial (HRPE) cells were significantly more sensitive than fibroblasts to the antiviral actions of ISIS 2922 and ISIS 12212. The data indicate that the anti-CMVR potency of the two oligonucleotides was similar. The enhanced potency of these oligonucleotides in HRPE cells may be associated with a delay in viral gene transcription and slow viral replication and spread in these cells (104). It was shown that following intravitreal injection, antisense oligonucleotides preferentially accumulate in the retinal pigment epithelium and remain present for an extended period of time. It was also demonstrated that the presence of one antisense oligonucleotide homologous to rat RPE cathepsin S (Cat 5) induced the accumulation of photoreceptor-derived debris, which was reversible and temporary (105). A number of antisense compounds have progressed to the level of Phase 3 clinical trials. Initial stability problems due to the activity of exo- and endo-nucleases have been largely overcome by chemical modification of the ON structure. These modifications, however, have resulted in a loss of selectivity and the development of cellular toxicity in some instances. In addition, antisense agents have been used in the diagnostic approaches to determine whether the c-myc proto-oncogene is involved in cell proliferation and glycosaminoglycan synthesis in cultured orbital fibroblasts (106). Table 3 illustrates the characteristics of the major classes of DNA and RNA oligonucleotides.

Table 3 Oligonucleotides Strategy

Type of oligonucleotide	Strands	Target	Strategy
RNA	Single	MRNA	Antisense
		MRNA	Ribozyme
		Cellular protein	Combinatorial
DNA	Single	DNA	Triple helix
	Single	mRNA	Antisense
	Single	Cellular protein	Combinatorial
	Double	Transcription factor	Aptamer

Source: Ref. 107.

A. Design of Oligonucleotides and Biological Stability

A number of factors have been determined to contribute to the efficacy of antisense ON therapeutics, each of which must be carefully examined, but at present there is no one method or rule for the successful design of an ON. One primary consideration is the length of the ON species. Lengths of 17–25 bases have been shown to be optimal, as longer ONs have the potential to partially hybridize with nontarget RNA species (108). The G-C content of the ON is an important factor, as a high percentage of these nucleotides may result in the formation of secondary or tertiary structure within the oligonucleotide (109), which may affect the target binding.

Biological stability is the major barrier to consider when delivering both DNA and RNA oligonucleotides to cells. Natural phosphodiester (PO) oligonucleotides offer the opportunity to selectively intervene in gene expression; however, they are rapidly degraded in biological fluids (110,111) and cells (112,113) by exo- and endonucleases, which hydrolyze the phosphodiester linkages in natural ONs. Thus, phosphodiester oligonucleotides, in their native form, are not suitable in vitro, especially in serum containing culture media, or in vivo following parenteral administration (114,115). Intracerebroventricular applied phosphodiester ONs have somewhat longer half-lives in the brain but still undergo extensive degradation.

Protection from nuclease action has been achieved by modification of phosphate backbones, sugar moiety, and bases (Fig. 4). Substitution of one of the nonbridging oxygen atoms on the phosphate groups with either a methyl group or a sulfur atom produces methylphosphonate (116) and phosphorothioates, respectively. Methylphosphonate oligodeoxynucleotides (Table 4) are uncharged and enter the animal cells rapidly without distinguishing even a single mismatch (119). Phosphorothioates possess a negatively charged backbone and a sulfur-modified phosphate linkage that is less sensitive to nucleases (120), but they display significant non–sequence-specific background inhibition (121,122), which may result mainly from the interaction with cellular proteins (123). Phosphorodithioate, which is prochiral like phosphodiester, still lacks antisense efficacy and specificity (124) and may have potential toxicity in CNS applications (125–128). Moreover, methylphosphonate and phosphorothioate derivatives often exert lower binding affinity to their target sequences, possibly due to diastereomer formation (129,130). $2'$-Methoxy, $2'$-aminopropoxy, and $2'$-fluororibose are examples of deoxyribose modifications, and inosine and 5-methylcytosine are examples of base modifications. All of these chemical changes have been shown to convey protection from exo- and endonuclease activity, thereby increasing the stability and half-life of the antisense compounds. Each modification presents its own type of drawback when compared to phosphodie-

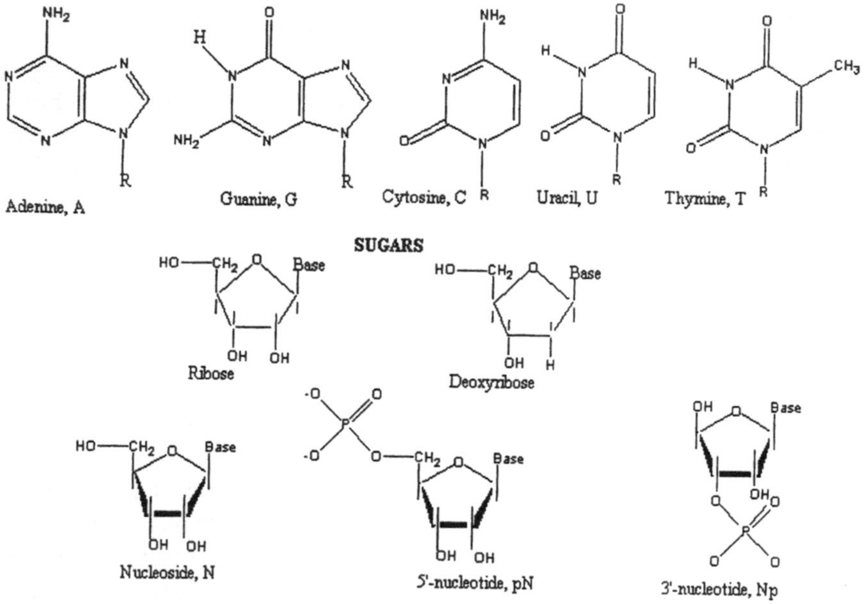

Figure 4 Nucleotide bases and sugars.

ster ONs, including issues of toxicity, targets selectivity, and cellular uptake. In spite of several disadvantages, these oligonucleotide modifications have thus far shown to be of utility (131).

In fact, the uptake of ONs in cells occurs in two steps: both charged and uncharged ONs are initially taken up by the process of endocytosis and accumulate in an endosomal-lysosomal compartment (132,133). In the second step, the ONs released from the endosomes enter the cytoplasm by an unknown mechanism and the transfer of ON to nucleus follows rapidly (134). One significant advantage of using oligonucleotides over gene therapy is that the transfer from cytoplasm to nucleus is faster with ONs than with larger DNA in gene therapy.

B. Cellular Uptake and Intracellular Fate

Cellular uptake of oligonucleotides has been a challenge, since only about 1–2% of the ONs may be taken up by cells (135). The uptake of ONs in the cells is dependent on time, concentration, energy, and temperature, indicating it to be an active process (136). As ONs are negatively charged the potential for diffusion across the lipid bilayer is extremely low. The length and sequence of ONs are determinants of their cellular uptake. Cell types,

Table 4 Important properties of Major Classes of Oligonucleotides Based on Chemical Structures

Oligonucleotide	Nuclease stability	Charge	Cellular uptake	Solubility
Phosphodiester (PO)	Poor	Polyanionic	Poor	Good
Phosphorothioate (PS)	Better than PO	Polyanionic	Worse than PO	Better than PO
Methylphosphonate (MP)	Better than PO	Neutral	Better than PO	Worse than PO

media, and culture conditions also affect uptake levels (137). A number of mechanisms have been identified for internalization of ONs. Receptor-mediated endocytosis of ON sequences occurs in a number of cell types. Proteins of 80 and 30 kDa have been identified to mediate ON uptake, while a simple charge association with the membrane may also be sufficient to trigger endo- or pinocytosis (138,139).

The pharmacological effects of ONs are dependent on the entry of ONs inside the cells and interaction with pre-mRNA or mRNA. The rate of permeation of both charged ONs and uncharged methylphosphonate compounds as well as alkyl-substituted phosphorothioate ONs across the lipid bilayers was found to be extremely slow (140,141). It is believed that there is binding of the oligonucleotide to the cell surface protein followed by internalization into the endocytic compartment (142), mainly by adsorptive endocytosis. It has been found that the oligonucleotides that adsorb best on the cell surface have better antisense activity. The release of antisense drugs from the endosomal compartment is the rate-limiting step for DNA trans-fection (143) as the antisense drug can be released by exocytosis or may be partially digested (144).

Zelphati and Szoka (145) proposed that, in a majority of the cell types, cationic lipids deliver oligonucleotides into the cell predominantly via an endocytic pathway rather than by fusion with the plasma mem-brane. The oligonucleotide is released from the complex when anionic lipids from the cytoplasm facing lipid monolayer of the cell flip into con-tact with the complex; the anionic lipids then laterally diffuse into the complex and form a charged neutralized ion pair with the cationic lipid, which leads to displacement of the oligonucleotide from the cationic lipids and its release into the cytoplasm (146,147) (Fig. 5). Recently, Wu-Pong discussed transporters involved in the nucleic acid transport and presented a hypothesis involving the porin-like transports in the internalization of oligonucleotides (148).

Once inside the cell, ONs can be distributed in various regions of the cell depending on the chemical modifications made to the ON. Phosphodiester and methylphosphonate ONs are sequestered within the nucleus in most cell types examined (149). Phosphorothioate derivatives remain in the cytoplasm in some cell lines but can enter the nucleus in others (150). Most ONs seem dependent on endocytotic processes, indicating that these molecules will enter the endosomal/lysosomal pathway. Interaction with the lysosomes results in the degradation of all types of ONs (151). Agents that disrupt endosomes can enhance the efficacy of some ONs (152). Therefore, circumventing the endosomal/lysosomal pathway is one possible mechanism to enhance the delivery and efficacy of antisense com-pounds.

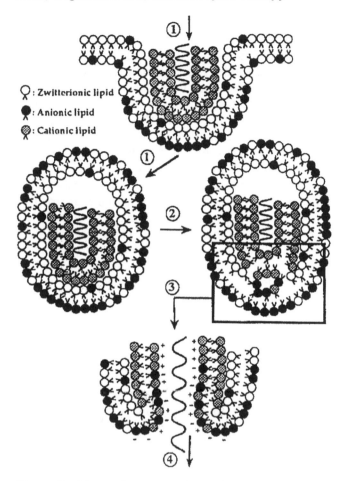

: Zwitterionic lipid

: Anionic lipid

: Cationic lipid

Figure 5 Oligonucleotide uptake pathway from cationic lipid complex. First the cell surface–associated complex is internalized via an endosome (step 1). The complex initiates a destabilization of the endosomal membrane that results in a flip-flop of anionic lipids (step 2), which are predominantly located on the cytoplasm face of the membrane. The anionic lipids laterally diffuse into the complex and form a charged neutralized ion pair with the cationic lipid (step 3). This displaces the oligonucleotide from the complex, and the oligonucleotide can diffuse into the cytoplasm (step 4).

C. Nonantisense Effects of Antisense Oligonucleotides

Although antisense technology has emerged as one of the latest advances in the development of biotechnology in therapeutics, its success is hampered by the nonspecific activity of antisense drugs. Based on the estimation of 3–4 billion base pairs in the human genome, assuming a random distribution, it is calculated that a minimum of 12–15 bases is required to recognize a single specific sequence of the genome. Interestingly, it has been pointed out that increasing the length of oligonucleotides may threaten its specificity, as it may hybridize to other mRNAs (153). It has been shown that changing the nature of phosphate linkage and the sugar moiety without changing the sequence of phosphorothioate and unmodified ONs may not affect the hybridization to target mRNA, but it may have an effect on binding to proteins (154). Phosphorothioate ONs (sulfated polyanions) have been shown to bind with a number of growth factors, including vesicular endothelial growth factor, and shown to inhibit protein kinase C or RnaseH. The interactions can be nonspecific, sequence specific, or structure specific. It was also shown that at a low concentration, these oligonucleotides could block their own uptake by the cells (155). The anticancer drugs that function as DNA intercalators can bind to certain oligonucleotides (156). A few motifs within the oligonucleotides could stimulate the immune response, and it has been suggested to avoid unmethylated CpGs in antisense drugs (157).

D. Delivery of Antisense Oligodeoxynucleotides

The major challenges in the delivery of antisense ONs are the stability of the drug in the body and transport through intercellular membranes. Natural phosphodiester oligonucleotides offer the opportunity to selectively intervene with gene expression, but they are rapidly degraded in biological fluids (158,159) and cells (160,161) by exo- or endonucleases, which hydrolyze the phosphodiester linkages in natural ONs. Except for methylphosphonate derivatives, ONs are polyanionic and hydrophilic in nature, which prevents their passive diffusion through the cellular and nuclear membranes (162–164). The extensively investigated phosphorothioate ONs may be more stable to endonuclease action and show improved transport properties (165).

One of the primary concerns of drug development is the ability to provide the drug in an oral dosage form to enhance patient compliance. Currently antisense ONs are primarily administered parenterally, with IV administration being the most often used method. Parenteral administration means that patients will likely be treated by a health care professional at a health care facility or by a home infusion specialist: this requirement may result in the cost of treatment becoming prohibitive. Such treatment regimens over the long term often result in a significant decrease in compliance as well. The development of delivery vehicles such as liposomes and microparticles may circumvent the problems of administration and distribution (166,167).

1. Polycations

As discussed in Sec. II, a number of polycations have been used to deliver oligonucleotides. Most common is DEAE-D (diethyl aminoethyl dextran), which complexes with RNA species (168) and enhances interferon induction (169). Poly(L-lysine) has been used to enhance transport of several drugs, including oligonucleotides (170,171). The rate and uptake of ONs were increased as demonstrated using flow cytometric analysis and fluorescent-labeled oligonucleotides (172). Highly specific delivery of ONs using positively charged poly(L-lysine) is attributed to its nonspecific interaction with negatively charged molecules on the cell surface and subsequent internalization by absorptive endocytosis (173). However, the use of poly(L-lysine) is limited due to its potential cytotoxicity, even at low concentrations (174), and nonspecific conjugation with cell membrane components. The recently introduced transfecting agent, polyethylenimine, has been showed to be effective in studying neuronal ion channel function with antisense oligonucleotides (175).

2. Lipid-Mediated Delivery

Cationic lipid-mediated transfection of DNA into cells is a well-documented approach in gene therapy protocols (176,177). A highly efficient DNA transfection technique, "lipofection," was introduced by Felgner et al. in 1987 (178). Commercially available Lipofectin^{TM} consists of a 1 : 1 weight mixture of positively charged quaternary amino lipid N-[1-(2,3-dioleyloxy)propyl]-N,N,N-trimethylammonium chloride (DOTMA) and neutral lipid dioleylphosphatidylcholine (DOPC). Complexes of oligonucleotides and the cationic lipid Lipofectin bind to and penetrate cellular membranes, and ONs are subsequently released into the cytoplasm (179). Zelphati and Szoka (180) reported that oligonucleotides are delivered by cationic lipids to the cytoplasm at an early stage of the endocytotic pathway that leads to a marked increase in antisense activity and oligonucleotide nuclear uptake. In recent years, several types of cationic lipids have been introduced, including quaternary ammonium compounds, lipid-conjugated polyamines, and cationic derivative of cholesterol-diacyl glycerol (for discussion and reviews, see Refs. 181,182).

Typical uptake studies are conducted in serum-free medium (OPTI-MEM^{TM}) as Felgner et al. first observed (183) and confirmed (184) that inclusion of serum during incubation of cationic lipid–nucleotide complex with cells reduces the transfection efficiency. In fact, the presence of only

20% serum could reduce the cellular binding/uptake of cationic lipid–oligo-nucleotide complex by 81% compared to that attained in serum-free medium. This effect may have been a result of negatively charged serum components possibly attaching to the complex and preventing cellular interaction (185). However, the serum has little effect on some cationic lipid-DNA formulations.

As carriers for the delivery of nucleic acids, liposomes offer a protective biocompatible and biodegradable delivery system that can enhance the cellular uptake of nucleic acids (186). Liposomes made of cationic lipids have been widely used to enhance cellular uptake of oligonucleotides. Jaaskelainen et al. (187) showed that the anionic and cationic charge ratio of liposomes is critical in fusion and aggregation of liposomes and that negative charge on the cell membrane is responsible for fusion of the lipid vesicles to cell membranes and the ability to transfer oligonucleotides (188). Hartmann et al. (189) reported that cationic lipids that form complexes with oligonucleotides markedly enhanced the amount of oligonucleotide uptake in all cells types and were most effective at a 1 : 1 positive-to-negative molar charge ratio.

pH-sensitive liposomes, consisting of dioleoyl phosphatidyl ethanolamine (DOPE) and a stabilizing acidic amphiphilic lipid, are another unique vehicle to deliver ONs to the cells. pH-sensitive liposomes bind to the cell membrane without any fusogenic peptide while the load is shielded from nuclease action and is delivered from the endocytic compartment before reaching the lysosomes. These liposomes collapse in the endosomes where the negative charges of their lipids become protonated (pKa 5.7–6.5) (190). Milhaud et al. (191) encapsulated a phosphodiester oligodeoxynucleotide to inhibit vesicular stomatitis virus in murine L929 cells. The liposomes were stable and remained pH sensitive for several hours; however, the higher concentrations of lipids caused toxicity. Immunoliposomes are specific means of delivering nucleic acids to targeted cells with specific receptors. pH-sensitive immunoliposomes could promote target-specific delivery of an exogenous gene in plasmid DNA to lymphoma cells (192,193) while reducing the degradation of the nucleic acids by lysosomes (194). Ma and Wei (195) demonstrated that anti-CD32 or anti-CD2 immunoliposomes improved the delivery of 18mer anti-myb oligo to leukemia cells carrying the appropriate receptor for the specific antibody-linked immunoliposomes and the uptake was twice that of the liposomes or nonspecific immunoliposome encapsulated oligos. A recent study by Brazeau et al. (196) demonstrated that cationic liposomes were less myotoxic than dendrimers and poly-(D,L-lysine). Myotoxicity was dependent on the type of cationic lipid macromolecule, concentration, molecular weight, and the presence of plasmid DNA, possibly due to the reduction of the net positive charge by the cationic lipid-plasmid DNA complex.

Recent reports by Filion and Phillips (197,198) suggest that the cationic liposomes should be used with caution to deliver gene or antisense oligonucleotides to mammalian cells. Irrespective of the DNA content, cationic liposomes downregulate the synthesis of the protein kinase C–dependent mediators NO, TNF-α, and PGE$_2$ by activated macrophages after in vitro incubation under nontoxic conditions or after in vivo treatment. Prolonged incubation (> 3 h) of macrophages with cationic liposomes induced high toxicity which was not observed with nonphagocytic T cells. The rank order of toxicity was DOPE/DDAB(dimethyl dioctadecylammoniumbromide) $>$ DOPE/DOTAP $>$ DOPE/Dc-Chol $>$ DOPE/dimyristoyltrimethylammonium propane (DMTAP). The replacement of DOPE by dipalmitoylphosphatidylcholine reduced the toxicity. On the other hand, anionic liposomes are safe and can be produced reproducibly. These liposomes are inactive in nature and are typically endocytosed, resulting in degradation of DNA fragments in lysosomal endosomes (199). The pharmaceutical production of liposomes is still a challenge in view of its short shelf life, scale-up problems, and absence of sufficient safety data for these carrier systems for chronic use (200).

Although there is growing interest in the ocular delivery of antisense drugs using liposomes, extensive work has not been done in this area. Couvreur et al. (201) reported the development and in vitro characterization of a model oligonucleotide in liposome dispersed in Pluronic 407 (a thermosensitive gel). It was observed that the system could be effective in slow delivery of antisense drugs to topical or intravitreal tissues. In addition to charged liposomes, water-soluble block polycations consisting of polyoxyethylene (POE) and polyspermine (PS) have been reported to increase the sequence-specific inhibition effect of oligonucleotide on the virus reproduction (202). Another interesting study shows that the use of hemagglutinating virus of fusogenic liposomes can transfer LacZ DNA and phosphorothioate oligonucleotides to adult rat and primate trabecular meshwork. This system may enable progress in glaucoma research and in the development of nonviral somatic gene therapy of the trabecular meshwork to treat glaucoma (203).

3. Biodegradable Microparticles

Recent cell culture and in vivo studies with antisense oligonucleotides have promoted the need for safe and effective delivery systems for such drugs. Microparticles and microspheres are monolithic, solid structures, distinguishable from fluid and vesicular structures like liposomes. For parenteral delivery of bioactive agents, microparticles smaller than 1 μm are used. A number of biodegradable biopolymers (gelatin, albumin, polysaccharides, etc.) and synthetic polymers [polyalkylcyanoacrylate, poly(lactide-co-glycolide), polycarprolactone, polyanhydride, polyorthoester, etc.] have been used to formulate microparticles for delivery of a diverse range of bioactive agents (204–208). Biologically active agents could be formulated to be entrapped in the matrix of the microparticles or simply be adsorbed on the surface. Release of the therapeutic agent from the microparticles could be based on diffusion of the drug through the matrix of the polymer, surface, and/or bulk erosion of the polymer matrix or desorption of the active agent from the surface. The use of biodegradable polymeric microparticles for delivery of oligonucleotides is a viable means to deliver the drug more efficiently and could be useful in promoting cellular uptake through endocytosis, as demonstrated by studies employing cells such as fibroblasts and macrophages (209,210).

The major advantage of biodegradable polyester poly(lactide-co-glycolide) (PLGA) polymer for parenteral oligonucleotide delivery systems is its ability to control the time and/or rate at which the incorporated material is released. This biodegradable system has been used to successfully deliver a number of bioactive materials (211–214), and the lack of toxicity of poly(-lactide-co-glycolide) polymers has been established by FDA and by years of their use as absorbable suture materials (215,216). PLGA undergoes random, nonenzymatic hydrolysis of its backbone ester linkages in vivo at a rate that is influenced by molecular weight, surface area, monomer stereoregularity, and the ratio of lactide to glycolide (217). The homopolymer itself is degraded very slowly when compared with PLGA and is most suitable for long-term delivery of bioactive agents (218). In addition to PLGA nanoparticles, aminoalkylmethacrylate nanoparticles have been extensively studied for stability and antisense efficacy in vitro (219).

In a recent review article, O'Donnell and McGinity (220) comprehensively discussed the pros and cons of preparation of microparticles by the widely used solvent evaporation technique. An interesting study by Akhtar et al. (221) showed that ultrasound caused maximum degradation of ONs at a lower pH, longer-chain-length ONs were more stable than the shorter ones, and the phosphorothioate ONs were more stable than phosphodiester during ultrasound exposure. This is an important parameter in the development of microparticle dosage forms as well as delivery of ON by phonophoresis. Akhtar et al. (222) incorporated ^{32}P-labeled oligonucleotides in poly(L-lactide) matrices and observed that the degradation of ON due to nuclease action is substantially reduced. They also observed that ON release from matrices was dependent on the oligomer chemistry (S-oligos were released more slowly than the D-oligos) and on the oligomer length (a 20-mer oligo was released more slowly than a 7-mer). The same group of workers (223) reported that cellular association of ONs entrapped within small microparticles was improved 10-fold in murine macrophages compared with free ONs. Uptake was enhanced when macrophages were activated with INF-γ and lipolysaccharide treatment but decreased significantly in the presence of metabolic and phagocytosis inhibitors.

Polyalkylcyanoacrylate microparticles have been shown to be promising in protecting the adsorbed ONs from nuclease action (224). Adsorbed ONs in such microparticles significantly increased the ON uptake in the human macrophage–like cell line U-937 as a result of the capture of microparticles by an endocytic/phagocytic pathway (225). Nakada et al. (226) showed that ON-adsorbed poly(isobutylcyanoacrylate) microparticles protected the ONs against nuclease action in vivo and deliver them to the liver. Godard et al. (227) observed that ONs covalently attached to a cholesterol moiety and adsorbed onto poly(isohexylcyanoacrylate) nanoparticles are more stable in biological media and better taken up by the eukaryotic cells. However, the use of poly(isohexylcyanoacrylate) and quaternary ammonium compounds as adsorbing agents has been criticized because of the cytotoxicity of poly(hexylcyanoacrylate) and general toxicity of quaternary ammonium compounds (228).

Among the polyester polymers, our previous studies using an 18-base deoxyribonucleic acid oligonucleotide (5′-CTGGTAGCATATGTAAGG-3′) of the rat serotonin transporter in the biodegradable poly(lactide-co-glycolide) 85:15 microparticles retained the stability of oligonucleotide and allowed a significant reduction in the rate of uptake of 5-HT without altering the affinity of 5-HT for the transporter in rat basophilic leukemia cells (229). The interaction of the particulate system with biological components, as well as its distribution and entry to the target cells, essentially depends on the hydrodynamic size and the particle charge. As discussed earlier, inherent negative charge of ONs significantly retards its delivery, and positively charged components in the matrix of the microparticles would promote efficient uptake of ONs in the target cells.

The biodegradable microparticles can also be used for delivery of ONs across the blood-brain barrier. Schroder and Sabel (230), and Kreuter (231) have discussed the delivery of drug-loaded polyalkylcyanoacrylate microparticles to the brain tissues. An interesting study by Quong et al. (232) discussed the encapsulation of DNA using alginate microparticles and the effect of calcium ion.

4. Physical Approaches

A more significant and efficient transfer of plasmid DNA, polynucleotides, and oligonucleotides can be achieved using the technique of electroporation. This system provides higher efficiency of transfer compared to other nonviral transfer systems, including cationic liposomes (233). Application of electroporation to cultured cells is well established, but the use of electroporation in vivo has received little attention (234,235). Electroporation or a change in the permeability of the cell membrane by electric current has achieved popularity in recent years due to its high efficiency of transfer of gene or oligonucleotides (236). Recently, Flanagan and Wagner (237) described efficient inhibition of gene using electroporation of antisense oligodeoxynucleotides. However, electroporation is not a viable technique for delivery of antisense drugs to ocular tissues.

IV. APTAMERS

Aptamers are artificial nucleic acid ligands, typically composed of RNA, single-stranded DNA, or a combination of these with nonnatural nucleotides that can be generated against amino acids, drugs, proteins, and other molecules. They are isolated from complex libraries of synthetic nucleic acid by an iterative process of adsorption, recovery, and reamplification. They bind with the target molecules at a very low level with high specificity. One of the earliest aptamers studied structurally was the 15 mer DNA aptamer against thrombin, d(GGTTGGTGTGGTTGG) (238). RNA aptamers, or nucleotides with predominantly RNA-like properties, are capable of adopting a greater variety of structures (239). The structures of protein-binding aptamers affects the function of aptamers. For example, aptamers that bind the HIV-1 regulatory protein, Rev, accommodate an alpha helix of their target within a modified major groove that is widened by the presence of a number of non–Watson-Crick base pairs (240). In contrast, a class of aptamers that bind the reverse transcriptase of HIV-1 possess a compact form of pseudoknot structure (241). Aptamers can show a great deal of specificity. For example, α-thrombin can be differentiated from γ-thrombin (242); two isozymes of protein kinase C differing in just 23 residues could be readily distinguished (243), as could the CD4 glycoproteins of rat and mouse (73% identity) (244). For the purpose of diverse application, it is necessary for the aptamer to be small, typically 10 kDa. Interestingly, aptamers can bind with small molecules, e.g., Zn^{2+} (245), to bigger ones like ATP (246), neutral disaccharides (247), dopamine (248), porphyrin (249), and aminoglycoside antibiotics (250), spanning a size range of 65–150 kDa or more.

Natural, 2'-OH RNA degrades very rapidly in human serum in vitro, but this process can be slowed at least 1000-fold by 2'-amino modification (135). In vivo studies on the $t_{1/2}$ of single-stranded DNA aptamers give values in the range of less than 2 to approximately 8 minutes (136–138). Conjugation of the aptamer to either lipids or polyethylene glycol has been reported to improve the stability and distribution kinetics of DNA aptamers sufficiently to produce therapeutic effects (139,140). Although there is no evidence regarding aptamers in ocular therapy, there has been promising research on thrombin aptamers (251–252) and angiogenin (253) (a DNA aptamer that prevents angiogenesis and cell proliferation) that indicates the possible application of aptamers in ocular applications in future.

In a healthy adult, angiogenesis occurs during the menstrual cycle and wound healing, but it is also a central feature of various disease states, including cancer and diabetic retinopathy. Recently it has been reported that an aptamer antagonist of vascular endothelial growth factor (VEGF) can inhibit blood vessel growth, or angiogenesis, in vivo. Data from in vitro experiments demonstrated that a liposomal formulation of VEGF aptamer bound with high affinity to VEGF and inhibited the growth of endothelial cells and cancer cells. In all experiments, the liposomal formulation substantially enhanced the inhibitory activity of the aptamer.

V. RIBOZYMES

An important development in the use of nucleic acid–related drugs in ocular tissues is the use of ribozymes. RNA enzymes or ribozymes are a relatively new class of single-stranded RNA molecules capable of assuming three-dimensional conformations and exhibiting catalytic activity that induces site-specific cleavage, ligation, and polymerization of nucleotides involving RNA or DNA (254). They function by binding to the target RNA moiety through Watson-Crick base pairing and inactivate it by cleaving the phosphodiester backbone at a specific cutting site. Three classes of natural ribozymes have been described based on their unique characters in the sequence and three-dimensional structure: (a) self-splicing introns of bacteria, mitochondria, (b) RNAase p, required for 5' trimming of tRNA precursors, and (c) self-cleaving viral agents, including the hepatitis delta virus ribozyme. Because of their small size, specificity for target sequence, and catalytic activity (can be effective in a low concentration), ribozymes have great potential for use in inhibiting viral replication or cell proliferation (255,256). They may catalyze self-cleavage (intramolecular or "in-*cis*" catalysis) as well as the cleavage of external substrates (intermolecular or "in-*trans*" catalysis) (257,258). The term "hammerhead ribozyme" reflects its structural similarity to a hammerhead. These are the best understood of all ribozymes. Some ribonucleotides within the sequence selectively form Watson-Crick base pairs with others to form a stem, while the rest stay in a single-stranded state called a loop. These loops and stems can be predicted at the secondary structure level using conformational energy analysis. Most ribozymes can be chemically engineered to cleave RNA in *trans* by separating the catalytic domain from ribozyme and attaching recognition (i.e., antisense) arms to the catalytic center in order to target a substrate. These *trans*-acting ribozymes can be very useful in the study of molecular biology and pharmaceutics.

The single-dose safety trial of the anti–hepatitis C ribozyme LY 466700 has been recently been completed in the first cohort of normal volunteers. Administration of LY466700 to chronic hepatitis C patients has now been initiated in a clinical trial designed to study safety and to assess the effect of the compound on HCV viral RNA levels following a 28-day dose-response regimen.

About 1 in 3000 Americans has retinitis pigmentosa, a degenerative disease, the symptoms of which generally first appear during adolescence. As the disorder progresses, night vision, peripheral vision, and ultimately all sight can be lost. Currently, there is no way to halt the deterioration. Autosomal dominated retinitis pigmentosa (ADRP) is caused by mutations in genes that produce mutated proteins, leading to the apoptotic death of photoreceptor cells (259). The pioneering work of Lewin and Hauswirth in the delivery of ribozymes in ADRP in rats shows promise for ribozyme therapy in many other autosomal dominant eye diseases, including glaucoma. They constructed ribozymes that would bind to the mutant forms of rhodopsin messenger RNA but not to normal (wild-type) rhodopsin mRNA. The most potent ribozymes were cloned (as DNA) in recombinant adeno-associated viral vectors and injected behind the photoreceptor layer of transgenic rats containing a mutated form of the rhodopsin gene with defective P23H (proline residue to histidine at 23—common form of ADRP in North America) and S334ter (serine for premature termination at 334—a representative of whole class of ADRP mutations). The ribozyme successfully slowed the rod cell apoptosis and maintained rod cell function for a minimum of 8 months after a single injection (260). In a recent study the P347S porcine hammerhead ribozyme cloned in rAAV vector and packaged into AAV was found to cleave the full length of P347S mRNA (261). Moreover, ribozymes can discriminate between the mutant and wild-type sequences of mRNA associated with autosomal dominant retinitis pigmentosa. The kinetics and specificity of ribozyme cleavage (Fig. 6) indicate that they should reduce the amount of aberrant rhodopsin in the rod cells and could have potential as therapeutic agents against genetic diseases. The most active ribozymes against P23H target were first hammerhead and then hairpin ribozyme (262). The same group also reported that ribozyme rescue appears to be a potentially effective long-term therapy for autosomal dominant retinal degeneration and is highly effective even when the gene transfer is done after significant photoreceptor cell loss (263).

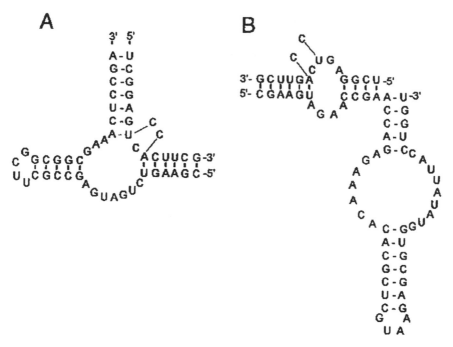

Figure 6 Hammerhead (A) and hairpin (B) ribozymes used to target P23H opsin mRNA. The positions of cytosine nucleotide in wild-type rhodopsin are indicated.

There are several advantages of using ribozymes over antisense RNA products (264):

1. Greater specificity of ribozymes—ribozymes inhibited viral replication 2- to 10-fold compared to a comparable antisense molecule (265).
2. Ribozymes are short, while antisense oligonucleotides could be long—ribozymes are more selective than antisense oligonucleotides. A single base mismatch in a ribozyme could produce a completely different effect, while the same type of mismatch in an antisense oligonucleotide could have little impact.

Mutation-independent hammerhead ribozymes targeting rhodopsin and peripherin have been screened in vitro and a number of extremely efficient ribozymes identified subsequent to detailed kinetic analyses, suggesting that these ribozymes may provide mutation-independent methods for treating ADRP. The reported ribozymes have potential for use in inherited retinopathies (266). The future of ribozymes in the management of wound healing in ocular diseases is still to be investigated. One group has demonstrated that ribozymes against TGF-β1 mRNA in vitro successfully reduce expression of TGF-β1 at both protein and mRNA levels within 3 days of application (267).

VI. CONCLUSION

A great number of eye diseases are currently difficult to treat with conventional medications due to the lack of target specificity of small molecule–based therapies and the propensity of these compounds to enter the general circulation. In addition, small molecules cannot restore the function of a missing gene or protein. As more information about the genetic basis of ocular disease is revealed, gene therapy and antisense oligonucleotide–based treatment strategies may afford a mechanism by which to alter or correct aberrant gene function in a highly selective manner. A great deal of progress has been made in the engineering of vector systems, but the classic issue of absorption and distribution, which exist with all drug development programs, remain a significant hurdle to the use of genetic material in the treatment of disease. Until effective mechanisms by which to deliver nucleotide-based materials are developed, the progress and utilities of these therapies will be limited. The ability to regain or specifically inhibit gene function, however, is a significant force in driving the continued development of this potentially powerful set of therapeutic tools.

REFERENCES

1. S. C. Hyde, D. R. Gill, C. F. Higgins, A. E. Trezise, L. J. MacVinish, A. W. Cuthbert, R. Ratcliff, M. J. Evans, and W. H. Colledge. (1993). Correction of the ion transport defect in cystic fibrosis transgenic mice by gene therapy. *Nature, 362*:250–255.
2. J. A. Roth and R. J. Cristiano. (1997). Gene therapy for cancer. What have we done and where are we going? *J. Natl. Cancer Inst., 89*:21–39.
3. D. J. Weatherall. (1995). Scope and limitations of gene therapy. *Br. Med. Bull., 51*:1–11.
4. N. Somia and I. M. Verma. (2000). Gene therapy: trials and tribulations. *Nat. Rev. Genet., 1*:91–99.
5. J. Stephenson. (2001). New therapies show promise for patients with leukemia, hemophilia and heart disease. *J. Am. Med. Assoc., 285*:153–155.
6. T. Sakamoto, H. Kimura, Z. Scuric, and C. Spee et al. (1995). Inhibition of experimental proliferative vitreoretinopathy by retroviral vector mediated transfer of suicide gene. *Ophthalmology, 102*:1417–1424.

7. A. F. Wright. (1997). Gene therapy for the eye. *Br. J. Ophthalmol., 81*:620–623.

8. P. V. Algvere, L. Berglin, P. Gouras, and Y. Sheng. (1994). Transplantation of fetal retinal pigment epithelium in age-related macular degeneration with subfoveal neovascularization. *Graefe's Arch. Clin. Exp. Ophthalmol., 232*:707–716.

9. W. W. Hauswirth and L. Beaufrere. (2000). Ocular gene therapy: Quo Vadis? *Invest. Ophthalmol. Vis. Sci., 41*:2821–2826.

10. W. F. Anderson. (1998). Human gene therapy. *Nature, 392*:25–30.

11. A. Rolland. (1993). *Pharmaceutical Particulate Carriers: Therapeutic Applications.* Marcel Dekker, New York.

12. A. D. Miller. (1992). Human gene therapy comes of age. *Nature, 357*:455–460.

13. W. F. Anderson, R. M. Blaese, and K. W. Culver. (1990). The ADA human gene therapy clinical protocol. *Hum. Gene Ther., 1*:327–362.

14. S. A. Rosenberg, P. Aebersold, K. Conetta, et al. (1990). Gene transfer into humans: Immunotherapy of patients with advanced melanoma, using tumor-infiltrating lymphocytes modified by retroviral gene transduction. *N. Engl. J. Med., 323*:570–578.

15. The Journal of Gene Medicine, John Wiley & Sons, 2001, www.wiley.co.uk/genmed.

16. G. Romano, C. Pacilio, and A. Giordano. (1999). Gene transfer technology in therapy: Current applications and future goals. *Stem. Cells, 17*:191–202.

17. J. Bennett, and A. M. Maguire. (2000). Gene therapy for ocular disease. *Mol. Ther., 1*:501–505.

18. J. M. Coffin. (1996). Retroviridae: The viruses and their replication. In *Virology*, Vol. 2 (B. N. Fields, D. M. Knipe, and P. M. Howley, eds.). Lippincott, Philadelphia, pp. 1767–1847.

19. D. G. Miller, M. A. Adam, and A. D. Miller. (1990). Gene transfer by retrovirus vectors occurs only in cells that are actively replicating at the time of infection. *Mol. Cell. Biol., 10*:4239–4242.

20. P. L. Stewart, R. M. Burnett, M. Cyrlaff, et al. (1991). Image reconstruction reveals the complex molecular organization of adenovirus. *Cell, 67*:145–154.

21. P. L. Stewart, S. D. Fuller, and R. M. Burnett. (1993). Difference imaging of adenovirus: Bridging the resolution gap between X-ray crystallography and electron microscopy. *EMBO J., 12*:2589–2599.

22. H. S. Ginsberg, and G. A. Prince. (1994). The molecular basis of adenovirus pathogenesis. *Infect. Agents Dis., 3*:1–8.

23. T. J. Wickham, P. Mathias, D. A. Cheresh, and G. R. Nemerow. (1993). Integrins alpha v beta 3 and alpha v beta 5 promote adenovirus internalization but not virus attachment. *Cell, 73*:309–319.

24. S. L. Brody and R. G. Crystal. (1994). Adenovirus-mediated in vivo gene transfer. *Ann. NY Acad. Sci., 716*:90–101.

25. M. Ali, N. R. Lemoine, and C. J. Ring. (1994). The use of DNA viruses as vectors for gene therapy. *Gene Ther., 1*:367–384.

26. S. Yei, N. Mittereder, K. Tang, C. O'Sullivan, and B. C. Trapnell. (1994). Adenovirus-mediated gene transfer for cystic fibrosis: Quantitative evalua-

tion of repeated in vivo vector administration to the lung. *Gene Ther.*, *1*:192–200.

27. M. D. Hoggan, N. R. Blacklow, and W. P. Rowe. (1966). Studies of small DNA viruses found in various adenovirus preparations: Physical, biological and immunological characteristics. *Proc. Natl. Acad. Sci. USA*, *55*:1467–1474.

28. H. Handa, K. Shiroki, and H. Shimojo. (1977). Establishment and characterization of KB cell lines latently infected with adeno-associated virus type 1. *Virology*, *82*:84–92.

29. K. I. Berns, T. C. Pinkerton, G. F. Thomas, and M. D. Hoggan. (1975). Detection of adeno-associated virus (AAV) specific nucleotide sequences in DNA isolated from latently infected Detroit 6 cells. *Virology*, *68*:556–560.

30. G. Podsakoff, K. K. Wong, Jr., and S. Chatterjee (1994). Efficient gene transfer into nondividing cells by adeno-associated virus-based vectors. *J. Virol.*, *68*:5656–5666.

31. R. M. Kotin, M. Siniscalco, R. J. Samulski, X. D. Zhu, L. Hunter, C. A. Laughlin, S. Mclaughlin, N. Muzyczka, M. Rocchi, and K. I. Berns. (1990). Site-specific integration by adeno-associated virus. *Proc. Natl. Acad. Sci. USA*, *87*:2211–2215.

32. J. Y. Dong, P. D. Fan, and R. A. Frizzell. (1996). Qualitative analysis of the packaging capacity of recombinant adeno-associated virus. *Hum. Gene Ther.*, *7*:2101–2112.

33. L. M. Hoffman, A. M. Maguire, and J. Bennett. (1997). Cell-mediated immune response and stability of intraocular transgene expression after adenovirus-mediated delivery. *Invest. Opthal. Vis. Sci.*, *38*:2224–2233.

34. K. Tsubota, H. Inoue, K. Ando, M. Ono, K. Yoshino, and I. Saito. (1998). Adenovirus-mediated gene transfer to the ocular surface epithelium. *Exp. Eye Res.*, *67*:531–538.

35. J. Guy, X. Qi, H. Wang, and W. W. Hauswirth. (1999). Adenoviral gene therapy with catalase suppresses experimental optic neuritis. *Arch. Opthalmol.*, *117*:1533–1539.

36. H. B. Oral, D. F. P. Larkin, Z. Fehervari, A. P. Byrnes, A. M. Rankin, D. O. Haskard, M. J. A. Wood, M. J. Dallman, and A. J. T. George. (1997). Ex vivo adenovirus mediated gene transfer and immunomodulatory protein production in human cornea. *Gene Therapy*, *4*:639–647.

37. A. Di Polo, L. J. Aigner, R. J. Dunn, G. M. Bray, and A. J. Aguayo. (1998). Prolonged delivery of brain-derived neurotrophic factor by adenovirus infected Muller cells temporarily rescues injured retinal ganglion cells. *Proc. Natl. Acad. Sci. USA*, *95*:3978–3983.

38. C. Jomary, J. Grist, J. Millbrandt, M. Neal, and S. E. Jones. (2001). Epitope-tagged recombinant AAV vectors for expressing neurturin and its receptor in retinal cells. *Mol. Vis.*, *7*: 36–41.

39. D. Lau, L. H. McGee, S. Zhou, K. G. Rendahl, W. C. Manning, J. A. Escobedo, and J. G. Flanner. (2000). Retinal degeneration is slowed in transgenic rats by AAV-mediated delivery of FGF-2. *Invest. Ophthalmol. Vis. Sci.*, *41*:3622–3633.

40. X. Liu, C. R. Brandt, B. T. Gabelt, P. J. Bryar, M. E. Smith, and P. L. Kaufman. (1999). Herpes simplex virus mediated gene transfer to primate ocular tissues. *Exp. Eye. Res., 69*:385–395.
41. C. R. Brandt, R. E. Kalil, and S. Agarwala. (2000). Replication competent, a virulent herpes simplex virus as a vector for neural and ocular gene therapy. US Patent 6,106,826, August 22, 2000.
42. E. L. Berson. (1994). Retinitis pigmentosa and allied diseases. In: D. M. Albert, F. A. Jakobiec, eds. *Principles and Practice of Ophthalmology*, Vol. 2. Saunders, Philadelphia, pp. 1214–1237.
43. S. L. Bernstein and P. Wong (1998). Regional expression of disease-related genes in human and monkey retina. *Mol. Vis., 4*:24.
44. D. T. Organisciak and B. S. Winkler. (1994). Retinal light damage: Practical and theoretical considerations. *Prog. Retin. Eye Res., 13*:1–29.
45. C. Grimm, A. Wenzel, F. Hafezi, and C. E. Reme. (2000). Gene expression in the mouse retina: The effect of damaging light. *Mol. Vis., 6*:252–260.
46. T. Murata, J. Cui, K. E. Taba, J.-Y. Oh, C. Spee, D. R. Hinton, and S. J. Ryan. (2000). The possibility of gene therapy for the treatment of choroidal neovascularization. *Ophthalmology, 107*:1364–1373.
47. R. Niven, J. Smith, and Y. Zhang. (1997). Toward development of a non-viral gene therapeutics. *Adv. Drug Deliv. Rev., 26*:135–150.
48. H. Pollard, J. S. Remy, G. Loussouarn, S. Demolombe, J. P. Behr, and D. Escande. (1998). Polyethylenimine but not cationic lipids promotes transgene delivery to the nucleus in mammalian cells. *J. Biol. Chem., 273*:7507–7511.
49. F. D. Ledley. (1995). Nonviral gene therapy: The promise of genes as pharmaceutical products. *Hum. Gene Ther., 6*:1129–1144.
50. J. W. Streilein. (1996). Ocular immune privilege and the Faustian dilemma. *Invest. Ophthalmol. Vis. Sci., 37*:1940–1950.
51. H. Kimura, Y. Ogura, T. Moritera, Y. Honda, Y. Tabata, and Y. Ikada. (1994). In vitro phagocytosis of polylactide microspheres by retinal pigment epithelial cells and intracellular drug release. *Curr. Eye Res., 13*:353–360.
52. J. Zabner, A. J. Fasbender, T. Moninger, K. A. Poellinger, and M. J. Welsh. (1995). Cellular and molecular barriers to gene transfer by a cationic lipid. *J. Biol. Chem., 270*:18997–19007.
53. Y. Xu. and F. C. Szoka. (1996). Mechanism of DNA release from cationic liposome/DNA complex used in cell transfection. *Biochemistry, 35*:5616–5623.
54. J. Flensburg, S., Eriksson, and H. Lindblom. (1988). Purification of supercoiled plasmid DNA by ion exchange chromatography. *DNA Protein Eng. Tech., 1*:85–90.
55. M. Cotten, A. Baker, M. Saltik, E. Wagner, and M. Buschle. (1994). Lipopolysaccharide is a frequent contaminant of plasmid DNA preparations and can be toxic to primary human cells in the presence of adenovirus. *Gene Ther., 1*:239–246.
56. M. A. Hickman, R. W. Malone, K. Lehmann-Buinsma, T. R. Sih, D. Knoell, F. C. Szoka, R. Walzem, D. M. Carlson, and J. S. Powell. (1994). Gene

expression following direct injection of DNA into liver. *Human Gene Ther.,* 5:1477–1483.

57. J. P. Yang and L. Huang. (1996). Direct gene transfer to mouse melanoma by intratumor injection of free DNA. *Gene Ther., 3*:542–548.

58. M. Kriegler. (1990). Gene transfer. In: *Gene Transfer and Expression: A Laboratory Manual.* W. H. Freeman and Co., New York, pp. 3–8.

59. J. Vacik, B. S. Dean, W. E. Zimmer, and D. A. Dean. (1999). Cell-specific nuclear import of plasmid DNA. *Gene Ther., 6*:1006–1014.

60. D. A. Dean, J. N. Byrd, and B. S. Dean. (1999). Nuclear targeting of plasmid DNA in human corneal cells. *Curr. Eye Res., 19*:66–75.

61. S. A. Johnston and D. C. Tang. (1994). Gene gun transfection of animal cells and genetic immunization. *Methods Cell Biol., 43*:353–365.

62. W. H. Sun, J. K. Burkholder, J. Sun, J. Culp, X. G. Lu, T. D. Pugh, W. B. Ershler, and N. S. Yang. (1992). In vivo cytokine gene transfer by gene gun reduces tumor growth in mice. *Proc. Natl. Acad. Sci. USA, 89*:11277–11281.

63. D. L. Tanelian, M. A. Barry, S. A. Johnston, T. Le, and G. Smith (1997). Controlled gene gun delivery and expression of DNA within the cornea. *Bio Techniques, 23*:484–488.

64. S. A. Konig Merediz, E. P. Zhang, B. Wittig, and F. Hoffmann. (2000). Ballistic transfer of minimalistic immunologically defined expression constructs for IL-4 and CTLA4 into the corneal epithelium in mice after orthotopic corneal allograft transplantation. *Graefes Arch. Clin. Exp. Ophthalmol., 238*:701–707.

65. A. Shiraishi, R. L., Converse, C. Y. Liu, F. Zhou, C. W. Kao, and W. W. Kao. (1998). Identification of the cornea-specific keratin 12 promoter by in vivo particle mediated gene transfer. *Invest. Ophthalmol. Vis. Sci., 39*:2554–2561.

66. P. L. Felgner. (1996). Improvements in cationic liposomes for in vivo gene transfer. *Hum. Gene Ther., 7*:1791–1793.

67. E. Tomlinson and A. Rolland (1996). Controllable gene therapy: Pharmaceutics of non-viral gene delivery systems. *J. Control. Rel., 39*:357–372.

68. T. S. Ledley and F. D. Ledley. (1994). Multicompartment, numerical model of cellular events in the pharmacokinetics of gene therapies. *Hum. Gene Ther., 5*:679–691.

69. S. T. Crooke. (1997). Advances in understanding the pharmacological properties of antisense oligonucleotides. *Adv. Pharmacol., 40*:1–49.

70. B. Tavitian, S., Terrazzino, B., Kühnast, S. Marzabal, O. Stettler, F. Dollé, J.-R. Deverre, A. Jobert, F Hinnen, B. Bendriem, C. Crouzel, and L. D. Giamberardino. (1998). In vivo imaging of oligonucleotides with positron emission tomography. *Nat. Med., 4*:467–471.

71. H. Farhood, S. Serbina, and L. Huang. (1995). The role of dioleoylphosphatidylethanolamine in cationic liposome mediated gene transfer. *Biochem. Biophys. Acta, 1235*:289–295.

72. A. Katchalsky. (1964). Polyelectrolytes and their biological interactions. *Biophys. J., 4*:9–41.

73. H. Moroson. (1971). Polycation-treated tumor cells in vivo and in vitro. *Cancer Res., 31*:373–380.

74. E. Mayhew and S. J. Nordling. (1966). Electrophoretic mobility of mouse cells and homologous isolated nuclei. *J. Cell Physiol., 68*:75–80.

75. P. Delpine, C. Guillaume, V. Floch, S. Loisel, J. J. Yaouanc, J. C. Clement, H. Des Abbayes, and C. Ferec. (2000). Cationic phosphonolipids as nonviral vectors: in vitro and in vivo applications. *J. Pharm. Sci., 89*:629–638.

76. D. L. Stull. (2000). New tools enable gene delivery: Companies improve existing technologies and offer new ones. *Scientist, 14*(24):30.

77. L. Vitiello, A. Chonn, J. D. Wasserman, C. Duff, and R. G. Worton. (1996). Condensation of plasmid DNA with polylysine improves liposome-mediated gene transfer into established and primary muscle cells. *Gene Ther., 3*:396–404.

78. G. Osaka, K. Carey, A. Cuthbertson, P. Godwoski, T. Patapoff, A. Ryan, T. Gadek, and J. Mordenti. (1996). Pharmacokinetics, tissue distribution, and expression efficiency of plasmid [P-33] DNA following intravenous administration of DNA/cationic lipid complexes in mice: Use of a novel radionuclide approach. *J. Pharm. Sci., 85*:612–618.

79. D. D. Lasic. (1997) *Liposomes in Gene Delivery*. CRC Press, Boca Raton, FL.

80. T. Matsuo, I. Masuda, T. Yasuda, and N. Matsuo. (1996). Gene transfer to the retina of rat by liposome eye drops. *Biochem. Biophys. Res. Commun., 219*:947–950.

81. K. Abul-Hassan, R. Walmsley, and M. Boulton. (2000). Optimization of nonviral gene transfer to human primary retinal pigment epithelial cells. *Curr. Eye Res., 20*:361–366.

82. M. Hangai, Y. Kaneda, H. Tanihara, and Y. Honda. (1996). In vivo gene transfer into the retina mediated by a novel liposomes system. *Invest. Ophthalmol. Vis. Sci., 37*:2678–2685.

83. T. Hara, F. Liu, D. Liu, and L. Huang (1997). Emulsion formulations as a vector for gene delivery in vitro and in vivo. *Adv. Drug Deliv. Rev., 24*:265–271.

84. C. Plank, W. Zauner, and E. Wagner. (1998). Application of membrane-active peptides for drug and gene delivery across cellular membranes. *Adv. Drug Deliv. Rev., 34*:21–35.

85. E. Wagner. (1999). Application of membrane-active peptides for nonviral gene delivery. *Adv. Drug Deliv. Rev., 38*:279–289.

86. L. Shewring, L. Collins, S. L. Lightman, S. Hart, K. Gustafsson, and J. W. Fabre. (1997). A nonviral vector system for efficient gene transfer to corneal endothelial cells via membrane integrins. *Transplantation, 64*:763–769.

87. E. Wagner (1999). Application of membrane-active peptides for nonviral gene delivery. *Adv. Drug Deliv. Rev., 38*:279–289.

88. M. X. Tang and F. C. Szoka. (1997). The influence of polymer structure on the interactions of cationic polymers with DNA and morphology of the resulting complexes. *Gene Ther., 4*:823–832.

89. O. Boussif, F. Lezoualc'h, M. A. Zanta, M. D. Mergny, D. Scherman, B. Demeneix, and J. Behr. (1995). A versatile vector for gene and oligonucleotide

transfer into cells in culture and in vivo: Polyethylenimine. *Proc. Natl. Acad. Sci. USA, 92*:7297–7301.

90. E. Chaum, M. P. Hatton, and G. Stein. (1999). Polyplex-mediated gene transfer into human retinal pigment epithelial cells in vitro. *J. Cell Biochemistry, 76*:153–160.

91. C. L. Bashford, G. M. Alder, G. Menestrina, K. J. Micklem, J. J. Murphy, and C. A. Pasternak. (1986). Membrane damage by hemolytic viruses, toxins, complement and other cytotoxic agents: A common mechanism blocked by divalent cations. *J. Biol. Chem., 261*:9300–9308.

92. S. Choksakulnimitr, S. Masuda, H. Tokuda, Y. Takakura, and M. Hashida. (1995). In vitro cytotoxicity of macromolecules in different cell culture systems. *J. Control. Rel., 34*:233–241.

93. M. X. Tang and F. C. Szoka. (1997). The influence of polymer structure on the interactions of cationic polymers with DNA and morphology of the resulting complexes. *Gene Ther., 4*:823–832.

94. J. C. Roberts, M. K. Bhagat, and R. T. Zera. (1996). Preliminary biological evaluation of polyamidoamine (PAMAM) Starburst dendrimers. *J. Biomed. Materials Res., 30*:53–65.

95. L. Qin, D. R. Pahud, Y. Ding, A. U. Bielinska, J. F. Kukowska-Latallo, J. R. Baker, Jr., and J. Bromberg. (1998). Efficient transfer of genes into murine cardiac grafts by Starburst polyamidoamine dendrimers. *Hum. Gene Ther., 9*:553–560.

96. T. Hudde, S. A. Rayner, R. M. Comer, M. Weber, J. D. Isaacs, H. Waldmann, D. F. P. Larkin, and A. J. George. (1999). Activated polyamidoamine dendrimers, a non-viral vector for gene transfer to the corneal endothelium. *Gene Ther., 6*:939–943.

97. A. Urtti, J. Polansky, G. M. Lui, and F. C. Szoka. (2000). Gene delivery and expression in human retinal pigment epithelial cells: effects of synthetic carriers, serum, extracellular matrix and viral promoters. *J. Drug Target., 7*:413–421.

98. M. A. Kay, D. Liu, and P. M. Hoogerbrugge. (1997). Gene therapy. *Proc. Natl. Acad. Sci. USA, 94*:12744–12746.

99. D. Pogocki and C. Schoneich. (2000). Chemical stability of nucleic acid-derived drugs. *J. Pharm. Sci., 89*:443–456.

100. I. Jaaskelainen, J. Monkkonen, and A. Urtti. (1994). Oligonucleotide cationic liposome interactions. A physicochemical study. *Biochem. Biophys. Acta, 1195*:115–123.

101. T. J. Anchordoquy, L. G. Girouard, J. F. Carpenter, and D. J. Kroll. (1998). Stability of lipid/DNA complexes during agitation and freeze-thawing. *J. Pharm. Sci., 87*:1046–1051.

102. S. D. Allison and T. J. Anchordoquy. (2000). Mechanisms of protection of cationic lipid-DNA complexes during lyophilization. *J. Pharm. Sci., 89*:682–691.

103. L. M. Crowe et al. (1993). Does the preferential exclusion hypothesis apply to hydrated phospholipid bilayers? *Cryobiology, 30*:224–225.

104. B. Detrick, C. N. Nagineni, L. R. Grillone, K. P. Anderson, S. P. Henry, and J. J. Hooks (2001). Inhibition of human cytomegalovirus replication in a human retinal epithelial cell model by antisense oligonucleotides. *Invest. Ophthalmol. Vis Sci., 42*:163–169.

105. P. E. Rakoczy, M. C. Lai, M. Watson, U. Seydel, and I. Constable. (1996). Targeted delivery of an antisense oligonucleotide in the retina: Uptake, distribution, stability and effect. *Antisense Nucleic Acid Drug Dev., 6*:207–213.

106. A. E. Heufelder and R. S. Bahn. (1995). Modulation of cellular functions in retroorbital fibroblasts using antisense oligonucleotides targeting the c-myc protooncogene. *Invest. Ophthalmol. Vis. Sci., 36*:1420–1432.

107. K. K. Jain. (1998). Antisense therapy. In: *Textbook of Gene Therapy*. Hogrefe & Huber Publishers, Kirkland, WA, pp. 73–99.

108. W. F. Lima, B. P. Monia, D. J. Ecker, and S. M. Freier. (1992). Implication of RNA structure on antisense oligonucleotide hybridization kinetics. *Biochemistry, 31*:12055–12061.

109. J. R. Wyatt, T. A. Vickers, J. L. Roberson, R. W. Buckheit, Jr., T. Klimkait, E. DeBaets, P. W. Davis, B. Rayner, J. L. Imbach, and D. J. Ecker. (1994). Combinatorially selected guanosine-quartet structure is a potent inhibitor of human immunodeficiency virus envelope-medicated cell fusion. *Proc. Natl. Acad. Sci. USA, 91*:1356–1360.

110. P. S. Eder, R. J. DeVine, J. M. Dagle, and J. A. Walder. (1991). Substrate specificity and kinetics of degradation of antisense oligonucleotides by a 3′ exonuclease in plasma. *Antisense Res. Dev., 1*:141–151.

111. J. Goodchild, B. Kim, and P. C. Zamecnik. (1991). The clearance and degradation of oligodeoxynucleotides following intravenous injection into rabbits. *Antisense Res. Dev., 1*:153–160.

112. A. Teichman-Weinberg, U. Z. Littauer, and I. Ginzburg. (1988). The inhibition of neurite outgrowth in PC12 cells by tubulin antisense oligodeoxynucleotides. *Gene, 72*:297–307.

113. T. Saison-Behmoaras, B. Tocque, I. Rey, M. Chassignol, N. T. Thuong, and C. Helene. (1991). Short modified antisense oligonucleotides directed against Ha-ras point mutation induce selective cleavage of the mRNA and inhibit T24 cells proliferation. *EMBO J., 10*:1111–1118.

114. Y. Rojanasakul. (1996). Antisense oligonucleotide therapeutics: Drug delivery and targeting. *Adv. Drug Delivery Rev., 18*:115–131.

115. S. T. Crooke. (1997). Advances in understanding the pharmacological properties of antisense oligonucleotides. *Adv. Pharmacol., 40*:1–49.

116. C. H. Agris, K. R. Blake, P. S. Miller, M. P. Reddy, and P. O. Ts'o. (1986). Inhibition of vesicular stomatitis virus protein synthesis and infection by sequence-specific oligodeoxyribonucleoside methylphosphonates. *Biochemistry, 25*:6268–6275.

117. F. Eckstein and G. Gish. (1989). Phosphorothioates in molecular biology. *Trends Biochem. Sci., 14*:97–100.

118. M. Matsukura, K. Shinozuka, G. Zon, H. Mitsuya, M. Reitz, J. S. Cohen, and S. Broder. (1987). Phosphorothioate analogs of oligodeoxynucleotides:

inhibitors of replication and cytopathic effects of human immunodeficiency virus. *Proc. Natl. Acad. Sci. USA, 84*:7706–7710.

119. E. H. Chang and P. S. Miller. (1991). Ras, an inner membrane transducer of growth stimuli. In: *Prospects for Antisense Nucleic Acid Therapeutics for Cancer and AIDS* (E. Wickstrom, ed). Wiley-Liss, New York, p. 115.

120. J. M. Campbell, T. A. Bacon, and E. Wickstrom. (1990). Oligodeoxynucleoside phosphorothioate stability in subcellular extracts, culture media, sera and cerebrospinal fluid. *J. Biochem. Biophys. Methods, 20*:259–267.

121. R. P. Erickson and J. G. Izant, eds. (1991). *Gene Regulation: Biology of Antisense RNA and DNA*. Raven Press, New York.

122. J. A. H. Murray, ed. (1992) *Antisense RNA and DNA*. Wiley-Liss, New York.

123. C. A. Stein (1996). Phosphorothioate antisense oligodeoxynucleotides: Questions of specificity. *Trends Biotechnol., 14*:147–149.

124. M. K. Ghosh, K. Ghosh, O. Dahl, and J. S. Cohen. (1993). Evaluation of some properties of a phosphorodithioate oligodeoxyribonucleotide for antisense application. *Nucleic Acids Res., 21*:5761–5766.

125. P. Yaswen, M. R. Stampfer, K. Ghosh, and J. S. Cohen. (1993). Effects of sequence of thioated oligonucleotides on cultured human mammary epithelial cells. *Antisense Res. Dev., 3*:67–77.

126. M. K. Ghosh, K. Ghosh, and J. S. Cohen. (1993). Phosphorothioate-phosphodiester oligonucleotide co-polymers: Assessment of antisense application. *Anticancer Drug Des., 8*:15–32.

127. C. A. Stein and A. M. Krieg. (1994). Problems in interpretation of data derived from in vitro and in vivo use of antisense oligodeoxynucleotides. *Antisense Res. Dev., 4*:67–69.

128. C. Waheslstedt. (1997). Modulation of receptors. Practical approaches to the regulation on antisense oligonucleotide gene knockout in the nervous system, March 16–19. Oxford University, UK.

129. R. S. Quartin and J. G. Wetmur. (1989). Effect of ionic strength on the hybridization of oligodeoxynucleotides with reduced charge due to methylphosphonate linkages to unmodified oligodeoxynucleotides containing complementary sequence. *Biochemistry, 28*:1040–1047.

130. C. A. Stein, K. Mori, S. L. Loke, C. Subasinghe, K. Shinozuka, J. S. Cohen, and L. M. Neckers. (1988). Phosphorothioate and normal oligodeoxyribonucleotides with 5′-linked acridine: Characterization and preliminary kinetics of cellular uptake. *Gene, 72*:333–341.

131. R. Zhang, Z. Lu, X. Zhang, H. Zhao, R. B. Diasio, T. Liu, Z. Jiang, and S. Agrawal. (1995). In vivo stability and disposition of a self-stabilized oligodeoxynucleotide phosphorothiote in rats. *Clin. Chem., 41*:836–843.

132. G. D. Gray, S. Basu, and E. Wickstrom. (1997). Transformed and immortalized cellular uptake of oligodeoxynucleoside phosphorothioate, 3′-alkylamino oligodeoxynucleotides, 2′-O-methyl oligoribonucleotides, oligodeoxynucleoside and methylphosphonates, and peptide nucleic acids. *Biochem. Pharmacol., 53*:1465–1476.

133. Y. Shoji, S. Akhtar, A. Periasamy, B. Herman, and R. L. Juliano. (1991). Mechanism of cellular uptake of modified oligodeoxynucleotides containing methylphosphonate linkages. *Nucleic Acids Res., 19*:5543–5550.

134. T. L. Fisher, T. Terhorst, X. Cao, and R. W. Wagner (1993). Intracellular disposition and metabolism of fluorescently-labeled unmodified oligonucleotides microinjected into mammalian cells. *Nucleic Acids Res., 21*:3857–3865.

135. S. Wu-Pong, T. L. Weiss, and C. A. Hunt. (1992). Antisense c-myc oligodeoxyribonucleotide cellular uptake. *Pharm. Res., 9*:1010–1017.

136. R. M. Crooke. (1991). In vitro toxicology and pharmacokinetics of antisense oligonucleotides. *Anticancer Drug Des., 6*:609–646.

137. R. M. Crooke, M. J. Graham, M. E. Cooke, and S. T. Crooke. (1995). In vitro pharmacokinetics of phosphorothioate antisense oligonucleotides. *J. Pharmacol. Exp. Ther., 275*:462–473.

138. L. A. Yakubov, E. A. Deeva, V. F. Zarytova, E. M. Ivanova, A. S. Ryte, L. V. Yurchenko, and V. V. Vlassov. (1989). Mechanism of oligonucleotide uptake by cells: Involvement of specific receptors? *Proc. Natl. Acad. Sci. USA, 86*:6454–6458.

139. R. M. Bennett, G. T. Gabor, and M. J. Merritt. (1985). DNA binding to human leukocytes. Evidence for a receptor-mediated association, internalization, and degradation of DNA. *J. Clin. Invest., 76*:2182–2190.

140. S. Akhtar, S. Basu, E. Wickstrom, and R. L. Juliano. (1991). Interactions of antisense DNA oligonucleotide analogs with phospholipid membranes (liposomes). *Nucl. Acids Res., 19*:5551–5559.

141. J. A. Hughes, C. F. Bennett, P. D. Cook, C. J. Guinosso, C. K. Mirabelli, and R. L. Juliano. (1994). Lipid membrane permeability of 2'-modified derivatives of phosphorothioate oligonucleotides. *J. Pharm. Sci., 83*:597–600.

142. R. M. Crooke, M. J. Graham, M. E. Cooke, and S. T. Crooke. (1995). In vitro pharmacokinetics of phosphorothioate antisense oligonucleotides. *J. Pharmacol. Exp. Ther., 275*:462–473.

143. J. Zabner, A. J. Fasbender, T. Moninger, K. A. Poellinger, and M. J. Welsh. (1995). Cellular and molecular barriers to gene transfer by a cationic lipid. *J. Biol. Chem., 270*: 18997–19007.

144. J. L. Tonkinson and C. A. Stein (1994). Patterns of intracellular compartmentalization, trafficking and acidification of 5'-fluorescein labeled phosphodiester and phosphorothioate oilogodeoxynucleotides in HL60 cells. *Nucleic Acids Res., 22*:4268–4275.

145. O. Zelphati and F. C. Szoka, Jr. (1997). Cationic liposomes as an oligonucleotide carrier: Mechanism of action. *J. Liposome Res., 7*:31–49.

146. O. Zelphati and F. C. Szoka. (1996). Mechanism of oligonucleotide release from cationic liposomes. *Proc. Natl. Acad. Sci. USA, 93*:11493–11498.

147. F. C. Szoka, Y. Xu, and O. Zelphati. (1997). How are nucleic acids released in cells from lipid-nucleic acid complexes? *Adv. Drug Deliv. Rev., 24*:291.

148. S. Wu-Pong. (2000). Alternative Interpretations of the oligonucleotide transport literature: Insights from nature. *Adv. Drug Deliv. Rev., 44*:59–70.

149. D. J. Chin, G. A. Green, G. Zon, F. C. Szoka, Jr., and R. M. Straubinger. (1990). Rapid nuclear accumulation of injected oligodeoxyribonucleotides. *New Biol., 2*:1091–1100.

150. M. Cerruzzi, K. Draper, and J. Schwartz. (1990). *Nucleos. Nucleot., 9*:679–695.

151. S. L. Loke, C. A. Stein, X. H. Zhang, K. Mori, M. Nakanishi, C. Subasinghe, J. S. Cohen, and L. M. Neckers. (1989). Characterization of oligonucleotide transport into living cells. *Proc. Natl. Acad. Sci. USA, 86*:3474–3478.

152. Y. Rojanaskul. (1996). Antisense oligonucleotide therapeutics: drug delivery and targeting. *Adv. Drug Delivery Rev., 18*:115–131.

153. T. M. Woolf, D. A. Melton, and C. G. B. Jennings. (1992). Specificity of antisense oligonucleotides in vivo. *Proc. Natl. Acad. Sci. USA, 89*:7305–7309.

154. R. C. Bergan, E. Kyle, Y. Connell, and L. Neckers. (1995). Inhibition of protein-tyrosine kinase activity in intact cells by the aptameric action of oligodeoxynucleotides. *Antisense Res. Dev., 5*:33–38.

155. C. A. Stein, J. L. Tonkinson, L. M. Zhang, L. Yakubov, J. Gervasoni, R. Traub, and S. A. Rotenberg. (1993). Dynamics of the internalization of phosphodiester oligodeoxynucleotides in HL60 cells. *Biochemistry, 32*:4855–4861.

156. R. A. Stull, G. Zon, and F. C. Szoka. (1993). Single-stranded phosphodiester and phosphorothioate oligonucleotides bind actinomycin D and interfere with tumor necrosis factor-induced lysis in the L929 cytotoxicity assay. *Antisense Res. Dev., 3*:295–300.

157. A. M. Krieg, A. K. Yi, S. Matson, T. J. Waldschmidt, G. A. Bishop, R. Teasdale, G. A. Koretzky, and D. M. Klinman. (1995). CpG motifs in bacterial DNA trigger direct B-cell activation. *Nature, 374*:546–549.

158. P. S. Eder, R. J. DeVine, J. M. Dagle, and J. A. Walder (1991). Substrate specificity and kinetics of degradation of antisense oligonucleotides by a 3′ exonuclease in plasma. *Antisense Res. Dev., 1*:141–151.

159. J Goodchild, B. Kim, and P. C. Zamecnik. (1991). The clearance and degradation of oligodeoxynucleotides following intravenous injection into rabbits. *Antisense Res. Dev., 1*:153–160.

160. A. Teichman-Weinberg, U. Z. Littauer, and I. Ginzburg. (1988). The inhibition of neurite outgrowth in PC12 cells by tubulin antisense oligodeoxyribonucleotides. *Gene, 72*:297–307.

161. T. Saison-Behmoaras, B. Tocque, I. Rey, M. Chassignol, N. T. Thuong, and C. Helene. (1991). Short modified antisense oligonucleotides directed against Ha-ras point mutation induce selective cleavage of the mRNA and inhibit T24 cells proliferation. *EMBO J., 10*:1111–1118.

162. C. A. Stein and Y. C. Cheng. (1993). Antisense oligonucleotides as therapeutic agents—is the bullet really magical? *Science, 261*:1004–1012.

163. D. M. Tidd. (1990). A potential role for antisense oligonucleotide analogues in the development of oncogene targeted cancer chemotherapy. *Anticancer Res., 10*:1169–1182.

164. C. A. Stein, and R. Narayanan (1996). Antisense oligodeoxynucleotides: Internationalization, compartmentalization and nonsequence specificity. *Perspect. Drug Discov. Design, 4*:41–50.

165. R. M. Crooke. (1991). In vitro toxicity and pharmacokinetics of antisense oligonucleotides. *Anticancer Drug Des., 6*:609–646.

166. Y. Rojanasakul. (1996). Antisense oligonucleotide therapeutics: drug delivery and targeting. *Adv. Drug Delivery Rev., 18*:115–131.

167. J. W. Jaroszewski, and J. S. Cohen. (1991). Cellular uptake of antisense oligodeoxynucleotides. *Adv. Drug Delivery Rev., 6*:235–250.

168. D. R. Tovell and J. S. Colter (1969). The interaction of tritium-labeled mengo virus RNA and L cells: the effects of DMSO and DEAE-dextran. *Virology, 37*:624–631.

169. F. Dianzani, S. Baron, C. E. Buckler, and H. B. Levy. (1971). Mechanism of DEAE-D-dextran enhancement of polynucleotide induction of interferon. *Proc. Soc. Exp. Biol. Med., 136*:1111–1114.

170. J. P. Leonetti, B. Rayner, M. Lemaitre, C. Gagnor, P. G. Milhaud, J. L. Imbach, and B. Lebleu. (1988). Antiviral activity of conjugates between poly(L-lysine) and synthetic oligodeoxyribonucleotides. *Gene, 72*:323–332.

171. M. Stevenson and P. L. Iversen. (1989). Inhibition of human immunodeficiency virus type 1-mediated cytopathic effect by poly(L-lysine)-conjugated synthetic antisense oligodeoxyribonucleotides. *J. Gen. Virol, 70*:2673–2682.

172. J. P. Leonetti, G. Degols, and B. Lebleu. (1990). Biological activity of oligonucleotide – poly(L-lysine) conjugates: Mechanism of cell uptake. *Bioconj. Chem., 1*:149–153.

173. H. J. P. Ryser and W. C. Shen. (1978). Conjugation of methotrexate to poly(L-lysine) increases drug transport and overcomes drug resistance in cultured cells. *Proc. Natl. Acad. Sci. USA, 75*:3867–3870.

174. J. P. Leonetti, B. Rayner, M. Lemaitre, C. Gagnor, P. G. Milhaud, J. L. Imbach, and B. Lebleu. (1988). Antiviral activity of conjugates between poly(L-lysine) and synthetic oligodeoxyribonucleotides. *Gene, 72*:323–332.

175. R. C. Lambert, Y. Maulet, J. L. Dupont, S. Mykita, P. Craig, S. Volsen, and A. Feltz. (1996). Polyethylenimine-mediated DNA transfection of peripheral and central neurons in primary culture: probing Ca^{2+} channel structure and function with antisense oligonucleotides. *Mol. Cell. Neurosci., 7*:239–246.

176. G. J. Nabel, E. G. Nabel, Z. Y. Yang, B. A. Fox, G. E. Plautz, X. Gao, L. Huang, S. Shu, D. Gordon, and A. E. Chang. (1993). Direct gene transfer with DNA-liposome complexes in melanoma: Expression, biological activity, and lack of toxicity in humans. *Proc. Natl. Acad. Sci. USA, 90*:11307–11311.

177. N. J. Caplen, E. W. Alton, P. G. Middleton, J. R. Dorin, B. J. Stevenson, X. Gao, S. R. Durham, P. K Jeffery, M. E. Hodson, and C. Coutelle. (1995). Liposome-mediated CFTR gene transfer to the nasal epithelium of patients with cystic fibrosis. *Nat. Med., 1*:39–46.

178. P. L. Felgner, Y. R. Gadek, M. Holm, R. Roman, H. W. Chan, M. Wenz, J. P. Northop, G. M. Ringold, and M. Danielsen. (1987). Lipofection: a highly

efficient lipid-mediated DNA transfection procedure. *Proc. Natl. Acad. Sci. USA, 84*:7413–7417.

179. C. F. Bennett, M. Y. Chiang, H. Chan, J. E. Shoemaker, and C. K. Mirabelli. (1992). Cationic lipids enhance cellular uptake and activity of phosphorothioate antisense oligonucleotides. *Mol. Pharmacol. 41*:1023–1033.

180. O. Zelphati and F. C. Szoka, Jr. (1996). Intracellular distribution and mechanism of delivery of oligonucleotides mediated by cationic lipids. *Pharm. Res., 13*:1367–1372.

181. P. L. Felgner. (1990). Particulate systems and polymers for in vitro and in vivo delivery of polynucleotides. *Adv. Drug Del. Rev., 5*:163–187.

182. H. Farhood, X. Gao, K. Son, Y. Y. Yang, J. S. Lazo, L. Huang, J. Barsoum, R. Bottega, and R. M. Epand. (1994). Cationic liposomes for direct gene transfer in therapy of cancer and other diseases. *Ann. NY Acad. Sci. USA, 716*:23–35.

183. P. L. Felgner, T. R. Gadek, M. Holm, R. Roman, H. W. Chan, M. Wenz, J. P. Northrop, G. M. Ringold, and M. Danielsen. (1987). Lipofection: A highly efficient, lipid-mediated DNA transfection procedure. *Proc. Natl. Acad. Sci. USA, 84*:7413–7417.

184. P. L. Felgner and G. M. Ringold. (1989). Cationic liposome-mediated transfection. *Nature, 337*:387–388.

185. D. C. Litzinger, J. M. Brown, I. Wala, S. A. Kaufman, G. Y. Van, C. L. Farrell, and D. Collins. (1996). Fate of cationic liposomes and their complex with oligonucleotide in vivo. *Biochem. Biophys. Acta, 1281*:139–149.

186. R. L. Juliano and S. Akhtar. (1992). Liposomes as a drug delivery system for antisense oligonucleotides. *Antisense Res. Dev., 2*:165–176.

187. I. Jaaskelainen, J. Monkkonen, and A. Urtti. (1994). Oligonucleotide-cationic liposome interactions. A physicochemical study. *Biochem. Biophys. Acta, 1195*:115–123.

188. S. Capaccioli, G. Di Pasquale, E. Mini, T. Mazzei, and A. Quattrone. (1993). Cationic lipids improve antisense oligonucleotide uptake and prevent degradation in cultured cells and in human serum. *Biochem. Biophys. Res. Commun., 197*:818–825.

189. G. Hartmann, A. Krug, M. Bidlingmaier, U. Hacker, A. Eigler, R. Albrecht, C. J. Strasburger, and S. Endres. (1998). Spontaneous and cationic lipid-mediated uptake of antisense oligonucleotides in human monocytes and lymphocytes. *J. Pharmacol. Exp. Ther., 285*:920–928.

190. C. J. Chu, J. Dijkstra, M. Z. Lai, K. Hong, and F. C. Szoka. (1990). Efficiency of cytoplasmic delivery of pH-sensitive liposomes to cells in culture. *Pharm. Res., 7*:824–834.

191. P. G. Milhaud, J. P. Bongartz, B. Lebleu, and J. R. Philippot. (1990). pH-sensitive liposomes and antisense oligonucleotide delivery. *Drug Delivery, 3*:67–73.

192. C. Y. Wang and L. Huang. (1989). Highly efficient DNA delivery mediated by pH-sensitive immunoliposomes. *Biochemistry, 28*:9508–9514.

193. S. Akhtar, S. Basu, E. Wickstrom, and R. L. Juliano. (1991). Interactions of antisense DNA oligonucleotide analogs with phospholipid membranes (liposomes). *Nucl. Acid. Res., 19*:5551–5559.
194. C. Ropert, M. Lavignon, C. Dubernet, P. Couvreur, and C. Malvy. (1992). Oligonucleotides encapsulated in pH sensitive liposomes are efficient toward Friend retrovirus. *Biochem. Biophys. Res. Commun., 183*:879–885.
195. D. D. F. Ma and A. Q. Wei. (1996). Enhanced delivery of synthetic oligonucleotides to human leukemic cells by liposomes and immunoliposomes. *Leukemia Res., 20*:925–930.
196. G. A. Brazeau, S. Attia, S. Poxon, and J. A. Hughes. (1998). In vitro myotoxicity of selected cationic macromolecules used in non-viral gene delivery. *Pharm. Res., 15*:680–684.
197. M. C. Filion and N. C. Phillips. (1997). Toxicity and immunomodulatory activity of liposomal vectors formulated with cationic lipids toward immune effector cells. *Biochem. Biophys. Acta, 1329*:345–356.
198. M. C. Filion and N. C. Phillips. (1998). Major limitations in the use of cationic liposomes for DNA delivery. *Int. J. Pharm., 162*:159–170.
199. Lasic, D. D. (1997). *Liposomes in Gene Delivery.* CRC Press, New York, p. 227.
200. G. Strom and D. J. A. Crommelin. (1998). Liposomes: Quo vadis? *Pharm. Sci. Technol. Today, 1*:19–31.
201. A. Bochot, E. Fattal, A. Gulik, G. Couarraze, and P. Couvreur. (1998). Liposomes dispersed within a thermosensitive gel: a new dosage form for ocular delivery of oligonucleotides. *Pharm. Res., 15*:1364–1369.
202. A. V. Kabanov, S. V. Vinogradov, Y. G. Suzdaltseva, and V. Yu Alakhov. (1995). Water-soluble block polycations as carriers for oligonucleotide delivery. *Bioconjugate Chem., 6*:639–643.
203. M. Hangai, H. Tanihara, Y. Honda, and Y. Kaneda. (1998). Introduction of DNA into the rat and primate trabecular meshwork by fusogenic liposomes. *Invest. Ophthalmol. Vis. Sci., 39*:509–516.
204. J. Kreuter. (1991). Nanoparticles preparations and application. In: *Microcapsules and Nanoparticles in Medicine and Pharmacy* (M. Donbrow, ed.). CRC Press, London, pp. 125–148.
205. J. Kreuter. (1978). Nanoparticles and nanocapsules—new dosage forms in the nanometer size range. *Pharm. Acta Helv., 53*:33–39.
206. J. Heller. (1993). Polymers for controlled parenteral delivery of peptides and proteins. *Adv. Drug Del. Rev., 10*:163–204.
207. W. Lin, A. G. Coombes, M. C. Davies, S. S. Davis, and L. Illum. (1993). Preparation of sub-100 nm human serum albumin nanospheres using a pH-coacervation method. *J. Drug Target., 1*:237–243.
208. A. Maruyama, T. Ishihara, N. Adachi, and T. Akaike. (1994). Preparation of nanoparticles bearing high density carbohydrate chains using carbohydrate-carrying polymers as emulsifier. *Biomaterials, 15*:1035–1042.

209. V. Guise, P. Jaffray, J. Delattre, F. Puisieux, M. Adolphe, and P. Couvreur. (1987). Comparative cell uptake of propidium iodide associated with liposomes or nanoparticles. *Cell. Mol. Biol., 33*:397–405.

210. P. Guiot and P. Couvreur. (1984). Quantitative study of the interaction between polybutylcyanoacrylate nanoparticles and mouse peritoneal macrophages in culture. *J. Pharm. Belg., 38*:130–134.

211. M. Singh, A. Singh, and G. P. Talwar. (1991). Controlled delivery of diphtheria toxoid using biodegradable poly(D,L-lactide) microcapsules. *Pharm. Res., 8*:958–961.

212. A. M. Hazrati, D. H. Lewis, T. J. Atkins, R. C. Stohrer, and L. Meyer. (1992). In vivo studies of controlled release tetanus vaccine. *Proc. Int. Symp. Control. Rel. Bioact. Mater., 19*:114.

213. I. C. Bathurst, P. J. Barr, D. C. Kaslow, D. H. Lewis, T. J. Atkins, and M. E. Rickey. (1992). Development of a single injection transmission blocking malaria vaccine using biodegradable microspheres. *Proc. Int. Symp. Control. Rel. Bioact. Mater., 19*:120.

214. J. H. Elridge, C. J. Hammond, J. A. Meulbroek, J. K. Staas, R. M. Gilley, and T. R. Tice. (1990). Controlled vaccine release in the gut associated lymphoid tissues I. Orally administered biodegradable microspheres target the Peyer's patches. *J. Control. Rel., 11*:205–214.

215. D. K. Gilding and A. M. Reed. (1979). Biodegradable polymers for use in surgery—polyglycolic/poly(lactic acid) homo- and copolymers. *Polymer, 20*:1459–1484.

216. D. L. Wise, T. D. Fellmann, J. E. Sanderson, and R. L. Wentworth. (1979). In: *Drug Carriers in Biology and Medicine.* (G. Gregoriadis, ed.). Academic Press, London.

217. M. Vert, S. M. Li, and H. Garreau. (1994). Attempts to map the structure and degradation characteristics of aliphatic polyesters derived from lactic and glycolic acids. *J. Biomater. Sci. Polymer Ed., 6*:639–649.

218. C. G. Pitt and A. Schindler. (1984). Capronor: A biodegradable delivery system for levonorgestrel. In: *Long Acting Contraceptive Delivery Systems* (G. I. Zatuchni, A. Goldsmith, J. D. Shelton, and J. J. Sviarra, eds.). Harper and Row, Philadelphia, pp. 48–63.

219. H. P. Zobel, M. Junghans, V. Maienschein, D. Werner, M. Gilbert, H. Zimmermann, C. Noe, J. Kreuter, and A. Zimmer. (2000). Enhanced antisense efficacy of oligonucleotides adsorbed to monomethylaminoethylmethacrylate methylmethacrylate copolymer nanoparticles. *Eur. J. Pharm. Biopharm., 49*:203–210.

220. J. W. McGinity and P. B. O'Donnell. (1997). Preparation of microspheres by the solvent evaporation technique. *Adv. Drug Del. Rev., 28*:25–42.

221. V. M. Meidan, D. Dunnion, W. J. Irwin, and S. Akhtar. (1997). Effect of ultrasound on the stability of oligodeoxynucleotides in vitro. *Int. J. Pharm., 152*:121–125.

222. K. J. Lewis, W. J. Irwin, and S. Akhtar. (1995). Biodegradable poly(L-lactic acid) matrices for the sustained delivery of antisense oligonucleotides. *J. Control. Rel., 37*:173–183.

223. S. Akhtar and K. J. Lewis. (1997). Antisense oligonucleotide delivery to cultured macrophages is improved by incorporation into sustained release biodegradable polymer microspheres. *Int. J. Pharm., 151*:57–67.

224. C. Chavany, T. Le Doan, P. Couvreur, F. Puisieux, and C. Helene. (1992). Polyalkylcyanoacrylate nanoparticles as polymeric carriers for antisense oligonucleotides. *Pharm. Res., 9*:441–449.

225. C. Chavany, T. Saison-Behmoaras, T. Le Doan, F. Puisieux, P. Couvreur, and C. Helene. (1994). Adsorption of oligonucleotides onto polyisohexylcyanoacrylate nanoparticles protects them against nucleases and increases their cellular uptake. *Pharm. Res., 11*:1370–1378.

226. Y. Nakada, E. Fattal, M. Foulquier, and P. Couvreur. (1996). Pharmacokinetics and biodistribution of oligonucleotide adsorbed onto poly(isobutylcyanoacrylate) nanoparticles after intravenous administration in mice. *Pharm. Res., 13*:38–43.

227. G. Godard, A. S. Boutorine, E. Saison-Behmoaras, and C. Helene. (1995). Antisense effects of cholesterol-oligodeoxynucleotide conjugates associated with poly(alkylcyanoacrylate) nanoparticles. *Eur. J. Biochem., 232*:404–410.

228. I. Aynie, C. Vauthier, E. Fattal, M. Foulquier, and P. Couvreur. (1998). Alginate nanoparticles as a novel carrier for antisense oligonucleotides. In: *Future Strategies for Drug Delivery with Particulate Systems* (J. E. Diederichs and R. H. Muller, eds.). MedPharm Scientific Publishers, Stuttgart, pp. 11–16.

229. S. K. Das, K. J. Miller, and S. C. Chattaraj. (1998). Facilitated delivery of oligonucleotides as inhibitor of serotonin reuptake. *Proc. Inter. Symp. Control. Rel. Bioact. Mater., 25*:350–351.

230. U. Schroder and B. A. Sabel. (1996). Dalargin loaded nanoparticles passed the BBB. *Proc. Int. Symp. Bioact. Mater., 23*:611–612.

231. J. Kreuter. (1996). Nanoparticles as potential drug delivery systems for the brain. *Proc. Int. Symp. Bioact. Mater., 23*:85–86.

232. D. Quong, R. J. Neufeld, G. Skjak-Braek, and D. Poncelet. (1998). External versus internal source of calcium during the gelation of alginate beads for DNA encapsulation. *Biotechnol. Bioeng., 57*:438–446.

233. T. Nishi, K. Yoshizato, S. Yamashiro, H. Takeshima, K. Sato, K. Hamada, I. Kitamura, T. Yoshimura, H. Saya, J. C. Kuratsu, and Y. Ushio. (1996). High efficiency in vivo gene transfer using intraarterial plasmid DNA injection following in vivo electroporation. *Cancer Res., 56*:1050–1055.

234. L. M. Mir, S. Orlowski, J. J. Belehradek Jr., and C. Paoletti. (1991). Electrochemotherapy potentiation of antitumor effect of bleomycin by local electric pulses. *Eur. J. Cancer, 27*:68–72.

235. A. V. Titomirov, S. Sukharev, and E. Kistanova. (1991). In vivo electroporation and stable transformation of skin cells of newborn mice by plasmid DNA. *Biochim. Biophys. Acta, 1088*:131–134.

236. K. E. Matthews, S. B. Dev, F. Toneguzzo, and A. Keating. (1995). Electroporation for gene therapy, *Methods Mol. Biol., 48*:273–280.

237. W. M. Flanagan and R. W. Wagner. (1997). Potent and selective gene inhibition using antisense oligodeoxynucleotides. *Mol. Cell. Biochem., 172*:213–225.

238. L. C. Bock, L. C. Griffin, J. A. Latham, E. H. Vermaas, and J. J. Toole. (1992). Selection of single-stranded DNA molecules that bind and inhibit human thrombin. *Nature, 355*:564–566.

239. A. R. Ferre-D'Amare and J. A. Doudna. (1999). RNA FOLDs: Insights from recent crystal structures. *Annu. Rev. Biophys. Biomol. Struct., 28*:57–73.

240. X. Ye, A. Gorin, A. D. Ellington, and D. J. Patel. (1996). Deep penetration of an alpha-helix into a widened RNA major groove in the HIV-1 rev peptide-RNA aptamer complex. *Nat. Struct. Biol., 3*:1026–1033.

241. D. H. Burke, L. Scates, K. Andrews, and L. Gold. (1996). Bent pseudoknots and novel RNA inhibitors of type 1 human immunodeficiency virus (HIV-1) reverse transcriptase. *J. Mol. Biol., 264*:650–666.

242. L. R. Paborsky, S. N. McCurdy, L. C. Griffin, J. J. Toole, and L. C. Leung. (1993). The single-stranded DNA aptamer-binding site of human thrombin. *J. Biol. Chem., 268*:20808–20811.

243. R. Conrad, L. M. Keranen, A. D. Ellington, and A. C. Newton. (1994). Isozyme-specific inhibition of protein kinase C by RNA aptamers. *J. Biol. Chem., 269*:32051–32054.

244. E. Kraus, W. James, and A. N. Barclay. (1998). Cutting edge: Novel RNA ligands able to bind CD4 antigen and inhibition CD4+ T lymphocyte function. *J. Immunol., 160*:5209–5212.

245. J. Ciesiolka, J. Gorski, and M. Yarus. (1995). Selection of an RNA domain that binds Zn^{2+}, *RNA, 1*:538–550.

246. M. Sassanfar and J. W. Szostak. (1993). An RNA motif that binds ATP. *Nature, 364*:550–553.

247. Q. Yang, I. J. Goldstein, H. Y. Mei, and D. R. Engelke. (1998). DNA ligands that bind tightly and selectively to cellobiose. *Proc. Natl. Acad. Sci. USA, 95*:5462–5467.

248. C. Mannironi, A. DiNardo, P. Fruscoloni, and G. P. Tocchini-Valentini. (1997). In vitro selection of dopamine RNA ligands. *Biochemistry, 36*:9726–9734.

249. Y. Li, C. R. Geyer, and D. Sen. (1996). Recognition of anionic porphyrins by DNA aptamers. *Biochemistry, 35*:6911–6922.

250. M. Famulok and A. Huttenhofer. (1996). In vitro selection analysis of neomycin binding RNAs with a mutagenized pool of variants of the 16S rRNA decoding region. *Biochemistry, 35*:4265–4270.

251. W. X. Li, A. V. Kaplan, G. W. Grant, J. J. Toole, and L. L. Leung. (1994). A novel nucleotide-based thrombin inhibitor inhibits clot-bound thrombin and reduces arterial platelet thrombus formation. *Blood, 83*:677–682.

252. M. F. Kubik, A. W. Stephens, D. Schneider, R. A. Marlar, and D. Tasset. (1994). High-affinity RNA ligands to human alpha-thrombin. *Nucleic Acids Res., 22*:2619–2626.

253. V. Nobile, N. Russo, G. F. Hu, and J. F. Riordan. (1998). Inhibition of human angiogenin by DNA aptamers: Nuclear colocalization of an angiogenin-inhibitor complex. *Biochemistry, 37*:6857–6863.

254. T. R. Cech and B. L. Bass. (1986). Biological catalysis by RNA. *Annu. Rev. Biochem., 55*:599–629.

255. A. Gervaix, L. Schwarz, P. Law, A. D. Ho, D. Looney, T. Lane, and F. Wong-Staal. (1997). Gene therapy targeting peripheral blood CD34+ hematopoietic stem cells of HIV-infected individuals. *Hum. Gene Ther., 8*:2229–2238.

256. N. Sarver, E. M. Cantin, P. S. Chang, J. A. Zaia, P. A. Ladne, D. A. Stephens, and J. J. Rossi. (1990). Ribozymes as potential anti-HIV-1 therapeutic agents. *Science, 247*:1222–1225.

257. H. Kijima, H. Ishida, T. Ohkawa, M. Kashani-Sabet, and K. J. Scanlon. (1995). Therapeutic applications of ribozymes. *Pharmacol Ther., 68*:247–267.

258. J. Ohkawa, T. Koguma, T. Kohda, and K. Taira. (1995). Ribozymes: From mechanistic studies to applications in vivo. *J. Biochem. (Tokyo), 118*:251–258.

259. T. P. Dryja and T. Li. (1995). Molecular genetics of retinitis pigmentosa. *Hum. Mol. Genet., 4*:1739–1743, 1995.

260. A. S. Lewin, K. A. Drenser, W. W. Hauswirth, S. Nishikawa, D. Yasumura, J. G. Flannery, and M. M. LaVail. (1998). Ribozyme rescue of photoreceptor cells in transgenic rat model of autosomal dominant retinitis pigmentosa. *Nat. Med., 4*:967–971.

261. L. C. Shaw, A. Skold, F. Wong, R. Petters, W. W. Hauswirth, and A. S. Lewin. (2001). An allele-specific hammerhead ribozyme gene therapy for a porcine model of autosomal dominant retinitis pigmentosa. *Mol. Vis., 7*:6–13.

262. K. A. Drenser, A. M. Timmers, W. W. Hauswirth, and A. S. Lewin. (1998). Ribozyme-targeted destruction of RNA associated with autosomal dominant retinitis pigmentosa. *Invest. Ophthalmol. Vis. Sci., 39*:681–689.

263. M. M. LaVail, D. Yasumura, M. T. Matthes, K. A. Drenser, J. G. Flannery, A. S. Lewin, and W. W. Hauswirth. (2000). Ribozyme rescue of photoreceptor cells in P23H transgenic rats: Long-term survival and late-state therapy. *Proc. Natl. Acad. Sci. USA, 97*:11488–11493.

264. W. W. Hauswirth and A. S. Lewin. (2000). Ribozyme uses in retinal gene therapy. *Prog. Retin. Eye Res., 19*:689–710.

265. R. Hormes, M. Homann, I. Oelze, P. Marschall, M. Tabler, F. Eckstein, and G. Sczakiel. (1997). The subcellular localization and length of hammerhead ribozymes determine efficacy in human cells. *Nucleic. Acids Res., 25*:769–775.

266. B. O'Neill, S. Millington-Ward, M. O'Reilly, G. Tuohy, A. S. Kiang, P. F. Kenna, P. Humphries, and G. J. Farrar. (2000). Ribozyme-based therapeutic approaches for autosomal dominant retinitis pigmentosa. *Invest. Opth. Vis. Sci., 41*:2863–2869.

267. X. Ren and G. Schultz. (1999). Reduction of transforming growth factor beta-1 protein in cells transfected with plasmids expressing hammerhead and hairpin ribozymes. *Invest. Ophthalmol. Vis. Sci., 40*(suppl.):46.

20
Regulatory Considerations

Robert E. Roehrs* and D. Scott Krueger
Alcon Research, Ltd., Fort Worth, Texas, U.S.A.

I. INTRODUCTION

The usual goal of ophthalmic drug delivery system research is to develop an improved therapeutic regimen. Some form of performance testing is necessary to determine if the goal has been met, and such testing may involve federal regulatory considerations. If the drug delivery researcher is only interested in the in vitro performance of his or her system and/or its in vivo performance in laboratory research animals for research and publication purposes, federal regulations can largely be ignored. However, if the delivery system is being developed for testing and use in human and/or veterinary medicine, a knowledge of the regulations governing animal and human testing and ultimately the application to market such a pharmaceutical drug product will be essential.

The commercial consideration for development of an ophthalmic drug delivery system is not limited to new therapeutic agents. Many existing ophthalmic drugs have inherent limitations due to poor bioavailability or short duration and are candidates for improved delivery systems. The current U.S. federal regulatory system offers some marketing incentives for these new dosage form improvements through a period of market exclusivity prior to generic competition. Obtaining a U.S. patent for the dosage form improvement can also provide a market extension for the drug and require competitors to delay market entry or develop a noninfringing improved dosage form.

---

*Retired

Drug regulation is not limited to the United States, and most commercial development programs have the objective to obtain approval in the major foreign markets as well as the United States. While regulatory requirements vary considerably around the world, there are harmonization efforts underway in the major countries, particularly between the United States, the European Union, and Japan, that hopefully will lead one day to a common marketing application for these countries if not mutually recognized approvals. This chapter will of necessity focus on the regulatory requirements in the United States.

II. OVERVIEW OF FEDERAL DRUG LAWS

Federal legislation regulating the importation of adulterated articles dates back to the Import Drug Act of 1848. The first significant federal legislation regulating the interstate shipment of food and drugs was enacted in 1906 and was known as the Pure Food and Drug Act. It prohibited the interstate shipment of adulterated or misbranded foods or drugs. In 1912 it was amended by Congress to include false statements or fraudulent claims as part of the definition of a misbranded product (1).

A. Federal Food, Drug & Cosmetic Act

In 1938, the Federal Food, Drug and Cosmetic Act (FD&C Act) was enacted in response to the elixir of sulfanilamide disaster in which the manufacturer of the first liquid form of a sulfa drug used diethylene glycol as the solvent and over 100 deaths were attributed to its poisonous nature (2). The 1906 Act did not require premarket testing for safety and did not allow the removal of unsafe drugs from the market. The "elixir" of sulfanilamide did not contain alcohol and, only because of this technical violation of labeling, was removed from the market as misbranded. The 1938 Act required drugs to be tested for safety and to provide this information prior to marketing. It contains a "grandfather" clause which exempts certain drugs on the market at that time, and some of these drugs are still legally marketed under this "old drug" provision of the Act.

The FD&C Act as amended is the primary federal law regulating the interstate shipment of food, drugs, medical devices, and cosmetics and is enforced by the U.S. Food and Drug Administration (FDA). It has been amended numerous times to add new regulatory provisions, and the most pertinent of these amendments are discussed below in chronological order.

B. Kefauver-Harris Amendments

The 1962 amendments required for the first time that the proof of efficacy as well as safety be submitted in a New Drug Application (NDA) for marketing approval. They also established the requirements for submission of a clinical investigational application (IND) to the FDA prior to initiating research on human subjects. These amendments also established Good Manufacturing Practice (GMP) regulations (21 CFR 210 & 211).

C. Environmental Policy Act

The National Environmental Policy Act of 1969, implemented by regulations of the Council on Environmental Quality, requires the FDA and other federal agencies to assess the possible environmental effects of their actions. As a result, FDA regulations (21 CFR 25) require that certain applications to market drug products contain environmental assessments (EA). The FDA reviews the EA information provided by the applicant as well as other information available to the agency to determine if the requested action will significantly affect the human environment. If there is a finding of no significant impact (FONSI), the FDA is required to prepare and publish the FONSI document. If there is a finding of possible significant impact, then a full environmental impact statement (EIS) is required of the applicant. The Act and the implementing regulations define certain low-risk actions as categorical exclusions that do not require the submission of an EA. The final revised regulation was published on July 29, 1997 (62 FR 40569). The FDA has published a guidance document on the preparation of environment assessments (3).

D. Orphan Drug Act

The Orphan Drug Act of 1983 was enacted to provide incentives for the research and development leading to market availability of drugs to treat rare diseases. Only about 10 such products had been marketed in the decade prior to the Act. The congressionally mandated R&D incentives include research grants to investigators for the conduct of necessary clinical testing to obtain FDA approval, tax credits for R&D, and significant market exclusivity for the applicant who is the first to obtain marketing approval for the drug and rare disease. The Act also encourages early availability of orphan drugs through open protocols, allowing patients to be added to ongoing studies. Since 1983, more than 200 orphan products have been brought to the market.

An application is required to be submitted to the FDA's Office of Orphan Products Development (OOPD) for designation of a drug as an orphan drug for a rare disease. A rare disease is defined as one where there are fewer than 200,000 patients in the United States diagnosed with the disease at the time of the application or one for which the company developing the product cannot recover the R&D costs necessary to bring the orphan product to the market. More than one drug can be designated as an orphan drug for the same rare disease, and more than one applicant can obtain designation for the same drug and rare disease. The drug must be designated as an orphan drug prior to submission of the marketing application. A list of orphan drug designations and marketing approvals is published by the FDA monthly as is an annual cumulative update (www.fda.gov/orphan).

The first marketing application to obtain approval for the designated drug and rare disease is awarded 7 years of marketing exclusivity as long as an adequate supply of the drug to the market is maintained. However, the final regulation provides that when a drug, otherwise the same as the approved orphan, is shown to be clinically superior for the rare disease, it can also be approved and marketed. Therefore, new modifications of the same active moiety (salts, esters, etc.) or the same drug in an improved delivery system which provides a significant therapeutic advantage over the approved orphan product can be approved prior to expiration of the original market exclusivity period. FDA final regulations (21 CFR 316) for the designation and approval of orphan drugs were published in 1992 (57 FR 62076).

E. Drug Price Competition and Patent Restoration Act

This amendment, also known as the Waxman-Hatch Act, was passed in 1984 to allow marketing of generic equivalents of pioneer NDA drugs approved since 1962 and thereby increase competition and lower drug prices. An abbreviated NDA (ANDA) is required to be submitted for approval and must demonstrate that the generic drug product is the "same as" the pioneer NDA product (21 CFR Part 314 Subpart C). The approval application is abbreviated in that the manufacturer does not have to repeat the expensive and time-consuming animal safety and human clinical studies but must instead demonstrate that the generic product is bioequivalent to the pioneer drug product. However, the generic applicant is required to meet the same FDA requirements for chemistry, manufacturing, and quality control. The Act also modified the patent law such that it is no longer an infringement to use the patented drug for experimental purposes related to obtaining U.S. regulatory approval. Thus, the development of a generic equivalent can be accomplished at any time prior to patent expiration.

The second part of the Act provides incentives to the pioneer industry to continue the costly R&D programs for new therapeutic agents by extending, or in effect restoring, a limited portion of the patent term for certain new drugs. The Act also established market exclusivity periods for new drugs during which generic applications cannot be approved. These provisions will be discussed in more detail in Sec. VI of this chapter.

The Act also requires the FDA to publish a list of approved drug products and update the list monthly. The FDA makes this list available along with additional information in the publication *Approved Drug Products with Therapeutic Equivalence Evaluations*, also known as the "Orange Book." The publication is an important information document for the pharmacist in selecting multisource drug products considered by the FDA as therapeutically equivalent when state law and the prescriber allow generic substitution. It also provides the pharmaceutical industry with therapeutic equivalence requirements as well as information on U.S. patents that potentially could be infringed by generic applicants and the patent term and/or market exclusivity period expirations. The Orange Book is also available electronically via the FDA website at www.fda.gov/cder/ob/default.htm.

F. FDA Export Reform and Enhancement Act

Prior to 1986 only drugs approved by the FDA could be legally exported. This placed the U.S. pharmaceutical industry at a competitive disadvantage since new drugs may sometimes be first approved overseas, requiring manufacturing plants to be located outside the United States to meet the need for drug substances and drug products in these markets prior to FDA approval. In 1986 Congress, recognizing the desire to retain jobs in the United States that might otherwise be lost to offshore manufacturing, amended the export law, allowing unapproved new drugs to be exported to 21 designated countries, under certain conditions, that have premarket approval systems comparable to the United States.

Ten years later, Congress amended the export act with further enhancements to facilitate new drug exports, including investigational new drugs for clinical testing overseas. It is now possible to export unapproved human drugs to any country in the world if the drug complies with the laws of the importing country, among other requirements, and it has been approved for marketing in any of the currently designated countries of Australia, Canada, Israel, Japan, New Zealand, Switzerland, South African, and countries in the European Union and European Free Trade

Association. The exporting company does not require prior FDA approval but must provide a notification to the FDA. The company must also maintain records of all drugs exported and the countries to which they were exported. There are additional requirements for good manufacturing practices and labeling.

Additional significant new export enhancements include the ability to export unapproved drugs to any of the designated countries to complete manufacturing, packaging, and/or labeling processes in anticipation of marketing approval. This allows expedited market availability once official marketing authorization is obtained. Also, shipment of new drugs to the listed countries for the purpose of clinical investigations may be made in accordance with the laws and requirements of the importing country, and such shipments are exempt from U.S. IND regulations. The early phases of human clinical research are sometimes conducted initially overseas, which previously required a U.S. IND or other approval to export the clinical supplies.

G. Prescription Drug User Fee Act

In 1992 Congress, after consultation with the FDA and the pharmaceutical industry, amended the FD&C Act to authorize the FDA to collect fees for the review of certain human drug and biological applications and other specific agency actions. Congress was reacting to the desire to speed approval of safe and effective new human drugs and biologicals and the need for additional resources at the FDA to accomplish this goal. The prescription drug user fee act (PDUFA) was authorized for a 5-year period, and during this period the agency was able to reduce the average review time from 30 months to 15 months, made possible by FDA managerial reforms and the addition of 700 employees financed by collection of $329 million in user fees from the pharmaceutical industry. Based on this success, PDUFA was reauthorized in 1997 for 5 more years (PDUFA II), and the FDA goal for review times for most new drug applications was shortened from 12 to 10 months. The one-time user fee for application review is now collected at the time of submission. The fee is partially refunded if the application is not accepted for filing and review. If accepted but not found approvable after a complete review, there is no refund, but the FDA must provide a listing of all deficiencies, which must be overcome for approval.

In addition to one-time fees for review of new human drug applications, user fees are also required on an annual basis for prescription drug manufacturing facilities and for approved prescription drug products prior to approval of a generic version. During the first 5 years of PDUFA, the approximate average user fee charged was $200,000 for each new drug application, $100,000 for each manufacturing facility, and $10,000 for each product dosage form and strength.

Human drug applications that are exempt from user fees include those for clinical investigations, generic drug approvals, over-the-counter drug approvals, orphan drug approvals, and pediatric use approvals. Fees may be waived in certain specified cases, including small businesses submitting their first approval application.

H. FDA Modernization Act

In 1997, Congress passed major legislation focused on reforming the regulation of food, drugs, devices, and cosmetics. One of the major provisions of the Act was the reauthorization of PDUFA for 5 years as described above. A number of the reforms affecting drug products were already FDA and industry initiatives to modernize and streamline the regulatory process for approval of new drugs as well as the postapproval requirements for marketed drugs without lowering the standards by which these medical products are introduced into the marketplace. These include measures to bring more harmony to the regulation of biological and human drugs, eliminating the batch certification procedures for insulin and antibiotics, eliminating the separate regulations for antibiotics and drugs, streamlining the approval process for biological and drug manufacturing changes, and reducing the need for environmental assessments as part of product applications. Also, the practice of allowing, in certain circumstances, one clinical investigation as the basis for product approval for drugs is now codified. However, the presumption that, as a general rule, two adequate and well-controlled studies are needed to prove the product's safety and effectiveness is preserved in the regulations.

The act also codified the FDA's regulations and practices to increase patient access to experimental drugs and medical devices and to accelerate the review of important new medicines. Additionally, the law provides for an expanded database on clinical trials accessible by patients, and with consent of the sponsor, the results of such trials will be included in the database. Also, patients will receive advance notice when a manufacturer plans to discontinue a drug on which they depend for life support or sustenance or for treatment of a serious or debilitating disease or condition.

III. FOOD AND DRUG ADMINISTRATION

The Food and Drug Administration is the federal agency with statutory authority to regulate the testing and marketing of new ophthalmic delivery systems based on the laws enacted by Congress. The FDA publishes the proposed and final regulations in the *Federal Register* (FR), and the implementing regulations are contained in Title 21 of the Code of Federal Regulations (CFR). The FR and the CFR documents are available on the Internet at www.access.gpo.gov.

The FDA is organized into various Centers, which have the primary responsibility for reviewing clinical trial and marketing applications. There is a Center for each major product category: Center for Drug Evaluation and Research (CDER), Center for Biologics Evaluation and Research (CBER), Center for Devices and Radiological Health (CDRH), Center for Veterinary Medicine (CVM), and Center for Food Safety and Applied Nutrition (CFSAN), which includes cosmetics and dietary supplements. Within each Center are review divisions, usually organized by therapeutic classes, which are staffed by scientists and support staff who review applications and make recommendations for acceptance or rejection to Division and Center management. Human ophthalmic drug products are reviewed within the CDER Division, which is staffed with ophthalmologists who review the human clinical data, chemists who review the chemistry, manufacturing, and controls, and pharmacologists who review the animal studies. Also included, as needed, in the application review team are microbiologists, statisticians, and biopharmaceutics reviewers.

The FDA maintains an informative website on the Internet at www.fda.gov, and each Center can be accessed through the site. The CDER site can be accessed directly at www.fda.gov/cder. The FDA also maintains a fax-on-demand system for access to guidance and information documents.

IV. REGULATORY CLASSIFICATION OF DELIVERY SYSTEMS

The regulatory requirements for each legally defined class of medical products vary, and so it is important to know how a potential new ophthalmic delivery system will be classified. Each FDA Center, in addition to statutory requirements, differs in its rules and procedures for submission and review of applications.

A. Drug Versus Device

A *drug* is legally defined as:

1. Articles recognized in the official *United States Pharmacopoeia* (USP), official *Homeopathic Pharmacopoeia of the United States* or the *National Formulary* (NF) and their supplements.
2. Articles intended for use in the diagnosis, cure, mitigation, treatment, or prevention of disease in man or other animals.
3. Articles other than foods intended to affect the structure or any function of the body of man or other animals.
4. Articles intended for use as a component of any article specified in the above three clauses.

A *device* is defined as an instrument, apparatus, implement, machine, contrivance, implant, in vitro reagent, or other similar or related article, including any component, part, or accessory which is:

1. Recognized in the official USP or NF or any supplements
2. Intended for use in the diagnosis of disease or other conditions, or in the cure, mitigation, treatment, or prevention of disease in man or other animals
3. Intended to affect the structure or any function of the body of man or other animals, and which does not achieve any of its principal intended purpose through chemical action within or on the body of man or other animals and which is not dependent upon being metabolized for the achievement of any of its principal intended purposes

While there are some similarities in the two definitions, there are also important differences. The definition of a device lists specific types of articles that are covered, and these are the articles that one would typically associate with the literal definition of a device. A device is also an accessory of one of these articles. For example, contact lens care products, which have compositions containing chemicals such as disinfectants, lubricant polymers, etc., are regulated as devices since they are considered necessary for the safe use of another device, a contact lens.

Another ophthalmic example is seen with the regulatory history of the Lacrisert,® a sterile rod-shaped solid consisting entirely of a cellulosic polymer intended for use in the eye to slowly erode and dissolve in the tear film to provide lubrication for painful dry eye conditions. The FDA initially approved it as a device and then changed its mind and reclassified it as a drug (4). In doing so, the FDA explained that the term article in the definition of a drug is a broad category in contrast with the specific types of articles listed in the device definition, and the Lacrisert is not one of those specific device articles. The FDA also stated that a drug is a chemical or a combination of chemicals in liquid, paste, powder, or other drug dosage form that is ingested, injected, or instilled into body orifices or rubbed or poured onto the body in order to achieve its intended medical purpose. Also, note that the legal definition of a drug does not require it to achieve its principal intended purpose through chemical action or by being metabolized.

B.   New Drug

A *new drug* is legally defined as one that is not generally recognized among experts qualified by scientific training and experience as safe and effective for use under the conditions prescribed, recommended, or suggested in its labeling (FD&C Act Section 201(p)). New drugs require INDs for conducting clinical investigations and NDAs for marketing approval. The terms drug and new drug are inclusive of the drug substance and the drug product.

It is important to understand that a new drug is not just a newly discovered chemical or biological compound. This can best be illustrated by several examples of when a drug can become a new drug for regulatory purposes:

1. The drug is a new derivative of a known molecule such as a prodrug of epinephrine.
2. A previously approved drug has been discovered to have a new therapeutic use such as a nonsteroidal anti-inflammatory agent used to inhibit miosis during cataract surgery.
3. A component of a drug is new for drug use such as an EVA polymer film to control the release of pilocarpine in the eye or a gel-forming polymer to extend the duration of IOP-lowering of timolol maleate.
4. Two or more approved drugs are combined for use such as a fixed combination of tobramycin and dexamethasone.
5. A change is made in the route of administration such as a topical ocular dosage form of acetazolamide for IOP reduction.
6. A change is made in the dosage or strength of an approved drug.
7. A change is made in the intended patient population such as the use of a drug, approved to lower IOP in glaucoma patients, to be used in normotensive patients prior to laser surgery to prevent IOP spikes.
8. The addition or deletion of an inactive component changes the risk-to-benefit ratio for an approved drug.
9. Radiation sterilization is used for a drug product (21 CFR 200.30).

C. Combination Drug and Device

It is possible to have as a new ophthalmic delivery system a combination of a drug and a device. For example, the system could contain the drug in aerosolized form, which is associated with a novel apparatus (device) to instill the drug directly onto the surface of the eye in a manner that avoids the blink response. The FDA product review jurisdiction would be determined by Intercenter agreements and usually assigned based on the primary mode of action of the product.

In this chapter, we will discuss the requirements for ophthalmic delivery systems in which a drug is incorporated in a carrier for its pharmacological effect on the human eye and is reviewed as a new drug product by the FDA's Drug Center (CDER).

V. CLINICAL TESTING OF NEW OPHTHALMIC DRUG DELIVERY SYSTEMS

A. Human Versus Animal Testing

Human drug products are often tested during development in animals for potential acute and chronic signs of toxicity as well as for their primary and secondary pharmacological effects. If the new drug is shipped interstate for the purpose of clinical investigation in animals, an exemption similar to a human IND is required, and the label must bear the following statement (21 CFR 511.1b): "Caution. Contains a new animal drug for use in investigational animals in clinical trials. Not for use in humans. Edible products of investigational animals are not to be used for food unless authorization has been granted by the U.S. Food and Drug Administration or by the U.S. Department of Agriculture." However, if the interstate shipment is intended solely for use in animals used only for laboratory research purposes, then it is exempted from the IND requirements if it is labeled as follows (21 CFR 312.160): "Caution. Contains a new drug for investigational use only in laboratory research animals or for tests in vitro. Not for use in humans." The exemption also requires that due diligence be used to assure that the consignee is regularly engaged in conducting such tests and shipment will actually be used as stated in the Caution. Records of the shipments must be kept for a period of 2 years after shipment and delivery and made available to an FDA inspector if requested.

B. Federal Versus State Regulation

Clinical investigations conducted solely intrastate do not escape federal regulation if the drug or dosage form or any components of these articles are obtained through interstate shipments.

C. IND Exemption for Clinical Investigations in Humans

The FD&C Act provides for an exemption from prior approval for interstate shipment of new drugs if the shipment is for the purpose of clinical testing in humans. The investigational new drug application (IND) is the notice of exemption that must be submitted prior to the shipment (21 CFR 312). The applicant agrees not to begin clinical use for 30 days or longer if so notified by the FDA. During the 30-day period, the FDA makes an initial assessment of the clinical testing plans and the data supporting safe use in human subjects. If the FDA has serious questions about the application, the investigations may be put on a clinical hold until the applicant removes the deficiencies. Beyond the initial 30-day review period, the FDA will conduct a more in-depth review of the data submitted and may from time to time notify the sponsor of the application regarding deficiencies that must be corrected prior to additional clinical investigations being undertaken. The sponsor is required to update the application with certain amendments to ongoing investigation protocols and all new testing protocols. Also, the sponsor is required to submit an annual progress report of the investigations and immediate reports of serious and unexpected adverse reactions in humans and certain serious findings in animal safety tests.

D. IND Application

FDA regulations specify the format and content requirements of an IND. This is shown in Table 1.

1. Clinical Testing

The first section of the IND informs the FDA as to what drug is to be tested, the objectives of the clinical experiments, and the scientific rationale and existing knowledge. The FDA uses this information to determine the adequacy of the technical data to support the proposed human experiments.

Clinical testing usually occurs in several phases, and an IND can be filed for one or more of these phases (Table 2). Typically, an IND would be filed with specific protocol(s) for Phase 1 and a general outline of the plan for Phase 2. The IND can be amended as necessary to add additional protocols and a revised clinical plan included in the annual report. The clinical

Table 1 IND—Format and Content Outline

Part 1	Form FDA 1571
Part 2	Table of Contents
Part 3	Introductory Statement—brief introductory statement to include:

a. Name(s) of the drug
   Drug's pharmacological class
   Drug's structural formula
   Dosage form and formulation
   Route of administration
   Broad objectives and planned duration of the proposed clinical
   investigations
b. Brief summary of previous human experience with the drug:
   Reference of other IND/NDAs, if pertinent
   Investigational or marketing experience in other countries that may
   be relevant to the safety of the proposed clinical investigation(s)
c. Identification of countries where drug has been withdrawn from
   investigation or marketing for any reasons related to safety or
   effectiveness and reasons for withdrawal

Part 4   General Investigational Plan—brief description of the overall plan for
investigating the drug product for the following year to include:
a. Rationale for drug study
b. Indication(s) to be studied
c. General approach to be followed in evaluating the drug
d. Kinds of clinical trials to be conducted in the first year (indicate if
   plans not developed for full year)
e. Estimate number of patients to be given the drug
f. Safety risks anticipated—any risks of particular severity or
   seriousness anticipated based on toxicology data or prior human
   experience with the drug or related drugs

Part 5   Investigator's Brochure—to contain the following information:
a. Brief description of the drug (include structural formula) and the
   formulation
b. Summary of the pharmacological and toxicological effects of the
   drug in animals and, to the extent known, in man
c. Summary of pharmacokinetics and biological disposition of the drug
   in animals and, if known, in man
d. Summary of information relating to safety and effectiveness in
   humans from prior clinical studies (can append reprints when
   pertinent and useful)
e. Description of possible risks and side effects to be anticipated based
   on experience with the drug or with related drugs. Precautions or
   special monitoring to be done as part of the investigations

Part 6   Clinical Investigation
a. Protocol for each planned study

Table 1 Continued

b. Investigators
Name, address and CV of each investigator
Name of each subinvestigator
Name and address of research facilities
Name and address of IRB
c. Monitor—name, title, and CV
(The person responsible for monitoring the conduct and progress of
the clinical investigations)
Safety Monitor(s)—name, title and CV
(The person or persons responsible for review and evaluation of
information relevant to safety of the drug)
d. Contract Research Organizations (CRO)
   i. Name and address of CRO used for any part of the clinical
studies
   ii. Identify the studies and CRO monitor
   iii. List sponsor obligations transferred to CRO, if any
e. Labeling for clinical supplies

Part 7   Chemistry, Manufacturing, and Controls Information
a. Drug Substance
   1. Description of physical and chemical characteristics
   2. Name and address of manufacturer
   3. Method of preparation
   4. Reference standard
   5. Specifications
   6. Methods of analysis
   7. Stability
b. Drug Product
   1. Components (reasonable alternatives)
      i. Inactive components—tests and specifications
   2. Composition (reasonable variations)
   3. Name and address of manufacturer
   4. Manufacturing and packaging procedure
   5. Specifications
   6. Methods of analysis
   7. Packaging
   8. Stability
   9. Labeling for clinical supplies
   10. Placebo—composition, manufacture, and control
   11. Environmental analysis—Claim for categorical exclusion

Part 8   Pharmacology and Toxicology
a. Pharmacology and drug disposition
   1. Section describing the pharmacological effects and mechanism(s)
of action of the drug in animals
   2. Section describing the ADME of the drug, if known

   b. Toxicology
      1. ID and qualifications of persons conducting and evaluating results of studies concluding reasonably safe to begin purposed investigations
      2. Statement where studies conducted and where records available for inspection
      3. Integrated summary of the toxicological effects of the drug in animals and in vitro
      4. Detailed tox study reports with full tabulations of data for each study primarily intended to support the safety of the proposed clinical investigation
      5. GLP Compliance Statement(s)

Part 9   Previous Human Experience
Summary of known prior human experience with the investigational drug to include:
   a. If previously investigated or marketed (anywhere):
      i.   Detailed information about such experience relevant to safety of proposed investigation or rationale
      ii. If drug has been subject of controlled clinical trials, detailed information on such trials relevant to an assessment of the drug's effectiveness for the proposed investigational use
      iii. Published material directly relevant to safety or effectiveness for the proposed investigational use—provide full copies
          Published material less directly relevant—bibliography
   b. For combination of drugs—Part 9a information for each drug
   c. Foreign marketing
      i.   List of countries where marketed
      ii. List of countries where drug has been withdrawn from marketing for reasons potentially related to safety or effectiveness

Part 10 Pediatric Studies—plans for assessing pediatric safety and effectiveness

Source: Adapted from 21 CFR 312.23

protocol is a critical element of the investigational phase for a new drug. FDA regulations establish requirements for the protocol (Table 3). The FDA medical officer reviewing the protocol will provide a critique as to its scientific and regulatory acceptability as well as the acceptability of the risk to human subjects. If the study is intended to be used as part of the NDA to establish safety and effectiveness, it would be important to know if the FDA has any serious questions about the protocol before proceeding.

Ophthalmic drug clinical development generally follows three phases, particularly if the drug is a new molecule and this is its first introduction into humans. Phase 1 for ophthalmic drugs usually is focused on the potential for

Table 2 Clinical Testing Phases

Phase 1: Initial introduction into man—closely monitored patients or normal volunteers. Primarily for side effects with increasing doses, ADME and clinical pharmacology and early readout on effectiveness. Used to design well-controlled, scientifically valid Phase 2 studies. Also used for structure-activity and mechanism of action studies as well as using drugs as research tool to explore biology and disease processes. Usually involve fewer than 100 subjects.

Phase 2: Controlled studies for effectiveness in patients and determination of common short-term side effects and risks. Well-controlled and closely monitored studies in usually no more than several hundred patients. Used to screen out drugs with limited potential for safety and/or effectiveness. Data critical to design Phase 3, particularly for dosage regimens and patient populations.

Phase 3: Expanded studies in patients both controlled and uncontrolled to gather data on safety and effectiveness needed to evaluate overall benefit-risk and provide basis for labeling. Usually involve several hundred to several thousand subjects.

Phase 4: Studies usually conducted after initial marketing. May be requested by FDA as condition of approval. May be used to examine specific patient subpopulations such as geriatric or pediatric or to increase exposure to further define benefit-to-risk ratio.

ocular toxicity in healthy subjects. Because of the potential for systemic absorption for ocular dosing, attention is also given to the possibility of systemic effects, and concurrently, or in separate studies, the extent of systemic absorption is determined.

In Phase 2 of clinical testing, the drug is usually first introduced into patients with the disease and a dose-response relationship is investigated.

Table 3 Clinical Protocol Requirements

Objectives and purpose of study
Identification of each investigator and subinvestigator, research facilities, and each IRB
Criteria for patient selection and exclusion and estimated number of patients
Study design including group (if any) and methods to minimize bias on part of subjects, investigators, and analysts
Method for determining doses to be used, the maximum dose and duration of patient exposure
Description of the observations and measurements to fulfill objectives of study
Description of clinical procedures, lab tests, or other measures to monitor drug effects in subjects and to minimize risk

For oral drugs, the dose-response testing is a crucial parameter; however, it has not been a rigorous part of most topical ophthalmic drug-development programs. The drug delivery researcher may find that these data are missing for his or her drug and needs to establish this relationship for optimization. An example of this occurred during the development of the Ocusert containing pilocarpine in which patients were given multiple micro doses of pilocarpine topically to establish the required release rate to provide the desired IOP-lowering response (5).

The final Phase 3 testing is essential for providing the substantial evidence from adequate and well-controlled studies required for proof of safety and effectiveness. It is particularly important that the endpoints used to measure the response of the delivery system be clinically relevant and that enough patients are included to detect a significant difference if one exists.

The FDA has established standards for the conduct of clinical studies in order to ensure the quality and integrity of the data on which the safety and effectiveness decisions will be based and also, importantly, the protection of the rights and health of the participating subjects. These are commonly referred to as Good Clinical Practices (GCPs) but are not embodied in one regulation. They are a combination of the Informed Consent regulation for clinical subjects (21 CFR 50), the Institutional Review Board (IRB) regulations (21 CFR 56), and the obligations of sponsors and investigators defined in the 1987 IND Rewrite regulations (21 CFR 312).

2. Preclincal Testing

The nonclinical or preclinical section addresses the biological data that support the pharmacological rationale for the intended use of the drug, the animal toxicology data to assess the safety risks for human exposure, and, if available, systemic and ocular pharmacokinetic data. These data may necessarily be limited at this point, particularly if the drug is a new molecule. If the delivery system is being developed with a known drug, then comparative tests will be useful to assess the risk. If the delivery system contains a new component, such as a polymer or surfactant to prolong ocular residence and/or enhance bioavailability, then additional safety testing may be required for the new component if the supplier has not already provided this information. In some cases this component may have already been used in other drug applications or sometimes for food or cosmetic uses and have established a generally recognized as safe (GRAS) status. The toxicologist will have to assess the relevance of these data to the intended topical application.

FDA does not have specific requirements or guidelines to answer the often asked question: How much animal safety data do I need for an ophthalmic IND? In general, to begin clinical testing, FDA will require at least the same duration of testing in animals as proposed for human exposure. The requirements will vary with the particular drug and the novelty of the particular delivery system. The approach of one company in establishing the safety/toxicity profile of ophthalmic drugs and devices has recently been published (6).

FDA implemented Good Laboratory Practice (GLP) regulations in 1976, which established standards for the conduct and reporting of all animal safety-related studies to be used in support of an IND or NDA. This was a reaction to the discovery that some industrial and contract toxicology testing labs were conducting studies in a sloppy manner and in instances had falsified data that were submitted to FDA. FDA now routinely audits on a periodic basis all labs conducting such studies. Therefore, if animal safety data are generated in an academic institution and the results are to be used in support of an IND, the studies must meet GLP regulations and any deviations from these requirements must be explained. A certification of GLP compliance is required in the IND for each safety study (21 CFR 58).

3. Chemistry, Manufacturing, and Controls

The next major section of the IND describes the chemistry of the drug substance and the composition, manufacturing, packaging, quality control, and stability of the dosage forms to be used in the clinical trials. Inadequacies in this section can cause FDA to withhold the approval to conduct the proposed clinical trials, particularly if the deficiencies cause a concern related to safety.

a. Drug Substance. The drug substance must be characterized as to its structure and adequate analytical procedures must be specified to analyze routinely the identity and purity of the drug. If the drug is in an official pharmacopeia, the monograph for the drug may be referenced; however, the FDA is not bound by these requirements and may require additional tests and specifications. For example, the assay method for the drug should be stability indicating, and some monographs may not meet this standard. Also, FDA will be interested in the major impurities and require specific tests and specifications for them, which may not be part of a monograph.

The supplier of the drug substance is required to be identified as well as the methods of synthesis and controls used by the manufacturer. This will also be required for compendial drugs. Since the information on synthesis is usually considered proprietary, FDA has established a mechanism by which this confidential information can be supplied for their review directly from the manufacturer through a Drug Master File (DMF) (7). The manufacturer will send the FDA a letter authorizing the IND sponsor to access this information in a specific DMF, and the sponsor is required to include a copy of this letter of authorization in this section of the IND.

An authentic reference standard is required for each drug substance. If not available from USP, it will have to be established independently, must be of the highest purity available, and the method of synthesis and purification must be included.

b. Drug Product. The dosage form containing the active drug substance and its vehicle or delivery system must be described in detail:

Components—Listing of all active and inactive ingredients that are used in preparation of the finished product.

Inactive Components—The quality standard which is used and, if other than compendial items, the actual tests and specifications.

Composition—The quantitative composition for the entire formula expressed in terms of percent, milligrams per milliliter, and a typical batch quantity.

Manufacture—The name and address of each firm involved in the manufacture, packaging, labeling, and testing of the drug product.

Method of Manufacturing—The method of manufacturing, packaging, and labeling the product and the controls used in these processes.

Packaging Components—The packaging is identified and the components are described and specified. The USP specifies tests required for suitability of plastics in ophthalmic containers, which are both physicochemical and biological. The tests should be conducted on the containers after they are cleaned and sterilized.

Stability—Sufficient stability data using stability-indicating methods should be submitted to assure a stable product for the duration of the clinical trials.

Labeling—Copy of the labels to be applied to the containers of the clinical supplies. These are usually multipart labels so as to provide complete labeling information during shipment, which can be removed before given to the patient to mask the identity of the product from the patient and the physician. The label must bear the statement: "Caution: New Drug Limited by Federal Law to Investigational Use."

Placebo—Many studies require the drug to be compared to a placebo, which is usually the vehicle or delivery system itself. The same information described above for the active drug product is provided for the placebo dosage form.

Environmental Assessment—The environmental regulations provide for a categorical exclusion from preparing an environmental assessment for clinical trials.

c. Sterilization. FDA regulation requires that all ophthalmic drug products be manufactured and packaged in a sterile manner. This can be accomplished in two ways: by terminal sterilization or by aseptic combination of sterile components. Terminal sterilization is preferred, since it provides the greatest assurance of final product sterility. Often this is not feasible because of the heat lability of the ingredients or the packaging system. Terminal sterilization is usually done by radiation or steam under pressure. Many drug products are made sterile by sterilizing the individual components, including the packaging materials, and then aseptically combining them in a sterile environment. The FDA has provided guidelines for the proper validation of the aseptic process for sterile products (8).

Because of the much greater sterility assurance offered by a terminal sterilization process, the FDA will require the applicant to justify the use of an aseptic process for sterilization (9). Data, therefore, should be generated during the development of the delivery system to determine the impact of a terminal sterilization process on the final packaged dosage form. This would usually involve chemical and physical analyses of the product for degradation products and any change in the toxicology profile.

d. Preservation. If the delivery system is a liquid in a multiple dose package, the requirement for addition of substance(s) to inhibit the growth of microorganisms during use needs to be considered. The regulation states that these substances must be added *or* the product packaged in such a manner that harmful contamination cannot reasonably occur during use (21 CFR 200.50). Therefore, the regulation does not absolutely require a preservative be used in all multidose packages. However, FDA has not given any published guidance as to their interpretation of what type of unpreserved multidose product would meet the requirements of this regulation.

The regulation specifically states a requirement for *liquid* products and provides no guidance for multidose semisolids such as aqueous gels. The drug delivery scientists should work closely with the microbiologist and packaging scientist to determine the best means to accomplish the safe administration of a sterile product.

New ophthalmic delivery systems in unit dose form offer the opportunity to improve the ability of the patient to comply with the prescribed dosage regimen and also obviate the need for the addition of a preservative agent.

e. Good Manufacturing Practices. Clinical supplies of the new ophthalmic drug delivery system should be manufactured in conformance with the GMP regulations. The pharmaceutical industry has recognized that the official GMP regulations are not always practical or suitable for clinical supplies. The quantities are usually small, and since this is a research and development process, changes will necessarily occur as experience is gained and the scale of manufacture increases. FDA has also recognized these facts and has issued guidelines that address the allowable differences in GMP compliance for clinical trial manufacture (10).

VI. MARKETING NEW OPHTHALMIC DRUG DELIVERY SYSTEMS FOR HUMAN USE

Once a manufacturer has obtained sufficient information from clinical trials in humans, safety testing in animals, and chemistry and manufacturing experience to establish that the new ophthalmic drug delivery system is safe and effective for its intended use, a New Drug Application is submitted to the FDA to obtain approval for distribution in interstate commerce.

Two types of NDAs for new drugs are recognized by the FD&C Act in Section 505(b):

1. A new drug requires full reports of investigations for safety and effectiveness among other requirements. For a new drug, first submitted for approval, the investigations providing the full reports will ordinarily have been conducted by the applicants or by others under contract with a full right of reference (21 CFR 314.3) to the results of the investigations for inclusion in the marketing application. This is the typical NDA for a new chemical entity (NCE) and is sometimes referred to as a "Full NDA."

2. The second type of NDA is one in which the applicant does not have a full right of reference for some or all of the investigations relied upon for demonstrating safety and effectiveness and is relying on data generated by others, for example, publicly available information. This has been termed a "paper NDA" but is now referred to as a 505(b)(2) NDA for the section of the Act.

The 505(b)(2) NDA is applicable to the development of a new ophthalmic delivery system for an already approved drug because once the new drug is approved, and any applicable patent protection and market exclusivity periods have expired, the safety and efficacy data become public information and can be referenced by another applicant as part of a subsequent application for a modification of the approved drug (21 CFR 314.430). For the new ophthalmic delivery system of an approved drug, the basic human clinical and animal safety studies would not have to be repeated but only referenced to the approved drug's NDA. Full reports would only be required for demonstration of safety and efficacy of the new delivery system, i.e., the changes made to the approved drug. A complete chemistry, manufacturing, and controls section would also be required as this is not public information (21 CFR 314.54). Additionally, for a Section 505(b)(2) NDA, a patent certification is required in the application for any patent that claims the drug, drug product, or method of use for which prior investigations are relied upon without a right of reference from the original applicant. In addition to any patent protection, the new ophthalmic delivery system may be eligible for 3 years of Waxman-Hatch market exclusivity (21 CFR 314.108).

A. NDA Content and Requirements

The format and content of an NDA is seen in Table 4. The FDA Form 356h is the official signed application form.

An index to the entire application is essential to direct the reviewer to the location of the contents by volume and page numbers.

A comprehensive summary of the entire application is written in the style of a review article. A copy of the index and summary is provided to each reviewer of the application. The summary begins with an annotated copy of the proposed labeling, i.e., the product's proposed package insert. The applicant must be able to justify each statement in the labeling which is annotated to the supporting information in the Summary and Technical sections.

There are six major technical sections comprising the data generated to support the approval for the claimed indication(s). FDA guidelines for the technical sections are included on the FDA's web site at www.fda.gov/cder/guidance/index.htm.

Chemistry, Manufacturing and Control—drug substance and drug product
Microbiology—applicable only if for an anti-infective drug
Human Pharmacokinetics—ADME data from human studies
Pharmacology—animal study data for pharmacology, toxicology, and ADME
Clinical—human data for safety and efficacy
Statistics—mathematical analysis of the human clinical data

There are several sections ancillary to the technical sections. A section containing documentation for the analytical methods validation, drug sub-

Table 4 NDA—Format and Content Outline

FDA Form 356h
Index to Entire Application
    Summary
    a. Labeling text annotated to both Summary & Technical Sections
    b. Pharmacological Class, Scientific Rationale, Intended Use(s), and
       Potential Clinical Benefits
    c. Foreign Marketing History—Applicant and others if known
       i. Countries in which marketed
       ii. Countries where withdrawn from market for safety or efficacy
       iii. Countries where marketing applications pending
    d. Summary of Chemistry, Manufacturing and Controls Section
    e. Summary of Nonclinical Pharmacology & Toxicology Section
    f. Summary of Human P-Kinetics & Bioavailability Section
    g. Summary of Microbiology Section
    h. Summary of Clinical Section including Statistical Analysis
    i. Concluding Discussion—Benefit/Risk Consideration
Chemistry, Manufacturing, and Controls Section
    a. Drug Substance
       i. Description of Chemical & Physical Characteristics
       ii. Stability
       iii. Source & Location of Manufacturer(s)
       iv. Synthesis, Purification, and Controls
       v. Specifications & Analytical Methods
       vi. Reference Standard
    b. Drug Product
       i. Components
       ii. Specs and Test Methods for Inactives
       iii. Composition
       iv. Name and Location of Each Manufacturer
       v. Manufacturing & Packaging Procedures & In-Process Controls
       vi. Acceptance Specifications for Each Batch
       vii. Analytical and Microbiological Test Methods
       viii. Packaging Container/Closure Systems
       ix. Stability Data & Protocols
       x. Proposed Expiring Dating & Storage Conditions
    c. Environmental Assessment of Manufacturing Process & Ultimate Use
Samples, Methods Validation, Labeling
    a. Description & assay results of samples for FDA validation
    b. Methods Validation Package (Regulatory Specs & Methods)
    c. Container Labels & Package Insert Labeling
Nonclinical Pharmacology & Toxicology
    a. Pharmacology Studies
    b. Toxicology Studies
    c. Animal ADME Studies
    d. GLP Compliance Statements

Table 4 Continued

Human Pharmacokinetics & Bioavailability
   a. Waiver for topical or injectable product bioavailability studies
   b. For each human bio- or pharmacokinetic study:
      i.   Study report including analytical and statistical methods
      ii. IRB/Informed Consent Compliance Statements
   c. For specs or methods to assure bioavailability of drug or product:
      i.   Rationale for establishing spec or method
      ii. Data and information supporting rationale
   d. Summary Discussion & Analysis of:
      i.   Pharmacokinetics & metabolism or active ingredient
      ii. Bioavailability and/or bioequivalence of drug product
Microbiology (for Anti-Infectives Only)
Clinical Data
   a. Clinical Pharmacology Studies
   b. Controlled Clinical Studies
   c. Uncontrolled Clinical Studies
   d. All other data and information relevant to evaluation of the safety
      and effectiveness of the drug product
   e. Integrated Summary of Effectiveness
   f. Integrated Summary of Safety
   g. Studies related to abuse potential or over dosages
   h. Integrated summary of Benefits and Risks
   i. Compliance Statements (IRB & IC) for each clinical study
   j. Contract Research Organizations & Obligations Transferred
   k. List of studies where original subject records were audited or reviewed
      to verify accuracy of case reports
Reserved for Safety Update Reports
   a. Required After NDA Filed at:
      i.   4 months
      ii. Approvable letter and whenever FDA requests update
   b. New Safety Information from any source that may reasonably affect
      the labeling
   c. Case Report Forms for patients who died or were adverse event
      dropouts
Statistical Section
   a. Copy of the following Clinical Data Sections
   i. Controlled Studies
      ii. Integrated Summary of Effectiveness
      iii. Integrated Summary of Safety
   b. Documentation and Supporting Statistical Analysis used to Evaluate
      each of the above Clinical Data Sections
Case Report Tabulations
Data on each patient from
   a. Each adequate and well-controlled study (Phase 2 & 3)

    b. Each Phase 1 Clinical Pharmacology study
    c Safety data from other clinical studies
Case Report Forms
    a. For patients who:
        died during a clinical study or did not complete study due to adverse event
          whether or not thought to be drug related including patients on reference
          drug or placebo
    b. Additional CRFs may be requested after submission and must be submitted
       within 30 days of FDA request
Pediatric Studies—Information on use in Pediatric Population unless
    Waived or Deferred
Patent Information—Listing of U.S. Patents that could be infringed
which claim
    a. Drug
    b. Drug product composition
    c. Intended use
Patent Certification—For 505(b)(2) Applications
Claimed Market Exclusivity
Financial Certification or Disclosure Statements

Source: Adapted from 21 CFR 314.50.

stance and drug product samples, and the container labels and package insert. The samples are submitted to one or more FDA district laboratories for validation of the regulatory analytical methods and to confirm the identity, purity, and strength of the drug and drug product. The FDA uses the regulatory analytical methods to periodically test the drug product from regular production batches after approval. A section is reserved for periodic updates of new safety information that may be obtained after the NDA is submitted while under review and just prior to approval.

    The case report tabulations contain the clinical data from each patient's case report form (CRF). This is the raw data from the clinical studies and is tabulated by entry into sophisticated relational databases for evaluation and mathematical statistical analysis. A copy of the actual CRFs is only required in the initial submission and periodic safety updates for all deaths and patients discontinued due to adverse medical events. However, the FDA may request additional patient CRFs during the review.

    Studies in pediatric patients (birth to 16 years) are required for all new drugs during development and for certain marketed drugs (21 CFR 314.55). The applicant may request a waiver or deferment of the studies. A waiver may be granted if the new drug may not provide a meaningful therapeutic benefit over existing pediatric treatments and is not likely to be used in a substantial number of pediatric patients. The scope of the regulation includes new active ingredients, new indications, new dosage forms, new dosage regimens, and new routes of administration. For marketed drugs, FDA can require pediatric studies for those that are used in a substantial number of pediatric patients for the claimed indications or would provide a meaningful therapeutic benefit over existing treatments and where the absence of adequate labeling could pose significant risks.

To provide adequate data to meet the requirements may not always require controlled clinical trials in pediatric patients and may not require separate studies. In some cases where the course of the disease and the product's effects in adults and children are similar, the FDA may accept an extrapolation from adult studies with additional data such as dosing, pharmacokinetic, and safety data in pediatric patients. Also, adequate data may sometimes be obtained by including sufficient pediatric patients as well as adults in the original clinical studies where appropriate. The pediatric data is only required for the indications claimed by the applicant.

Since the Waxman–Hatch Act of 1984, NDAs must contain information of all unexpired U.S. patents for the drug substance, drug product, and methods of use (21 CFR 314.53). The applicant certifies the validity of the patent information and the FDA, without verification, upon NDA approval publishes the information in the Orange Book so that subsequent applicants are put on notice as to the patents that may be infringed and delay their entry into the marketplace.

For each patent that claims the drug, drug product, or method of use for which prior investigations are relied upon without a right of reference from the original applicant, a patent certification must be included (21 CFR 314.50(i)). The certification must show that there is no patent information filed with the FDA, that the patent has expired or the date the patent will expire, or that the patent is invalid or will not be infringed. If the certification that the patent is invalid or not infringed is made, notice must be given to the patent and NDA holder, who have 45 days to bring an infringement action in court, which enjoins the FDA from approving the application for 30 months or until the case is resolved by the court, whichever is shorter (21 CFR 314.52).

The Act provides for periods of market exclusivity upon approval of most NDAs. The exclusivity period must be requested by the applicant and if granted by the FDA will be published in the Orange Book for notice to generic applicants (21 CFR 314.50(j)). A 5-year period of market exclusivity is provided for the first approval of a new chemical entity and a 3-year period for all others, such as new uses and new dosage forms. Certain criteria must be met for the grant of market exclusivity, primarily the requirement for the conduct of clinical studies essential to approval as well as criteria for their financial support. During the exclusivity period, generic equivalent products cannot be marketed; however, during the 3-year period a generic application may be submitted. For the 5-year period, a generic application cannot be submitted during the first 4 years and during the last year of exclusivity can be submitted only if there is a patent challenge.

Congress included economic incentives for conducting pediatric studies in the Modernization Act of 1997 for drugs that are eligible for marketing exclusivity or patent protection under the Waxman-Hatch Act of 1984. The legislation makes available a 6-month extension of existing market exclusivity on drug products that the FDA has made a written request for pediatric studies and the manufacturer has conducted such studies meeting the requirements.

A long-standing requirement of clinical studies is that they are designed, conducted, analyzed, and reported in a manner that minimizes bias. One element that could introduce bias is the financial arrangements between the sponsor of the study and the clinical investigator. Since 1999, the FDA has required certain financial disclosure information for designated clinical studies be included in NDAs for their use in assessing data reliability in making the final approval decision (21 CFR Part 54).

The FDA is interested in certain financial arrangements for clinical studies that are relied on for proof of efficacy, including comparisons to effective products, and those that make a significant contribution to the demonstration of safety. Specific financial arrangements that must be disclosed for each such clinical investigator are those where the compensation of the clinical investigator is affected by the outcome of the study, or where there is significant equity interest in the sponsoring company, or compensation is tied to product sales, or a proprietary interest in the product, or receives significant payments from the sponsor such as for grants to fund ongoing research, compensation in the form of equipment, retainer for ongoing consultation or honoraria, and any steps taken to minimize the potential for bias due to these financial arrangements. If none of the above financial arrangements were in effect for the clinical studies, then the company may submit a certification attesting to this fact for each such clinical investigator.

B. Electronic Submission

The FDA has encouraged submission of parts or all of an NDA in electronic form to expedite the review of large datasets such as clinical, animal safety, biopharmaceutics, and chemistry sections. These computer-assisted NDAs (CANDA) have been adopted by most pharmaceutical companies in the anticipation that they will expedite the review and approval of their submissions. However, until recently, they could not be used to replace the official paper copy version of the NDA, which can involve more than 100 volumes. In March 1997, a new Electronic Records regulation was promulgated, allowing acceptance of documents entirely in electronic format with a certifying electronic signature. The FDA has been active in providing guidance to industry so that regulatory submissions can increasingly be made in electronic format with the hope that entire regulatory submissions can be paperless. The FDA provides updated information and guidance for electronic submissions on their website (www.fda.gov/cder/guidance/index.htm).

C. Patent Term Extension

The Waxman-Hatch Act makes available the possibility of extending the term of one unexpired patent for the drug, drug product, or use but only upon the first NDA approval for a new chemical entity. This provision was enacted to partially restore the effective patent life that is lost during the time required to meet FDA approval requirements. The patent holder must apply within 60 days of NDA approval to the U.S. Patent and Trademark Office (PTO) for extension of the selected unexpired patent. The PTO and FDA cooperate to determine the eligibility of the patent and the period of time for the extension. The extension is determined by a formula based on the amount of time diligently pursuing development under the IND and the amount of time from NDA filing until approval. The term extension is subject to the limitations of a maximum of 5 years and a maximum of 14 years patent term remaining with the extension (21 CFR 60).

D. Accelerated Availability of Certain New Drugs

The acquired immunodeficiency syndrome (AIDS) crisis focused attention on the drug development and regulatory processes for making new therapies available for life-threatening and severely debilitating conditions, particularly where no approved therapy or suitable alternative therapies exist. FDA instituted new procedures to make promising new drug therapies available to treat patients as early in the drug development process as possible, whereas at the same time obtaining data on the drug's safety and effectiveness in clinical trials.

The treatment IND regulations finalized in 1987 (21 CFR 312.34) make it possible for patients to receive promising new drugs for certain serious and life-threatening conditions as early as Phase 2 or 3 while controlled clinical trials are still underway to make a final determination on the new drug's safety and effectiveness. In some cases the manufacturer may charge for the investigational new drug product if necessary to undertake or continue the clinical trials. The sponsor of the new drug must apply to FDA for treatment use and provide available data supporting the drug's potential efficacy and safety. FDA may deny the request if the available scientific evidence, taken as a whole, is insufficient to support a reasonable conclusion that the drug may be effective for its intended use or would expose patients to unreasonable and significant additional risk of illness or injury. Also, clinical trials must be continuing to complete development and submission of an application to market the drug.

FDA also instituted accelerated drug development and review programs for certain serious or life-threatening conditions so that approval can be obtained for marketing at the earliest possible point that safety and efficacy are reasonably established (21 CFR Part 312 Subpart E). The FDAMA of 1997 essentially codified these programs for certain new drugs designated as "fast track" products (FD&C Act Section 506). The fast track programs of FDA are designed to facilitate the development and expedite the review of new drugs that meet certain requirements as treatments for serious or life-threatening conditions and that demonstrate potential to address unmet medical needs. For these fast track products, FDA may approve an NDA using a clinical endpoint or a surrogate endpoint that is reasonably likely to predict clinical benefit. Also, FDA can accept for review portions of a marketing application prior to receipt of the complete application (21 CFR Part 314 Subpart H).

In addition to the fast track programs accelerating development and market availability of certain new drugs, the FDA, working with industry and Congress, has established NDA review time goals for all NDAs as part of the quid pro quo for payment of user fees. Priority applications are to be reviewed within 6 months of filing and all other applications (standard) are to be reviewed within 10 months. The review classification as a priority or standard NDA is established at the time the NDA is filed and is based on FDA's estimate of the drug product's medical value, compared to already available products, using the safety and effectiveness submitted in the original application. To be designated for a priority review, the FDA must consider the drug product to be a significant improvement compared to marketed products as demonstrated by such elements as increased effectiveness, elimination or substantial reduction of an adverse drug reaction limiting use, documented enhancement of patient compliance, or evidence of safety and effectiveness in a new subpopulation.

VII. INTERNATIONAL HARMONIZATION

The technical requirements for registration of human pharmaceuticals vary throughout the world, which makes global development more expensive and delays introduction of new products in many markets while studies are being repeated to meet local requirements. In 1990, a unique project was undertaken to bring together the regulatory authorities of the United States, the European Union, and Japan along with scientific and regulatory experts from these three regions with the aim to produce a single set of technical requirements for the registration of new drug products and hence streamline the development process while maintaining the necessary safeguards to protect public health. The International Conference on Harmonization (ICH) is the driving force behind the project with representatives from the three major market regions and where most of the new drug development originates. The output of ICH are tripartite guidelines in the major areas of drug development: efficacy, safety, and quality. As of January 2000, 37 guidelines have been finalized and adopted as tripartite guidelines after rigorous scientific review and modification by the expert working groups. The efficacy topics cover clinical testing programs and safety monitoring, the safety topics cover preclinical toxicity and related tests, and the quality topics are concerned with chemistry and control specifications. Harmonized guidelines are also being developed for products of biotechnology.

In addition to differing technical requirements in the three ICH regions, the requirements for the technical sections of registration applications also differ, and a separate document must be prepared for each region. The concept of a Common Technical Document (CTD) for each of the three major topics has been adopted by ICH along with a standardized terminology for the reporting of adverse reactions in the *Medical Dictionary for Regulatory Activities* (MeDRA). Also being explored by ICH is harmonization of electronic information transfer standards (ESTRI) so that the CTD can be established eventually as an electronic document.

The ICH guidelines and additional information on the ICH process can be obtained from the ICH Secretariat website at www.ifpma.org/ ich1.html. The FDA publishes the ICH guidelines in the *Federal Register* at the draft stage for public comment and the finalized guidelines upon adoption. They can be obtained from the FDA web site at www.fda.gov/ cder/guidance/index.htm.

REFERENCES

1. Nielsen, J. R. (1986). *Handbook of Federal Drug Law*. Philadelphia, Lea & Febiger.
2. J. L. Fink, et al., eds. (1991). *Pharmacy Law Digest*. Facts and Comparisons, Inc., p. DC-4.
3. *Guidance for Industry, Environmental Assessment of Human Drugs and Biologics Applications* (Rev. 1), July 1998.
4. *Fed. Reg., 47*(200):46139, October 15, 1982.
5. Lerman, S., and Reininger, B. (1971). *Can. J. Ophthalmol., 6*:14.
6. Hackett, R. B. (1990). Non clinical study requirements for ophthalmic drugs and devices in the United States. *Lens & Eye Toxic. Res., 7*(3&4):181.
7. *Guideline for Drug Master Files* (Sept. 1989). Center for Drug Evaluation and Research, FDA.
8. *Guidelines on Sterile Drug Products Produced by Aseptic Processing* (1987). June, FDA.
9. *Fed. Reg., 56*(198):51354, October 11, 1991.
10. *Guideline on the Preparation of Investigational New Drug Products (Human & Animal)* (1991). March, FDA.

21
Patent Considerations

Robert E. Roehrs*
Alcon Research, Ltd., Fort Worth, Texas, U.S.A.

I. INTRODUCTION

A patent is the legal instrument by which inventors protect their substantial investment in time, effort, and money to create new technology and new products. Patents are a form of intellectual property with rights afforded by the U.S. constitution in Article I, Section 8: "The congress shall have the power . . . to promote the progress of science and the useful arts by securing for limited times to . . . inventors the exclusive right to their . . . discoveries."

Patents may be viewed as a contract between the inventor and the government under which the inventor is granted a limited monopoly to exclude others from making, using, selling, offering to sell the claimed invention in the United States, or importing it into the United States for a limited period of years. In return for this grant, the inventor agrees to disclose to the public via the patent the complete invention. Patents are an important public source of technological information, and studies show that a majority of patents contain information that is not published elsewhere. This public disclosure promotes the progress of science by allowing others to begin using the information to make their own improvements, which may also be patentable and thus disclosed to the public. This is quite common in the pharmaceutical field, where many patents are improvements on earlier discovered drugs and their medical uses and dosage forms.

Patents are a synthesis of law and science. The legal issues involved in protecting inventors' rights can be as complex as the subject matter of the invention. The pharmaceutical scientist needs legal expertise to fully protect

*Retired

695

his or her inventions. Although patent law allows inventors to represent themselves in obtaining a patent, it is advisable that they work closely with a patent legal specialist, such as a registered patent attorney or agent, to obtain an issued patent with the broadest legal protection that the law allows. It is helpful if the inventor has some understanding of the basic legal requirements for patenting inventions to work effectively with the legal expert who will prepare and prosecute the patent application. This overview refers only to U.S. patents and patent law requirements unless otherwise indicated.

II. UTILITY PATENTS

There are three types of patents: utility, design, and plant patents. Each has its own legal requirements for obtaining patent protection. Pharmaceutical patents for drugs and their delivery systems and uses are considered utility patents. In this chapter we will be discussing the requirements and uses of utility patents exclusively.

A patent consists of several parts that will be referred to in subsequent sections. Two major parts of a patent that the drug delivery researcher should become familiar with are the specification and the claims. The specification is the written description of the invention that concludes with one or more claims that define and delineate the scope of the rights granted to the inventor. Patent claims are often compared to the description of real property contained in a deed that sets the boundaries for the property. For a patent, everything contained within the boundaries of the claims is the exclusive right granted to the inventor.

III. PATENT RIGHTS

A. Right to Exclude

A U.S. patent gives the inventor the right to *exclude others* from making, using, selling, or offering for sale his claimed invention within the United States or importing the invention into the United States. If the U.S. patented invention is a process, the right to exclude also prevents others from using, offering for sale, or selling in the United States, or importing into the United States, products made by that process. These infringing acts are sometimes referred to as "practicing" the invention. In this chapter, the terms "practice" or "use" of the patented invention are used as shorthand for any and all of the statutory infringing acts. Along with this exclusionary right is the right to bring legal action in the courts when others practice the patented invention prior to its expiration without permission from the patent owner.

The right to exclude (a negative right) means that the inventor may in some cases be excluded from practicing his own patented invention. This occurs when there exists an unexpired U.S. patent that is broader in claims than the inventor's patent. The concept of "freedom to practice" or dominant/subservient patent claims is important for the drug delivery researcher to understand, since he may consider incorporating patented drugs into his new delivery system to improve their therapeutic benefits. The owner of the unexpired drug patent can exclude others from using the drug and therefore has a dominant exclusionary right over subsequent patents that include the drug as part of their claimed invention. Also, patentable improvements may in some cases be subservient to the original invention's patent claims. On the other hand, the inventor of the drug or earlier delivery system cannot use the drug in the separately patented delivery system or use the improved version without permission.

B. Right to Assign

The inventor is the owner of the patent rights, and he or she may assign, i.e., transfer his or her interest in the patent, either the exclusive rights to the whole patent or an undivided part or share of these rights. Employers may require their employees (inventors) to assign their exclusive rights to inventions conceived as part of their employment. The assignment is recorded in the United States Patent and Trademark Office (USPTO). Upon assignment, the employer owns the property rights inherent in the patent.

C. Right to License

The patent owner may license, i.e., transfer some or all of the patent rights; however, title is retained by the patent owner. A license may be exclusive or nonexclusive, and the licensee may be given the right to sublicense. The commercial value of a drug delivery system patent often involves the ability to license the technology to owners of patented drugs with limitations in their pharmacokinetics or duration of effect. Companies such as Alza have become successful using this corporate strategy.

IV. PATENT TERM

The patent grant is for a limited term, which in the United States is now 20 years from the earliest effective filing date for applications filed beginning June 8, 1995. Prior to the new law, patents had a term of 17 years from issue. In the transition to the new patent term, there are issued patents in effect with expiration dates of 17 years from issue, or 20 years from the earliest effective filing date, or various dates depending on certain patent term extensions that have been enacted by Congress. Patent maintenance fees are required at 3.5, 7.5, and 11.5 years after issuance (subject to a grace period), and failure to pay the required fee will result in premature expiration of the patent term.

Patent expiration dates for FDA-approved drugs are published in the FDA "Orange Book." These dates are provided to FDA by the company submitting the NDA and are not validated by FDA or the USPTO. (Patent term extensions for FDA-approved drugs are discussed in Chapter 20.) Patent terms may also be extended by the USPTO in certain cases where delays in patent application review would provide the inventor with less than a 17-year patent term. The new minimum patent term guarantee applies only to delays by the USPTO during examination of the application and not to delays caused by the applicant.

V. PATENTABLE INVENTIONS

Congress has defined patentable inventions in four broad categories: "Whoever invents or discovers any new and useful process, machine, manufacture, or composition of matter, or any new and useful improvement thereof may obtain a patent therefor, subject to the conditions and requirements of this title."

Ophthalmic drug delivery systems (ODDS) typically are claimed in a patent as compositions of matter and/or processes. Compositions of matter include chemical compounds and physical mixtures. Drug delivery system dosage forms are usually a combination or association of ingredients that cooperate to produce a unitary result exhibiting properties different from those possessed by the individual ingredients. One of the ingredients may be a drug molecule, which, in association with the ingredients of the delivery system (vehicle), is delivered in a new or improved manner to the eye. Drug molecules sometimes are developed specifically for ocular drug delivery purposes, i.e., prodrugs such as dipivefrin or the carbonic anhydrase inhibitors dorzolamide and brinzolamide, and are claimed as compositions of matter.

A patentable process consists of an act, operation, step, or series of steps performed upon specified subject matter to produce a physical result. A patentable process includes the method of making and method of using a substance, e.g., a pharmacologically active ingredient. Method of use or treatment claims often are recited in drug delivery patents. These so-called "use patents" also can include new uses for old products.

A patentable invention must contain claim(s) to statutory subject matter that are novel (new), useful (utility), and nonobvious among other requirements for specificity of the claims and adequacy of disclosure of the invention.

A. Utility

This is perhaps the easiest of the three statutory requirements to satisfy for patentability, particularly for most pharmaceutical inventions. Only useful inventions may be patented, i.e., inventions providing a beneficial use in society. A useful invention does not have to provide an advantage or an advance in the art to be considered to meet the utility requirement, nor does it have to necessarily provide the best or even a commercially feasible product or process. Issues of utility may arise if the usefulness is not apparent or credible. A patent usually states under the objectives of the invention one or more intended purposes for the invention. These statements of specific utility are usually sufficient unless there is a reason for one skilled in the art to question the truth of the statement of utility or its scope. The invention must be operable for at least one of the intended purposes to meet the utility requirement.

For pharmaceutical inventions, issues can arise if the utility alleged has never before been demonstrated or there are no in vitro tests that correlate with a practical utility or animal tests with recognized relevance to human utility. If human use is not alleged, it need not be proved, veterinary utility being sufficient. Also, FDA requirements for safety and efficacy are not patent law requirements for utility. Indeed, patent protection is often obtained prior to completion of human clinical trials, and it is the patent rights that provide the economic incentive to complete FDA's marketing requirements.

B. Novelty and Loss of Right to Patent

Useful statutory subject matter may be patented if it meets the legal requirements of novelty and nonobviousness, and these two requirements essentially define the limits of what may be protected for a particular invention. Novelty is relatively straightforward, i.e., if the claimed subject matter has been done before in exactly the same manner, then it is old (lack novelty) and is not patentable. However, even if the invention is new, further inquiry is required to determined whether it is nonobvious, i.e., not obvious to one of ordinary skill in the art to which it pertains. The patent law also defines certain circumstances where acts by the inventor or others may prevent a patent from being obtained, i.e., so-called statutory bars, even though the invention may meet all other requirements.

The novelty provisions of patent law prevent an inventor from obtaining a patent for subject matter that was known, used, patented, described, or made by another prior to the applicant's invention. The novelty requirement is one of strict identity, i.e., a *single* reference must contain all the limitations of the claimed subject matter and in the same order (steps) in which they are arranged in the claim. This is termed "anticipation," and for meeting the novelty requirements, the USPTO cannot combine more than one reference to show anticipation of the claimed subject matter.

Patent law prescribes the following conditions, which if are found to have occurred *prior to the invention* prevent a patent from issuing for lack of novelty:

1. The invention was known or used by others in this country, or patented or described in a printed publication in this or a foreign country
2. The invention was described in a patent granted on an application for patent by another filed in the United States or on an international application by another fulfilling certain requirements
3. The invention was made in this country by another who had not abandoned, suppressed, or concealed it

Note that knowledge or use by others outside of this country does not prevent a patent unless the invention has been published or patented anywhere in the world. Knowledge or use in this country refers to that which is accessible to the public. The terms "others" and "another" refer to any entity different from the so-called inventive entity, i.e., single inventor or joint inventors.

Certain acts by the inventor may cause a loss of rights and bar the issuance of a patent:

1. The invention was patented or described in a printed publication in this or a foreign country or in public use or on sale in this country, more than one year prior to the filing date of the U.S. patent application.
2. The invention was abandoned.
3. The invention was first patented or caused to be patented in a foreign country prior to the filing date of the U.S. patent application on an application in the foreign country filed more than 12 months before the filing of the U.S. patent application.

United States patent law provides a 1-year grace period for filing a patent application in this country when the invention has been patented or published anywhere in the world or for public use or sale in this country.

Thus it is important that the inventor recognize when the 1-year grace period may be triggered and keep the patent legal specialist informed of all potential public disclosures, uses, and offers for sale of the invention so that a timely application may be filed to prevent a statutory bar. It is also important that the inventor not try to second-guess the meaning of these legal conditions since they have been and are subject to various legal interpretations by the courts based on specific set of facts and circumstances. For example, what is considered "printed" is certainly now more complex than when it was first promulgated and has been interpreted to mean all material accessible to the public in tangible form, including a single copy of a thesis indexed and catalogued in a university library. The conduct of tests in the public eye to perfect an invention or the sale of an invention for the sole purpose of experimental use may or may not trigger the 1-year grace period, and legal advice should be obtained in advance.

C. Nonobviousness

A new and useful invention must also meet the statutory requirement for nonobviousness. The patent law states that "if the differences between the subject matter sought to be patented and the prior art are such that the subject matter as a whole would have been obvious at the time the invention was made to a person having ordinary skill in the art to which the subject matter pertains," then the invention is considered obvious and a patent cannot be granted.

The determination of whether a particular invention is or is not obvious is largely subjective, although the courts have established some guidelines and tests for its determination as a matter of law. Obviousness does not hinge on the manner in which the invention was made, i.e., there is no requirement for "a flash of genius." Many inventions are made after considerable experimentation or even by error or accident and rarely by revolutionary imagination. The test of obviousness of an invention is not whether it would have been "obvious to try" the combination of steps or elements that led to the invention. In hindsight, it may seem like it would have been obvious to try certain experiments leading to the claimed subject matter, but the focus of the patent law is on the level of knowledge and skill in the art at the time the invention was made.

To ascertain if the nonobviousness requirement has been met, the USPTO and the courts examine the following:

1. The scope and content of the prior art
2. The differences between the art and the claims at issue

3. The level of ordinary skill in the art
4. Whatever objective evidence may be present

The prior art is the body of knowledge or information that is publicly available or accessible at the time of the invention. Patent law presumes that the inventor and the person of ordinary skill have full and comprehensive knowledge of the prior art pertinent to the invention. For determining obviousness, reference is made to the scope and content of the art relevant to the subject matter of the invention as well as to so-called analogous art. This is different from the requirement for novelty where anticipation is not restricted to the prior art of the invention but includes all prior art. Analogous prior art is that art that may be outside the field of the invention but that the inventor would examine to solve a problem or obtain a result leading to the invention. Analogous art is said to be art that is reasonably pertinent to the particular problem the inventor was involved with, and there is a similarity of elements, problems, and purposes.

The content of the prior art is examined for what it teaches about the claimed subject matter. Does the prior art teaching render it obvious to one of ordinary skill in the art, or does it teach away, i.e., discourage one of ordinary skill from following the path taken by the inventor or suggest that it would be unlikely to be productive? Prior art that "teaches away" can be evidence of nonobviousness.

If the invention is novel, then there must exist some difference from that found in the prior art, and it is this difference that has sometimes been termed the "invention" or "inventive step." What matters is not necessarily the degree of difference, but whether or not the difference is obvious to the one ordinarily skilled in the art at the time the invention was made. However, the degree of difference can be a factor, particularly if it causes disproportionate, unexpected, surprising, or unusual results. The difference from the prior art is examined for the invention's "subject matter as a whole." This means that the inherent properties of what is claimed and disclosed in the patent's specification are also part of the comparison to the teachings of the prior art. If the invention produces certain advantages or unexpected results and these might be crucial to a determination of nonobviousness, they should be included in the patent specification.

The person of ordinary skill in the art is a hypothetical person and is usually considered to be one who follows conventional wisdom in the art rather than one who is an innovator in the art. The level of ordinary skill is ascertained at the time the invention was made, not at a later time when advances in the art could have made the original invention obvious, particularly if the advances were made possible by the claimed invention. Certain factors may be considered in determining the level of ordinary skill, including the education level of active workers in the art, the types of problems encountered and the prior art solutions to those problems, the sophistication of the technology, and the rapidity with which innovations are made.

Objective evidence of nonobviousness usually comes as proof or evidence of what are called "secondary considerations." The most common type of secondary considerations include the commercial success of the invention, the satisfaction of a long-felt need, the failure of others to find a solution to the problem the invention addresses, copying of the invention by others, unexpected results, and expression of disbelief or praise by experts. While the absence of such secondary considerations does not necessarily indicate that an invention is obvious, their presence in an invention is not always conclusive of nonobviousness.

VI. INVENTORSHIP AND PRIORITY OF INVENTION

Only the true and original inventor may obtain a U.S. patent. The inventor cannot have derived the invention from someone else. If more than one independent inventor applies for a patent on the same invention, it will be awarded to the first inventor. Although we speak of the inventor, it is more correct to speak of the "inventorship entity" since there may be more than one inventor. Where there is more than one inventor, the inventorship entity is spoken of as joint inventors or co-inventors. Joint inventorship is quite common in the pharmaceutical field where several scientists collaborate on a project. A patent can be invalidated if more or fewer than the correct number of co-inventors is named in an application, but the law presumes that the listing of inventors in an issued patent is correct. Legal remedies are available to correct a mistake in the inventorship entity as long as it was made without intent to deceive.

Each inventor owns an equal and undivided interest in the patent rights and, absent an agreement to the contrary, can individually assign or license their property rights to different parties. In most cases the joint inventors work for the same organization and assign their patent rights to their employer. However, if a project involves collaboration with scientists outside of the organization and there is the possibility of joint inventorship, the question of the ownership of property rights between the two organizations should to be addressed prior to applying for a patent.

A joint invention occurs when more than one person contributes something meaningful to the conception of the claimed invention. The contribution must be more than a mere suggestion of a desired result or must do more than merely follow the instructions of another. Someone preparing a composition provided by his or her supervisor and submitting it for testing does not rise to the level of an inventor. However, if in so doing he or she makes a contribution, such as a modification in the composition that allows it to achieve its intended purpose, then he or she could become a joint inventor. According to U.S. patent law, joint inventors may obtain a patent even though they did not physically work together or at the same time, each did not make the same type or amount of contribution, or each did not make a contribution to the subject matter of every claim of the patent.

United States patent law is a "first-to-invent" system, as opposed to other countries, which have "first-to-file" systems. The priority of invention is an issue when more than one inventorship entity submits a patent application for the same claimed subject matter. The priority contest (interference) is invoked to determine who was the first to invent. Invention is considered the acts of conception and reduction to practice. The patent will be awarded to the first to conceive the invention even if last to reduce it to practice as long as he or she was reasonably diligent in pursuing the reduction to practice from the time prior to conception by the other inventorship entity. Conception is considered the mental part of inventing. The inventor forms in his or her mind the complete form of his or her part of the invention. In some cases, conception may not be complete until after some experimentation has taken place. Reduction to practice is the demonstration that the invention works for its intended purpose, but the act of filing a patent application is recognized in patent law as a constructive reduction to practice. Scientists are taught to keep records of their experimental work, and it is important to record the conception of an invention in a timely manner and keep timely records of the acts taken to reduce it to practice. The conception and reduction to practice records should be witnessed by someone other than another co-inventor. The witness should have sufficient knowledge or qualifications to understand the technical information regarding the invention records.

VII. PATENT APPLICATIONS

A. Provisional Application

Since 1995, a provisional patent application may be filed with the USPTO for the purpose of establishing priority of invention and the benefit of an earlier filing date but not starting the 20-year patent term. A patent does not issue from filing a provisional application, and the application automatically becomes abandoned after 1 year from filing. To obtain the benefit of an earlier filing date, a regular or nonprovisional patent application must be filed before the end of the 1-year period. The provisional application need only contain a written description of the invention, drawings (if needed) and the name of the inventor(s) along with some formal requirements and a fee.

No claims are required in the application, but the invention must be fully disclosed to support the claims of a subsequent regular application, otherwise the benefit of the earlier filing date would only apply to the claims supported by the disclosure in the provisional application.

B. Nonprovisional Application

A regular application submitted to the USPTO to obtain a patent consists of a number of parts prepared by a patent legal specialist with the aid of the inventor(s). The following sections will focus on two major parts of the application that are incorporated into the issued patent. These parts are the patent specification and the claims.

VIII. PATENT SPECIFICATION

The specification is the written description of the invention that concludes with one or more claims that define the exclusive rights granted to the inventor. The specification is usually presented in several subparts:

1. *Title of the Invention.* A short and specific description of the nature of the invention.
2. *Cross-Reference to Related Applications, if any.* These are prior filed applications of the same applicant and, if certain requirements are met, establish the earliest effective filing date for some or all of the claimed subject matter. Several types that may appear in the patent are:

    a. Continuation—for the same invention but may be used to add claims to subject matter disclosed but not claimed in the earlier application.
    b. Continuation-in-part—contains some or all of the prior application plus new information disclosed (new matter) to support new claims.
    c. Divisional—filed for distinct or independent inventions than cannot be claimed in the same application.
    d. Provisional—previously discussed. For benefit of earlier filing date.
    e. Foreign or international application—Establish priority (earlier) filing date.

3. *Background of the Invention.* Consists of two parts—a brief statement of the field of art to which subject matter pertains, and a

description of the relevant prior art including problems, limitations, disadvantages in the prior art and those that have been solved or overcome by the applicant's invention.

4. *Summary of the Invention.* A brief summary that presents the substance or general idea of the invention and may include the objective's of the invention and may point out advantages and how it solves problems presented in the Background.

5. *Brief Description of the Drawings.* Drawings are not always required unless they are needed for a full understanding of the claimed subject matter. Drawings are more commonly used in mechanical and electrical patents. However, graphical presentations of experimental data are also considered drawings and sometimes are used in composition of matter patents.

6. *Detailed Description.* This section presents the invention described in sufficient detail to support the scope of the claimed subject matter and distinguish it from other inventions and what is old (prior art). It is also used to meet the patent law requirements to describe the method of making and using it in sufficient detail to allow a person skilled in the art to make and use the invention without undue experimentation, and the best mode (preferred embodiment) contemplated by the inventor for practicing the invention at the time of filing the application. If there are drawings, each element should be described. For improvement inventions, it points out specifically the part or parts of the statutory subject matter such as a composition of matter that is the improvement. It is understood in patent law that the inventor is his own lexicographer and has latitude in choosing the terminology to describe and claim his invention, but there must be correspondence in terminology between the description, claims, and drawings.

7. *Abstract of the Invention.* A brief statement of the technical disclosure in the patent so as to enable the patent office and the public to determine quickly from a cursory inspection the nature and gist of the invention. The abstract appears on the front page of the published patent.

IX. PATENT CLAIMS

The patent concludes with one or more claims that define the physical extent or boundary of the exclusionary rights granted by the government to the patent owner. The claims also serve notice on the public as to what acts will violate the personal property rights (infringement) as well as the physical embodiments of the new knowledge that will come into the public domain upon expiration of the patent's term.

The language of the claims follows certain prescribed rules. Each claim is one sentence as the object of the introductory "I (We) claim:" and contains three parts: the preamble, the transition and the body. The *preamble* is an introductory phrase that introduces the name of the subject matter and may include the purpose, object, or intended use of the invention. The preamble may also in some cases include elements of the prior art to segregate what is new or modified by the invention recited in the body of the claim. The claimed invention in this Jepson-type claim consists of the preamble elements combined with the new or improved elements for operability. Ordinarily, the preamble does not limit the scope of the claims and most patent practitioners avoid such limiting preambles. However, in some circumstances a preamble has been deemed by a court to be significant to claim scope where terms appearing in a preamble gives meaning to the claim and properly defines the invention.

The second part of the claim, the *transition*, is the bridge between the preamble and the body of the claim and plays a major role in the interpretation of the scope of the claim. Specific terminology for the transition has been adopted in patent practice to indicate whether the body of the claim should be read as open-ended or closed:

1. When the transition used is *"comprises"* (or "comprising, including, containing"), the claim is to be interpreted as open-ended, i.e., the claim covers the elements (components, ingredients, steps) recited in the body of the claim as well as additional elements. Thus the legal boundary is not limited only by the recited elements in the claim. A competitor cannot merely add an additional element and avoid infringement. The term comprises can be read as "having at least."

2. The transitional phrase *"consisting of"* indicates a closed-ended claim and the narrowest scope of coverage as the claim covers only the recited elements. A competitor can add an additional element and avoid literal infringement. This type of claim would only be used if necessary for operability or to avoid a novelty or obviousness rejection.

3. The transitional phrase *"consisting essentially of"* is intermediate in scope and is intended to exclude additional unspecified elements that would affect the basis and novel characteristics of the subject matter recited in the body of the claim.

The *body* of a claim recites the necessary elements required for the invention to be operable and patentable over the prior art. Each element usually includes a well-defined name distinguishing it from other elements, distinctive features, or properties of the element necessary for operability and patentability, such as concentration range, and nature of cooperation, if any, with the other elements. The body of the claim can vary in scope as to how the elements are claimed: the narrowest scope names one specific component (ingredient) per element; an intermediate scope names a group of similar functionally equivalent components as the element; and the broadest scope names only the function that the element performs. These variations of course can be used only in light of their operability and patentability. The use of alternative expressions (Markush groups) can be a defined genus such as "halogen" or a homemade generic expression such as "chlorine or bromine." The use of these groupings is considered closed-ended and is preceded by the use of "consisting of." An example of a functional claim element used in pharmaceutical compositions would be the element: "a pH-adjusting substance in an amount sufficient to adjust the pH to a value of from about 4 to 5.5." The specification would contain examples describing a range of pH adjusting substances contemplated but not limiting in the practice of the invention.

A patent usually includes multiple claims, some of which are independent and some dependent. The claims are numbered consecutively, and the first claim is an independent claim of the broadest scope of the claimed invention, i.e., it contains the fewest limitations. It has the fewest elements in the broadest language consistent with operability and patentability. The dependent claims add an additional element or limitation and refers back to another claim or claims that it so modifies. If the invention covers a commercial product, there usually is a claim that is narrowed to recite all the specific elements of the product.

There may be claims to more than one statutory class of subject matter. It is typical for drug delivery system patents to claim the delivery system (vehicle) as a composition of matter, claim the vehicle plus a pharmacologically active drug, and also claim a method for using the delivery system to administer the drug. For claims reciting a drug as an element of the composition of matter or method of use, it has become judicially acceptable to refer to the concentration of the drug as "a therapeutically effective amount." For drug molecule patents, claims are usually included covering the drug, the drug in dosage form(s) usually claimed broadly as "pharmaceutically acceptable carriers," and methods for using the drug. Composition of matter claims are preferred over method of use claims since they would be in a dominant position to later patented new uses. Also, the person infringing a method of use claim is usually a customer.

X. PATENT EXAMINATION AND PROSECUTION

Applications for U.S. patents are filed with the USPTO and examined by a patent examiner in the art class to which the invention pertains. The examiner searches the prior art including U.S. patents, foreign patents, printed publications as well as his or her own personal knowledge of the art. The examiner is looking for references that show the identical invention or prior art that can be combined or modified to demonstrate that the claimed subject matter would be obvious and thus unpatentable over the prior art.

The patent application will most likely contain pertinent prior art known to the inventor. In fact, each individual associated with the filing and prosecution of a patent application has a duty to disclose to the USPTO all information known to that individual to be material to patentability with respect to each pending claim. This duty of disclosure extends not only to the inventor(s) and the legal representative(s) but also to every other person substantially involved in the preparation and prosecution of the application and who is associated with the inventor, with the assignee, or with anyone to whom there is an obligation to assign. Individuals other than the inventor and legal representative can comply by disclosing the information to the inventor or legal representative. The information may be disclosed in the patent specification or in a separate Information Disclosure Statement (IDS). An IDS is not construed as a representation that a search of the prior art was made or that no better art exists. This duty to disclose is satisfied if all information known to be material to patentability of any claim issued in a patent was cited by the patent office or submitted to the patent office. The front page of an issued patent contains a listing of references cited by the patent office as to U.S. patents, foreign patents, and other publications. The front page of the patent also lists the classification of the patent's subject matter and the field of search, i.e., the various subject matter classifications searched by the examiner.

The examiner will most likely issue an Office Action (OA) that sets forth any deficiencies in the application and allow or reject some or all of the claims. The examiner is required in the OA to set forth the basis and cite the best art available and how it applies to the claims that are rejected. The applicant can respond usually in the form of an amendment to traverse the rejections. This give and take with the examiner is termed "prosecution" of the application. The amendment may include an affidavit or declaration to remove a prior art reference used by the examiner to reject claims or to provide data and information as objective evidence of invention. Often the claims will be modified or narrowed to traverse a rejection and obtain an allowance. The prosecution continues until claims are allowed or a final rejection is issued or the inventor abandons the application. In the case of a final rejection, the inventor may appeal within the patent office and if unsuccessful to the courts.

The prosecution of the application is conducted largely ex parte, i.e., in confidence between the USPTO and the inventor(s). The record of the prosecution, i.e., the examiners papers as well as the application and the inventors responses to the patent office are kept in a folder that is termed a "file wrapper." This file wrapper does not come with the printed patent but may be obtained separately from the patent office. It is often useful to obtain to determine what information the inventor provided that may not be a part of the patent and what modifications may have been made to the claims during prosecution.

The first public knowledge of a U.S. patent application, unless disclosed by the applicant or referred to in a published foreign patent application, had been the notification of an issued patent in the weekly *Official Gazette* published by the USPTO. However, since March 15, 2001, and subject to certain exceptions, regular nonprovisional utility patent *applications* filed in the USPTO and also filed in a foreign country are being published 18 months after the effective U.S. filing date beginning with qualifying applications filed on or after November 29, 2000, and those pending on that date that request and qualify for voluntary publication. This change in U.S. patent law brings U.S. practice in alignment with most European countries and Japan that publish patent applications. To avoid publication of a pending U.S. patent application, the applicant must specifically request that the application not be published and certify that no foreign counterpart application will be filed. Certain applications subject to a secrecy order will not be published. The exception to publication of a patent application does not exist in European countries and Japan.

Once an application is published, the application and the complete file wrapper are publicly available. This provides the public with an early notice of potentially patentable subject matter, although it is no guarantee that a patent will be issued or the scope of the claims finally allowed. Also, it allows members of the public such as competitors to monitor patent prosecution and to submit pertinent prior art for consideration by the patent examiner. The benefit to the inventor of having his or her pending patent applications published is the additional grant of so-called "provisional rights" to collect reasonable royalties for infringing acts prior to grant of a patent as discussed in the next section.

XI. PATENT INFRINGEMENT

The patent owner's exclusive property rights may be violated (infringed) by one or more of the acts of making, using, selling, offering to sell in the United States, or importing the patented invention into the United States. Some exceptions of interest to the pharmaceutical scientist are discussed below. The act of making or using the subject matter of at least one claim of a patent is sufficient for infringement. There does not have to be commercialization or intent to commercialize to commit an infringing act, but these are the usual reasons that a patent owner would sue for infringement. What is infringed is one or more claims of the patent, i.e., an embodiment of the invention and not the invention as a whole.

The question of whether an infringing act has been committed or whether infringement can be avoided is answered by focusing on the patent claims and their language in light of the patent specification, the prior art, and the prosecution history (file wrapper) of the patent. Literal infringement is determined by applying the claims to the suspect infringing product or process. If each and every element (limitation) of a claim exists in the suspect product or process, then there may be literal infringement. In patent jargon, the claim "reads on" the suspect product or process. If there are more elements in the suspect product or process and the claim is closed-ended by the transitional phrase used, then there may not be literal infringement.

The apparently straightforward interpretation of infringement can be complicated by the application of the judicially created Doctrine of Equivalents. Courts have in some cases, where the accused infringing product or process does not contain a limitation exactly as stated in a claim, extended the scope of the claim to interchangeable equivalents. Their reasoning is one of equity to the patent owner, who must find language to describe the various embodiments of the invention as best he or she can while what is protected is the actual physical structure of the invention and not merely the words used in the patent. This judicial doctrine is somewhat controversial and can be legally complicated in its application. Courts usually apply a tripartite test when applying the doctrine in a specific case to determine if the element in issue performs substantially the same function in substantially the same way to achieve substantially the same result as the claimed element. The substantially equivalent element does not necessarily have to be described in the patent but may be something that the hypothetical person skilled in the art would consider interchangeable. The range of interchangeable equivalents may be determined from those available at the time of the infringement and not just at the time of the invention.

When analyzing a patent for determining infringement or development of a non-infringing product or process, the prosecution history in the patent office (file wrapper) should be examined. During prosecution of the patent application, the claims may have been modified or certain arguments may have been put forth to avoid a rejection of the claimed subject matter. In subsequent enforcement of patent rights, the patent owner cannot try to recapture subject matter relinquished during prosecution or change his position as to arguments made to avoid rejection. Subject matter relinquished such as by adding further elements or limitations to a claim is not part of the patent property and cannot be recaptured by the Doctrine of Equivalents.

With the publication of pending patent applications, provisional rights are granted that enable the patent owner to collect reasonable royalties for infringement during the period beginning on the date of publication of an application until the date the patent issues. However, these provisional rights are only available if the invention as claimed in the issued patent is substantially similar to the invention as claimed in the published patent application and proof is available that the alleged infringing party had actual notice of the published patent application.

Several specific exceptions to the law of infringement have been enacted by Congress. As discussed in Chapter 20, development and testing to obtain data for submission to FDA for marketing approval is not an act of infringement. This exception was made so that a drug patent's limited monopoly would not, in effect, be extended if development of a generic product had to await patent expiration. The law makes the submission of the marketing application prior to patent expiration the infringement act.

Methods of diagnosis and treatment such as medical and surgical procedures performed on a body can and are patented as they qualify as statutory processes. Patent law was amended in 1996 (applies to patents granted on or after September 30, 1996) to preclude any remedy for infringement against a medical practitioner for his or her performance of a medical or surgical procedure. However, the exempted medical activities do not include use of a patented machine, article of manufacture or composition of matter in violation of the patent, or the practice of a patented use of a composition of matter in violation of the patent, or the practice of a process in violation of a biotechnology patent. Also, the term "patented use of a composition of matter" does not include a claim for a method of performing a medical or surgical procedure on a body that recites the use of a composition of matter where the use of the composition of matter does not directly contribute to achievement of the objective of the claimed method. Thus, the exception is directed primarily to pure medical and surgical procedures where it is in the public interest not to limit the use of innovative procedures because of the health care professional's concern for being sued for infringement.

XII.O PATENT SEARCHING

In researching the patentability of an invention, it is important to know the state of the prior art to which the invention pertains. Searching the prior art includes patents that have issued as well as printed publications in the non-patent prior art. While it is required to disclose to the USPTO material prior art known at the time the application is filed, it is not required by patent law that a search of prior art be made. However, it is beneficial to conduct as thorough a search of prior art as time and resources will allow. There are limitations on a patent search such that even the most thorough may not be 100% reliable in discovering all pertinent patented subject matter. Most patent searches focus on U.S. patents but may miss pertinent foreign patents, although the ability to search certain foreign patents using online databases is improving. There may be patent applications that have not been published, and patent databases that are searched may not be complete or some patents may have been misclassified.

In addition to searching for patentability, patent searches are undertaken to ascertain validity of issued patents such as in defense of an infringement suit or to determine the right to use a prospective product (avoid infringement). Patentability and validity searches focus on expired and unexpired patents and published applications with a worldwide perspective while a right-to-use search focuses on unexpired patents and published applications in the United States and other countries of marketing interest. Another type of patent search is a state-of-the-art or collection search in which all patents and published applications in a particular area of technology are reviewed. The state-of-the-art search is particularly useful when beginning research in a new product area and can aid in avoiding duplication of patented technology and focus efforts on improvements and new approaches.

Patent searching is usually conducted manually or electronically and increasingly by a combination of both methods using online patent databases. The availability of patent databases accessible through the Internet make it possible for the inventor to conduct at least a preliminary search for U.S. patents while in his or her lab or in the company or university library, just as he or she would conduct a literature search. These databases make it possible to keep up to date on new U.S. patents published on a weekly basis and published patent applications as well as some international applications and foreign patents. Specialized patent and research databases are being developed in areas such as AIDS and biotechnology.

The traditional manual method involves determining the most likely classification by the USPTO of the invention and then searching in these classes and subclasses for pertinent patents. This search may be done at the USPTO in Arlington, Virginia, where more than 6 million patents issued since 1790 are filed and can be manually examined. There is also a network of more than 80 Patent and Trademark Depository Libraries (PTDL) throughout the United States, most of which maintain a complete patent image collection on microfilm which is available for public patent searching. A list of the locations of these PTDLs is available on the USPTO website at www.uspto.gov/go/ptdl. These patent libraries have complete information on U.S. patent classifications including a computer search system known as CASSIS on CD-ROMs from which a list of patents issued in each patent classification can be obtained. The bibliographic data from the front page of a patent can also be accessed from CASSIS for utility patents issued since 1969. The front page of each patent includes the title of the invention as well as the patent abstract, which is often used to classify the subject matter of the invention. The front page also contains the patent classification, both U.S. and international, as well as references cited by the examiner. The references include U.S. patents, foreign patent documents, and printed publications cited by the examiner as prior art. Some of the patent libraries also have access to the APS (Automated Patent System) text search program. The APS is connected by computer terminal to the patent database at the USPTO and enables searching the entire text of patents issued since August 1971. Several of these libraries also have an enhanced version of APS that allows viewing of patent images as well as text. Patent images are necessary to view the drawings contained in an issued patent.

The basic method for using the U.S. patent classification system to conduct a patent search involves compiling a list of classes and subclasses to search. This is done by making lists of words (terms) describing the important structural and functional features of the invention and first looking up the terms in the *Index to the U.S. Patent Classification Manual* (Index). The Index is an alphabetical listing of technical and common terms with corresponding U.S. patent classifications used by the USPTO. The classes and subclasses are numerical and written as, for example, 514/772, which signifies Class 514 and its subclass 772. Second, once a list of potential classes and subclasses has been compiled, the *Manual of Classification* (Manual) is consulted, which lists all subclasses in an indented fashion under each main class in numerical order. The Manual aids in narrowing the classification to the most relevant subject matter. The *Classification Definitions* manual should then be consulted to further determine the relevance of the chosen classes and subclasses for searching as it contains a description of the subject matter for each class and subclass used by the USPTO. It also contains a cross-reference to other classification for similar subject matter and search notes explaining the scope and limits of a particular class or subclass.

If an inventor already has one or more patents in the same subject area as the prospective invention, he can begin classification searching using the U.S. classification(s) and Field of Search information listed on the front page of a patent. However, it is advisable to consult the USPTO classification documents referred to above, particularly for older patents, since the classification numbers may have changed or new class/subclass combinations may have been established. If the new invention contains new or different components, searching in additional classes and subclasses may be required.

Once a list of the most relevant class/subclass combinations has been obtained, the next step is to generate a list of patents issued in each class. The patent lists can be obtained using the CASSIS system or from online patent databases such as the USPTO. The lists contain the patent number and the patent title. It is usually necessary to review more than just the patent title to determine the most relevant patents that should be obtained for further review. The online databases usually have a link to the full text of the patent and a link to view the patent image (each page of the issued patent). Another means to review each patent from the list that may be relevant is the use of the *Official Gazette* that contains an exemplary claim and a representative drawing (if any) for each issued patent.

In reviewing a number of ophthalmic drug delivery patents, U.S. Classes 424 and 514 are frequently cited on the front page. The title of both classes is identical—"Drug, Bio-Affecting and Body Treating Compositions"—so these would be good places to begin a search. However, we need to narrow the search to specific subclasses, and we find in the Manual that classification 424/78.04 is listed as ophthalmic preparations. Obtaining a list of patents in this classification indicates that of January 2002 there are 238 U.S. patents cited. In class 514 in the Manual we find that subclass 912 contains ophthalmic subject matter involving the treatment of an ophthalmic disorder, and a list of patents in classification 514/912 reveals 739 patents as of January 2002. Some of the ophthalmic patents in both classifications are obviously the same, but this example points out that there is no single classification for all ophthalmic drug delivery patents. For example, Class 427 is titled "Coating Processes," and a number of pharmaceutical patents are contained in this class including ophthalmic drug and ocular devices. Also, Class 604, the Surgery classification, and subclass 890.1 include some patents directed to controlled release therapeutic devices or systems, a number of which relate to ophthalmic applications. Once relevant patent classifications have been established, the search can continually be updated by periodically obtaining new lists of patents issued and published applications in these classifications. New patents are issued on a weekly basis, and these updates can easily be obtained by online patent database, discussed in the next section.

Another use of the online patent databases is to monitor competitor activity. Periodic updates of issued patents can be obtained for patent classifications of research interest by searching in the current U.S. classification field. Monitoring can be enhanced by access to published foreign patent applications and the U.S. applications that are published. If there are certain companies and/or inventors that you want to monitor, this can be done by searching for issued patents for the company in the assignee field and the inventor (full name) in the inventor's field. These fields are found on the front page of a patent.

The USPTO maintains an online patent database that can be searched without charge. The patent database contains full text of U.S. patents issued since 1790 hyperlinked to their full-page images. The database can be accessed from the Home page of the website at www.uspto.gov. The database can be searched in specific blocks of years or for all years (1790 to present). For the years 1790–1976, the database can be searched only by patent number and current U.S. classification. For patents issued from 1976 to present, keyword searches can be conducted on the full text. Advanced Boolean searches can be done in selected patent fields as well as multiple fields. Patent number searching is also available. Searching in specific class/subclasses provides a list of issued patents with links to full-text and full-page images. The access to the image of each page of a patent allows examination of the drawings as well as the text. Special browser plug-ins or applications may be necessary to view the page images. The database contains a section that explains the contents and recent changes as well as missing or withdrawn patent numbers. It has Help functions that assist in most efficient use of the search functions and an Index to the site from which additional information available on the site can be obtained, for example, links to the three patent classification documents explained above. Patent documents can be ordered online for delivery in various forms for a fee.

Since March 15, 2001, the USPTO has been publishing certain patent applications, and these are available on their website in a separate database from issued patents. The published application database can be searched in essentially the same manner as the issued patent database. The published application database contains full-text and full-page images.

The Delphion Intellectual Property Network (formerly IBM) at www.delphion.com is a commercial online patent database. Due to a change in their business model in 2001, searching free of charge is now limited to

U.S. granted patents for certain years, and the free search is only conducted on the front page (bibliographic information) of the patent. More extensive searching capabilities including published U.S. patent applications and certain foreign published applications and granted patents are available now only by purchase of subscription packages. Copies of patent documents can be ordered online and delivered in various forms for a fee. Many of the searching features are the same as at the USPTO site, but Delphion and other commercial fee–based patent databases have an advantage because they contain collections of certain foreign-published patent applications and issued patents, and the searching can be done in certain cases across the United States and international collections. The commercial sites may also offer prior art searching capabilities using technical journals and magazines. Commercial online patent databases include Micropatent (www.micropatent.com), LexPat (www.lexis – nexis.com), and QPAT (www.qpat.com).

BIBLIOGRAPHY

The following publications were consulted in the preparation of the information presented in this chapter:

1. The Patent Act of 1952, as amended, codified in Title 35 United States Code.
2. Title 37 Code of Federal Regulations. USPTO Rules and Regulations.
3. Manual of Patent Examining Procedure, USPTO, 1997.
4. Patent Law Basics, Rosenberg, Peter D., West Group, Release #9, July 2001.
5. The Law of Chemical and Pharmaceutical Invention, Rosenstock, Jerome, Aspen Law and Business, Second Edition, 2001 Supplement.
6. Patent Practice Handbook, Canelias, Peter S., Aspen Law and Business, 2001.

Index

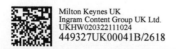